HIGHER CORTICAL FUNCTIONS IN MAN

PREFACES TO THE ENGLISH EDITION BY

HANS-LUKAS TEUBER

and KARL H. PRIBRAM

AUTHORIZED TRANSLATION FROM THE RUSSIAN

by BASIL HAIGH

HIGHER CORTICAL FUNCTIONS IN MAN

Second Edition, Revised and Expanded

ALEKSANDR ROMANOVICH LURIA

CONSULTANTS BUREAU *New York*

The original Russian text was published by
Moscow University Press in 1962

Library of Congress Catalog Card Number: 77-20421
ISBN: 0-306-10966-2

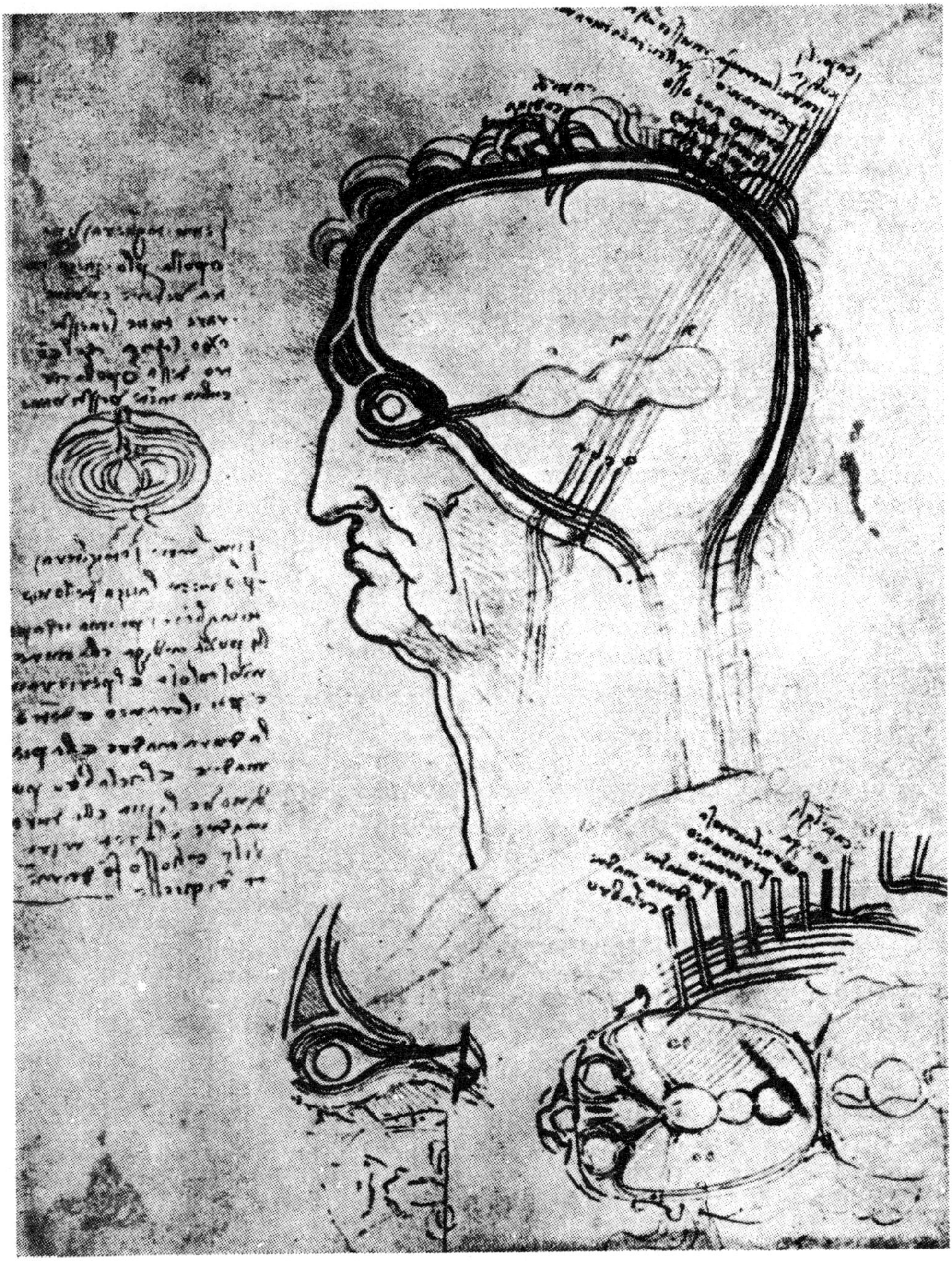

Drawing by Leonardo da Vinci illustrating the Renaissance view of the structure of the brain and of the three cerebral ventricles

Contents

II

DISTURBANCES OF THE HIGHER CORTICAL FUNCTIONS IN THE PRESENCE OF LOCAL BRAIN LESIONS

III

METHODS OF INVESTIGATING THE HIGHER CORTICAL FUNCTIONS IN LOCAL BRAIN LESIONS (SYNDROME ANALYSIS)

Preface

This full-length translation of Professor Luria's book introduces to the English-speaking world a major document in neuropsychology, summarizing Professor Luria's earlier contributions to that area for nearly a third of a century. It is a monumental contribution. Nothing of this scope exists in the Western literature of this field, with the possible exception of Ajuriaguerra and Hécaen's book (in French) on the cerebral cortex. Professor Luria's book thus marks a further and decisive step toward the eventual coalescence of neurology and psychology, a goal to which only a few laboratories in the East and West have been devoted over the last decades.

The book is unique in its organization. The first half deals with observations and interpretations concerning the major syndromes of man's left cerebral hemisphere: those grievous distortions of higher functions traditionally described as aphasia, agnosia, and apraxia. There is also a detailed and brilliant analysis of the syndrome of massive frontal-lobe involvement. The entire second half of the book is given over to a painstaking description of Professor Luria's tests, many of them introduced by himself, and set out in such detail that anyone could repeat them and thus verify Professor Luria's interpretations.

The two halves of the book are equally challenging and original. In the first, more theoretical, section, Professor Luria gives an account of the major syndromes in terms that reject with the same force the traditional localizationist view—the notion of discrete centers for different aspects of language, of calculation or writing—and the opposite view of holistic function of the cerebral hemisphere, a view clearly incompatible with clinical and experimental fact. In a similar way, Professor Luria's re-analysis of agnosia and apraxia reveals inadequacies of these clinical shorthand expressions; he points out that more elementary sensory and motor changes shade into the allegedly isolated aspects of distorted "higher" function, whether of recognition or skilled movement. As a result of this balanced approach, a further traditional distinction falls by the wayside—the traditional opposition in the description of aphasia between the "instrumental" and "noetic" views, that is, between those who believe that language is merely disturbed as a tool, with intelligence essentially intact, and those who believe that the trouble with language is simply one of several manifestations of an underlying change of intelligence.

The theoretical position adopted by Professor Luria himself in the face of these incredibly perplexing syndromes is most intriguing. He invokes cerebral reflexes as the basic elements of behavior. Yet careful reading reveals a remarkable restraint in the postulation of specific interruption of normal connections between different brain regions as the origin of major syndromes. In point of fact, he rejects the concept of conduction aphasia, preferring instead a carefully descriptive approach. Yet there is boldness too, as Professor Pribram stresses in his companion preface to this remarkable book: Professor Luria invokes again and again a principle of re-afference, in the tradition of Orbeli and Anokhin, and—one might add—of von Holst, modifying traditional reflex views and emphasizing the all-pervasive influence of self-produced stimulation (such as proprioceptive feedback) which the organism must compare continuously with its intended output in order to assess the success of its own movements. This sort of approach to sensorimotor coordination requires a new way of looking at the major brain syndromes in man. It becomes particularly fruitful in dealing with the baffling changes in human behavior after lesions of the frontal lobes, an area of furious controversy where Professor Luria reaches conclusions (he claims there is an essential disturbance of "intention") which are identical with those reached in our own laboratory on the basis of quite different clinical and experimental data.

The second half of the book with its rich descriptions of tests will be at least as influential as the first. Here one is struck primarily by the disarming simplicity of methods, nearly all suitable for bedside conditions, few requiring more than the examiner's voice, a few blocks, or paper and pencil. If one has had the privilege of observing Professor Luria and his staff in action at the Burdenko Institute in Moscow, one doubly appreciates the choice of his tasks, because he deals with large numbers of brain tumor cases, week after week; his assessment of these cases—the "neuropsychological" report—goes onto their clinical charts, together with other diagnostic techniques such as X-ray evaluations and electroencephalograms.

Where the situation demands it, Professor Luria is quite willing to employ more elaborate experimental techniques, such as the recording of eye movements, especially in cases of frontal-lobe involvement. Yet the emphasis remains on bedside tests, and a great many of them. It is here that the Western reader will be impressed by a difference in approach: neuropsychological laboratories in the West tend to be more quantitative.

The contrast is instructive, since one of the liberating effects of scientific exchange is to make one look at one's own work in a new and different way, as if one were permitted to look at it for a moment from the outside. Quantification is a major strength of the British and American tradition in psychology. If a book like Professor Luria's had been written here, it would teem with means and standard deviations, not to speak of analyses of variance and covariance. Yet the sobering fact is that most of Professor Luria's conclusions would not be changed if he had chosen to use these refinements. His own enormous clinical experience and his intuitive sense for what are reasonable interpretations are playing for him the role of large-sample statistics.

But there is a further and more important aspect to the difference in style of work: Much analysis in current neuropsychology in the United States (though much less in England and France) makes large-scale use of standard tests of intelligence, often at the expense of more versatile, qualitative tasks of the kind employed by Professor Luria. Here is a serious danger. By relying on routine psychometrics, one often loses crucial opportunities for the analysis of altered performance in the presence of brain lesions. Professor Luria's restraint in the use of psychometrics seems to me a major strength in his approach.

One of the most serious indictments of such psychometric tests comes from studies that permitted direct comparison of intelligence test scores obtained before, and again, in the same subjects, *after* a penetrating brain injury. In our own experience with such comparisons, two-thirds of an unselected group of brain-injured men have improved their scores from test to retest, even though the brain injury had intervened. Many of these patients increased their scores just as much as their controls. Yet most of the patients would have done poorly on a number of Professor Luria's informal, qualitative tasks, which are directly geared to the detection of specific change after cerebral lesions, while routine tests of intelligence are not.

The ingenious and abundant "little" tests employed by Professor Luria will undoubtedly find their uses here, and norms will be obtained in a number of laboratories. It will be of particular interest to see how his interpretations will hold up on cross-validation to other populations of patients, particularly those with selective removals of cortex for relief of epilepsy, or to those who have penetrating trauma in the absence of other complicating factors. Principal reliance on tumor cases, as in Professor Luria's work, entails certain risks of which Professor Luria is quite aware. His patients, on the whole, are more gravely ill than those studied in the neuropsychological program of, say, the Montreal Neurological Institute, where behavioral analyses are concentrated on cases of selective cortical removals for treatment of epilepsy, or in our own laboratory, with its major emphasis on the studies of late aftereffects of penetrating missile wounds of the brain. The more serious involvement in brain tumor cases is particularly apparent in patients with frontal-lobe tumors, since these tumors often grow undetected for considerable periods, as compared with those in other regions of the brain, where specific symptoms are more rapidly evident.

Yet Professor Luria makes the point that certain essential local symptoms are often brought out best against the background of more general changes in the brain, those due to pressure, vascular disturbance, or diffuse toxic effects

The touchstone will be cross-validation and, as regards frontal syndromes, the agreement between his conclusion and ours is simply astonishing, considering the vast difference in patients and in methods.

In this connection, a last word of caution, not so much to the physicians who will read and use this book, but to the psychologists, who will receive it with equal eagerness: Professor Luria's techniques, in their intent and in their application, are extensions of the classical neurological examination—major extensions, to be sure, but extensions nevertheless. This means that we must use his techniques just as he does—in conjunction with the standard neurologic examination, and not in its stead. In this way, the maximal benefit will accrue to the diagnosis of the patient's condition, and to an understanding of the roots of his difficulties. For it should be remembered that the central task of neuropsychology is always twofold: to help the patient by understanding his disease, and to understand the disease, in turn, as an experiment of nature, an experiment that, if properly used, may provide us with essential insights into the physiologic basis of normal function. In that sense, any contribution to neuropsychology attempts to tell us how the brain does work—by carefully observing how it sometimes does not.

Here then is the book, written by a master in his chosen field. Its translation marks a further step in the mutual recognition of common values in the scientific endeavors of East and West, a recognition which has at times been easier in the physical than in the behavioral and medical sciences, but is needed in every respect. And since it is the rapid development of physics that has made us so dangerous to one another, is it not fitting that we should get together over the great problem of detecting what makes us so frail and to join hands in the healing of the sick?

Hans-Lukas Teuber
Cambridge, Massachusetts
June, 1965

Preface

Higher Cortical Functions in Man marks an important accomplishment. Luria has, with one well-aimed stroke, managed to bring clinical neuropsychology back into the mainstream of scientific endeavor, while at the same time guarding the spirit and substance of the Soviet experience in this area of science. The volume is a documentary of bedside observation and experiment in the tradition of von Monakov and Goldstein—but the observations and the experiments are made in the image of Sechenov, Vigotsky, and Pavlov instead of Külpe, Brentano, and Wertheim. The reflex is regnant—but not the reflex arc. The volume is replete with evidence that reflex organization invariably involves a comparison between current input and residues of experience. Reflex organization is everywhere conceived and shown to be a two-way street whose traffic pattern is built of feedback between the central nervous system and peripheral sensory and motor structures. These are indeed current views; yet, as portrayed by Luria, they fall into place as naturally as if neurologists and psychologists had been groping in their various ways toward just this resolution of their dilemmas.

Higher Cortical Functions in Man is notable for another reason. These are the years when reticular systems, hypothalamic mechanisms, and other "diffuse," "facilitatory," and "inhibitory" processes are of central concern. Here, on the other hand, is a strong and sophisticated statement that does not flinch at complexities. This strength of statement is derived not from preconceived prejudice but flows from observation and experiment. Differences between neural systems and subsystems and their hierarchical relationships are spelled out. The hierarchical principle is then applied to unravelling disturbances of cognitive processes. But perhaps the most important achievement concerns the communicative behavior which ceases when the cortical mantle is destroyed: Here Luria applies the fruits of recent linguistic research to the problem of centrally-produced speech disorders.

In each chapter the historical context in which Luria's own and other current investigations are rooted is clearly spelled out for the reader; should, perchance, prejudice inadvertently be perpetrated it is openly declared for all to see. We are indeed fortunate to have available in English such a readable translation of an important contribution to neuropsychological knowledge by one of the outstanding Soviet scientists of our time.

Karl H. Pribram
Stanford University
May, 1965

Foreword

The purpose of this book is to analyze the disturbances of higher mental functions caused by local lesions of the brain.

The term "higher cortical functions" is a generally accepted one in the neurological literature, and it is used both in the title and in the text of this book. This has been done deliberately, although it is obvious that the higher mental processes are functions of the brain as a whole and that the activity of the cerebral cortex can be examined only in conjunction with that of nervous structures at lower levels.

Although the generalizations in this book are based on observations made during the past 25 years, and although an attempt has been made to correlate our findings with those presented in the literature, it cannot be said that this survey of the subject is exhaustive. An evaluation of the progress made in this area of study shows only too clearly that we are still only in the infant stages of the investigation of this complex field.

In describing disturbances of the higher cortical processes in their most general form, the author has drawn from the wide range of clinical phenomena encountered in neurology and neurosurgery and has disregarded findings pertaining to the pathogenesis, development, and clinical manifestations of the disturbances occurring with different types of brain lesions. This book is documented with very few actual case reports; a special book would be required to deal adequately with this additional material.

Another feature of this book has largely been determined by the present state of research into disturbances of the higher cortical functions in man in the presence of local brain lesions. A wealth of clinical material is available as a source of descriptions of such disturbances. After a careful clinicopsychological study of these disturbances, it is often possible to identify the underlying factors and to study important aspects of the cerebral organization of complex forms of mental activity. For this reason, the psychological study of the cortical functions has become an indispensable part of the clinical investigation directed at diagnostic localization of a lesion and restoration of the disturbed brain functions, and this aspect of the subject receives due attention herein.

Foreword

In contradistinction to the abundance of clinical data, accurate physiological investigation of the abnormal dynamics of the nervous processes accompanying local brain lesions is only in its infancy. Although extensive material is presently available on the pathophysiology of higher nervous activity in the presence of generalized organic brain lesions and psychoneuroses, it is only recently that careful physiological investigations have begun to be made in patients with local brain lesions. That is why the results of neurodynamic investigations of cases of circumscribed brain lesions could not be presented as fully as would have been liked, and to remedy this deficiency is an important task for the future.

The author has been greatly helped by many colleagues and associates in the writing of this book. He is particularly indebted to A. N. Leont'ev, F. V. Bassin, G. I. Polyakov, S. M. Blinkov, M. B. Eidinova, B. V. Zeigarnik, Y. V. Konovalov, and T. O. Faller and his collaborators N. A. Filippycheva, E. N. Pravdina-Vinarskaya, and E. P. Kok.

The author is grateful to G. I. Polyakov for accepting the task of writing the chapter dealing with modern views on the structural organization of the brain, in which he incorporated the results of his many years of experience (Part I, Section 2).

The assistance given to the author in the preparation of this book by his close collaborator E. D. Khomskaya has been especially valuable. The principal propositions in this book were formulated jointly with her, and it can rightly be said that this book is largely the result of our combined activity.

The author wishes to express his gratitude to the staff of the N. N. Burdenko Institute of Neurosurgery of the USSR Academy of Medical Sciences, Moscow, with whom he has been actively associated for nearly a quarter of a century, and to its Director, B. G. Egorov, who has done so much to facilitate our investigations of patients with local brain lesions.

The author is greatly indebted to Dr. Basil Haigh for the translation of the book, and especially to Professor Joseph Wortis for his invaluable help in editing the English text of the volume.

The author first began his clinicopsychological investigations of cases of local brain lesions more than 30 years ago under the guidance of his friend and teacher L. S. Vygotskii. Much of what is written in the following pages may therefore be looked upon as a continuation of Vygotskii's ideas, and this book is dedicated to his memory.

Foreword to the Second Edition

A second edition of *Higher Cortical Functions in Man* was called for soon after publication of the first edition. This is a measure of the current importance of the matters discussed in it and the wide interest in the problem of higher cortical functions shown by psychologists, neurologists, and physiologists; interest in this field has grown considerably as a result of progress in bionics and the theory of self-regulating systems, on which attention has recently become focused.

The discussion which the book has provoked in the press has not called any of its basic propositions into question, and the author does not consider that any substantial corrections are necessary. However, progress in the science of the brain and its neuronal organization in recent years has necessitated a number of additions, and these and others have been included by the author in the new edition.

Much has been written in recent years on the functions of the limbic systems of the brain and disturbances of the emotions and memory that arise in lesions of those systems. A short section devoted to research in this field has accordingly been introduced into the book. The author realizes that this section cannot hope to cover completely all the evidence that has accumulated in recent years on this subject; however, the basic theme of the book, the study of higher cortical functions, can allow only the most cursory examination of the data relating to the functions of this region.

Investigations of the functions of the components of nerve tissue conducted at the single neuron level have of late made rapid development. These investigations, published in several different countries, have yielded new and invaluable material, and indeed it would seem that within the lifetime of the present generation, the science of the functional organization of the cerebral cortex will undergo a radical change and assume a totally different form.

Since this new field of research lies outside the author's field of competence, he is deeply grateful to O. S. Vinogradova for undertaking the task of describing, in a short section, the results of recent research at the neuronal level in laboratories in the West and in E. N. Sokolov's laboratory at Moscow University, where she has been directly involved in this activity.

The section on the functions of the frontal lobes has been rewritten, drawing heavily on data obtained by E. D. Khomskaya and her colleagues, who have contributed much valuable material to this problem in recent years. The book also includes material from the author's friends and colleagues that is published in the complete form in the book *The Frontal Lobes and Regulation of Psychological Processes,* edited by E. D. Khomskaya.

Neuropsychology, the basic facts of which are dealt with in this book, has developed in recent years into a widely branching field of research. The author hopes that this second edition of his book will be useful to workers in this new branch of science.

Preface to the Second American Edition

A long time has elapsed since the publication of the first edition of this book, in which I attempted to lay the foundations of neuropsychology as a new branch of science. Indeed, it is already a fair time since the publication of the second Russian edition, which was prepared 10 years ago and published in 1969.

In the intervening decade some really important work has been done by the author and his group, and the same can be said for the whole wide field of neuropsychology. The old topics of neuropsychology, already studied in the past, have been probed to a much greater depth; new problems not hitherto investigated have appeared. The literature analyzing higher cortical functions in man from the standpoint of neuropsychology and its allied disciplines has grown enormously.

These developments have compelled the author to look carefully at the previous text of this book and, while retaining its basic features, to rewrite some sections and to add information on new problems not previously mentioned.

In the present edition, which differs substantially from the first Russian and first American editions of this book, and which is also substantially enlarged compared with the second Russian edition, the author has added new and very important data.

The section dealing with the psychophysiological mechanisms of activation, which is particularly afflicted by lesions of the frontal lobes, has been fully revised. This section is written by one of the author's closest colleagues, E. D. Khomskaya, whose investigations have developed particularly actively in the last decade: the results have been summarized in her book *The Brain and Activation*, published (in Russian) in 1972, and in many papers with her colleagues.

A new chapter on disturbances of higher cortical functions in deep brain lesions has been added.

Important additions reflecting the work of the author and his collaborators in the last decades have been made in the section on memory processes, methods of their investigation, the forms of their disturbances, and the mechanisms lying at the basis of these disturbances.

A new section on interaction between the hemispheres, and the role which each plays in the course of complex types of psychological activity, has been introduced. This section was deliberately left out of earlier editions of the book, but recent investigations by the author's colleague E. G. Simernitskaya have taken the first steps toward the analysis of the internal mechanisms of this interaction. Consequently, despite the very incomplete studies which have so far been made of this problem, the many articles which have been published demanded that a place be found for its discussion in this edition.

The author has deliberately decided to include only data obtained in the last 10 to 12 years in his laboratory and has not attempted to cover the vast literature on problems in neuropsychology containing the results of research in many different countries. These results have been published both in special monographs and in articles appearing in specialized journals such as *Neuropsychologia, Cortex,* and *Brain and Language,* not to mention many collections and periodicals devoted to advances in neurology and neurophysiology. The writer also decided with regret that he could not do justice to the work of his physiologist colleagues, who, during the last 10 to 15 years, have made tremendous advances and have opened up new and hitherto inaccessible ways of analyzing the intimate mechanisms of the working of the human brain.

To deal adequately with all these matters and to review in a succinct form the whole of the vast literature in this field would be far beyond the author's capacity. The author strives to maintain a modest outlook on his abilities and, more than anyone else, he is aware of the deficiencies of this book.

If, despite all that has been said, the decision is taken to publish the extended edition of *Higher Cortical Functions,* its purpose is simply to reflect a stage in the development of neuropsychology in which the author has participated directly, and which, of course, will see considerable progress as a result of future research currently taking place in many different countries by a large army of workers.

When presenting this revised version of the book for publication the author would like to extend his thanks once again to the staff of the N. N. Burdenko Institute of Neurosurgery, Academy of Medical Sciences of the USSR, with whom he has been connected now for 40 years, and to the publishers Basic Books and Plenum, for deciding to publish the new edition.

A. R. Luria
Moscow
June, 1977

I

THE HIGHER MENTAL FUNCTIONS AND THEIR ORGANIZATION IN THE BRAIN

1. *The Problem of Localization of Functions in the Cerebral Cortex*

Many generations of research workers have given their attention to the problem of the brain as the seat of complex mental activity and to the associated problem of the localization of functions in the cerebral cortex. Nevertheless, the solution of these problems has depended not only on the development of technical methods of studying the brain, but also on the theories concerning mental processes predominant at any particular time. For this reason, endeavors to localize cerebral cortical functions were for a long time restricted to futile attempts to "fit the system of abstract concepts of modern psychology into the material structure of the brain" (I. P. Pavlov, *Complete Collected Works*, Vol. 3. p. 203).* While these attempts yielded much valuable empirical material, they naturally failed to provide a scientific solution to the problem. It is only in recent years that, because of advances in modern (especially Russian and Soviet) physiology and materialistic psychology, there has been a breakthrough in the approach to this problem, new principles for its solution have evolved, and new evidence has accumulated to enrich our ideas of the functional organization of the human brain in health and disease.

A. PSYCHOMORPHOLOGICAL CONCEPTS AND THEIR CRISIS—A HISTORICAL SURVEY

The more important ideas regarding mental functions and their localization will be very briefly considered. These ideas are being outlined only to show how long in the history of science the view persisted that mental phenomena are specific properties of consciousness, incapable of further analysis, and

*The literature references cited throughout the book are listed in *two* bibliographies, Russian and non-Russian, at the end of the book.

how wide of the mark were the parallel views of their relationship to the brain structure. For a detailed account of the history of the study of localization of functions in the brain, see the writings of Head (1926), Ombredane (1951), and Polyak (1957).

Attempts to discover a material substrate for mental phenomena were undertaken in the very earliest days of philosophy, when they had no basis in positive fact. Gradually, the naive materialistic concept of the mind as the *pneuma* was supplanted by attempts to relate the complex mental functions to the material structures of the brain.

In the fifth century B.C., Hippocrates of Croton claimed that the brain is merely the organ of the "intellect," or the "guiding spirit" (ἡγεμονικόν), and that the heart is the organ of the senses. However, a few centuries later Galen (second century B.C.) offered a more precise explanation of the relationship between mental life and the brain. His system may be regarded as one of the first attempts to actually localize mental phenomena in the structures of the brain. He assumed that the impressions received by man from the outside world enter the ventricles of the brain through the eyes in the form of humors. Further, he suggested that the θαλαμος οπτικος, or internal chamber, containing these humors is the "temple" (θαλαμος) in which they meet the vital humors (πνευμα ζωοτικον) coming from the liver and are transformed by means of a network of vessels into the psychic humors (πνευμα ψυκικον or πνευμα λογιστικον). The notion that the cerebral ventricles (or, more precisely, the fluids that they contain) are the material substrate of the mental processes was destined to last for another 1500 years. In the sixteenth century A.D., Vesalius made the first detailed study of the solid structure of the brain. Nevertheless, Soemmering (1796) continued to believe that mental processes are brought about by "*spiriti animales*" running along the nerves.

With the passage of time the view that the cerebral ventricles *in toto* are the seat of the mental processes gradually was refined, with structural differentiation of these ventricles and ascription of special functions to the various parts. Nemesius (fourth century A.D.) was the first to propose that the "anterior ventricle" of the brain be regarded as the seat of perception or imagination ("*cellula phantastica*"), the "middle ventricle" as the seat of the intellect ("*cellula logistica*"), and the "posterior ventricle" as the seat of the memory ("*cellula memorialis*"). This notion of the "three ventricles of the brain" as the direct substrate of the principal mental abilities was handed on from century to century. It was still generally accepted in the Middle Ages (Fig. 1), and it is interesting to remember that even Leonardo da Vinci, as shown in an original drawing of his (Frontispiece), maintained the belief that the principal mental "faculties" are localized in the "three cerebral ventricles."

The subsequent history of concepts of cerebral localization of mental processes was associated with the development of psychology (which for a long time remained a branch of philosophy), on the one hand, and with the beginnings of descriptive anatomy of the brain, on the other. The conception of mental functions began to become less rigid, and the image of the structure of the brain began to grow clearer. Nevertheless, the basic premise of direct superposition of nonmaterial psychological principles on the material structure of the brain continued unchanged for many years. This explains why the first steps in the development of the science of anatomy in the new era were marked by the search for the particular part of the solid tissue of the "cerebral organ" that could be regarded as the material substrate of mental processes. Different investigators gave different answers to this question. Descartes (1686) considered this organ to be the pineal gland, situated in the center of the brain; by virtue of its position, in his opinion, it possesses the necessary qualities to serve as the carrier of mental functions. Willis (1664) was inclined to locate this organ in the corpus striatum; Vieussens (1685), in the mass of white matter of the cerebral hemispheres—the centrum semiovale; Lancisi (1739), in the corpus callosum, the structure joining the two hemispheres. Despite the many solutions that were offered to this problem, a common feature of the work of all investigators at this early stage was the desire to localize mental phenomena in one particular part of the brain.

These attempts to find a single "cerebral organ" for all mental processes comprised only the first step in the investigation of functional localization. Psychology was now no longer dominated by the view that consciousness was an indivisible whole. A school of psychology developed that subdivided mental

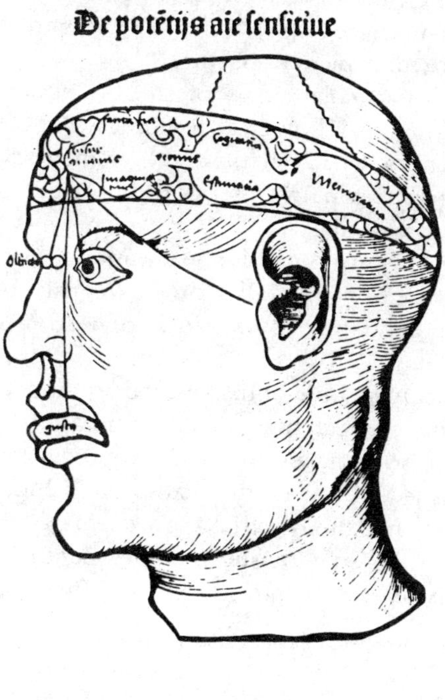

FIGURE 1 Diagram of the three "cerebral ventricles" from Reisch's (1513) treatise, *Margarita Philosophica.*

processes into separate, specialized "faculties," and this led to a search for the material substrate for these faculties. The brain was now regarded as an aggregate of many "organs," each of which was supposed to be the material carrier of one particular "faculty."

The investigators of that era related the contemporary picture of a "psychology of faculties" to the current knowledge of the structure of the brain. The initial attempts at cerebral localization of the mental faculties were therefore made by the leading anatomists and were highly speculative in nature. The first to adopt a differential approach to the localization of faculties in the brain was the German anatomist J. H. Meyer (1779), who, in his treatise on the anatomy and physiology of the brain, suggested that memory is localized in the cerebral cortex, imagination and reason in the white matter, and apperception and will in the basal portions of the brain, and that integration of all these mental functions is effected by the corpus callosum and the cerebellum. This attempt to relegate individual mental functions to isolated parts of the brain was carried to the limit by Gall, whose ideas were widely accepted at the time.*

Gall was one of the leading anatomists of the brain of his time. He was the first to recognize the importance of the gray matter of the cerebral hemispheres and its relationship to the fibers of the white matter. However, in his treatise on the functions of the brain (1825) he accepted the contemporary "psychology of faculties" as the starting point. He was, in fact, the author of the concepts that each mental faculty is based on a definite group of brain cells and that the whole cerebral cortex (which he was the first to regard as the more important part of the cerebral hemispheres, responsible for mental functions) is an aggregate of individual "organs," each of which is the substrate of a particular mental "faculty."

The faculties that Gall relegated to particular areas of the brain were simply taken by him from contemporary psychological teachings. Besides assigning such relatively simple functions as visual or auditory memory, orientation in space, and a sense of time to separate areas of the cortex, he also localized "instinct for continuation of the race," "love of parents," "sociability," "courage," "ambition," "aptitude for education," etc. Figure 2 is a phrenological map compiled in Gall's time. We may be justified in regarding it as the first depiction of the idea of restricted localization.

Gall's ideas need not have been included in a book devoted to modern views of higher cortical functions and cortical functional organization in man, for his phrenological views were so fantastic that they aroused sharp opposition as soon as they were published. However, they had been included for two reasons. First, the suggestion that the cerebral cortex is a system with various functions, even if offered in so fantastic and prescientific a form, was to some degree progressive, for it introduced a differential

* Gall's importance as an anatomist has recently been examined by Glezer (1959).

approach to an apparently homogeneous brain mass. Second, Gall's idea of "brain centers" housing complex mental functions was based on such solid principles that it endured in the psychomorphological thinking, in which "narrow localization" was taken for granted, until a much later time, or until the investigation of the cerebral organization of mental processes acquired a more realistic scientific basis. These ideas determined the nature of the investigation of cerebral localization of functions for almost a century.

Nevertheless, there was considerable opposition to the ideas of "localizationalism." The view that the brain is an aggregate of separate organs, put forward by Meyer and Gall, was rejected by some physiologists of that time, who supported the opposite, or antilocalization, theory.

Haller (1769), although not denying that different parts of the brain may be involved in different functions, postulated that the brain is a single organ, transforming impressions into mental processes, and that it is composed of parts of equal importance ("*sensorium commune*"). He felt that the validity of this hypothesis was proved by the fact that a single focus may cause a disturbance of various faculties and that the disabilities resulting from such a focal disturbance may, to some extent, be compensated for.

Half a century later a similar hypothesis based on the results of a physiological experiment was advanced by Flourens (1824). He observed

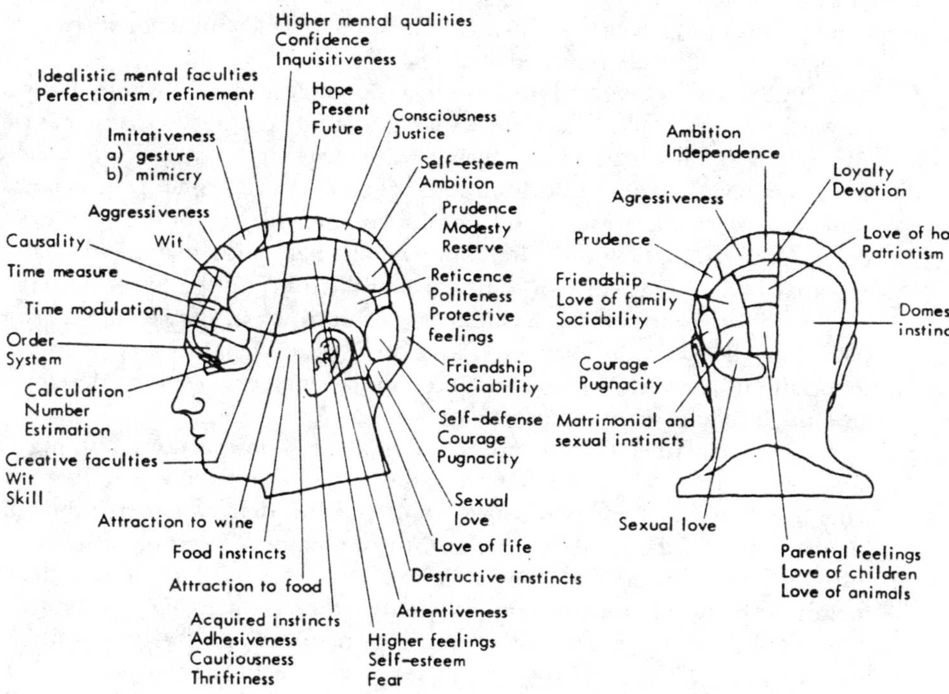

FIGURE 2 A phrenological map of the localization of mental faculties taken from a paper contemporary with Gall.

that a short time after destruction of isolated areas of the cerebral hemispheres in birds, behavior of the birds is restored, and, moreover, there is approximately the same degree of recovery regardless of which part of the cerebral hemispheres was destroyed. Although not yet aware that in the lower vertebrates the cerebral cortex has a very low level of differentiation and that functioning is inadequately corticalized, he concluded that even if the brain as a whole is a complex organ, its cortex acts as a homogeneous entity, whose destruction leads to a uniform disturbance of "sensation and intellectual faculties." Hence, the gray matter of the cerebral hemispheres as a whole is that *ἡγεμονικόν* described by the Greek writers. These hypotheses were confirmed by experiments in which the extensor and flexor innervation of the wing was crossed in a cock. Since wing function was restored to its original state, Flourens (1842) considered the premise of the homogeneity of the brain as a whole to be conclusively confirmed, declaring that "the mass of the cerebral hemispheres is physiologically just as homogeneous and uniform in its importance as the mass of any gland, for example the liver."

The experiments of Flourens marked a considerable advance from Gall's theoretical arguments. They replaced speculative presumption by scientific experimentation and directed attention to the plasticity and interdependence of the functions of the cerebral hemispheres. Further, they anticipated the conceptions of the dynamic activity of the brain to which subsequent scientific thought has frequently returned.

Although the concept of the brain as a single dynamic whole was put forward by physiologists, seemingly on the basis of accurate experimentation, the evidence that accumulated during subsequent decades tipped the scales once again in favor of localization. This evidence came from clinical observations on patients with circumscribed lesions of the brain, on the one hand, and from the rapid development of anatomical and physiological research into the structure of the brain, on the other. It led to the adoption of new views regarding the localization of functions in the cerebral cortex. The new theory of localization was closely connected with the theory of associationism, which, from its inception in the eighteenth century, developed into the foremost school in psychology.

At the same time that Flourens published his observations refuting all notions of structural differentiation in the cerebral cortex, Bouillaud (1825*b*), later head of the Paris Medical School, concluded from observations on patients that "if the brain did not consist of separate centers . . . it would be impossible to understand how a lesion of one part of the brain causes paralysis of some muscles of the body without affecting others" (pp. 279—280). Bouillaud believed that the principle of localization could be extended to the more complex processes of speech. In 1825, a year after the appearance of Flourens' account of his research, Bouillaud confirmed Gall's opinion on the localization of articulated speech. In this paper (1825*a*) he postulated the division of speech activity into an intellectual process, a process involving the use of signs, and the process of articulation of words, and mentioned the possibility of their dissociation. He argued that articulated speech is a function of the anterior portions of the brain. Thus, opposition to the view that the cerebral cortex is a homogeneous structure was based on the deduction from clinical observations on human patients that the cortex exhibits differentiation.

These hypotheses of the localization of functions in the cerebral cortex remained unconfirmed and were finally overthrown as a result of the observations of Dax (1836) and of Broca's (1861*a* and *b*) world-famous discovery.

In April, 1861, Broca exhibited the brain of a patient who had developed a disturbance of articulated speech during life before the Paris Anthropological Society. Postmortem examination of this patient revealed a lesion in the posterior third of the inferior frontal convolution of the left hemisphere. In November of the same year Broca conducted a similar demonstration of the brain of another patient with the same syndrome. He concluded from these observations that articulated speech is localized in a well-demarcated area of the brain and that this particular area is the "center of motor forms of speech." He then went on to make the bold assertion (while, in principle, continuing to assign psychological functions to definite areas of the brain) that the cells of a given area of the cerebral cortex constitute a "depot" of images of the movements composing articulated speech. Broca concluded his address on a somewhat pathetic note with the words: "No sooner will it be shown that intellectual function is associated with a localized area of the brain, than the view that intellectual functions are bound up with the brain as a whole will be rejected, and it will become highly probable that each convolution has its own special functions."

Broca's discovery stimulated clinical research, and this resulted in the accumulation of many more findings and observations supporting the views of the localizationists. A decade after Broca's demonstration, Wernicke (1874) described a case in which a lesion of the posterior third of the superior temporal gyrus of the left hemisphere caused a disturbance in speech comprehension. Wernicke's conclusion that the "sensory images of speech" are localized in a zone of the cortex of the left hemisphere (which he described) has become firmly entrenched in the literature.

The descriptions of two isolated areas of the brain in which corresponding lesions led to disturbances of such different functions caused unprecedented activity on the part of investigators of cerebral localization. These cases provoked the suggestion that other mental processes, even the most complex, may be localized in comparatively small areas of the cerebral cortex and that, in fact, the cortex is an aggregate of separate "centers" whose cell groups are "depots" of different mental faculties. All the attention of the neurologists of that time was therefore directed toward describing cases in which a lesion of a circumscribed area of the cerebral cortex caused a disturbance of mainly one form of mental activity. Having obtained such clinical findings and verified them with anatomical findings, these writers took little pains to study their cases carefully. They did not analyze the complex of symptoms lying outside the confines of the disturbance of a single function, and they made no attempt to accurately describe the functional disturbance they had identified. Like Broca and Wernicke, they immediately concluded from a discovery of a lesion in a particular area of the brain in an individual with a concomitant definite type of disturbance that the area containing the lesion is the "center" for the "function" that had been impaired and that the cells composing these areas are the "depots" of highly specialized "memory images." For example, during the two decades following the discoveries of Broca and Wernicke, together with their connections, the following centers were described: "centers of visual memory" (Bastian, 1869), "writing centers" (Exner, 1881), and "centers of ideas" or "centers of ideation" (Broadbent, 1872, 1879; Charcot, 1887; Grasset, 1907). Very soon, therefore, the map of the human cerebral cortex was filled with numerous schemes reflecting the ideas of the associative psychology dominant at that time. These schemes were considered by their authors to be the true explanation of all the mysteries surrounding the functional organization of the cortex, and the compiling of such schemes occupied a considerable portion of time in the clinical effort to develop ideas on the working of the brain.

The view that complex mental processes can be narrowly localized in circumscribed areas of the cerebral cortex would not have spread so widely or proved so successful had it not been for certain circumstances. The success of this theory was predetermined by the propositions of the contemporary psychology, which by that time had become an independent branch of science. According to the prevalent school of thought, human mental activity is based on the association of sensations and ideas.

Another and no less important factor in the favorable reception of the ideas of the localizationists of the second half of the nineteenth century, and without which these ideas would not have gained such wide acceptance, was the contemporary progress made in anatomy and physiology. It was at this time that Virchow (1858) put forward the notion that the organism can be regarded as a "cell state" consisting of units that are the primary carriers of all its properties. Virchow's ideas were taken up by Meynert (1867–1868), who gave the first accurate account of the cell structure of the cerebral cortex. In the face of the tremendous complexity of the structure of the human cerebral cortex, Meynert felt that the concepts in the field of cellular physiology could be transferred to this new field, and he began to regard the cortical cells as carriers of particular mental processes. "The cortical layer contains more than 1000 million cells," he wrote. "Each new impression meets a new, still vacant cell. With the existence of such vast numbers of these vacant cells, impressions arriving in succession find carriers in which they will remain for ever in the same close order . . . ." (1885 [Rus.], p. 166).

The time with which we are concerned was one of great and decisive scientific achievement. In the 1870's, which Pavlov called "an outstanding epoch in the physiology of the nervous system" (*Complete Collected Works*, Vol. 3, p. 202), two closely related scientific discoveries were made. In 1870, Fritsch and Hitzig, by stimulating the cerebral cortex of a dog with an electric current, showed for the first time that stimulation of certain cortical areas (subsequently found to be those containing pyramidal Betz cells) was followed by contraction of certain muscles. These experiments demonstrated that the cerebral cortex contains isolated "motor centers," a finding that was later confirmed by experiments on monkeys and, finally, by investigations in man. Almost simultaneously with this research, the Kiev anatomist Betz (1874) discovered giant pyramidal cells in the cortex of the anterior central gyrus, and he associated them with the motor function. The presence of these cells sharply distinguishes the structure of the motor cortex from that of the postcentral sensory cortex.

The discoveries of Fritsch and Hitzig, on the one hand, and of Betz, on the other, providing a factual basis for clinical observations, prompted a series of physiological experiments in which various areas of the cerebral cortex were extirpated in animals and the subsequent behavioral changes studied. Among these investigations were the well-known ones of Munk (1881), who found that after extirpation of the occipital portion of the brain a dog could still see but had lost the power of visual recognition of objects, and those of Hitzig (1874), Ferrier (1874, 1876), Bianchi (1895), and others who observed gross disturbances of "attention" and of "intellectual activity" in animals after extirpation of the anterior divisions of the brain.

The discovery of the highly differentiated structure of the cerebral cortex and of the possibility of strict differentiation of function between its various parts may be counted among the great achievements of science. Accepting these discoveries as proof of the existence of distinct cortical "centers" for various motor or sensory functions, research workers now began to relate more complex mental functions to particular areas of the cortex with far more confidence than hitherto. At the close of the nineteenth and the beginning of the twentieth centuries, the neurological literature was replete with case reports of disturbances in complex mental processes of circumscribed areas of the cerebral cortex, produced by lesions. The observers of these cases did not content themselves with describing the symptoms but also concluded that the corresponding areas of the cerebral cortex are the "centers" for the corresponding impaired functions. In this way it began to be taught that not only are visual, auditory, and tactile perception localized in the cerebral cortex, but that such complex mental processes as "number sense," "counting," "reading," "active ideation," and "volitional action," as well as even more complex forms, obviously social in origin, such as the "personal and social ego," are also localized. The fruit of these attempts to localize complex mental processes in circumscribed areas of the cerebral cortex was used until comparatively recently as the basis of fundamental treatises on psychiatry, such as the textbook of Kleist (1934), whose chart on cerebral localization (Fig. 3) was widely acclaimed. He sided with the "topistic" teaching of O. Vogt (1951), the founder of modern cytoarchitectonics, who postulated that the brain as a whole is composed of small organs ("*Kleinorgane*"), and that each organ is the seat of a particular faculty. These views were subsequently embodied in the basic textbooks on neurology, such as that of Nielsen (1946) published in the United States.

The suggestions that different areas of the cerebral cortex are highly differentiated in their structure and that complex mental functions are not uniformly related to the various areas of the brain were basically very progressive. They stimulated the more careful study of the brain and its functions. Nevertheless, the idea that highly complex mental phenomena may be localized in circumscribed areas of the cerebral cortex and that the circumscribed area responsible for a particular function can be directly deduced from a symptom naturally continued to arouse deep misgivings. For this reason, a century after the impact of the views of Meyer and Haller

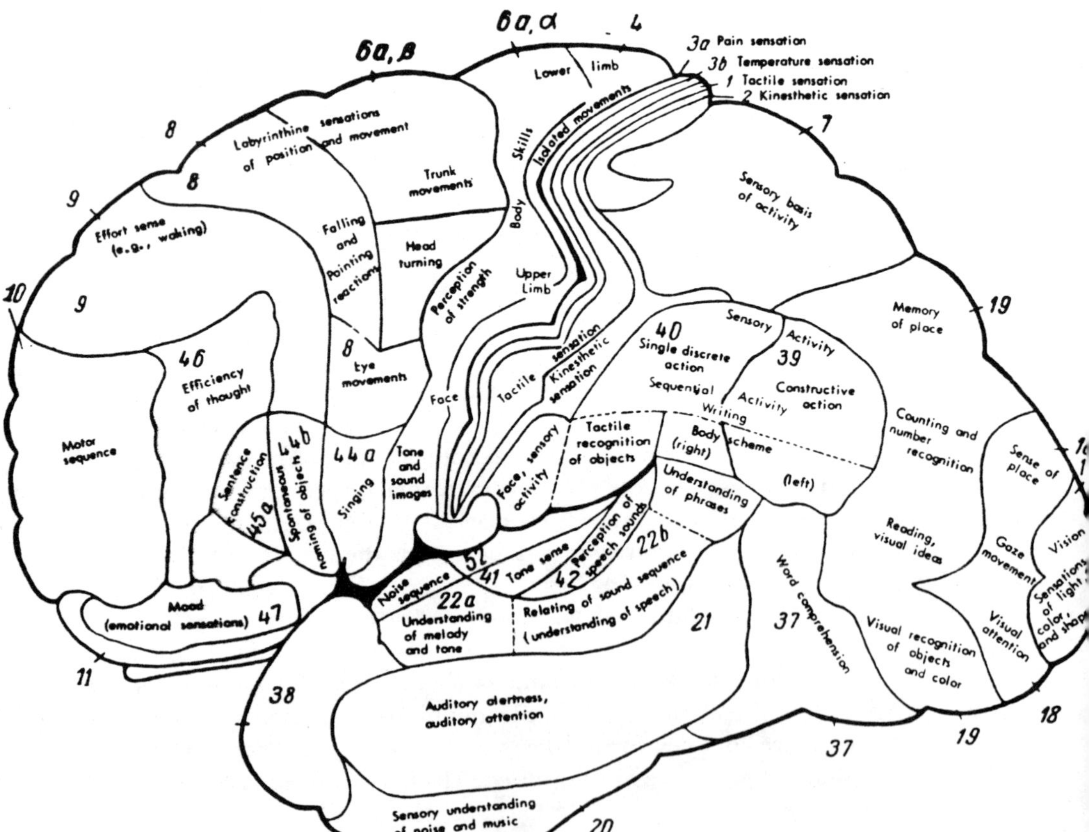

and half a century after the discussions of Gall and Flourens, the debate between the localizationists and the antilocalizationists was resumed, but this time for different reasons.

At the time that Wernicke demonstrated the importance of the cortex of the left temporal lobe in man for speech, that Fritsch and Hitzig obtained a specific effect from stimulation of the motor area of the cortex, and that Munk observed a disturbance in visual recognition after destruction of the occipital region in a dog, the eminent German physiologist Goltz (1876–1881) conducted a series of new experiments in which he extirpated different areas of the cerebral cortex in dogs. Goltz determined the results of his experiments by observing the changes in the animals' general behavior. After extirpation of different areas of the cerebral hemispheres, the animals developed marked disturbances of behavior, which Goltz interpreted to be the reaction of the brain as a whole. These disturbances subsequently disappeared, the functions were restored, and only a slight awkwardness of movement and lack of coordination remained, the latter being regarded by Goltz as a manifestation of a "general lowering of intellect." The conclusions drawn by Goltz from his experiments were similar to those of

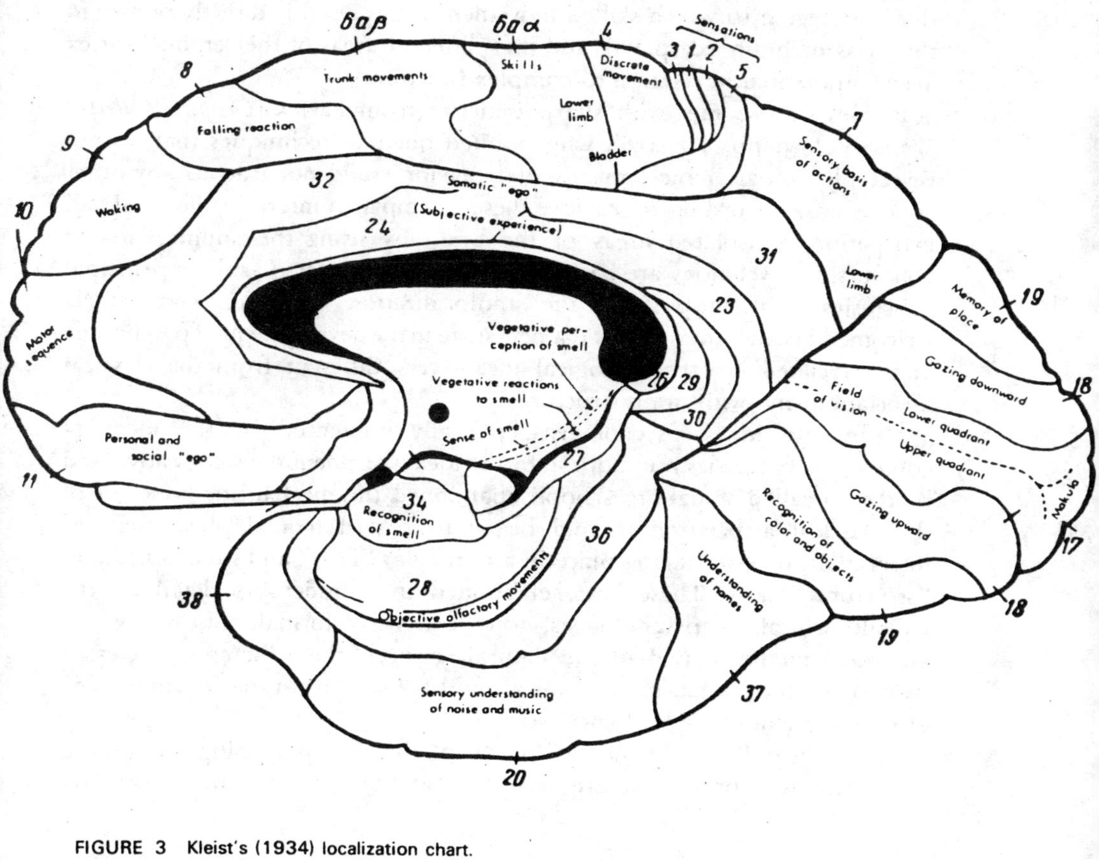

FIGURE 3 Kleist's (1934) localization chart.

Flourens, working with birds, namely, that any part of the brain is associated with the formation of will, sensations, ideas, and thoughts, and that the degree of loss of function is directly and entirely dependent on the size of the lesion.

As stated, Goltz limited his observations to the animal's general response to extirpation, without differentiating among the defects that developed. Moreover, he used psychological terms of excessively broad meaning, such as "will" and "intellect." It was therefore inevitable for him to reach the conclusions that he did. Nevertheless, his great merit lies in the fact that by referring to dynamic factors such as the "general reaction of the brain" and recognizing the great plasticity of the brain substance at a time when the concept of narrow localization was flourishing he directed attention to the activity of the brain as an entity.

It is interesting that Goltz's conclusions did not arouse much sympathy at the time of their publication, yet half a century later almost the same arguments were employed by Lashley (1929). After extirpating different areas of the brain in rats and observing the changes in their behavior while they were in a maze, Lashley concluded that a particular type of behavioral disturbance cannot be ascribed to a defect of a particular area of the brain, that the degree to which skilled movement is impaired is directly related to the mass of brain extirpated, and that different areas of the cerebral cortex are equipotential in relation to complex functions.

Lashley's views met with sharp criticism from Pavlov (*Complete Collected Works*, Vol. 3, pp. 428–456), who pointed out that techniques that do not reveal physiological mechanisms of behavior could not lead to any other conclusions. According to Pavlov, these attempts to interpret the results of extirpation of isolated areas of the brain by using the undifferentiated concepts of psychology are basically unsound. However, Lashley's principal conclusions, in support of the antilocalization doctrine, were widely welcomed because they reflected a new stage in the development of psychology and correlated new psychological ideas—very different from the classical associationism—with brain structure.

Meanwhile many psychologists, partially influenced by the ideas of contemporary physics but more so by the idealistic phenomenology advanced by the so-called Würzburg school, abandoned the mechanistic concepts of the classical associationism and began to regard mental phenomena as integrated processes taking place in a particular "field" and subordinated to "structural" laws. These laws, elaborated in considerable detail by the Gestalt school of psychologists, were extremely formal. Discarding the analytical methods used in the natural sciences, the adherents of Gestalt psychology took what, in fact, was a step backward from the previous stage of development of psychological science.

The "integral" or "dynamic" ideas of the new psychology, requiring correlation with brain structure, took support from Lashley's antilocalization hypotheses. In these hypotheses, functions labeled on the basis of generalized psychological concepts were correlated as before, directly and without physiological analysis, with brain structure. It is true that "integrated behavior" was correlated with the "integrated brain." The latter was now regarded as a homogeneous mass, acting in accordance with the integral laws of the field. Any suggestion of a differential anatomic-physiological analysis of the structure of the brain was rejected just as decisively as had been the differential analysis of the animal's skills or habits. Rather than make a detailed study of the cerebral apparatus, these investigators were content to use analogies on the relationships of structure and substrate as formulated in physics and the general morphogenic principles embodied in embryology.

The new form of antilocalizationism quickly spread beyond the confines of research on the cerebral mechanisms of animal behavior to clinical medicine. It gradually developed into an important force opposing the classical ideas of localization. It is therefore necessary to consider their development in greater detail.

During the 1860's, the celebrated English neurologist Hughlings Jackson, who gave the first account of epileptic fits arising on a localized basis, formulated a series of principles in sharp opposition to the contemporary ideas of narrow localization. These principles, destined to play an important role in the subsequent development of neurological thinking, were enunciated by Jackson in the course of a discussion with Broca soon after the latter had published his observations. During the following decades, however, these principles were overshadowed by the successful progress of the localizationist's views, and it was not until the first quarter of the twentieth century that these ideas came to be widely accepted. It should be noted that Jackson's investigations, which were cited some 50 years after they were performed by Pick (1913), Head (1926), and Foerster (1936), were first published in summary form only in 1932 (in England) and again in 1958 (in the United States).

The occurrences on which Jackson based his theories were irreconcilable with Broca's fundamental ideas and with the concepts proceeding from the belief in the cellular localization of functions. During his studies of motor and speech disturbances accompanying local brain lesions, Jackson observed a phenomenon that, at first glance, appeared paradoxical, namely, that a lesion of a circumscribed area of the brain never leads to the complete loss of a function. A patient with a lesion of a particular zone of the cortex frequently cannot perform a desired movement or repeat an arbitrarily given word, although he may be able to do so involuntarily, i.e., he may be able to reproduce the same movement or pronounce the same word when in a state of emotion or by habit. A case later described by Gowers—in which a patient, when asked by the doctor to say the word "no," replied: "No, doctor, I never can say 'no'!"—was used by Jackson as the starting point for his neurological analysis.

On the basis of occurrences such as these, Jackson elaborated a general theory of the neurological organization of functions that differed sharply from the classical views. In his opinion, every function performed by the central nervous system is not the domain of a narrowly circumscribed group of cells that serve as what might be termed a "depot" for this function. Rather, each function has a complex "vertical" organization. It is first represented at a "low" (spinal or brain-stem) level, re-represented at the "middle" level of the motor (or sensory) divisions of the cerebral cortex, and represented for the third time (re-re-represented) at a "higher" level, which Jackson considered to be the frontal divisions of the brain. Hence, according to Jackson, the *localization of a symptom* (the impairment of a particular function) accompanying a lesion of a circumscribed area of the central nervous system cannot in any way be identified with the *localization of the particular function.* The latter may emanate from the central nervous system in a much more complex manner and may have a completely different cerebral organization.

Jackson's contemporaries took an incorrect and biased view of his ideas. His hypothesis pertaining to the complex character and vertical organization of functions was many decades ahead of the development of science at that time, and for a long time it remained forgotten, having been confirmed only very recently. On the other hand, his declarations against the concept of narrow localization of functions in circumscribed areas of the cerebral cortex and his claims regarding the complex "intellectual" or "voluntary" character of higher psychological processes were soon adopted by the most idealistically oriented workers, who regarded these viewpoints as support in their stand against the materialistic sensualism of classical neurology. In the period after 1870, attempts were made to have mental processes be regarded as essentially complex, "symbolic" functions. The opinions held by the adherents of this doctrine clashed with the views inherent in narrow localizationism. Mental processes were looked upon as products of the activity of the brain as a whole, with cerebral localization entirely rejected. All that could be said about human mental life was that it is a new, "abstract" type of activity, performed by the brain as the "instrument of the spirit."

One member of this group of investigators was Finkelburg (1870), who, in contrast to Broca and Wernicke, regarded speech as a complex, "symbolic" function. A similar attitude was taken by Kussmaul (1885), who rejected the view that the material basis of memory is a special depot in the cerebral cortex, where images and ideas lie "neatly arranged on the shelves." He believed that the "symbolic function" is the basis of mental life and suggested that every complex disturbance of the brain leads to "asymbolia." In his own words: "We good-humoredly reject all naive attempts to localize speech in one or the other convolution of the brain."

Although at the end of the nineteenth century few voices were raised against the sensualistic approach to the activity of the brain and in support of the "symbolic function" of the brain and its complex anatomic basis, at the beginning of the twentieth century their number began to swell as a result of the revival of idealistic philosophy and psychology and they soon were in the forefront of the study of higher mental processes.

It was at this time that Bergson (1896), seeking to justify his frankly idealistic approach to mental activity, suggested that active dynamic schemes are the basic motive force of the mind, and contrasted them with material "brain memory." The beginning of this century was also marked by the psychological research of adherents of the Würzburg school, who concluded that abstract thought is a primary, independent process, not reducible to sensory images and speech, and who advocated a return to Platonism.

These ideas also spread to neurology. They came to the fore in the writings of the noetic school of neurologists and psychologists (Pierre Marie, 1906; van Woerkom (especially), 1925; Bouman and Grünbaum, 1925; and Goldstein, 1934, 1942, 1948). The followers of this school held that the principal form of the mental process is "symbolic activity," put into operation as "abstract" schemes, and that every disease of the brain is manifested, not so much by a loss of the ability to carry out specialized processes as by a depression of this symbolic function or abstract orientation.

These assertions brought about radical changes in the problems confronting neurologists at this later stage of scientific development. The analysis of the material basis of individual functions as the primary task of research was replaced by the description of the forms of depression of symbolic function or abstract behavior arising from any disease of the brain. In practice, the investigation of the cerebral mechanisms of these disturbances now took second place. Once again having adopted the view that the brain works as a single entity and having related disturbances of the higher mental processes primarily with the size of the lesion and not with its location, these writers made a valuable contribution to the psychological analysis of the changes in cognitive activity accompanying local brain lesions; on the other hand, they greatly impeded research into the material basis of the cerebral mechanisms of mental processes.

These attempts to deflect neurology into the idealistic channel of interpretation of disturbances of mental activity encountered appreciable opposition. The position of certain leading neurologists, notably Monakow (1914, [and Mourgue] 1928), Head (1926), and, above all, Goldstein (1934, 1942, 1948), was particularly complicated, for they more or less supported the noetic doctrine and had to harmonize the localizationists' views hitherto accepted in neurology with the new, antilocalizationists' views. Each of these neurologists found his own way out of the difficulty. Monakow, one of the leading authorities on the cerebral localization of elementary neurological symptoms and signs, refused to adopt the same principle of localization when analyzing the cerebral basis of disturbances of symbolic activity, which he called "asemia." In an article written jointly with Mourgue (1928), he was forced to give an idealistic explanation of the cause of these disturbances; he stated that they are due to changes in deep "instincts." Head, whose secure place in neurology rests on his investigation of sensation, limited his attempts at understanding complex speech disorders to describing disturbances of specific aspects of the speech act; he very conventionally ascribed these individual disturbances to lesions of large areas of the cerebral cortex. Without giving any neurological explanation of these phenomena, he resorted to using a general factor of "vigilance" as the ultimate explanatory principle.

The position of Goldstein, one of the leading neurologists of the present time, proved very constructive. While maintaining allegiance to the classic views on elementary neurological processes, he accepted the new, noetic ideas in respect to complex human mental processes. He classified the latter processes as manifestations of one of two forms of mental activity—"abstract orientation" and "categorical behavior." Goldstein believed that every brain lesion gives rise to a disturbance of abstract orientation or categorical behavior. This assertion forced him to adopt a unique position in regard to disturbances of elementary and higher mental functions. In an attempt to elucidate the cerebral mechanisms of these processes, Goldstein distinguished between the "periphery" of the cortex, in regard to which he retained the structural localization viewpoint, and the "central part" of the cortex, which, in contrast to the periphery, he regarded as "equipotential" and functioning in accordance with the principle of the creation of "dynamic structures" against some form of "dynamic background." Lesions of the periphery of the cortex lead to disturbances of the "means" of mental activity *(Werkzeugstörung)* but leave abstract orientation intact. A lesion of the central part of the cortex causes a profound change in both abstract orientation and categorical behavior, in accordance with the law of mass (the greater the mass of brain substance affected by a lesion, the greater the interference with the formation of complex dynamic structures and the less the differentiation between the structures and the background). In Goldstein's opinion, this differentiation constitutes the neurological basis of this complex categorical behavior. Having adopted a Gestalt psychological viewpoint, and a naturalistic interpretation of the complex forms of human behavior, Goldstein, in fact, repeated Laheley's mistakes in trying to use elementary concepts of the diffuse and equipotential properties of the brain substance to explain the most complex forms of intellectual activity. In other words, in practice Goldstein combined the classical postulate of narrow localization with the new antilocalizationist ideas.*

The history of the problem of the localization of functions in the cerebral cortex thus reached the present time. It was characterized by attempts to identify complex mental processes with the material structure of the brain and by the struggle between two apparently opposite factions, with the

*A critical analysis of Goldstein's views was made by Vygotskii in 1960 (pp. 374–386); this analysis remains one of the most exhaustive in the literature.

formulation of a theory mechanically combining the extremes of localizationism and antilocalizationism, it thus demonstrates what difficulties of principle bar the way to progress in psychomorphology.

This has been a very brief outline of the complex manner in which a solution has been sought to one of the most difficult problems in modern science—the problem of the cerebral mechanisms of mental activity, or, what amounts to the same thing, the problem of the localization of mental functions in the cerebral cortex.

We have seen that from earliest antiquity, all attempts at solution have had to contend with two opposing schools of thought, one attempting to relate mental processes to circumscribed areas of the brain, with the brain regarded as an aggregate of separate organs, and the other assuming that mental activity is a single, indivisible phenomenon, a function of the whole brain working as a single entity. Each of these schools of thought has made its contribution to the development of scientific ideas regarding the brain and the principal forms of its activity. It cannot be denied that the localizationists' views, allowing for their occasionally grossly mechanistic, even fantastic, form, reflected what, for that time, was a progressive tendency, i.e., to regard the brain as a differentiated organ. They also reflected the premature attempts of scientists to approach mental life and the structure of the brain analytically, attempts that subsequently led to the modern, precise sciences of anatomy of the brain and neurology.

Nor can we overestimate the importance of the clinical discoveries of the localizationists, not only for neurological practice, but also for the detection of areas in the apparently homogeneous mass of the brain that are especially significant in the performance of various forms of mental activity. Without these achievements it would have been impossible to formulate any truly scientific theory of the functional organization of the cerebral cortex. Although not equipped with modern scientific methods for the study of their problems, the localizationists made a great contribution to the understanding of the differential working of the brain, and, in this respect, their research must not be underestimated.

At the same time, it cannot be denied that the antilocalizationists also made a substantial contribution to the development of modern ideas on the working of the brain. By insisting that the brain, although a highly differentiated organ, always functions as a whole, by stressing the fact that the brain tissue is highly plastic and that the brain is thereby able to recover its functions, and finally, by emphasizing that the tone of cortical activity is important for perfect functioning of the brain, the followers of the antilocalization school formulated hypotheses that were later (after development and modification) incorporated into modern neurophysiological concepts. It must be remembered that, long before modern ideas on the working of the brain were evolved, members of the antilocalization school had introduced the concept of the vertical organization of functions, stressing the need for analysis of the hierarchal relationships of the different levels of the nervous system.

We must now consider with the greatest attention the stages in the development of research into this highly complex problem, choosing what may be used by modern science. The entire history of the attempt to localize mental processes in the cerebral cortex, whether these attempts were made from the standpoint of localizationism or antilocalizationism, betrays one false assumption, and this led to the most serious misconceptions. However much the two concepts that have been described may differ from each other, they share a common psychomorphological feature: They both look upon mental functions as phenomena to be directly correlated with the brain structure without intermediate physiological analysis. In other words, they both attempted to "superimpose the nonspatial concepts of contemporary psychology on the spatial construction of the brain" (Pavlov) and they continued to regard mental processes as properties incapable of further analysis, to be understood only as the direct product of the activity of cerebral structures. In fact, the belief in the material basis of mental activity, which had been openly incorporated in the medieval notions of the "faculties of the mind," persisted unchanged in all these theories, and the true scientific analysis of the mechanisms by which the brain adequately reflects the outside world was replaced by parallelistic views that complex mental functions correspond to circumscribed or extensive areas of the brain.

Psychomorphological attempts to localize function in a particular area of the brain were natural at a time when in psychology, just as in physiology, the word "function" was taken to mean the function of a particular organ and when the complex structure of the brain and of the physiological processes carried on by the brain had not yet become appreciated. Since then, however, there have been radical changes.

In modern psychology and physiology, new and incomparably more complex ideas on the forms of human activity and of the reflex mechanisms by means of which the organism maintains its equilibrium with the environment have been elaborated. In neuroanatomy, new concepts of the structure of the brain, advocating a material basis for the aforementioned physiological reflex processes, was elaborated. In the light of these achievements of modern science, the very important task of "identifying dynamic phenomena (taking place in the nervous system) with the finer details of brain structure" (Pavlov, *Complete Collected Works*, Vol. 6, p. 437) is incomparably more complex than the simple association of mental functions with circumscribed areas of the cerebral cortex. The task of creating a truly scientific approach to the localization of functions in the cerebral cortex was not tackled realistically until the work of Sechenov, followed by that of Pavlov, had created a new chapter in physiology—the reflex basis of mental processes and the reflex laws governing the activity of the cerebral cortex. Not only did this new teaching provide a new method to objectively analyze the more complex mechanisms of human and animal behavior, but it also led to a radical revision of the concept of function whereby function began to be regarded as an aggregate of complex temporary connections; further, this teaching introduced the view of the cerebral cortex as a collection of central apparatuses for the analysis and synthesis of external and internal stimuli and for the formation of temporary connections. It was as a result of the advances in contemporary physiology made by Pavlov that ideas on the dynamic localization of functions in the cerebral cortex were founded, displacing the older, prescientific, psychomorphological concepts. These new ideas initiated a new epoch in the study of the most complex functions of the brain and permitted a new approach to problems that had remained without adequate solution for centuries.

The development of a theory on the dynamic localization of functions in the cerebral cortex calls, first, for a radical revision of the actual concept of function or, in other words, of the concept of what it is that must be related to the structures of the brain. Second, it calls for the rejection of the elementary notion of centers as large or small cell groups directly responsible for particular mental processes.

Without such a re-examination, there can be no resolution of problems surrounding the subject of the localization of functions in the cerebral cortex, and, consequently, no progress can be made in the study of higher human cortical functions and of their disturbance in the presence of local brain lesions.

B. RE-EXAMINATION OF THE CONCEPT OF FUNCTION AND OF THE PRINCIPLES OF ITS LOCALIZATION

An important advance in modern physiology has been the radical revision of the concept of function, for this has led to new views concerning localization. In the light of modern data, function has ceased to be understood as a direct property of a particular, highly specialized group of cells of an organ. Since Pavlov advanced his reflex theories, the word "function" has come to mean the product of complex reflex activity comprising: uniting excited and inhibited areas of the nervous system into a working mosaic, analysing and integrating stimuli reaching the organism, forming a system of temporary connections, and thereby ensuring the equilibrium of the organism with its environment. This is why the concept of localization of functions has also undergone a radical change and has come to mean a network of complex dynamic structures or combination centers, consisting of mosaics of distant points of the nervous system, united in a common task (Pavlov, *Complete Collected Works*, Vol. 3, pp. 253, 288, etc.). Pavlov's views on localization have been summarized by Ivanov-Smolenskii (1949, pp. 19–62).

This change in our concept of function and localization is so important that special attention must be paid to it. One of the leading Soviet physiologists, Anokhin (1935, 1940), pointed out that "function" is usually employed in two completely different senses. On the one hand, it can mean the activity performed by a given organ or tissue; for example, the function of the liver cells is to secrete bile and the function of the cells of the pancreas is to secrete insulin. In this sense it may be said that the cells of the retina possess the function of light sensitivity and that the cells of the occipital region of the cortex possess the function of analysis and integration of the excitation caused by light stimulation. On the other hand, in biology, in the physiology of higher nervous activity, and in psychology "function" is very often used in a quite different sense. By "function" an organism's complex adaptive activity, directed toward the performance of some physiological or psychological task, is frequently meant. It is in this sense that we speak of the function of respiration, the function of locomotion, the function of perception, and even of the intellectual functions. In all these instances we are concerned with some form of activity that may be performed in various ways, with the requirements of the organism determining the means of execution.

The latter concept of function, which in the history of the study of localization has frequently been confused with the former, differs from it radically in implication and calls for a completely different view of both the structural and the anatomical-physiological basis of functions. Nearly a century ago, Jackson repeatedly declared that functions such as voluntary movement are multiple (nowadays we would say "multistage"*) in their representation in the central nervous system. Although this concept of function remained unnoticed for several decades, it has since gained wide recognition and is now accepted by all physiologists.

According to this view, a function is, in fact, a functional system (a concept introduced by Anokhin,) directed toward the performance of a particular biological task and consisting of a group of interconnected acts that produce the corresponding biological effect. The most significant feature of a functional system is that, as a rule, it is based on a complex dynamic "constellation" of connections, situated at different levels of the nervous system, that, in the performance of the adaptive task, may be changed with the task itself remaining unchanged. As Bernshtein (1935, 1947, etc.) pointed out, such a system of functionally united components has a systematic, not a concrete, structure, in which the initial and final links of the system (the task and the effect) remain constant and unchanged and the intermediate links (the means of performance of the task) may be modified within wide limits.

*So far as I know, the term "multistage representation" of a function was introduced by Filimonov (1940).

Functional systems such as these, complex in composition, plastic in the variability of their elements, and possessing the property of dynamic autoregulation, are apparently the rule in human activity. Pavlov referred to such a system as "... a system on its own, possessing the highest level of autoregulation ..." (*Complete Collected Works*, Vol. 3, p. 454). Examples of systems whose functions require the participation of various levels of the central nervous system are the respiratory system, studied in detail by Anokhin (1935, etc.), and the system of motion, studied in no less detail by Bernshtein (1935, 1947, etc.).

Stimulation of the cells of the medulla by an increased concentration of carbon dioxide in the blood sets in motion a whole system of nervous connections that, by means of the corresponding cells situated at a lower level in the spinal cord, cause contractions of the diaphragm and intercostal muscles; these contractions continue to increase in strength until the oxygen concentration in the blood rises, at which time respiration becomes slow and rhythmic in character. However, as Anokhin showed, the component links of this particular functional system do not form a fixed and constant chain of reactions but are adaptable to a good deal of substitution. For example, severance of the motor nerve of the diaphragm leads to increased activity of the intercostal muscles and inactivation of the intercostal muscles may be followed by other types of activity, even by swallowing, which normally is part of the system of digestion. In such special conditions, swallowing may be appropriated to the functional system of respiration by means of a new act, that of aerophagy.

If respiration is such a complex and plastic functional system, the localization of this function in any circumscribed area of the brain is naturally out of the question. What used to be called the "respiratory center" now acquires a completely different meaning. The situation was well summarized by Pavlov when he wrote: "From the very beginning it was thought that this [the respiratory center] was a point the size of a pin head in the medulla. Now, however, it has shifted around a great deal, climbing up into the brain and moving down into the spinal cord, so that nobody knows its precise limits ...." (*Complete Collected Works*, Vol. 3, p. 127). Thus, such an apparently simple function as respiration is actually a complex functional system, effected by a differential dynamic arrangement of nerve cells belonging to different levels of the nervous system.

The situation is still more complex in respect to voluntary movement, which cannot in any way be considered to be a function of only the giant pyramidal cells situated in the motor zone of the cerebral cortex.

Bernshtein's (1926, 1935, 1947, 1957, etc.) careful investigations showed that, in principle, it is impossible for the motor systems to be regulated only by efferent impulses arising in the cells of the anterior central gyrus. The motor act is not the "function" of any one localized group of nerve cells situated in the cerebral cortex but is a complex functional system, whose working is controlled by many factors. This system actually consists of many links with differentiated roles, and it is capable of the highest degree of autoregulation. Bernshtein showed that movement is primarily determined by the "motor task", which, in locomotion, goal-directed activity, or a symbolic act (e.g., a descriptive movement and writing), is formed at different levels and with the participation of different afferent systems. It is carried out not only by the cortical apparatuses, but also by the subcortical nuclei, which provide the tonal background and coordination without which the movement would be impossible. Finally—a particularly important feature—the regulation of voluntary movement requires a continuous afferent feedback in the form of constant proprioceptive signals from the moving muscles and the joints. Without these signals the correction of movement would be impossible. To this description of the systems of voluntary movement should be added the fact that every time there is the slightest change in the situation the act has to be carried out by a different set of muscles and a different series of motor impulses. For instance, if the initial position of the hand is changed, a simple blow with a hammer requires completely different motor innervations, sometimes even different muscles. In other words, as previously stated, the motor system is constructed according to a systematic, not a concrete, principle. Therefore, voluntary movement is least likely to be a fixed or stable "function" carried out only by efferent impulses arising from the giant pyramidal cells. The structural basis of voluntary movement is a whole system of afferent and efferent links, situated in different parts and at different levels of the central nervous system. Each link of this system plays its own differential role (providing the "motor task," the spatial or kinetic scheme of the movement, the tone and coordination of the muscle groups, the feedback of signals from the effect of the completed action, etc.). It is only by the close interaction of the elements of this functional system that its essential plasticity and self-regulation can be assured.

These investigations led to a radical revision of the concept of function. Function no longer was considered the "business" of some particular cerebral organ or group of cells, but began to be understood as a complex and plastic system performing a particular adaptive task and composed of a highly differentiated group of interchangeable elements. At the same time, they also led to a radical revision of views on the nature of *localization* in the central nervous system of any function, even the relatively simple ones. Localization ceased to be understood as the assignment of a function to a particular area of the brain or to an isolated group of nerve cells. This simplified and obsolete view was replaced by what the eminent Soviet neurologist Filimonov (1940, 1944, 1951, 1957) has called the principle of "graded localization of functions." Filimonov closely associated this principle with that of "functional pluripotentialism" of the cerebral components. Because of the importance of these principles, they must be discussed in greater detail.

Nowadays, with the modern view of function, nobody believes that phenomena such as the patellar reflex or, still less, voluntary movement may be localized in circumscribed areas of the brain. The smooth execution of each act requires a series of both simultaneously and successively excited connections. Analysis of the individual links of the patellar reflex or of a simply voluntary movement discloses the nerve elements that successively and simultaneously contribute to the achievement of the end result. The loss of any one link of this system immediately affects the end result and leads to the reorganization of the whole system, with the object of restoring the disturbed act. It is for this reason that Filimonov points out that a function cannot, by its nature, be associated with any single "center," and he suggests that the principle of "successive and simultaneous gradations in the localization of functions" replace the old view of isolated, static centers.

This concept of successive and simultaneous stages is closely connected with the concept of functional pluripotentialism of the cerebral structures. Filimonov (1951, 1957) introduced the principle of functional pluripotentialism in opposition to the ideas of narrow localizationism and equipotentialism of the brain tissue. In essence, it implies that no formation of the central nervous system is responsible for solely a single function; under certain conditions, a given formation may be involved in other functional systems and may participate in the performance of other tasks. These concepts have both a morphological and physiological basis.

When studying the olfactory structures of the cerebral cortex, Filimonov found that they also exist in anosmatics (for example, the dolphin); he concluded that these structures must also have other functions. Similar conclusions were reached by Lashley (1930–1942), who demonstrated the pluripotentialism of the visual cortex and by several other workers (e.g., Penfield and Jasper, 1954), who discovered sensory functions in the motor zone and motor functions in the sensory zone. In Grinshtein's (1956) opinion, the concept of cortical functional pluripotentialism is supported by Pavlov's view that the cerebral cortex contains a diffuse periphery, and that, as a result, individual zones of the cortex may be components of different systems and take part in different functions.

The functional pluripotentialism of cerebral structures was confirmed physiologically by the observation (Hess, 1954) that salivation, usually induced by stimulation of the appropriate nuclei of the brain stem, may be a product of thermoregulatory or digestive activities. It was previously mentioned that the act of swallowing may be induced by both the digestive and the respiratory systems.

The concepts of graded localization of functions and pluripotentialism of the brain structures, in which both narrow localization of function in a particular, special structure and homogeneity and equipotentialism of the brain tissue were rejected, are fundamental to the new principle of dynamic localization formulated by Pavlov (*Complete Collected Works*, Vol. 3, pp. 127,

233, 436, etc.) and Ukhtomskii (1945, pp. 101–102, etc.). According to this principle, functions are localized, not in fixed centers, but in dynamic systems whose elements maintain strict differentiation and play a highly specialized role in integrated activity. Ukhtomskii formulated his concept of a center as follows: "The center, or aggregate of central apparatuses necessary and adequate for the function, consists, in most cases, of cycles of interaction between more or less widely separated ganglion cells . . . . The 'center' of a complex function is a constellation of harmoniously working ganglionic areas, mutually exciting one another." He goes on to say: "Coordination in the time, speed, and rhythm of action, and, indeed, in the periods at which the various moments of the reaction occur creates a functionally unified 'center' from spatially different groups. . . ." (1945, p. 102).

The dynamically systematic structural basis of functions is confirmed by anatomical facts. Subsequently (Part I, Section 2) we shall see how complex is the system of connections in the apparatus of the central nervous system.

In man the zones in which there is "overlapping" of the cortical boundaries of different analyzers (i.e., regions in which, according to the modern view, combined activity of different cortical areas takes place) comprise 43% of the total mass of the cortex, so that it appears that the evolution of the cortex proceeds mainly on the basis of formations responsible for this integrative activity of the central nervous apparatus in relation to particular functional systems. This evidence fundamentally contradicts the idea of isolated centers and confirms the belief that the brain functions as a series of systems. The anatomical fact that the fibers of the pyramidal tract originate not only in the motor zone of the cortex, but also in areas far beyond its limits (Lassek, 1954; Grinshtein, 1946, etc.), is further confirmation. Likewise, the sensory fibers emerging from the associative nuclei of the thalamus extend not only to the sensory area of the cortex, but also to distant parts of the frontal, parietal, and temporal regions (Grinshtein, 1946, 1956) and thus allow for the wide regulation of movements. Finally, in recent decades (Polyak, 1932; Walker, 1938; Lindsley *et al.*, 1952; Magoun, 1958; Moruzzi, 1954; Jasper, 1954; etc.) the important role played in the whole apparatus of the brain by vertical centrifugal-centripetal connections has been demonstrated: They are present in every area of the cortex and connect it to the secondary nuclei of the thalamus and to the structures of the nonspecific activating formation. This evidence compels the re-examination of many previously held ideas on the structure of the brain and the adoption of views fundamentally different from those previously accepted.

The concept of the systematic structure and dynamic localization of functions also clarifies several observations that were difficult to explain on the basis of the previous concept of isolated, stable centers in the cerebral cortex.

For instance, we can understand more clearly the experimental results obtained many years ago by Brown (1915, 1916), Grünbaum and Sherrington (1901, 1903), and Leyton and Sherrington (1917). By stimulating the same point of the motor cortex, these workers elicited diametrically opposite effects, the nature of the effe . depending on the strength of stimulation and on previous stimuli. These results also help to explain the experiments described by Penfield and his co-workers (Penfield and Ericson, 1945; Penfield and Rasmussen, 1950; Penfield and Jasper, 1954), showing that motor effects may be obtained by stimulating the posterior central gyrus and that sensory changes may be obtained by stimulating the anterior segments of the cerebral cortex. Finally, the concept of the systemic structural organization of functions also explains the different results obtainable by stimulation of a particular area of the cortex with an electric current and with strychnine and the finding that extirpation of a particular area of the cerebral cortex may not be followed by the loss of the functions of those muscle groups that contract when the same area is stimulated (Ward, 1948, and Denny-Brown *et al.*, 1948: cited by Bassin, 1956).

Head (1926) was able to declare long before all the findings just described had been obtained that "... cortical activity, even when aroused by electrical stimulation, is revealed as a march of events with a definite temporal relation. The response obtained from any one point, at a particular moment, depends on what has happened before ...." (Vol. 1, p. 434).

The phenomena just considered seem to suggest that individual areas of the cerebral cortex cannot be regarded as fixed centers but, rather, that they are "staging posts" or "junctions" in the dynamic systems of excitation in the brain and that these systems have an extremely complex and variable structure.

From the standpoint of the concept of the systematic structure of functions and the pluripotentialism of the cortical structures, we may also gain a better understanding of facts relating to the disturbance of functions after local brain injuries or after extirpation of circumscribed areas of the brain. For many years, ever since the experiments of Leyton and Sherrington (1917), it has been known and repeatedly confirmed that in many cases total extirpation of a particular cortical center in an animal leads to only an initial loss of the corresponding function; the disturbed function is gradually recovered and, if any isolated part of the cerebral cortex is subsequently extirpated, it does not cause the secondary loss of this restored function. It was concluded from these findings that the cerebral cortex does not consist of separate, isolated centers and that the recovery of a function must not be attributed to transfer of the function to a new, vicarious center but rather, to a structural reorganization into a new, dynamic system widely dispersed in the cerebral cortex and lower formations.

We still know very little about the systems in which the restored function is accommodated. We do know that after injury to isolated areas of the cerebral cortex and, still more important, at different levels on the evolutionary scale, i.e., in animals differing in their degree of corticalization of functions and of cortical differentiation, the disturbed function may not recover to the same extent. We also know that some components of a disturbed function recover more easily than others. Finally, and we must emphasize this point particularly, clinicopathological investigations on human patients have shown that the restoration of a disturbed function is more correctly defined as the reorganization of that function, with the formation of a new functional system; the laws governing this reorganization have recently been studied in greater detail than was the case two decades ago. The present author has discussed these problems separately elsewhere (Luria, 1948). It may therefore be concluded that functions are not wholly associated with particular, isolated areas of the cerebral cortex and that the restoration of functions never takes place by transfer to equipotential areas of brain tissue.

Finally, by regarding functions as complex functional systems with dynamic levels of localization in the brain, light is shed on certain clinical phenomena long inexplicable on the basis of narrow, stable localization. For instance, Jackson's fundamental discovery that a local brain lesion may cause a disturbance of the voluntary, conscious performance of a function while leaving its involuntary performance intact is thus explained. This concept of function also explains the fact, which we shall discuss again, that a local brain lesion is hardly ever accompanied by total loss of a function but usually by its disorganization, with the latter leading to an abnormal performance and rarely to a complete loss. (The classical descriptions of total loss of functions in the presence of local brain lesions are, in many cases, oversimplifications of the observed facts.) As we shall see, the concept of functions as complex functional systems explains the basic fact, too often ignored by the older authorities in neurology and to which we shall pay particular attention, that the disturbance of a particular function may arise in association with lesions in very different parts of the cerebral cortex and that, in practice, a circumscribed focus leads to the disturbance of an entire complex of apparently very different functions (Part I, Section 3).

The foregoing shows that a radical re-examination of the concept of function and of the principles of localization in the cerebral cortex leads to a modification of our previous ideas and presents new opportunities for research into the functional organization of the brain.

C. THE HIGHER MENTAL FUNCTIONS IN MAN

We have seen that revision of our views on the structure of even relatively simple biological functions (not to mention the more complex ones, such as movement) has led to a radical modification of the principles of their localization in the brain. How does this affect the problem of the localization of the higher mental functions, which has always been foremost when considering the activity of the brain as the organ of mental function?

After what has been said, we have no grounds for localizing complex processes like object perception and logical thinking in circumscribed areas of the cerebral cortex or for reverting to the naive belief that the cerebral cortex contains innate centers of the will or of abstract thinking. Does this mean, however, that we must completely reject the differential analysis of the material basis of these more complex processes and merely assert that the higher mental functions are carried on by the brain as a single entity? Or, on the other hand, must we claim that these mental processes cannot, in general, be localized, i.e., agree with Sherrington (1940) that "between reflex action and mind there seems actual opposition. Reflex action and mind seem almost mutually exclusive . . . . The more reflex the reflex, the less does mind accompany it." (These are not the only remarks to this effect made by Sherrington. Similar ones may be found in several of his more recent publications [1946, 1948].) To answer these questions we must analyze the changes that have taken place in the understanding of higher mental functions during recent decades and consider the advances made during this period in the science of psychology.

The principal achievement of modern psychology may be considered to be the rejection of both the idealistic notion that higher mental functions are manifestations of a certain "mind" principle, distinct from all other natural phenomena, and the naturalistic assumption that these functions are natural properties bestowed by nature on the human brain. One of the major advances in modern materialistic psychology has been the introduction of the *historical method* by means of which higher mental functions are regarded as complex products of sociohistorical development. This viewpoint, connected above all with the names of Soviet psychologists (Vygotskii, 1956, 1960; Leont'ev, 1959, 1961, etc.) and to a certain extent with those of progressive non-Soviet workers (Janet, 1928; Wallon, 1942; etc.), is vitally important to the problem we are now considering.

Modern psychology has completely abandoned the previous conceptions of complex mental processes as "faculties" incapable of further analysis or as primary "properties" of human cerebral processes. It has totally rejected the view that human conscious processes must be interpreted as manifestations of a "mind" principle incapable of further elucidation.

Following the theories of Sechenov and Pavlov, the modern science of psychology regards the higher mental processes as a complex reflex activity, responsible for reflecting the outside world. It does not accept the belief in the existence of "purely active" volitional processes or "purely passive" sensations and perceptions. In adopting a deterministic approach to voluntary movement and activity, it always seeks their afferent basis. In studying sensation and perception as reflex processes, it attempts to describe the effector components of receptor activities; the effectors are considered responsible for the active "tuning" and participation of the receptors in the mechanism of formation of the "image" of the objective world. (The efferent organization of the receptor apparatus has recently been described by Granit [1955], Kvasov [1956], and others and also in works dealing with the study of reception as a complex orienting activity [Sokolov, 1957, 1958, etc., and Leont'ev, 1959].)

From the standpoint of modern psychology, the localization of such processes as visual or auditory perception in circumscribed sensory areas of the cerebral cortex, like the localization of voluntary movement and activity in circumscribed areas of the motor cortex, appears, not less, but actually more improbable than the localization of respiration or of the patellar reflex in a single, isolated area of the brain.

However, the mere fact that we recognize the reflex character of all mental processes and can relate psychology to the physiological theories of higher nervous activity does not in itself reveal the specific features distinguishing human higher mental functions.

From the point of view of modern psychology, the higher human mental functions are complex reflex processes, social in origin, mediate in structure, and conscious and voluntary in mode of function. We must pause here to consider this definition in more detail.

Modern materialistic psychology considers that the higher forms of human mental activity are sociohistorical in origin. In contrast to the animal, man is born and lives in a world of objects created by the work of society and in a world of people with whom he forms certain relationships. From the very beginning, this milieu influences his mental processes. The natural reflexes of the child (sucking, grasping, etc.) are radically reorganized as a result of the handling of objects. New motor patterns are formed, creating what is virtually a "mold" of these objects, so that the movements begin to match the properties of the objects. The same applies to human perception, formed under the direct influence of the objective world of things, themselves of social origin and the product of what Marx broadly called "industry."

The highly complex systems of reflex connections which reflect the objective world of products created by the practical efforts of society require the combined working of many receptors and the formation of new functional systems.

However, the child does not live entirely in a world of ready-made objects, produced by the work of society. From the very beginning of his life he must always be in contact with other people, and, in so doing, he must objectively master the existing language system and, with its aid, profit from the experience of other generations. This contact becomes the decisive factor in his future mental development, the decisive condition for the formation of the higher mental functions distinguishing man from animals.

Janet (1928) pointed out that the roots of processes such as voluntary memorizing, in daily use by everybody, are quite irrationally sought in the natural, distinctive features of the human brain; rather, in order to discover the origin of these complex forms of conscious mental activity it is necessary to turn to social history. The development of the higher forms of mental activity in the course of ontogenesis was studied by Vygotskii (1956, 1960), who showed that social contact between the child and adults always lies at the root of such forms of activity as paying attention or voluntary movement. By initially carrying out the adult's verbal command—pointing out a certain object or aspect of an object, suggesting a certain movement, etc.—and then reproducing the activity suggested by this verbal instruction and initiating it himself, the child gradually forms a new voluntary action that, in time, becomes a part of his individual behavior. Vygotskii's supposition that an action initially shared by two people later becomes an element of individual behavior has, as a corollary, the social origin of the higher mental functions and points to the social nature of those psychological phenomena that have usually been regarded as purely individualistic. The historical approach to the higher mental processes, revealing their social nature, thus eliminates both the spiritualistic and the naturalistic interpretations of these processes.

The social genesis of the higher mental functions—their formation in the process of objective activity and social communication—determines the second fundamental characteristic of these functions, *their mediate structure.* Vygotskii (1960) repeatedly declared that mental faculties do not evolve along "pure" lines, i.e., a particular property gradually perfecting itself, but, rather, develop along "mixed" lines, i.e., the creation of new, intermediate structures of mental processes and new "interfunctional" relationships directed toward the performance of previous tasks by new methods. The concept of "pure" and "mixed" evolution was introduced by the Russian psychologist, Vagner (1928), who conducted important research in the field of comparative psychology.

As examples of the mediate structure of higher mental functions, we may use any performance of a practical task by means of tools or solution of an internal, psychological problem by means of an auxiliary sign in order to organize the mental processes. When a person ties a knot in his handkerchief or makes a note in order to remember something, he carries out an operation apparently quite unrelated to the task in hand. In this way, however, the person masters his faculty of memory; by changing the structure of the memorizing process and giving it a mediate character, he thereby broadens its natural capacity. Mediate memorizing illustrates the structural principles of the higher mental functions. A closer analysis shows that this mediate structure is a characteristic feature of all higher mental processes.

Speech plays a decisive role in the mediation of mental processes. By being given a name, an object or its property is distinguished from its surroundings and is related to other objects or signs. The fact that "every word is a generalization" (Lenin) is vitally important to the systematic reflection of the outside world, to the transition from sensation to thinking, and to the creation of new functional systems. Speech not only gives names to the objects of the outside world; it also distinguishes among their essential properties and includes them in a system of relationships to other objects. As a result of language, man can evoke an image of a particular object and use it in the absence of the original. At the same time, speech, differentiating among the essential signs and generalizing on the objects or phenomena denoted, facilitates deeper penetration of the environment. Human mental processes are thereby elevated to a new level and are given new powers of organization, and man is enabled to direct his mental processes.

The reorganization of mental activity by means of speech and the incorporation of the system of speech connections into a large number of processes, hitherto direct in character, are among the more important factors in the formation of the higher mental functions, whereby man, as distinct from animals, acquires consciousness and volition.

The fact that the speech system is a factor in the formation of the higher mental functions is their most important feature. Because of this, Pavlov was justified in considering the "second signal system," which is based on speech, not only "an extraordinary addition, introducing a new principle of nervous activity," but also "the highest regulator of human behavior" (*Complete Collected Works*, Vol. 3, pp. 476, 490, 568–569, 577).

It would be wrong to suppose that the mediate structure of the higher mental functions, formed with the intimate participation of speech, is characteristic only of such forms of activity as memorizing, voluntary attention, or logical thinking. Recently reported investigations showed that even such mental processes as high-tone hearing, which have always been considered relatively elementary and apparently unrelated to the features described, are, in fact, formed under the influence of the prevalent social conditions and, above all, of language. The research of Leont'ev (1959, 1961) showed that high-tone hearing is one of the "systematic functions" formed in man with the close participation of language, the specific features of which cannot be understood without knowledge of the characteristic signs of the language in whose system human speech is formed. These investigations are not merely of great special interest, but are also of decisive general importance, for they demonstrate the social nature and systematic structure not only of complex, but also of relatively simple, human mental processes. Consequently, when considering the cerebral organization of higher mental functions, we must always take into account the factors just enumerated.

What conclusions can we reach from these remarks in regard to the main problem concerning us here—the localization of the higher mental functions in the cerebral cortex?

The first possible conclusion is obvious. If the higher mental functions are complex, organized functional systems that are social in origin, any attempt to localize them in special, circumscribed areas ("centers") of the cerebral cortex is even less justifiable than the attempt to seek narrow, circumscribed "centers" for biological functional systems. The modern view regarding the possible localization of the higher mental functions is that they have a wide, dynamic representation throughout the cerebral cortex, based on constellations of territorially scattered groups of "synchronously working ganglion cells, mutually exciting one another" (Ukhtomskii, 1945). Hence, the higher mental functions are accommodated in the brain in systems of "functional combination centers," as Pavlov called them (*Complete Collected Works*, Vol. 3, p. 288). The fact that systems of speech connections are necessary components of the higher mental functions makes the cerebral organization of these functions an exceptionally complex matter. We therefore suggest that *the material basis of the higher nervous processes is the brain as a whole* but that *the brain is a highly differentiated system whose parts are responsible for different aspects of the unified whole.*

The second conclusion is that the complex functional systems of conjointly working cortical zones, which, it might be assumed, are their material basis, are not found ready-made in the child at birth (as in the case of respiratory and other systems) and do not mature independently, but are formed in the process of social contact and objective activity by the child, gradually acquiring the character of the complex intercentral connections that Leont'ev (1959, pp. 466–468) called "functional brain organs." These intercentral systems, or functional brain organs, arise under the influence of the child's practical activity and are extremely stable. It will be sufficient to analyze the interactions between the cortical systems that are necessary for speaking, writing, for practical operations with objects, for the hearing of speech, reading, and so on to appreciate the enormous complexity of these systems and their exceptional stability. Naturally, these functional systems can exist only in the presence of an apparatus allowing for the formation of new, dynamically variable, yet enduring intercentral connections. As we shall show later (Part I, Section 2), the upper associative layers of the cerebral cortex, the vertical connections arising in the secondary associative nuclei of the thalamus, and the overlapping zones uniting different boundaries of cortical analyzers evidently constitute the apparatus that performs this highly complex task. It is in man that this apparatus of the brain has attained its highest development, sharply distinguishing the human brain from that of animals. We, therefore, agree with the view that evolution, under the influence of social conditions, accomplishes the task of conversion of the cortex into an organ capable of forming functional organs (Leont'ev, 1961, p. 38) and that the latter property is one of the more important features of the human brain.

We have indicated the highly differentiated nature of the intercentral dynamic connections comprising the cerebral basis of the higher mental functions. As previously stated, the higher mental functions have as their basis relatively elementary sensory and motor processes. Investigations in the field of child psychology (Zaporozhets, 1960; Gal'perin, 1957, 1959; Él'konin, 1960; etc.) have shown that in the early stages of development this connection between the higher mental processes and their objective (sensory and motor) basis stands out particularly clearly but that during later development these objective components, although continuing as components, gradually diminish in importance.

We are indebted to Vygotskii (1960, pp. 375–393—especially 384–393) for his detailed analysis of the hypothesis that higher mental functions may exist only as a result of interaction between the highly differentiated brain structures and that individually these structures make their own specific contributions to the dynamic whole and play their own roles in the functional system. This hypothesis, intrinsically opposed to both narrow localization and diffuse equipotentialism, is a thread running through the whole of this book.

It remains for us to draw the last conclusion from this account of the genesis and structure of the higher mental functions. It has already been pointed out that the higher mental functions are formed in the process of ontogenesis, passing through several successive stages. Leont'ev (1931, 1959) and Vygotskii (1956, 1960) showed that during the early stages the higher mental functions depend on the use of external evocative signs and that their pattern is one of a series of unfolding operations. Only when this is complete do they gradually consolidate, so that the whole process is converted into a concise action, based initially on external and then on internal speech. During recent years these ideas have been reflected in the investigations of Piaget (1947, 1955) and, in the Soviet Union, in a series of investigations conducted by Gal'perin (1957, 1959, etc.). It may be concluded that at successive stages of their development the structure of the higher mental functions does not remain constant but that they perform the same task by means of different, regularly interchanging systems of connections.

To give a specific example of this point of view, we may compare the process of writing as carried out during the first stages of training, when it consists of a complex cycle of unconnected acts (converting sound elements into visual images, drawing the separate graphic components of the letters), with its execution when it has become a highly automatized skill. Other skills, such as reading and calculating, whose psychological composition is totally different at different stages of training, take a similar course. In respect to the higher mental functions, these hypotheses side with the systemic rather than the concrete view of the structure of activity; important conclusions may be drawn from this viewpoint in connection with the cerebral organization of the higher mental functions.

The structural variation of the higher mental functions at different stages of ontogenetic (and, in some cases, functional) development means that their cortical organization likewise does not remain unchanged and that at different stages of development they are carried out by different constellations of cortical zones.

It is difficult to overestimate the importance of this concept to the correct diagnosis of brain lesions and to the understanding of the qualitative modifications that the higher mental functions undergo in the course of restoration. The essential thing to remember, however, is that this change in the character of localization (or, more accurately, cortical organization) of the higher mental functions is strictly regular, conforming to a pattern ascertained by Vygotskii (1960, pp. 390–391). This section of the book will be concluded with a brief account of his formulation.

Observations have shown that the relationships between the individual components of the higher mental functions do not remain the same during successive stages of development. In the early stages, relatively simple sensory processes, which are the foundation for the higher mental functions, play a decisive role; during subsequent stages, when the higher mental functions are being formed, this leading role passes to more complex systems of connections that develop on the basis of speech, and these systems begin to determine the whole structure of the higher mental processes. For this reason, disturbance of the relatively elementary processes of sensory analysis and integration, necessary, for example, for the further development of speech, will be decisively important in early childhood, for it will cause underdevelopment of all the functional formations for which it serves as a foundation. Conversely, the disturbance of these forms of direct sensory analysis and integration in the adult, in whom the higher functional systems have been formed, may have a more limited effect, compensated for by other differentiated systems of connections. This concept implies that *the character of the cortical intercentral relationships does not remain the same at different stages of development of a function and that the effect of a lesion of a particular part of the brain will differ at different stages of functional development.*

Vygotskii (1960) formulated the following rule of the different influence of a local lesion at different stages of the development of a function: In the early stages of ontogenesis, a lesion of a particular area of the cerebral cortex will predominantly affect a higher (i.e., developmentally dependent on it) center than that where the lesion is situated, whereas in the stage of fully formed functional systems, a lesion of the same area of the cortex will predominantly affect a lower center (i.e., regulated by it). This rule, whose importance is hard to overestimate, shows how complex are the intercentral relationships in the developmental process and how important it is to take into account the laws of formation of the higher mental functions when analyzing the sequelae of circumscribed lesions of the cerebral cortex.

We shall endeavor to make use of all these principles when we analyze actual cases of disturbance of the higher mental functions resulting from local brain lesions.

• • •

We have seen the complex way in which the functional systems usually referred to as the higher mental functions are formed, encompassing a wide range of phenomena from the relatively elementary processes of perception and movement to the complex systems of speech connections acquired by training and of higher forms of intellectual activity. We have repeatedly mentioned that these higher mental processes are based on the conjoined working of functional combination centers of the cerebral cortex.

However, a question arises that, if left unanswered, will prevent continuance without description of cortical functioning and discussion of the pathology of the cerebral systems: How is the cerebral cortex—the organ of mental life—actually constructed? What modern ideas can help us take a more concrete approach to an understanding of how these complex systems really work, and what are the actual apparatuses on which we can base this dynamic localization of the higher mental functions in the cerebral cortex?

This problem requires special consideration, and such consideration will be given to it in the next section of this book.

2. *Modern Data on the Structural Organization of the Cerebral Cortex**

A. ORIGINAL CONCEPTIONS

Progress in our knowledge of the microscopic structure of the cerebral cortex and of the functional significance of the various groups of neurons *from* which it is formed has largely been determined by the historical development of our conceptions of the nature of functional localization in the brain as has been outlined. A particularly important role in the development of modern ideas on the localization of functions in the cerebral cortex has been played by the discovery of a highly intricate differentiation of the cortex into cyto-architectonic and myeloarchitectonic areas and fields. The diagrams of the architectonic fields of the cerebral cortex composed by Campbell (1905), Brodmann (1909), C. and O. Vogt (1919–1920), and others, as well as reports on findings pertaining to the organization of the connections between the different cortical divisions and between the cortex and the subcortical cerebral formations of the brain, have provided an accurate guide for the understanding of the anatomical basis of the complex functional systems of the cortex.

The subdivision of the cerebral cortex into numerous formations, differing in the architectonics of their cells and fibers (Figs. 4 and 5), was used by the psychomorphologists and adherents of narrow localization in their attempts to ascribe the more complex brain functions to isolated areas of the cortex. Among the leading exponents of these doctrines were Kleist (1934), Henschen (1920–1922), and C. and O. Vogt (1919–1920). They regarded each field as the material basis of a separate function and as independent of the functions of other fields. Brodmann's (1909) views on this matter were more moderate, for, besides agreeing with the concept of absolute localization of functions

*This section was written by G. I. Polyakov.

in cortical fields clearly demarcated from neighboring areas, he also accepted that of the relative localization of functions in fields morphologically showing gradual transformation into other fields.

A correct understanding of the nature of the interrelationships and the functional significance of the cortical areas, and, in turn, regions, became possible only after the decline of the old, obsolete conceptions of both the equipotentialists and the narrow localizationists. With the passing of the concept of the brain as a static aggregate of organs or centers in which the faculties, independent in character, are localized, there developed the view that the cerebral cortex is a dynamic association of formations, distinguished by their high plasticity, unification into mobile, dynamic complexes, and joint participation, in varying degrees, in the various stages of the foundation, development, and perfection of the different forms of cortical activity.

The reflex principle, the basis of the theory of comprehensive multistage localization of functions, allows the various fields of the cortex together with their systems of connections to be regarded as highly specialized elements of a functionally single but structurally complex entity. The increasingly intricate subdivision of the cortex into architectonic areas and regions occurring in the course of phylogenesis is brought about by the increasing complexity of the reflex arcs established under various circumstances and the resultant increasing complexity of the functional differentiation of the cortex.

Our ideas on the functional significance of the various elements of cortical organization have undergone further development as a result of application

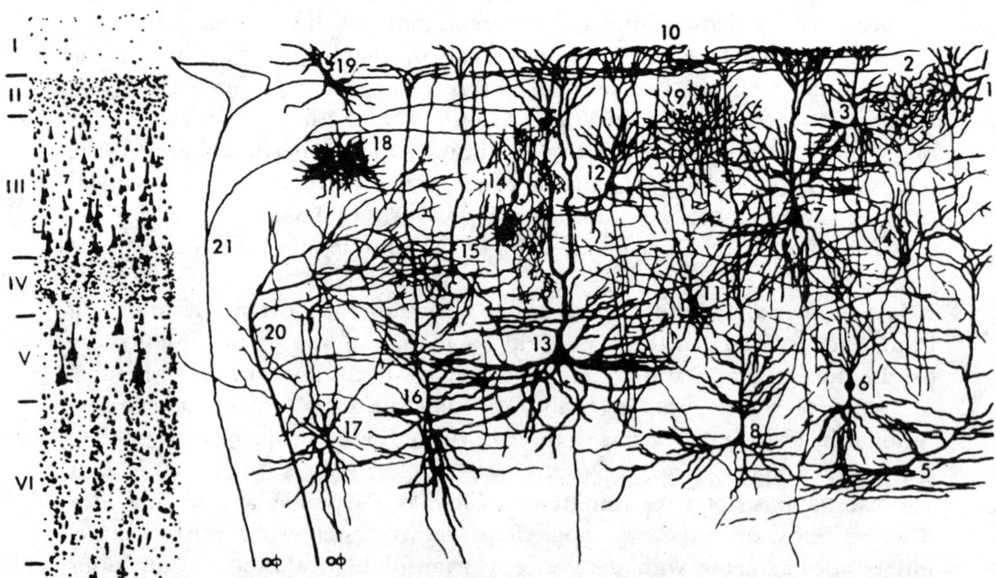

FIGURE 4 Scheme of the neuronal and architectonic structure of the cerebral cortex. The cytoarchitectonic layers of the cortex are shown on the left and the various shapes of the cortical neurons (pyramidal, fusiform, and stellate) on the right. (*After Polyakov, 1959.*)

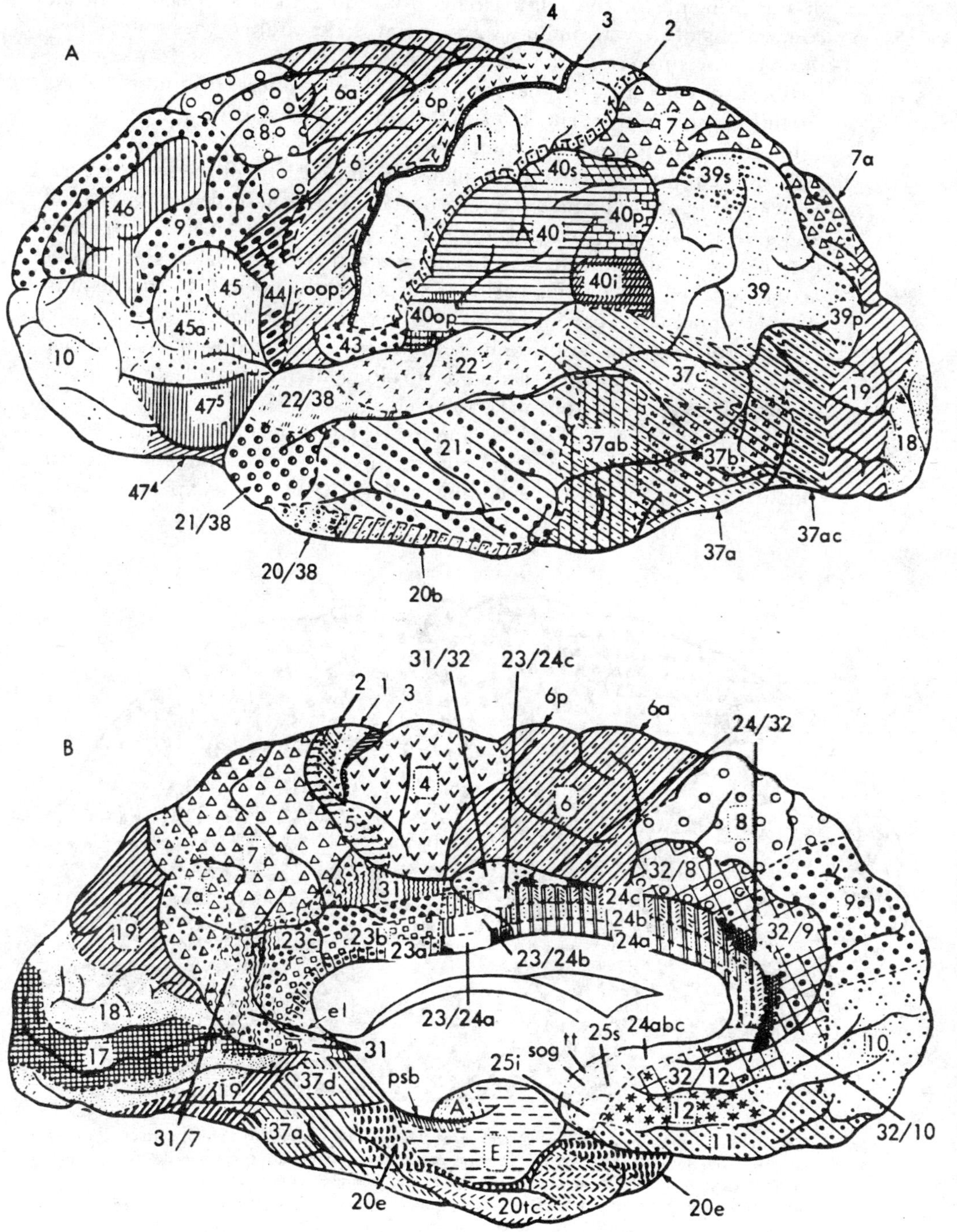

FIGURE 5 Scheme of the cytoarchitectonic fields of the cerebral cortex (*a*) Convex surface of the cortex. (*b*) Medial surface of the cortex. (*Based on the records of the Moscow Brain Institute.*)

of the principle of the reflex circuit. According to this principle, all the connections of nervous impulses arriving at the central nervous system from the receptor surfaces of the organism are carried out by the formation of feedback circuits (i.e., on the basis of antidromic afferent impulses); these circuits constitute an essential link in the system of centripetal and centrifugal connections of the brain and spinal cord.

The cerebral cortex, the most highly organized part of the entire central nervous system, has come to be regarded as a higher-level center for analysis and integration of signals received by the organism from its internal and external environments. It may be supposed that the programs of definite actions worked out on this basis are subsequently integrated with the antidromic signals ("signals of effect," i.e., of success or failure of the action carried out). As a result of comparing what was planned with what, in fact, takes place, the initiated action is prolonged, terminated, or modified (Anokhin, 1955; Pribram, 1959*b*, 1960).

The principle of feedback is universal in the operation of the central nervous system. In the cerebral cortex, this principle is put into effect in singularly complex forms, depending on the actual functional purpose of the

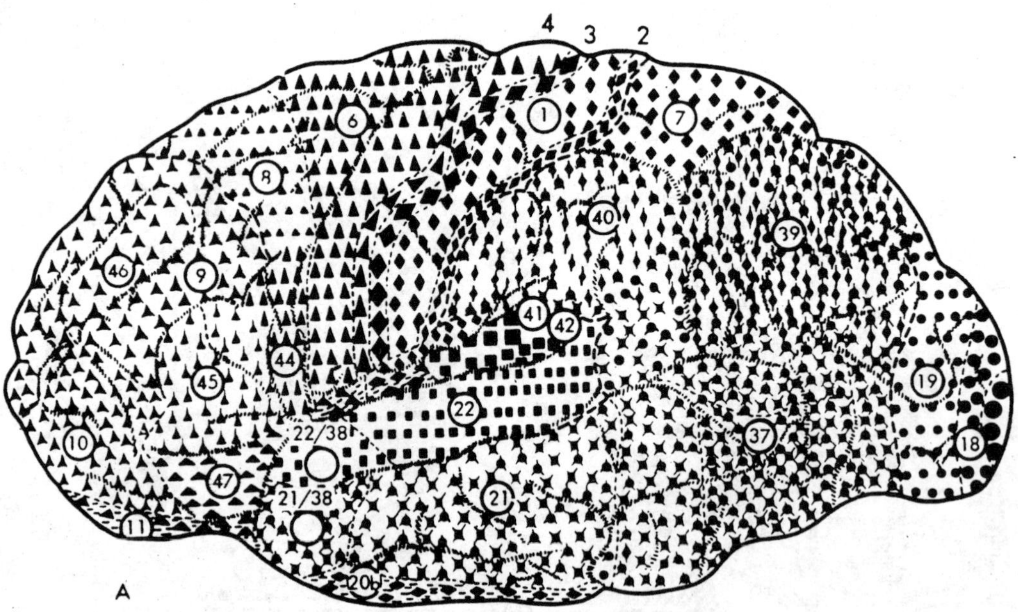

FIGURE 6 Nuclear and extranuclear zones of the cerebral cortex. (*A*) Lateral surface. (*B*) Medial surface. The nuclear zones of the cerebral cortex are denoted by circles (visual zone), squares (auditory zone), rhombi (general sensory zone), and triangles (motor zone); the central fields are demarcated by larger symbols. Overlapping zones of analyzers in the posterior divisions of the

cortical-subcortical mechanisms responsible for the various aspects of the organism's reflection of the outside world and its internal environment.

If we examine these actual mechanisms we start from Pavlov's fundamental idea of systems of analyzers and of nuclear zones of analyzers in the cerebral cortex (Fig. 6). By the term "nuclear zones of analyzers" Pavlov meant particular areas of the cortex in which the concentration of the specific elements of the analyzers and their corresponding connections is maximal. Pavlov regarded these zones as being associated with the most highly differentiated manifestation of the activity of individual analyzers yet, at the same time, carrying out an integrative function.

Numerous physiological, clinical, and anatomical investigations undertaken recently have confirmed the correctness of this concept, which was originally formulated on the basis of experimental extirpation of particular regions of the cerebral cortex in dogs and detailed studies of the ensuing changes in conditioned-reflex activity. That the cerebral cortex of all mammals is composed of circumscribed areas, receiving the bulk of the afferent impulses from the corresponding sensory organs and having special importance in relation to the analysis and integration of the stimuli arriving from the

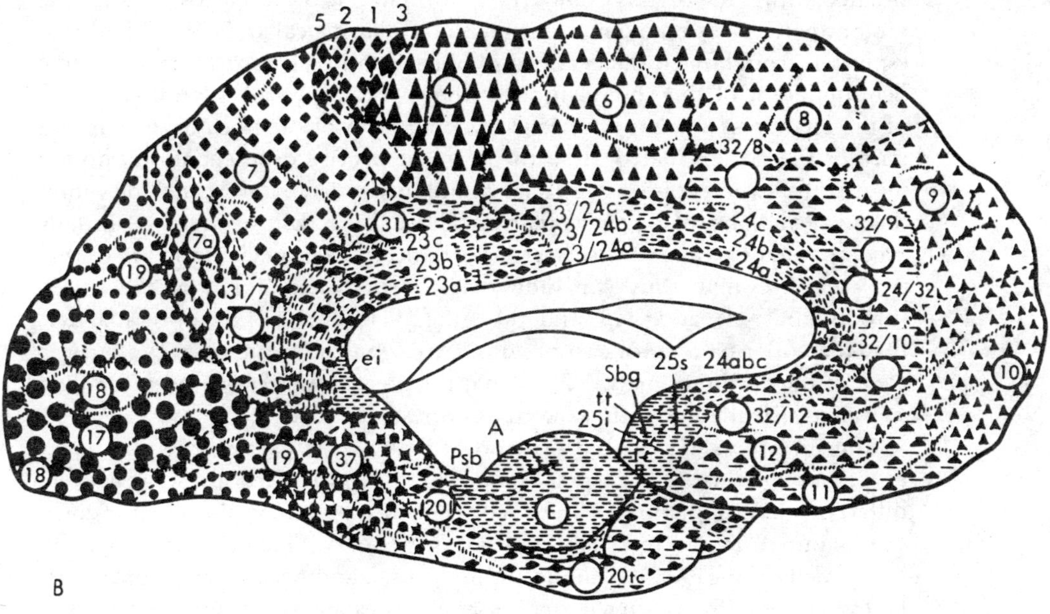

B

hemisphere (parietotemporal-occipital and inferior parietal regions) are denoted by mixed symbols and the anterior divisions of the hemisphere (frontal region) by modified triangles; the limbic and insular regions and the phylogenetically old zones of the cortex are shaded with broken lines. (*After Polyakov.*)

receptor surfaces of the organism, may be regarded as an established fact. However, the greatest difficulty arises when we try to match the cortical endings of the various analyzers with particular cortical fields in the various stages of mammalian phylogenesis. The distribution and topographical interrelationships of the cortical ending of the analyzers on the surface of the cerebral hemispheres can be comprehended only by considering the whole system of discrimination and integration both within the individual analyzers and between the analyzers at different levels of the central nervous system.

B. STRUCTURAL ORGANIZATION OF THE POSTERIOR CORTICAL DIVISIONS

As a result of physiological experiments and clinical observations made during the second half of the nineteenth century, regions were discovered in the posterior divisions of the cerebral cortex (Fig. 7) into which are projected the receptor surfaces both of the sensory organs concerned with the outside world (vision, hearing, cutaneous sensation) and of those actually situated within the organs of movement (kinesthetic or, in Pavlov's words, the motor analyzer). Subsequent experimental physiological and clinical findings, especially from large numbers of cases of head injury, led to the more accurate determination of the composition of the cortical fields of the nuclear zones of the analyzers. Starting with Pavlov's definition of the nuclear zone as that part of the cortex that deals with the most precise differentiation and the most complex integration of special stimuli, we must therefore include within the nuclear zone of a given analyzer those fields whose injury is usually accompanied by various forms of disturbance of the special function of that analyzer. We may thus conclude that the occipital region of the cortex (Brodmann's* Areas 17, 18, and 19) is the nuclear zone of the optic analyzer, that the superior temporal subregion (Areas 41, 42, and 22) is the nuclear zone of the auditory analyzer, and that the postcentral region (Area 3, 1, and 2) is the nuclear zone of the cutaneous-kinesthetic analyzer.

Clinical observations over a period of many years have shown that injury to different fields of the cortical nucleus of an analyzer gives rise to very different clinical pictures. One field, centrally placed in the nuclear zone, stands out from the rest. This central, or primary, field consists of Area 17 in the visual zone, Area 41 in the auditory zone, and Area 3 in the cutaneous-kinesthetic zone. It is after injury to these central areas that the most marked manifestations of a decrease in the power of direct perception and of accurate differentiation of the corresponding stimuli appear. This phenomenon (which we shall refer to repeatedly) has recently been confirmed by the experiments

* Henceforth, numbered cortical areas refer to those in the scheme devised by Brodmann.

of Penfield and Jasper (1954). During electrical stimulation of these fields while the patient is on the operating table, isolated sensations of light, color, sound, or touch are aroused.

The central fields of the nuclear zones are sharply distinguished by their unique cytoarchitectonic picture (coniocortex). The small granular cells of Layer IV, relaying impulses arriving via the powerfully developed projection fibers from the subcortical divisions of the analyzers to the pyramidal neurons of Layers III and V of the cortex, are particularly numerous in these fields. Besides these elements, grouped together in the three sublayers of Layer IV, conspicuous features of the primary visual Area 17 are the very

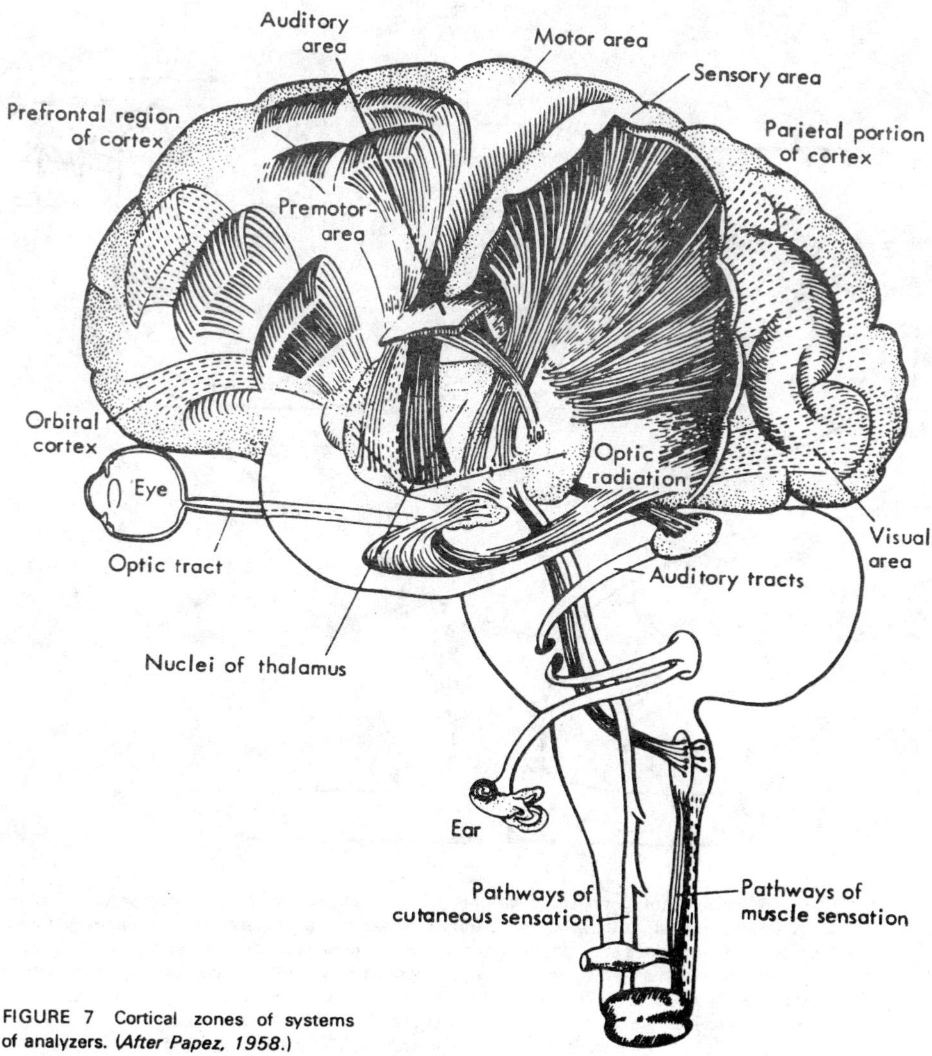

FIGURE 7 Cortical zones of systems of analyzers. (*After Papez, 1958.*)

large stellate cells of Layer IV and the pyramidal cells of Layer V (the cells of Cajal and Meynert), giving origin to descending projection fibers directed toward the eye-movement centers in the mesencephalon. These formations comprise the primary projection neuronal complex of the cortex (Fig. 8, I).

It can be seen from the unique neuronal structure of the primary fields that the complex of neurons adapted to provide bilateral cortical-subcortical connections by the most direct and the shortest route (i.e., with the fewest relays in the subcortex), thereby connecting the cortex to the receptor surfaces of the corresponding sensory organs, reaches its highest relative development here (Fig. 9).

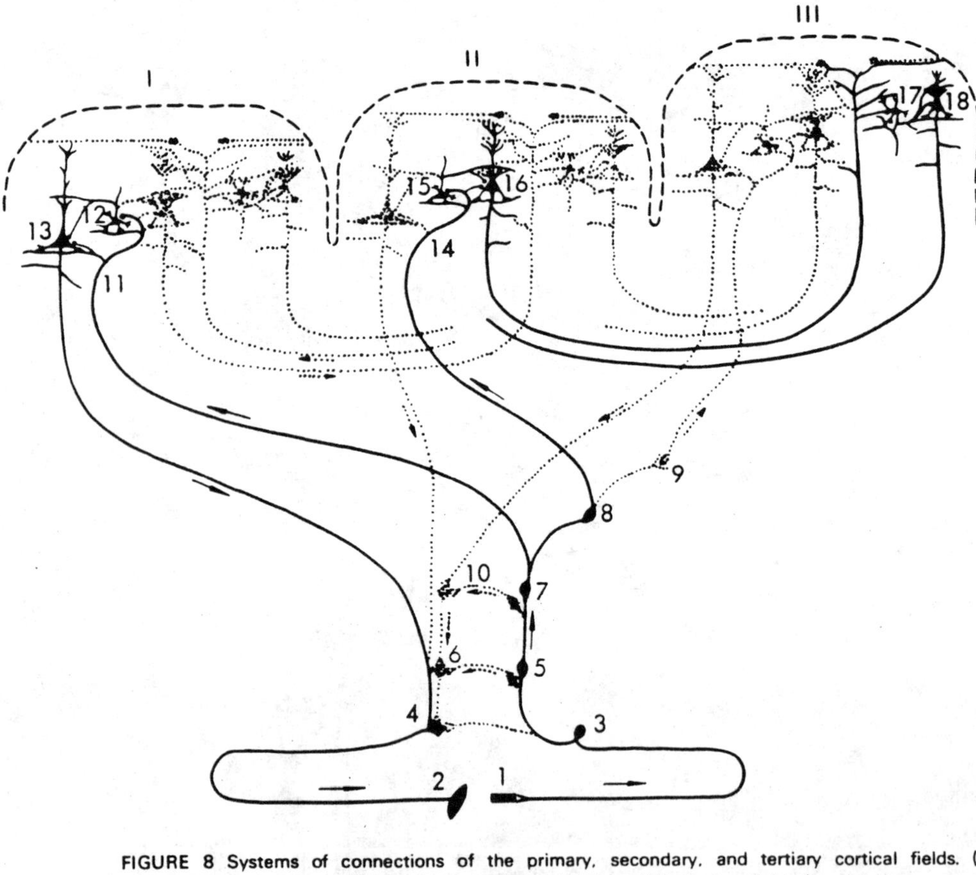

FIGURE 8 Systems of connections of the primary, secondary, and tertiary cortical fields. (*I*) Primary (central) fields. (*II*) Secondary (peripheral) fields. (*III*) Tertiary fields (overlapping zones of analyzers). The thick lines indicate: (*I*) system of cortical projection (cortical-subcortical) connections; (*II*) system of cortical projection-association connections; (*III*) system of cortical association connections. (*1*) Receptor; (*2*) effector; (*3*) neuron of sensory ganglion; (*4*) motor neuron; (*5, 6*) collateral neurons of the spinal cord and brain stem; (*7–10*) collateral neurons of the subcortical formations; (*11, 14*) afferent fibers from the subcortex; (*13*) pyramid of Layer V; (*16*) pyramid of Sublayer III^3; (*18*) pyramids of Sublayers III^2 and III^1; (*12, 15, 17*) stellate cells of the cortex. (*After Polyakov.*)

As a result of the formation of numerous afferent connections and feedbacks with the subjacent relay stations of the analyzers, the primary cortical fields can discriminate very finely between stimuli, and by means of effector adaptations to the sensory organs they can ensure that the receptors are capable of optimal perception of the corresponding stimuli. This is done by means of the "local" reflexes of the particular analyzer, whose connections lie in the cortex.

A very important common feature of the structural and functional organization of the primary fields is their well-defined somatotopic projection, by means of which individual points at the periphery (skin surface, skeletal muscles of the body, retina, cochlea) are projected into strictly demarcated, corresponding points in the primary cortical fields. In accordance with this property, these fields were named the "projection areas" of the cortex. It is important to note that the somatotopic projection of the receptor surface on the central cortical field is not geometrical (mirror-image) in structure but is based on function. In other words, the various parts of the body are not represented in the primary fields of the cortex in proportion to their size but, rather, in proportion to their physiological importance. Hence, in the central visual zone a disproportionately large area is occupied by the projection of the central part of the retina (the macula), responsible for the most acute vision; the areas of projection of the skin and muscle receptors of the fingers and hand, receptors having the greatest power of discrimination among weak stimuli of those in this group, are the largest in the cutaneous-kinesthetic zone (Fig. 10).

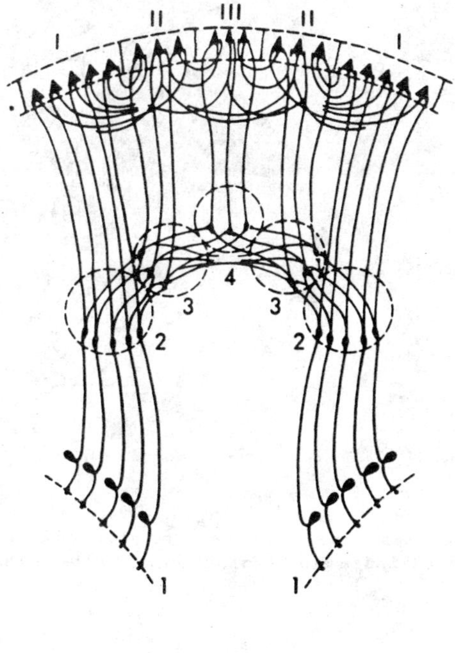

FIGURE 9 Scheme of relays in systems of analyzers. (*1*) Peripheral receptor surfaces of analyzers: (*2, 3, 4*) relays in the subcortical divisions of the analyzers: (*I, II, III*): as in Fig. 8. (*After Polyakov.*)

It is clear from what has been said that the primary fields of the nuclear zones in man are highly specialized areas of the cortex, capable of minute differentiation of stimuli. This is an indispensable property for the integrated perception of complex groups of stimuli reflecting the diversity of the outside world.

The strictly demarcated, isolated projection points within these primary areas must be understood as having, not a static, but a dynamic construction. This is particularly notable in the primary motor area of the cortex (precentral giant pyramidal Area 4). As previously mentioned, the earlier investigations of Foerster (1936), Brown and Sherrington (1912), and others showed that electrical stimulation of the same point of the motor cortex may give rise to different effects, the nature of the effect depending on the intensity of the current applied and on the previous state of the particular part of the cortex. For example, during repeated stimulation of the centers of the flexor muscles, flexion may alternate with extension.

The peripheral, or secondary, fields, situated in the peripheral segments of the nuclear zones, show characteristic differences from the central, or primary, fields in their physiological manifestations and in the details of their architectonic and neuronal organization. The effects of a lesion or of electrical stimulation of these fields mainly pertain to the more complex forms of mental processes. In cases of injury to the peripheral fields of the nuclear zones, the ability to experience elementary sensations is left relatively

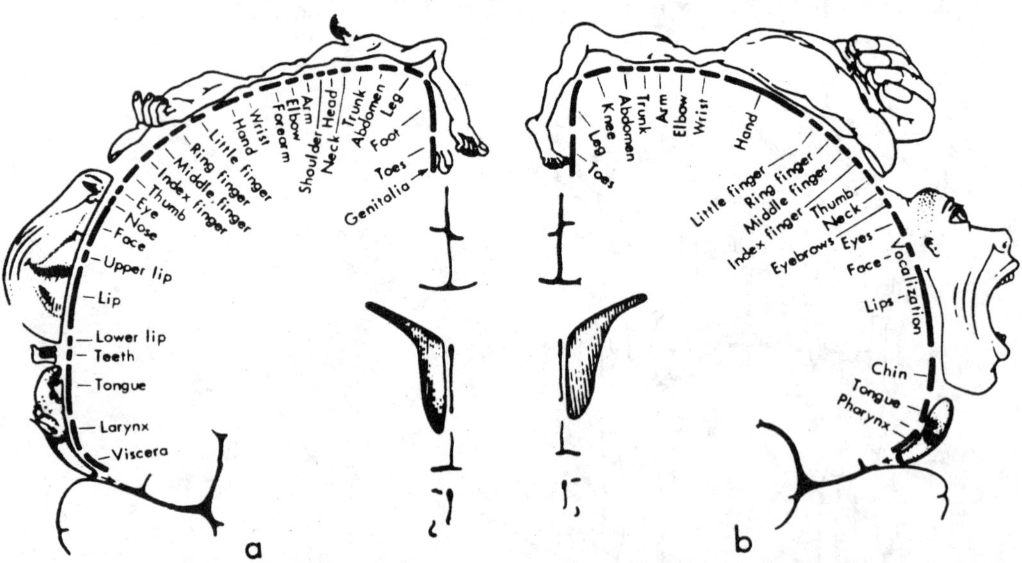

FIGURE 10 Scheme of the somatotopic projection in the cerebral cortex. (*a*) Cortical projection of sensation; (*b*) cortical projection of the motor system. The relative size of the organs reflects the area of the cerebral cortex from which the corresponding sensations and movements may be evoked. (*After Penfield and Rasmussen, 1950.*)

intact, and it is the power of adequate reflection of complex groups of stimuli and of the relationships between the components of the perceived objects that is principally disorganized.

Stimulation of the peripheral fields of the visual and auditory cortex by an electric current or by agents evoking epileptic fits is accompanied by visual and auditory hallucinations that follow each other in a definite space-time sequence. These phenomena shall be referred to subsequently (Part II, Section 3B).

The most prominent cytoarchitectonic features of the secondary fields of the cortical nuclear zones are those elements of their neuronal structure that are adapted for relaying the afferent impulses coming from the subcortex. These impulses come through the granular cells of Layer IV to the large pyramidal cells of the lower level of Layer III (Fig. 11). These structural characteristics are responsible for the most powerful system of associative connections of the cortex (the secondary projection-association neuronal complex, shown in Fig. 8, II). As a result of this unique mode of construction, the secondary fields of the nuclear zones play a highly important part in relaying the individual stimuli differentiated by the primary fields and in functionally integrating the nuclear zones of different analyzers and of the groups of impulses arriving from the receptors in the different analyzers. Hence, these fields are mainly involved with the relatively more complex forms of coordinated mental processes associated with detailed analysis of

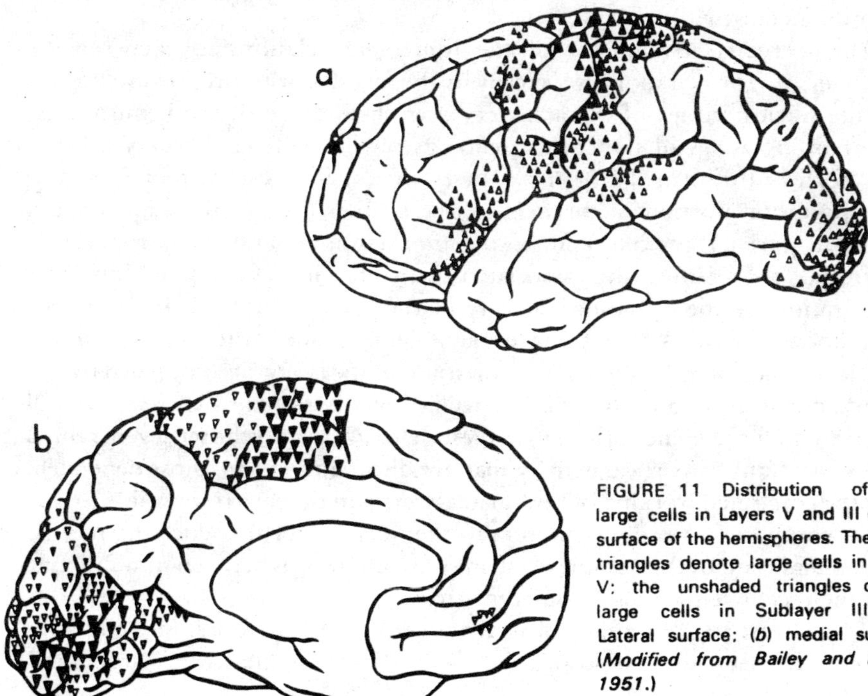

FIGURE 11 Distribution of the large cells in Layers V and III on the surface of the hemispheres. The black triangles denote large cells in Layer V: the unshaded triangles denote large cells in Sublayer III[3]. (*a*) Lateral surface: (*b*) medial surface. (*Modified from Bailey and Bonin, 1951.*)

the relationship between concrete objective stimuli and with orientation in relation to a concrete spatial and temporal environment.

This feature of the neuronal organization of the peripheral fields of the nuclear zones is illustrated by neurophysiological findings. Experiments using the technique of neuronography (McCulloch, 1943) showed that excitation arising as a result of stimulation of the primary fields of the cortex has only a comparatively limited spread and is confined to the corresponding nuclear zones. On the other hand, excitation arising in the secondary fields has a tendency to spread over much wider areas of the cortex and outside the nuclear zone of origin (Part II, Section 3B and 4B).

In conformance with the greater complexity of the association connections, the projection connections of the secondary cortical fields have a more complex system of relays in the subcortical internuncial neurons of the analyzers than the primary fields (Fig. 9). Afferent impulses traversing to the cortex from the receptor surfaces of the sensory organs reach these fields through a larger number of additional relays in the associative nuclei of the thalamus than do the afferent impulses traveling to the primary fields via the shorter path through the thalamic relay nuclei. Thus, the receptor impulses reaching the peripheral fields and utilized for wide associations, both within the corresponding zones and between the different zones of the cortex, undergo some degree of preliminary integration while still at the subcortical level. This applies not only to the system of the particular initial analyzer but also to that of other analyzers contributing to the process of coordinated activity.

The increased complexity of the functional relationships between the analyzers is reflected morphologically by the fact that with progressive growth of the nuclear zones of the analyzers over the surface of the hemispheres, overlapping zones of the cortical endings of the analyzers (tertiary fields of the cortex) are formed (Fig. 12). These cortical formations, represented in the posterior portion of the hemisphere by the fields of the superior and inferior parietal regions and of the mid-temporal and temporoparietal-occipital subregions, are associated with the most complex forms of integration of the conjoined activity of the visual, auditory, and cutaneo-kinesthetic analyzers. Since the tertiary fields of the cortex lie outside the nuclear zones proper, their injury or stimulation is not accompanied by any marked loss or modification of the specific functions of the analyzers. As shall be seen, in the presence of lesions in these fields it is mainly the most generalized manifestations of cortical activity that are disorganized, i.e., those dependent on the combined working of several analyzers and that are responsible for the most complex forms of orientation to the outside world and for the analysis and integration of the complex systems of relationships between stimuli acting on the receptive part of the different analyzers.

In contrast to the groups of neurons of the nuclear zones, the numerous groups of neurons composing the tertiary fields of the cortex are almost completely lacking in specific analyzer functions, having made the complete functional transition to the adequate reflection of the most complex forms of spatial and temporal relationships between groups of actual stimuli and

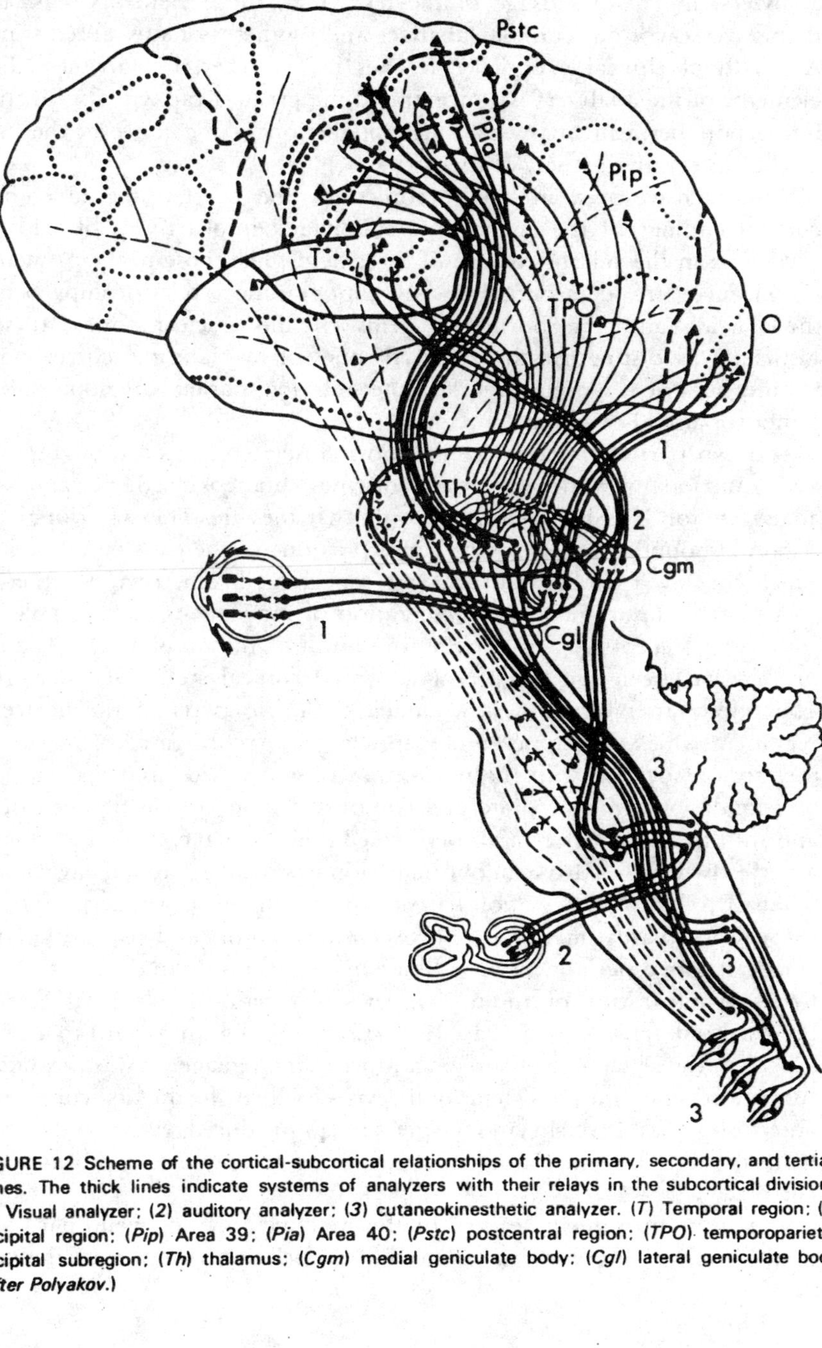

FIGURE 12 Scheme of the cortical-subcortical relationships of the primary, secondary, and tertiary zones. The thick lines indicate systems of analyzers with their relays in the subcortical divisions. (*1*) Visual analyzer; (*2*) auditory analyzer; (*3*) cutaneokinesthetic analyzer. (*T*) Temporal region; (*O*) occipital region; (*Pip*) Area 39; (*Pia*) Area 40; (*Pstc*) postcentral region; (*TPO*) temporoparietal-occipital subregion; (*Th*) thalamus; (*Cgm*) medial geniculate body; (*Cgl*) lateral geniculate body. (*After Polyakov.*)

to the handling of these relationships during the organism's active response to the outside world. From this point of view, the tertiary cortical fields can be looked upon as a collection of the "diffuse" elements of the analyzers, in Pavlov's usage of the term (i.e., those elements that cannot themselves carry out complex analyses and syntheses of specialized stimuli). A wealth of clinical experience teaches us, however, that in these diffuse elements of the analyzers is concentrated the greatest capacity for functional interaction between analyzers, such interaction taking place at the higher level of integrative activity of the cortex.

The extensive area in man occupied by the overlapping zones of the cortical endings of the analyzers is subdivided into a series of fields. The variations in the microstructure of these fields, like those in their functional significance, are determined by the topographical relationships between these fields and the bordering fields of the nuclear zones. It seems justifiable to distinguish three special zones of overlapping, corresponding to the superior parietal region, the inferior parietal region, and the temporoparietal-occipital subregion.

The two parietal regions are the most closely connected topographically and functionally with the zones of the cutaneokinesthetic and visual analyzers, for it is between these zones that they lie. The superior parietal region is bounded anteriorly by those portions of the postcentral region in which the lower limbs and trunk are represented. This region is therefore particularly important for the integration of movements of the whole body with visual reception and for the formation of the body image. The latter process has been the subject of a special clinical study (Schilder, 1935). The inferoparietal region is bounded by those parts of the postcentral region in which the upper limbs and face are represented. This region is therefore associated with the integration of generalized and discrete forms of stimulation, with accurate and complex discrimination between objects and with the act of speech, all performed under visual control and requiring a perfectly developed system of orientation toward the external environment.

Finally, clinical observation has shown that the temporoparietal-occipital subregion, an area intermediate between the auditory and visual zones of the cortex, has an especially intimate functional relationship to the most complex forms of integration of auditory and visual reception, particularly, as shall be discussed subsequently (Part II, Sections 2 and 3), in regard to a specific aspect of the semantics of spoken and written language. It was through this subregion and the mid-temporal gyrus, which forms its continuation anteriorly, that Penfield and Jasper (1954) produced visual and auditory hallucinations by stimulating isolated points of the cortex with an electric current.

The most prominent feature of the architectonic and neuronal pattern of the overlapping zones is the tertiary association complex of the cortex

(Fig. 8, III), represented by the pyramidal and stellate cells of the highest layers and sublayers of the cortex—the last to become differentiated in the evolution of the mammals—namely, the middle and upper sublayers of Layers III and II. The neurons of this part of the cortical gray matter dispatch, receive, and relay the most intricate and subtly differentiated streams of impulses responsible for the functional integration of the neurons of the nuclear zones into unceasingly diverse and differentiated working constellations corresponding to the higher mental functions to be carried out.

Besides having these highly differentiated, multilateral associative connections, the tertiary cortical fields are distinguished from the primary and secondary fields by the presence of extremely complex chains of projection relays into the subcortical divisions of the analyzers. In conformity with their high-level capacity of generalization and abstraction from actual, concrete stimuli, the tertiary cortical formations are connected in the most indirect manner, through the largest number of successive relays in the subcortex, with the peripheral endings of the analyzers (Fig. 9). The cortical overlapping zones form bilateral connections with the pulvinar group of thalamic nuclei—the last to differentiate in the course of evolution—which, in turn, are connected with the relay nuclei proper of the thalamus through a complex chain of internal relays in the thalamus itself. Hence, impulses sent to these cortical areas from below undergo the most complex processing in the subcortex and are passed on to the cortex as integrated signals resulting from the interaction between the sensory messages provided by the different analyzers.

In summary, it should be emphasized that in the normally acting brain the three groups of cortical fields, along with their systems of relays and connections, both among themselves and between them and the subcortical divisions of the analyzers, work together as a single elaborately differentiated whole.

C. STRUCTURAL ORGANIZATION OF THE ANTERIOR CORTICAL DIVISIONS

The primary, secondary, and tertiary fields of the occipital, temporal, and parietal regions of the cortex, which we have been discussing so far, are concentrated in the posterior portion of the hemispheres, behind the central sulcus. The cortical fields of the frontal lobe of the brain, situated anteriorly to this sulcus and including the precentral region and the frontal region proper, have a number of functional and structural features that distinguish them essentially from the part of the cortex posterior to the central sulcus.

In principle, we can distinguish the same three main groups of fields in the frontal lobe of the brain as in the regions previously considered. The precentral region, bounded anteriorly by the postcentral region, has been known ever since the time of Fritsch and Hitzig (1870) by neurophysiologists and clinicians as the motor zone of the cortex. In the course of phylogenesis this region became differentiated from the single sensorimotor cortex and was divided into two fields: a primary, giant pyramidal or motor zone, known as Area 4 (the central motor area), and the secondary premotor zones, known as Areas 6 and 8 (the peripheral motor areas). The general structural and functional features of these fields and their connections with the subcortical divisions of the brain have much in common with those of the primary and secondary fields of the occipital, temporal, and postcentral cortex. Nevertheless, as already stated, there are important differences, due to the fact that in the cortical organization of the whole frontal lobe, in contrast to that of the posterior portion of the hemisphere, the accent is on the performance of coordinated and goal-directed acts by the organism in relation to the external world in response to perceived groups of stimuli.

The most obvious features of the microscopic structure of the primary giant pyramidal Area 4 in the adult human brain that distinguish it from other areas are the absence of a clearly identifiable Layer IV and the presence of strongly developed giant Betz cells in Layer V. The latter send off the largest fibers of the pyramidal tract, conveying impulses of voluntary movement to the motor centers of the skeletal muscles situated in the brain stem and spinal cord. These two distinctive structural features constitute evidence that in the central motor area the elements of the neuron group adapted for the fastest and shortest path for conducting voluntary impulses to the effector neurons of the central nervous system attain their greatest comparative development. Conversely, the elements of cortical organization adapted for the perception of afferent impulses from the subcortex, and concentrated in large numbers in the fields of the posterior divisions of the hemisphere in Layer IV, are more widely scattered in the giant pyramidal area and do not form a clearly identifiable layer.

Hence, it may be concluded that the projection afferent fibers, strongly developed in Area 4, and bringing impulses from the subcortical formations, relay most of the impulses reaching the giant efferent pyramidal cells of Layer V. This structural arrangement is particularly favorable for the rapid rebound to the motor periphery of the body of all the signals arriving at this part of the cortex from the subcortical levels of the central nervous system and, likewise, from other divisions of the cortex.

Those microscopic structural features of the giant pyramidal Area 4 that characterize it as central are completely consistent with its physiological and clinical characteristics, for in man the movements of individual muscle groups are represented in this area with an exceptionally fine degree of differentiation.

The secondary premotor Area 6, as may be deducted from physiological and clinical data (Part II, Section 4E), has as its principal function the performance and automatization of the more complex coordinated movements, i.e., those taking place over a period of time and requiring the joint activity of various groups of muscles. Although it is basically similar in structure to the giant pyramidal area, it is cytoarchitectonically characterized by the absence of Betz cells and by a more marked development of large pyramidal cells in Layer III (especially in its deep sublayer). The projection links between the premotor cortex and the subcortical formations constitute an important part of the extrapyramidal systems of the cortex, which, in contrast to the direct pyramidal tract, reach the terminal motor centers of the brain and spinal cord through a series of relays in the subcortical levels of the central nervous system (Fig. 13).

Area 8, in which eye movements are represented, is also the place of origin of one of the extrapyramidal projection systems of the cortex. It may be classed as a peripheral (secondary) division of the motor zone of the cortex, although in its cytoarchitectonic structure this formation shows signs of transition to the area of the frontal cortex proper. The province of Area 8 is the performance of coordinated eye movements during the fixation of attention

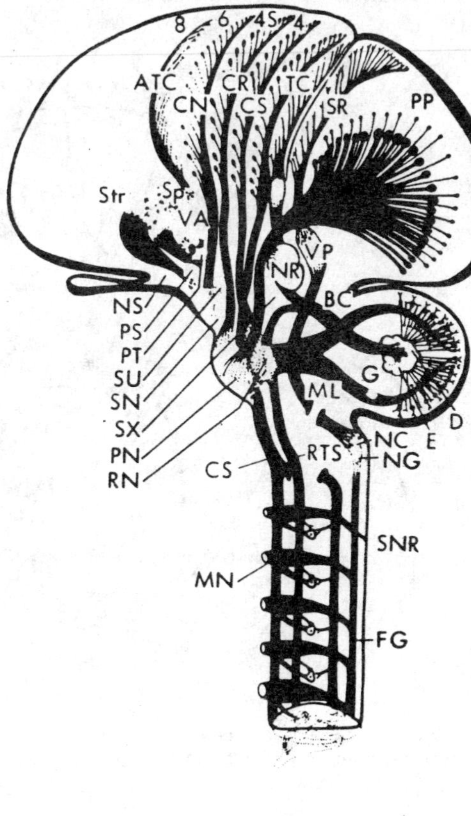

FIGURE 13 Scheme of the pyramidal and extrapyramidal systems. *FG–NG–ML–VP–SR*: Conducting pathways and relays of the cutaneokinesthetic receptors. *(FF/PP)*) *D–BC–NR–VL–TC*: Connections between the cerebral cortex and cerebellum. *CS–MN*: Corticomotor pyramidal tract. *CS–RN–RTS*: Connections between the cortex and the nuclei of the reticular formation. *CR–SN*: Connections between the cortex and the substantia nigra. *Str*: Subcortical ganglia of the cerebral hemispheres. (*After Papez.*)

and manipulation of objects under visual control. Disturbances of eye movements accompanying lesions of this area will be discussed subsequently (Part II, Section 4E).

The motor and premotor fields of the precentral region, forming a single kinesthetic complex in the cortex, possess a well-developed projection and association afferent system of bilateral connections of the fields with each other, with the other cortical fields, and with the subcortical formations. However, the streams of afferent impulses arriving in the motor field of the cortex originate from sources different from those of the impulses reaching the nuclear zones of the analyzers and the internuclear zones of the cortex of the posterior portion of the hemisphere (Fig. 14). It is in the latter, as has been mentioned, that the main conductors of impulses from the receptors of the sensory organs to the cortex are gathered and form the trunks of the systems of analyzers and their supplementary relays in the portion of the subcortex nearest the cortex (certain nuclei in the thalamus and geniculate bodies).

The afferent impulses directed toward the motor and premotor cortex relay in a different group of nuclei in the thalamus from the afferent impulses directed toward the cortical formations of the posterior part of the hemisphere. The channels of transmission of the impulses reaching the fields of the precentral region are mainly tracts leading from the cerebellum through the

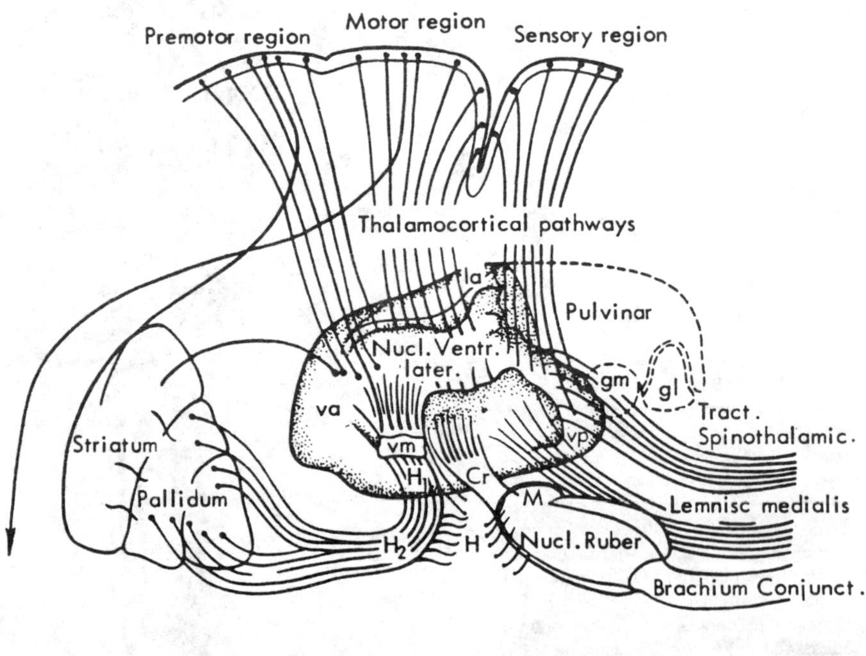

FIGURE 14 Scheme of the various afferent systems of the sensory and motor (kinesthetic and kinetic) segments of the cortex. (*After Papez and others.*)

red nucleus and the thalamus to the cortex (Fig. 14). A large portion of this afferent system serves for the feedback of streams of impulses circulating in the extrapyramidal cortical-subcortical systems of the brain (cortex–subcortical ganglia of the cerebral hemispheres–thalamus–cortex; cortex–cerebellar system–thalamus–cortex; pathways of superficial and deep sensations–thalamus–subcortical ganglia of the cerebral hemispheres–thalamus–cortex).

Recognition of the unique qualitative composition of the projection afferent system serving the motor cortex is of fundamental importance for the proper interpretation of the functional role of this portion of the cortex in the integrated activity of the cortical endings of the analyzers. It has been stated that the feedback mechanism is applied universally in the reflex activity of the whole central nervous system and, in particular, of the cerebral cortex. In the nuclear zones of the analyzers, however, feedback from overlapping zones is put into operation mainly during the perception by the analyzers of stimuli of different complexity, coming from the outside world. The physiological mechanism of this function involves the integration and correspondence of the appropriate analyzers to produce an adequate reflection of the changing picture of the outside world.

The principle of feedback is applied quite differently in the activity of that part of the cortex responsible for the organization, programming, and execution of voluntary motor activity, for in this realm it becomes the main source of information on the effect of the movements and actions performed. The physiological role of the motor cortex essentially consists of matching the "assigned program" of a motor act, formed mainly on the basis of the analytical and integrative cortical activity of the posterior divisions of the hemispheres, with the actual course of its performance, i.e., in detecting signals of success and signals of error (agreement or disagreement between the program and the performance) and in making the required corrections at the right time in the course of the actions (Bernshtein, 1947; Pribram, 1959*b*, 1960, etc.). In view of what has been said, it will be apparent that both centrifugal and centripetal (responsible for the feedback) chains of relays of impulses, connecting the motor cortex to the subcortical formations, are included in the extrapyramidal systems of the brain, which are known to be of essential importance to the coordination of voluntary movement.

The subdivisions of the motor zone of the cortex into a motor area and premotor areas was the result of progressive structural differentiation of the originally single cortical anlage in the course of evolution in response to the growing complexity of the range of cortically directed active movements. The higher development and perfection of the whole sphere of voluntary, goal-directed acts was associated with the formation of the tertiary fields of the frontal region proper. These fields, occupying in man about one quarter of the entire surface of the cortex, belong to the phylogenetically youngest divisions of the neocortex. They were formed as a result of the growth, anteriorly, of elements of the same type of neuronal organization as lies at the basis of the motor zone of the cortex.

In the frontal region there is a closer arrangement of the small cells at the level of Layer IV, receiving afferent impulses from the subcortex; for this reason, the fields of the frontal region, in contrast to those of the motor area, possess a more clearly defined Layer IV. This suggests a rather compact character of the afferent information directed to the frontal portion of the cortex from the corresponding group of nuclei in the thalamus.

Just as the tertiary fields of the posterior part of the hemisphere are related to the most highly generalized and integrated forms of perception of the external world, so also the tertiary fields of the prefrontal part of the hemisphere are related to the most highly integrated forms of goal-directed activity. This will be treated in greater detail subsequently (Part II, Section 5).

The projection centripetal and centrifugal connections of the frontal portion of the cortex include many of the subcortical formations (a definite group of the medial nuclei of the thalamus and the subcortical ganglia of the cerebral hemispheres). In man, the connections with the cerebellar system are particularly highly developed, owing to the assumption of erect posture and the importance of cerebellar coordination in the performance of goal-directed actions. Besides projection connections, the frontal fields possess extensive bilateral associative connections with the fields of the precentral region and of cortical regions lying posterior to the central sulcus and on the medial and inferior surfaces of the hemisphere.

As a result of these associative connections, as well as of those connections functionally uniting the various divisions of the cortex through the subcortical formations, the activity of all sections of the cortex of the anterior and posterior parts of the cerebral hemispheres is integrated. Functional unity of all the higher mental processes is thereby achieved. Information from the sensory organs, reaching the nuclear zones of the analyzers and analyzed and integrated in their overlapping zones, is then transmitted to the motor and frontal regions, where it is recoded into a series of motor impulses, organized in space and time and under the constant control of impulses passing back both from the effectors themselves and from the sensory organs perceiving the movement.

D. PROGRESSIVE DIFFERENTIATION OF THE CORTICAL REGIONS AND FIELDS IN THE COURSE OF PHYLOGENESIS AND ONTOGENESIS

The topographical representation of the subdivision of man's cerebral cortex into regions and fields reveals an extreme degree of differentiation, resulting from the prolonged and progressive development of what initially was a simple, undifferentiated cortical organization without clearly localized representation.

In the lower mammals only a few of the principal analyzer zones (visual, auditory, cutaneokinesthetic), although not yet differentiated internally into fields and only very indistinctly demarcated from each other, can be distinguished (Fig. 15). At higher stages of mammalian evolution, the nuclear zones of the analyzers in the posterior part of the hemisphere are more clearly demarcated and there is differentiation into central and peripheral fields. Parallel with this process, there is an increasing tendency for one zone to extend into another, with the formation of overlapping zones, because of intensive growth of the nuclear zones over the surface of the hemisphere (Fig. 16). These are still ill defined in the carnivores and ungulates but are clearly distinguishable in the primates. In the anterior part of the hemispheres, the

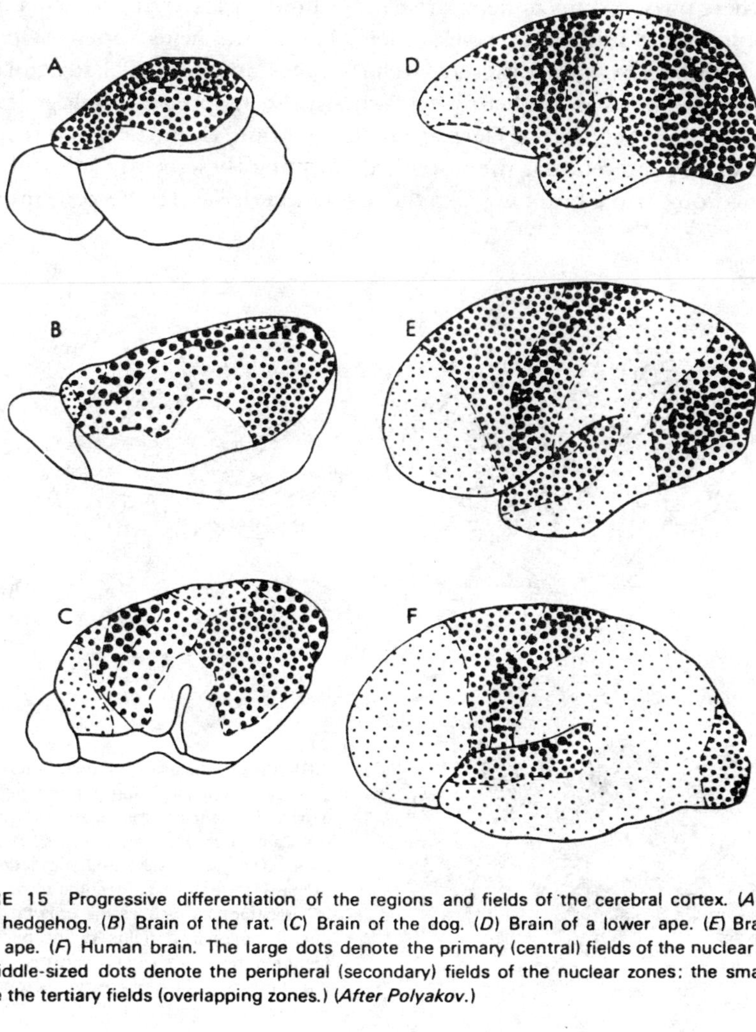

FIGURE 15 Progressive differentiation of the regions and fields of the cerebral cortex. (*A*) Brain of the hedgehog. (*B*) Brain of the rat. (*C*) Brain of the dog. (*D*) Brain of a lower ape. (*E*) Brain of a higher ape. (*F*) Human brain. The large dots denote the primary (central) fields of the nuclear zones; the middle-sized dots denote the peripheral (secondary) fields of the nuclear zones; the small dots denote the tertiary fields (overlapping zones.) (*After Polyakov.*)

progressive cortical differentiation gives rise to a distinct motor zone of the cortex, subsequently dividing into motor and premotor fields, and to the intensive growth of the area occupied by the fields of the frontal region proper. In the anthropoid apes nearly all the fields present in man can be distinguished; only in man, however, is the qualitative differentiation of the structure of these fields perfected and their final topographical relationships established.

In man, the territory occupied by the tertiary fields grows enormously, to over half the total surface area of the cortex. Parallel with this growth, the area of the peripheral fields compared with that of the central fields, which occupy a relatively small area in man, increases sharply (Fig. 17); in absolute terms, the central fields, too, are much more extensive than in monkeys.

These three groups of fields arise in a definite order during both mammalian evolution and individual development. The central fields appear first and can be identified by their different architectonics and neuronal structure; these differences develop both in phylogenesis and in prenatal ontogenesis. The original investigations of Flechsig (1920, 1927) and C. and O. Vogt (1919–1920) and others showed that the systems connecting these fields to the subcortical formations of the brain are also the first to mature and to become myelinated

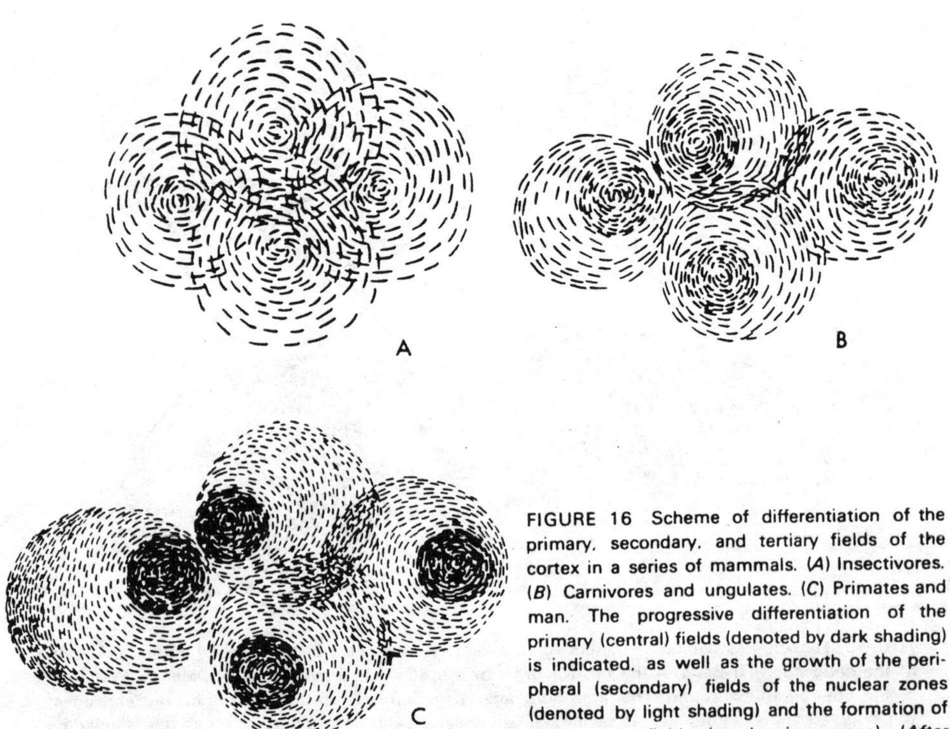

FIGURE 16 Scheme of differentiation of the primary, secondary, and tertiary fields of the cortex in a series of mammals. (*A*) Insectivores. (*B*) Carnivores and ungulates. (*C*) Primates and man. The progressive differentiation of the primary (central) fields (denoted by dark shading) is indicated, as well as the growth of the peripheral (secondary) fields of the nuclear zones (denoted by light shading) and the formation of the tertiary fields (overlapping zones). (*After Polyakov.*)

(Fig. 18). The peripheral fields of the nuclear zones attain their period of intensive development rather later than do the central fields. In human ontogenesis this period coincides with the first weeks and months of life. The process of myelination of the conducting pathways connected with these fields takes place at correspondingly later periods. The latest of all to mature are the overlapping zones of the analyzers and the formations of the frontal region; this process occupies the first few years of life. The connections of these cortical areas are also the last to complete their cycle of development.

The important transformations of cortical organization caused by the appearance of the second signal system, associated with man's productive activity, speech, thought, and consciousness, are a specifically human feature. The transformations referred to affect all the groups of cortical fields that have been under consideration. They are especially marked in relation to the secondary and tertiary cortical fields.

It is only in man, in the peripheral segments of the nuclear zones of the analyzers and of the motor cortex, that structural and functional differentiation into highly specialized, distinct areas, concerned with the analysis and integration of stimuli of especial importance to the various aspects of speech, took place. For instance, a special area in the posterior segment of the peripheral field of the auditory cortex (Wernicke's "center") is concerned with the analysis and integration of the receptive elements of spoken language or phonemes, and an area in the peripheral fields of the visual cortex is concerned with the analysis and integration of the visual elements of receptive language. In areas of the inferior segments of the parietal region, situated next to the cutaneokinesthetic zone and in direct contact with the sensory "centers" of the arm, lips, tongue, and larynx, the analysis and integration of cutaneokinesthetic reception fundamental to articulation takes place. A certain portion of the periphery of the motor cortex, the inferior segments of the

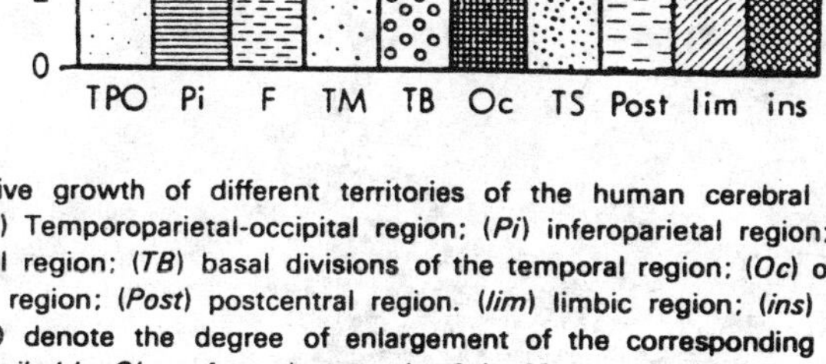

FIGURE 17 Relative growth of different territories of the human cerebral cortex in postnatal ontogenesis. (*TPO*) Temporoparietal-occipital region; (*Pi*) inferoparietal region; (*F*) frontal region; (*TM*) mid-temporal region; (*TB*) basal divisions of the temporal region; (*Oc*) occipital region; (*TS*) superior temporal region; (*Post*) postcentral region. (*lim*) limbic region; (*ins*) insular region. The numbers 0 to 10 denote the degree of enlargement of the corresponding region in postnatal ontogenesis. (*Compiled by Glezer from the records of the Moscow Brain Institute.*)

premotor zone (Broca's "center"), is the seat of the neurodynamic processes involved in the synthesis of the individual sounds of spoken speech into complex, successive units. In another portion of the premotor zone, adjoining the motor "centers" of the upper limb (in the posterior segment of the mid-frontal gyrus), are located the cortical mechanisms for the programming and performance of the complex systems of successive movements and motor skills. Much more will be said about this subject in special sections of this book.

As a result of the segregation of specialized speech areas of the cortex in the peripheral fields of the nuclear zones, the neuronal structure of the central fields of these zones becomes perfected and capable of perceiving the elements of speech and of differentiating their sensory and motor components with a high degree of precision. This process is particularly conspicuous in the central auditory field. The work of Blinkov (1955) has shown that in man this field is much more extensive than in the monkey, both absolutely and relatively, and has undergone further differentiation into a series of subsidiary fields. These progressive structural changes reflect the fundamental role of spoken language in the entire system of verbal communication.

The upshot of the qualitative transformation undergone by the overlapping

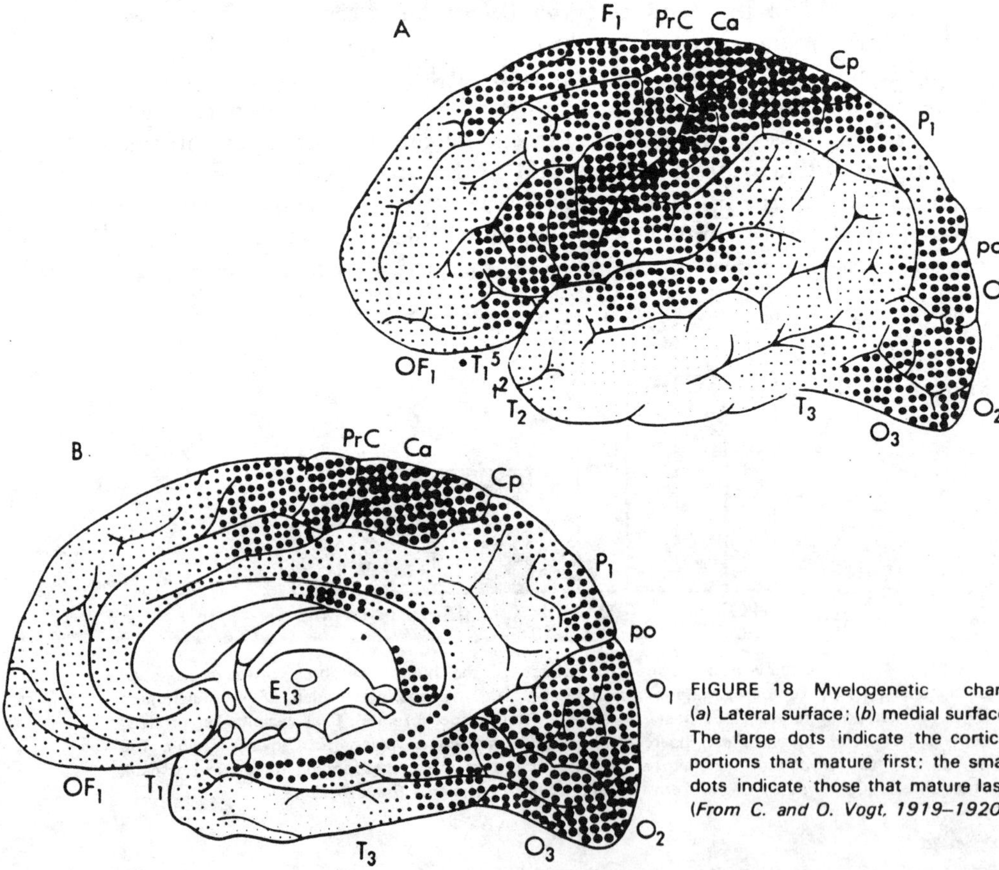

FIGURE 18 Myelogenetic chart. (*a*) Lateral surface; (*b*) medial surface. The large dots indicate the cortical portions that mature first; the small dots indicate those that mature last. (*From C. and O. Vogt, 1919–1920.*)

zones of the analyzers in the frontal portion of the cortex following the formation of the second signal system is that all of man's conscious mental processes, governing his actions, involve the participation of the system of verbal communication and, indeed, are under its domination, as will be shown in more detail in subsequent chapters of this book.

With the differentiation and qualitative specialization of the elements of all the layers in the course of mammalian phylogenesis, in particular that of the primates, Layer III of the cortex became especially well developed; its neurons send, receive, and analyze the greater part of the association impulses of the cortex. The width of this layer gradually increases from the lower to the higher members of the primates, and its division into sublayers becomes increasingly evident. A similar process takes place throughout ontogenesis. Figure 19 shows that the increase in width of Layer III takes place relatively faster than that of the other layers of the cortex, so that in the adult human brain it occupies about one third of the total width of the cortex.

At this juncture another feature of the neuronal organization, common to all three groups of cortical formations and of considerable importance to the understanding of their physiological role in integrated cortical activity, must be mentioned, namely, that the entire neuronal organization undergoes a definite change in character with transition from the primary to the secondary and from the secondary to the tertiary fields (Fig. 20). The central cortical fields, which handle the most highly concentrated streams of impulses and connect the cortex in the most direct manner with the sensory organs and the peripheral motor organs, are distinguishable from the other fields by the "coarseness" of their neuronal structure, which is adapted for the reception and return of intensive flows of excitation. It is the tertiary fields of the cortex that possess the finest neuronal structure, and this may be interpreted as the morphological

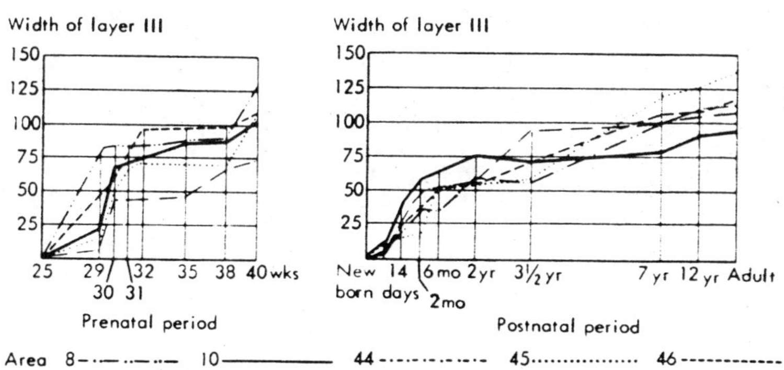

FIGURE 19 Diagrams showing the ontogenetic increase in width of the third layer in various fields of the cortex. The numbers on the right side of each diagram denote the corresponding fields; the numbers on the left side indicate the degree of increase in width of Layer III. (*Based on the records of the Moscow Brain Institute.*)

expression of the particular precision and complexity of the functional differentiation of these fields, which are responsible for the most highly specialized functional connections and interactions between the analyzers. In this respect, as in all of their characteristics, the secondary fields are intermediate between the primary and tertiary fields.

In the course of human ontogenesis the difference between the structural differentiation of the fields in the posterior divisions of the hemispheres, principally responsible for the organization of the various forms of sensation and for the perception of external stimuli, and that of the fields in the anterior divisions of the hemispheres, principally responsible for the organization of actions, also stands out clearly. Starting with the early stages of embryonic cortical development, the process of subdivision into layers and the formation of neurons with their connections are different in different parts of the hemispheres. In the posterior part of the cortex the development of the layers proceeds according to a clear-cut, typically six-layered plan, with a separate, concentrated Layer IV as the main receiver of afferent impulses from the subcortical divisions of the analyzers. Brodmann (1909) described this part of the cortex as "homotypical." In the anterior part of

A

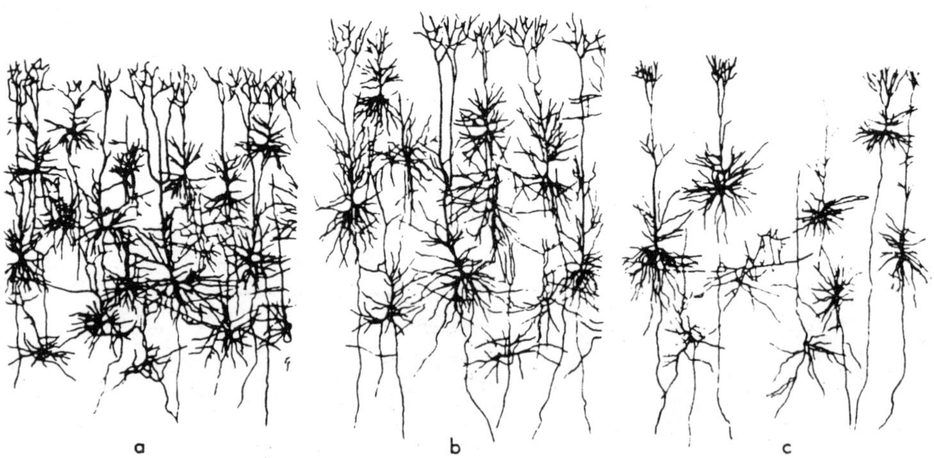

FIGURE 20 Illustrations of the relative widths of the neuronal structure of the primary, secondary, and tertiary fields of the cortex, showing decreasing width from primary to tertiary fields. (*A*) Neuronal structure of the fields of the posterior divisions of the hemisphere: (*a*) Primary field of the postcentral region; (*b*) secondary field of the postcentral region; (*c*) tertiary field (inferior parietal region).

the cortex, especially the primitive motor cortex, the formation of vertical layers is much less intensive, with the structure corresponding to the more diffuse arrangement in this portion (as in the adult human brain) of the elements receiving subcortical impulses. In the primitive portion of the cortex there is a curious arrangement of groups of neurons (undulation), presumably caused by the pattern of development of the interneuronal connections (Fig. 21).

E. STRUCTURAL ORGANIZATION AND CONNECTIONS OF THE MEDIOBASAL CORTICAL DIVISIONS

All of the foregoing descriptions have been concerned with those cortical territories that reach their highest degree of development and their most complex structural differentiation in man and that, with their connections, occupy the entire convex superolateral surface of the hemispheres. We have not yet considered those cortical formations situated on the medial and

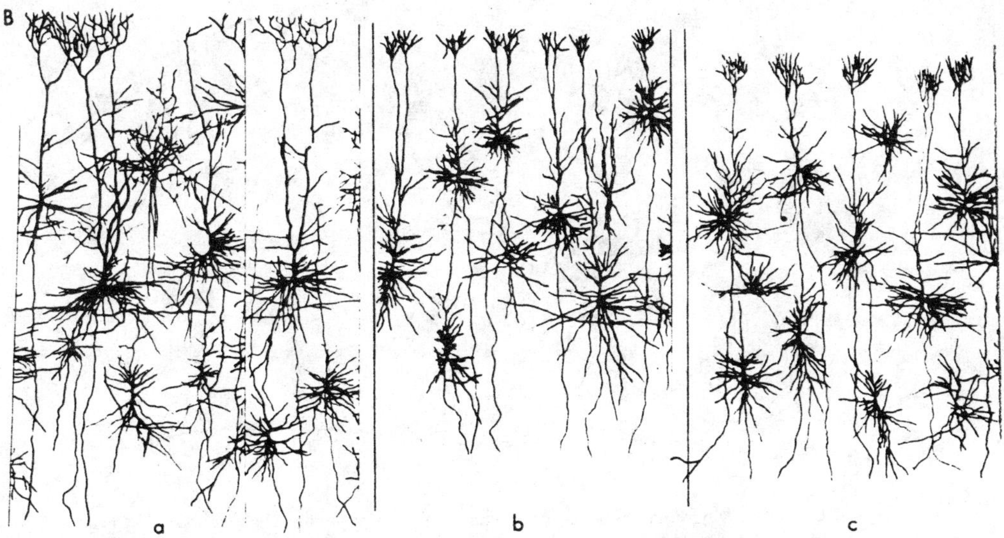

FIGURE 20 (*B*) Neuronal structure of the fields of the anterior divisions of the hemisphere: (*a*) Primary giant pyramidal field (motor area): (*b*) secondary field (premotor area): (*c*) tertiary field (frontal region). (*After Polyakov.*)

inferior surfaces of the hemisphere (the mediobasal portion of the cortex) and those adjoining the subcortical formations (Figs. 6*B* and 22). Anatomically, one segment of the mediobasal portion of the cortex is part of the neocortex—the two marginal zones, the limbic lobe and insula, together with those sections of the neocortex of the basal and part of the medial surfaces of the frontal and temporal lobes that are specially related to the marginal zones functionally and topographically (Areas 11, 12, 20, 31, and 32). Also located in the mediobasal portion of the cortex are the phylogenetically older cortical formations (according to Filimonov's classification)—the archicortex, paleocortex, and intermediate cortex, the hippocampus and the adjacent formations of the entorhinal cortex, and the olfactory tubercle and the adjacent semicortical structures (i.e., not yet completely detached from the subcortical groups of neurons lying within the wall of the hemisphere). The first of the subcortical formations to engage our attention are the amygdaloid complex of nuclei, the phylogenetically older portions of the thalamic nuclei (the anterior and part of the medial groups of nuclei), and the subcortical ganglia of the cerebral hemispheres. Most of the enumerated formations were included by the older neuroanatomists under the general heading of the rhinencephalon, and they were regarded as being mainly involved in the analysis and integration of olfactory stimuli. The results of more recent investigations have greatly broadened the classical ideas on the functional

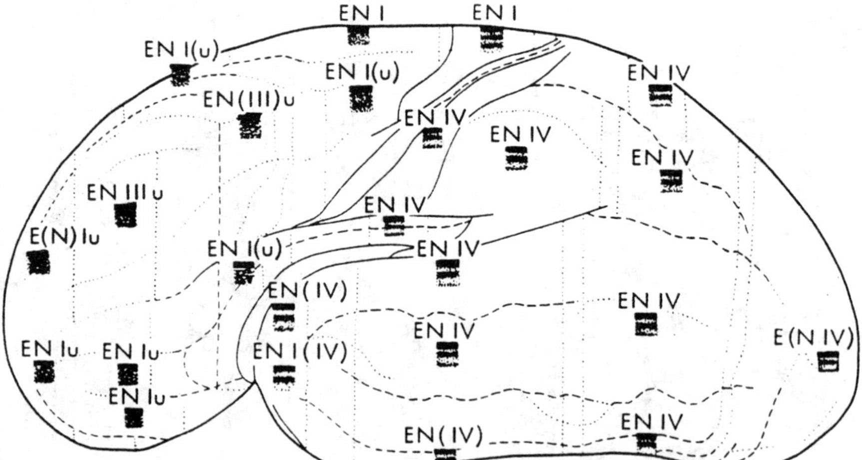

FIGURE 21 Difference between the structural differentiation of the cortex of the anterior and posterior divisions in early human ontogenesis. The diagram shows two types of cortical differentiation on the surface of the hemispheres. In the occipital, temporal, and parietal regions the six-layered structure is clear cut; in the frontal region differentiation of the layers follow another plan. (*E*) Embryonic type of cortex; (*N*) condensed Layer II; (*u*) undulation; (*I*) absence of differentiation in depth; (*II*) separation into superior and inferior "stories"; (*III*) separation of inferior "story" into layers; (*IV*) separation of superior "story" into layers. (*After Polyakov.*)

significance of these regions, showing that these regions are involved in many different functions. Experiments on various animals have clearly shown that the regions under review are essential to the formation of behavior and to the determination of the character of the reactions to stimulation effected through the cortex.

Observations have shown that electrical stimulation of these regions does not give rise to fast discharges of excitation obeying the "all or nothing" rule but, rather, that it causes slow waves of excitation that rise and fall gradually. Furthermore, these waves are concerned more with modifying the state of the nervous tissue of the brain than with producing isolated reactions of individual muscles or secretory organs. These divisions of the central nervous system are particularly important for the realization of the influence of reinforcement—positive or negative—on the higher nervous activity of the animal. This is apparently the place where one can note the effects of both positive reinforcement, associated with the satisfaction of the demands of the organism and leading to a lowering of stress, and negative reinforcement impelling the animal to seek new methods for obtaining positive reinforcement and for relieving stress.

Experimental studies of the limbic lobe have been particularly revealing in this respect. By recording the potentials from the limbic lobe it was found that each positive or negative reinforcement produced electrical discharges in this region. If the limbic lobe was injured, these reactions were disturbed, in that the discharges continued irrespective of whether the particular action was reinforced or not. This question will be reconsidered subsequently (Part II, Section 5B).

Experiments using extirpation and electrical stimulation have shown that the cortical and subcortical regions under discussion are concerned, not merely with the perception of smell and, to some extent, of taste, but also

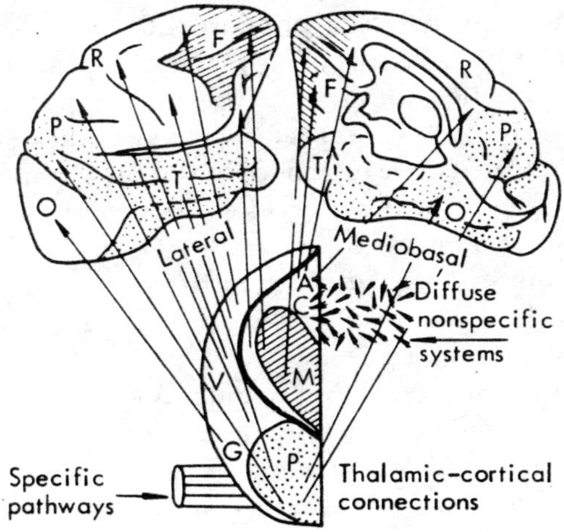

FIGURE 22 Diagram of the connections of the lateral and mediobasal regions of the cortex. (*M*) Medial nucleus of the thalamus; (*V*) ventral nucleus of the thalamus; (*P*) pulvinar; (*G*) geniculate bodies; (*O*) occipital cortical region; (*T*) temporal cortical region; (*R*) central cortical region; (*F*) frontal cortical region. (*After Pribram.*)

with the perception, analysis, and integration of the many varieties of stimuli arriving from the internal environment of the organism, i.e., from the different internal organs and systems. Subsequent anatomical and physiological investigations demonstrated the particularly close relationship between these regions of the telencephalon not only with each other (especially, between the limbic lobe and the basal portion of the frontal portion of the cortex), but also with the hypothalamic structures of the diencephalon; the latter constitute a group of centers that coordinate the autonomic and endocrinal regulatory systems and direct the trophic and metabolic processes in the tissues. Because of these findings, the concept of "rhinencephalon" has been replaced by that of "visceral brain."

It is important to emphasize that the formations of the visceral brain, in particular the limbic lobe, are very intimately connected, both directly and through the hypothalamic region, with the formations of the brain stem associated with the various autonomic functions of the organism. This is especially so with regard to the reticular formation of the brain stem, now regarded as the principal physiological apparatus for maintaining the tonus of the cortical neurons at the required level and thereby exerting a direct influence on the integrative functions of the cortex and on the alternation of the waking and sleeping states.

For instance, the investigations of Penfield and Jasper (1954) and others demonstrated that the taste analyzer, the organs of mastication, deglutition, and salivation, and the alimentary tract are represented in the insula and the adjacent opercular divisions of the anterior and posterior central gyri. Stimulation of different points of the limbic lobe in animals produced changes in cardiac activity, in the blood pressure, and in the cycle of sleeping and waking and provoked jaw movements characteristic of the act of seizing food, etc. Reactions of sham rage and sham fear with distinct and appropriate autonomic changes were repeatedly produced by stimulation of particular nuclei in the hypothalamus and the adjacent primitive portions of the telencephalon. In the experiments of Olds (1955, 1959) and Olds and Olds (1958) on rats, electrodes were inserted in specific areas of the primitive regions of the telencephalon and the rats repeatedly pressed the lever switching on the current that stimulated these regions of the brain; apparently positive reinforcement was achieved in this way. After destruction of the amygdaloid complex of nuclei in the monkey (Weiskrantz, 1956), biochemical changes that interfered with the normal regulation of the food requirements of the organism were observed; the animal ceased to feel hungry or, conversely, continued eating whether satisfied or not.

Experiments of particular interest are those conducted on the hippocampal portion of the cortex and on the formations of the neocortex lying at the base of the frontal and temporal lobes. Stimulation or extirpation of these areas caused profound emotional disturbances, such as changes in temperament, the development of affective crises and aggressiveness in hitherto tranquil animals, and, conversely, the development of undue submissiveness in hitherto aggressive animals. Electrical stimulation of these areas resulted in a series of reactions associated with various drives and instinctive forms of behavior.

These reactions, all revealing profound changes in the physiological mechanisms regulating the animal's normal behavior, show beyond doubt that the mediobasal divisions of the neocortex, together with the associated group of phylogenetically primitive cortical, subcortical, and brain-stem formations, are intimately involved in the regulation of the internal states of the organism. They receive stimuli giving information about these states or changes taking place in them, and they suitably modify or reconstruct the animal's actions in regard to its external environment. Because of the close links between these formations, especially between the limbic lobe and the basal frontal portion of the cortex, the general conclusion may be reached that two of the more important forms of impulse feedback are brought together and are functionally integrated in the frontal region. This applies, on the one hand, to impulses derived from the motor activity of the organism, directed toward the outside world and formed under the influence of information on events taking place in the external environment, and, on the other hand, to impulses arriving from the internal environment of the organism. A comprehensive analysis of all that takes place outside and inside the organism as a result of its own activity is thus made possible. As the morphological and physiological basis of the most complex forms of man's mental activity, the frontal portion of the cortex, in which external and internal information is integrated and transformed into definitive motor acts that determine the behavior of the organism as a whole, may be considered to have become of cardinal importance in man. This will be demonstrated subsequently (Part II, Section 5).

F. FUNCTIONAL PROPERTIES OF CORTICAL NEURONS *

So far we have confined our attention to the structure and functional organization of the various regions of the cortex, using information obtained mainly by morphological methods and to some extent by stimulation of localized areas of the cortex or extirpation of certain parts of the cerebral hemispheres.

In the last decade, however, the first steps have been taken toward probing into the most delicate and intimate mechanisms of brain activity. As a result of advances in experimental techniques, scientists now find it possible to analyze the activity of single neurons by recording potentials arising in

* This section was written by O. S. Vinogradova.

them under various conditions which alter the animal's behavior. This new field of research will undoubtedly yield valuable information on the intimate mechanisms of the activity of nerve tissue and, with the passage of time, it will compel a revision of many of the ideas that are held at present on functional organization in local areas of the cortex.

We must begin by stating that nearly all the available data on unit activity in the cortex has been obtained from rabbits or cats, with the exception of a few investigations on monkeys. This means that the information we have is only of the most primitive kind, and it can be extrapolated to man only with the utmost caution. Nevertheless, research at the neuronal level has already yielded important material that can serve to elucidate the general principles of functional organization of the cortical centers and the main tendencies of their development.

The visual cortex

Investigations of the primary visual cortex in Jung's laboratory (1958, 1961) have demonstrated the presence of different types of neurons, which can be found with the aid of diffuse light. Jung distinguished 5 principal types: (A) neurons not responding to light; (B) neurons giving an on-response to light consisting of a volley of spikes; (C) neurons with an inhibitory on-response to light; (D) neurons with an off-response to light; (E) on- and off-responding neurons. The type A neurons, according to Jung's observations, account for about 50% of all visual cortical neurons.

Other workers have found that the number of neurons not responding to diffuse illumination is even greater. As Hubel (1962) showed, it is possible to obtain responses from all visual neurons by specially choosing visual stimuli of a definite shape or structure. Hubel demonstrated that this depends on the particular organization of the receptive fields of the visual cortical cells. He first described cells with "simple receptive fields." By contrast with neurons of the lateral geniculate body, with their concentric fields, these cells have extensive active fields that depend on the size, shape, position, and direction of motion of the stimulus. Each such active zone is surrounded by a region with an antagonistic, inhibitory influence on responses evoked from the central zone. In this way, diffuse illumination excites the neuron's active center as the inhibitory periphery of the receptive field simultaneously prevents its response. Besides these neurons, Hubel also found cells with "complex receptive fields." These fields are more extensive and less dependent on the precise shape and size of the stimulus. Active stimuli for some neurons are an edge or outline that is light on one side and dark on the other. Active stimuli for neurons of this type can vary in size and angle of inclination within wide limits. However, the general shape and direction of motion of the stimulus continues to be significant. With increasing distance from the region of projection of the macula, the fields of the neurons increase in size. Hubel regards these neurons as integrators on which several cells with "simple fields" converge to give an "abstraction of direction and shape irrespective of the precise position of the object in the visual field."

The cortical projection of the retina (Area 17), according to the results of unitary studies, can thus no longer be regarded as a simple topographical point-by-point mosaic; rather, it is an organ of integration of a high order, specially adapted for visual perception of objects.

It is interesting to note that during displacement of an electrode held strictly perpendicular to the cortical surface all neurons lying one beneath the other have similar receptive fields. This has led to enunciation of the principles of organization of the cortical analyzer zones as "functional columns"; the same principle will be found later when the organization of other regions is examined.

The neurons described above are not the only ones in the functional mosaic of the visual cortex. Neurons responding only to monochromatic sources of light within a narrow band of the spectrum (60–100 nm) are also found there (Andersen, Buchman, and Lennox, 1962). These neurons, which account for one-third of all cells, do not respond to white light, and their response is independent of brightness. They distinguish the quality of the light within wide limits regardless of the other characteristics of the stimulus. Burns (1964) also has shown that some cells do not change their activity in response to various changes in the properties of the stimulus, but they respond to all changes in their intensity.

Many neurons of the primary visual cortex respond to vestibular stimulation (Jung, 1961). In these cases convergence of visual and vestibular influences on the same neuron is observed; vestibular influences, moreover, can modulate responses to visual stimuli to a considerable degree. Jung points out not only are discrete forms of visual information received on the same neuron, but this information is also integrated with vestibular and optokinetic stimuli. The primary visual cortex has also been shown to contain a very few (not more than 5%) neurons with binocular convergence. When convergence was found, responses arose to local stimulation of homotopical areas of the retina of the two eyes. Under these circumstances the influences were usually antagonistic: for example, the contralateral eye became excited, and the ipsilateral eye became inhibited. True summation of binocular stimuli has been observed so infrequently that most workers have concluded that the seat of the mechanisms of binocular vision is not, at least, in the primary visual cortex.

Finally, a frequent observation by different researchers must be mentioned. A fairly large number of neurons of the primary visual cortex respond to acoustic, tactile, olfactory, and nociceptive stimuli. These responses are more variable than response to light, their latent periods are longer, and they often converge on neurons which do respond to light. Their functional role is not quite clear; all that can be said is that most of them have no connection with the orienting reflex or attention, for their activity continues with no tendency toward weakening during prolonged application of the stimulus.

Auditory cortex

A tonotopical organization is observed in the primary auditory cortex of the cat at the single neuron level, although results obtained by different workers on this question do not always agree fully. Katsuki (1962) notes that mainly cells responding to high tones are located in the anterior part of the ectosylvian gyrus, cells responding to tones of average frequencies in the middle part, and cells responding to low tones in the posterior part. Other workers (Evans, Ross, and Whitefield, 1965) conclude from their observations that cells responding to high tones (over 10 kHz) in fact lie in the anterior part of Area A1, but cells responding to lower tones are uniformly distributed over the whole of the auditory cortex, so that a truly tonotopic organization does not exist. Whatever the case, one thing is certain: at the neuronal level this organization is much more complex, for neurons of the auditory cortex are characterized not simply by particular parameters of pitch, but by much more complex functional attributes. The situation is similar to that described above for neurons of the visual cortex.

Suggested classifications of auditory neurons are very complex and varied (Oonishi and Katsuki, 1965), and for that reason only some of the types of responses observed mainly in the auditory cortex of the cat will be described.

Most neurons in Area A1 respond to sounds (short or long) by short phasic on-responses. Less frequently neurons are observed with a tonic type of response, in the form of a long increase or decrease in the level of activity throughout the period of action of the stimulus. Some neurons have a narrow optimal frequency * and do not respond to other adjacent frequencies, or else they respond to them much more weakly and with much higher thresholds. Galambos and co-workers, for example, have described a neuron in the cat auditory cortex which responded to a tone of 235 Hz, but not to tones of 234 or 236 Hz, indicating extremely high precision of auditory analysis. However, cells with very wide bands of optimal frequencies, much wider than the characteristic parameters for cells of the medial geniculate body, are most typical of the auditory cortex. As Katsuki considers, this indicates that the full course of tonal analysis in all probability terminates at the thalamic level and that auditory cortical neurons act as integrators on

* "Optimal frequency" is a concept corresponding to "receptive field" in the visual and somesthetic systems; it means the frequency which evokes the maximal response of a neuron with the lowest threshold.

which several cells of the medial geniculate body converge. This view is supported by the fact that cells are found in the cortex with several peaks on their reactivity curve (i.e., they have several optimal frequencies in different parts of the tonal scale, something never observed at lower levels of the auditory system). The important point is that Katsuki did not observe in cortical neurons what is a characteristic feature of all of the remaining auditory systems, namely a relationship between the response parameters and sound intensity described by an S-shaped curve. Only very sudden and sharp changes in a sound can be reflected in cortical unit responses (which are usually depressed), and changes of intensity within the range of average are not so reflected.

Consequently, the function of intensity is encoded by cells at the lower level, and the task of the cortical neurons is to distinguish the more informative and the finer characteristics of the sound.

Responses of auditory cortical neurons are considerably augmented if two different sounds are applied simultaneously. Under these circumstances particularly clear responses are observed if the sounds bear a harmonic ratio to one another (i.e., their frequencies are in the ratio of 1:2, 1:3, and so on) and they form beats. In such cases short phasic on-responses to a tone are converted into long rhythmic responses. Katsuki links this phenomenon with the perception of the complex characteristics of the timbre of a sound at the cortical level. It has been shown that 10% of auditory cortical neurons respond only to frequency-modulated tones. Many of them have a frequency orientation, i.e., they respond only to an increase or decrease in frequency of a tone.

It is, of course, even more difficult to draw conclusions from data obtained on animals in the field of hearing. Yet the facts described suggest that individual neurons which, in the cat, are already able to distinguish such varied and complex characteristics of a sound, may have undergone further differentiation in man in the analysis of individual phonemes and the complex acoustic parameters of the sounds of speech. Galambos and coworkers (1958) have described a group of neurons in the cat auditory cortex (about 10%) which responds only to complex meaningful sounds (a call, mewing, the squeak of a mouse). These results are capable of widely different interpretations: they are not necessarily the result of specific cortical integration, but they could equally well be the result of convergence of influences from activating and "emotional" systems (the nonspecific thalamus, limbic formations) on these neurons.

As Katsuki has found, the principal neurons of the auditory cortex, with their relatively wide frequency characteristics, have an anatomical organization in vertical columns with identical functional properties. Single neurons responding to stimuli of nonacoustic modalities are also found here.

Somatosensory cortex

The postcentral cortex in the region corresponding to the somatotopical projections of somatic sensation has been investigated in cats and monkeys by Mountcastle and co-workers (1957, 1959, 1966). This region is occupied mainly by cells with local receptive fields and with a sufficiently precise somatotopical arrangement. The receptive fields may sometimes be very limited in extent (2–8 cm^2 at the periphery), but as a rule the receptive fields in the cortex are from 15 to 100 times larger than the fields of first-order somatic afferent neurons. The overwhelming majority of cells in this cortical region respond only to stimulation of the contralateral half of the body. The excitatory receptive field of these neurons is surrounded by a zone, often with complex and irregular configuration, from which inhibition of the cell response to stimulation of the center of the receptive field can be induced. In the region anterior to the somatosensory area, at the boundary with the motor cortex in the anterior part of the hemisphere, the number of neurons with very large, diffuse receptive fields increases steadily—a response of these cells can often be evoked from all four limbs or from the whole of one half of the body—and ipsilateral and contralateral stimuli converge on one neuron. Latent periods here are longer, and the fields themselves are more labile, than in the central part of the somatic analyzer. These neurons can be regarded as integrators of receptive fields of neurons in the central zone.

The characteristics of somatic neurons are not, however, limited to their topical representation. Some cells respond only to stimuli of certain submodalities: to touching the skin, pulling the hair, pressure on deep tissues, or movement of a limb at a joint. The relationship between stimuli of different modalities may be reciprocal, and the response to one submodality (touch) may be inhibited by the application of a different stimulus to the same receptive field (pressure). In experiments on monkeys, Mountcastle discovered a selective location of principal submodalities in cytoarchitectonic areas (cutaneous sensation in Area 3, deep sensation in Area 2, the transition from one to the other in Area 1). However, at the same time there are neurons on which different types of sensation converge, so that one cell can respond to flexion of the fingers, to pressure on the skin, and to pulling on the hair.

Several responses may be phasic or tonic. For example, when a limb is rotated at the joint some cells respond with a short volley of spikes at the time of rotation whereas others maintain a higher level of activity as long as the limb remains in its altered position. Some units thus provide information about movement, others about the maintenance of posture. However, even in units with wide stimulus convergence, some investigators consider that different submodalities or different points on the surface can be encoded in cell discharge patterns, as a result of which the specificity of information is partly preserved despite its extensive convergence.

The principle of vertical organization of the cortex was first demonstrated by Mountcastle in the somatosensory region. He showed that there is considerable similarity between receptive fields in columns of neurons as the recording microelectrode, held perpendicular to the surface of the cortex, is inserted into its depth. He found functional columns of this sort not only for tonic fields, but also for characteristic submodalities. Mountcastle accordingly regards vertical columns as integral functional units of the cortex responsible for the discrete analysis and synthesis of corresponding stimuli.

Secondary zones of analyzers

Information on areas outside the primary zones of the cortical analyzers is much less abundant and definite than that described above for the primary projection zones. The reason for this is perfectly clear, for in certain experimental animals (rabbits) these areas themselves are poorly developed and are defined differently by different experimental physiologists. On the other hand, as was pointed out above, in order to investigate the primary zones themselves the experimenter is faced with the need for a careful choice from a number of very complex and special stimuli. When studying cortical areas outside the projection zones the search for adequate stimuli is even more difficult, and the various investigations of neurons from these regions leave the impression that the results are oversimplified to some degree because of the inadequacy of the stimuli used. For this reason only a list of the more general distinguishing features of the secondary areas, as revealed by the work of different investigators, will be given here.

In the anterior part of the lateral, suprasylvian, and ectosylvian gyri, when integral-evoked potentials were recorded, secondary responses to photic, acoustic, and cutaneous stimuli were found to be equally represented. Microelectrode studies in these regions revealed a high percentage of neurons with broad multisensory convergence. The percentage of responding neurons was usually lower here than in the projection areas, but most neurons responded to two or three modalities. At the same time, unitary studies demonstrate the absence of that homogeneity that is apparent when evoked potentials are recorded. For example, in the anterior lateral gyrus of the cat the neurons respond preferentially to acoustic stimuli and to a lesser degree to photic and tactile stimuli, whereas in the suprasylvian gyrus responses to photic stimuli predominate, and so on. Each region thus has its own set of sensory integration and, correspondingly, its own specific functions (Dubner, 1966).

The most penetrating investigation of specific sensory functions of nonprimary areas of the visual cortex (Brodmann's Areas 18 and 19) has been carried out recently by Hubel and Wiesel (1965). According to their observations these areas, like the primary zone, possess topographical organization; however, the peripheral regions of the retina are perhaps not represented at all in them. A progressive increase in complexity of the receptive fields of the neurons is found in Areas 18 and 19, and the change in functional characteristics corresponds exactly to the cytoarchitectonic boundaries between areas. In Area 18 simple fields (see above) are almost absent, and 90% of neurons have complex fields. Cells with hypercomplex fields (5–10%) also appear here. Hypercomplex cells of the lower order respond to visual complexes ("a moving boundary" and "a moving line of limited length" and "a moving line limited in length in both directions"); the situation can be expressed rather more simply by saying that they respond to angles and rectangles, strictly in the size and width of the surrounding "limiting edge," and the orientation and direction of movement. Hypercomplex "higher order" cells respond to two groups of visual stimuli with orientation differing by 90°. By their properties, their fields are clearly characterized as a result of synthesis of several complex or hypercomplex lower-order fields. Cells of this type count for more than half of the cells in Area 19. Individual cells of this area have complex fields, and in the vertical columns complex and hypercomplex cells with an identical field orientation are often found, forming discrete functional systems.

At the neuronal level, a generalized reception of complex visual information thus predominates in Areas 18 and 19, with distinction not of the outline (as in Area 17), but of disturbance of the continuous outline (breaks in lines, curvature, rotation, a change in the direction of movement). Besides this, binocular synthesis of information evidently also takes place largely in Area 18. The second somatic area, where the topical organization of somatosensory representation is preserved to some extent but, by contrast with the primary area, the two halves of the body (ipsilateral and contralateral) are superposed one above the other in this representation, possesses a special feature of its own. The physiological importance of this fact is not quite clear. Here also there are many neurons with very large receptive fields, and they often respond also to sound (Mountcastle, 1962; Carreras and Andersson, 1963).

Neurons of the second auditory area (A II) often have no optimal frequency whatsoever and respond to sounds regardless of its physical characteristics (Katsuki, 1962). In the secondary zones of the auditory cortex a significantly higher proportion of neurons have responses of tonic type. These responses arise after a longer latent period, but they are maintained throughout the action of the stimulus and frequently persist for some time after its end, whereas in the primary zone phasic on-responses of the cells to acoustic stimulation predominate.

Neurons of the secondary areas have much more labile responses, and they are variable with respect to their receptive fields and to reproduction of the response structure (temporal discharge pattern). These responses are the first to disappear after administration of small doses of narcotics, evidence of their multisynaptic nature (Carreras and Andersson, 1963).

It follows from the facts described above that the functions of analysis of elementary physical characteristics of stimuli are in any event much less pronounced in the secondary areas. On this basis some workers have ascribed to the multimodal cells of secondary areas the role of diffuse activators, receiving influences from the nonspecific activating systems of the brain and controlling the general level of brain activity (including organization of orientation and attention) on the spot. The apparent "simplicity" of the integral responses of these cells is, as was said above, the result of the use of primitive and inadequate forms of stimulation. Analysis of interneuronal connections and data on the structural organization of these areas given in the preceding section suggests that neurons of the secondary areas are true integrators, generalizing information after its primary analysis by one or more analyzers.

The motor cortex

The data on neurons of the motor cortex (Areas 4–6) obtained by different workers are very similar. Responses in this region are recorded usually at a considerable depth (more than 1000μ from the surface), and on this account the cells from which activity is recorded are usually identified as the large pyramids of Betz in Areas 5–6. Of the total number of cells, three-quarters responded to somatic stimulation of more than two limbs. Responses to stimulation of deep tissues, to stretching and to pricking the muscles, and flexion of the limbs at the joints are predominant. However, many neurons also respond to tactile stimulation of the skin. Stimuli from the vestibular system and cerebellum converge here. All writers are agreed that there is wide convergence of auditory and visual excitation (Albe-Fessard, 1964; Buser and Imbert, 1961; Sokolova, 1966). The activity of some neurons is considerably quickened during a movement. Experiments on unanesthetized monkeys have shown that in some cases neurons whose response is definitely activated during an active limb movement do not change their spontaneous firing pattern during passive movements of the same limb (Evarts, 1965). In other cases an increase in firing rate is observed before the movement takes place, to coincide with the general cortical activation response.

These observations suggest that neurons of the motor cortex are elements of the true "final path" or a general zone of sensomotor integration. Universal convergence of this sort is not found in any of the posterior zones of the hemispheres. The final results of the analytical and synthetic activity of the posterior zones are evidently sent out to the motor pyramids in order to regulate the voluntary motor response of the organism.

Unfortunately, no information is available at the present time on unit activity in the premotor and frontal zones of the brain.

Dynamic characteristics of cortical neurons

Many workers who have studied neurons of a primary sensory area have emphasized that their characteristics are strictly constant. The stimulus evoking a response from a neuron in a projection area is usually encoded in a particular sequence of discharges, which changes only with a change in some of the properties of the stimulus. The receptive fields of the neurons are also strictly constant. Unfortunately, it is not yet possible to record single unit responses for long periods of time (several days), but in the overwhelming majority of cases recording for 8–10 h shows no change in the characteristics of the unit responses. It is therefore assumed that these characteristics are determined by the anatomical connections of the neurons and in the initial stages of their functioning (Hubel and Wiesel, 1963), after which they are consolidated as functional units forming the analyzer systems.

However, the cortex has always been regarded as the principal apparatus of learning, attention, memory, and individual experience. It is therefore natural that investigators should wish to find correlates of these dynamic processes in cortical neurons.

Experiments have shown that single unit responses change their characteristics during stimulation of the activating reticular formation and the nonspecific thalamus (Jung, 1958; Fuster, 1961). Previously inactive cells thereupon begin to respond, the likelihood of responses is increased, and the critical flicker fusion frequency rises in the visual cortical neurons. These phenomena can be regarded as analogs of the mechanisms of attention. It has also been shown that the responses of auditory neurons are increased during attentive examination of a source of sound. Looking at the mouse evokes a general increase in discharge frequency in the visual cortex of a cat, accompanied by a simultaneous decrease in unit responses to a diffuse flash. Neurons responding only if a stimulus is new or unfamiliar ("novelty detectors") have been found in the visual, auditory, somatosensory, and motor areas. On repetition of the stimulus, the responses of such neurons rapidly diminish and then disappear completely, but they can be restored by a change in any one aspect of the stimulus (Hubel, Galambos, et al., 1959; Vinogradova and Lindsley, 1963; Murata and Kameda, 1963). The activity of these neurons can be regarded not only as an analog of the orienting reflex or of sensory attention, but also as a correlate of fixation of the trace of a stimulus in the system of memory.

After the initial investigations of Jasper and co-workers (1958), who demonstrated the complex redistribution of activity in neurons in the various cortical areas of monkeys during motor conditioning, very recently many papers have been published on the formation of conditioned reflexes to single neurons. In response to a combination of stimuli, one of which ("reinforcing") evokes the initial response, a "conditioned" response can be obtained to a hitherto inactive stimulus. In essence, the "conditioned" response to the combination in no way reproduces the response to the "reinforcing" stimulus; this suggests that the integration thus formed is complex in character.

Although at present there are nothing more than a few hints, it can be postulated that the elements of dynamic transformation will be more marked in the secondary and tertiary formations of the cortex. In the primary areas these processes are the exception rather than the rule. For instance, the number of "novelty detectors" in the visual and auditory areas is only 4–5%. The impression is that functions in the primary areas are so arranged as to create maximal stability of the information received and transmitted, as the "objective" reflection of external influences, largely independent of attitude or interest or the significance and emotional tinge of the stimulus. Secondary processing, namely the selection of information on the basis of its individual significance, fixation in the memory, and so on, takes place later, in topographically different regions, on the basis of this stable reflection. In some respects this processing may perhaps also take place in nonprimary cortical areas.

There are good grounds at present for considering that the oldest region of the cortex, the hippocampus, plays some part in these processes. Investigations of hippocampal neurons have revealed the extraordinarily wide convergence of stimuli of different sensory modalities. However, all these stimuli evoke distinctive tonic unit responses only if they possess the quality of novelty. The responses quickly become adapted and can be restored by a change in any of the parameters of the stimulus. Neurons with this dynamic response pattern constitute about 80% of all reactive hippocampal neurons, a fact which suggests that the hippocampus plays a special role in the processes of distinguishing between familiar and unfamiliar stimuli, fixation of novel stimuli, and the inhibition of responses to stimuli already fixed in the past experience of the organism (Vinogradova, 1965).

This concludes our brief survey of the facts marking the first steps in the creation of the functional cytoarchitectonics of the cortex.

3. *Disturbances of Higher Mental Functional Systems in the Presence of Local Brain Lesions*

The systematic principle of the structure of the higher mental functions and of their graded localization have been explained, and the complexity of organization that distinguishes the human cerebral cortex has been discussed. What bearing have these matters on the disturbances of higher mental functions in the presence of circumscribed brain lesions? What principles must guide the approach to the local pathology of the cerebral cortex? These are crucial questions, and they must be examined closely before the concrete facts pertaining to the pathology underlying higher human cortical functions are analyzed.

We have previously mentioned the assertion, first made by Jackson, that the localization of a symptom in no way coincides with the localization of the function that has been impaired. It cannot be deduced from the fact that a lesion of a circumscribed area of the cerebral cortex causes a disturbance of a particular function, for example that of writing or calculation, that writing or calculation are "localized" in that part of the brain. The principles of the systematic organization of functions and of their graded localization are compatible with the proposition that for a function to be disturbed it is sufficient, in practice, for any one link in a complex functional system to be broken. In other words, if any link essential for the performance of the function is removed, the functional system as a whole will either collapse or, in accordance with the systematic and not the discrete principle of its organization, is reorganized to perform the required function by means of a new chain of mechanisms. However, the fact that a disturbance of a functional system may, in practice, result from a lesion affecting any of its links does not mean that the function is disturbed equally by any lesion of the brain and that the antilocalizationists are right in their belief that the brain works as a homogeneous, equipotential entity. We need only remember how complex and highly differentiated a structure the brain is in order to see how groundless such views are.

A fundamental principle, to serve as a guide throughout the subsequent analysis, has been formulated. It may be stated as follows: *The higher mental functions may be disturbed by a lesion of one of the many different links of the functional system; nevertheless, they will be disturbed differently by lesions of different links.* To analyze how the higher mental functions are, in fact, disturbed by lesions situated in different parts of the brain is the main task in studying the functional pathology of circumscribed brain lesions.

Let us consider this point in more detail. It has previously been stated that every higher mental function, in our interpretation of this term, is composed of many links and depends for its performance on the combined working of many parts of the cerebral cortex, each of which has its own special role in the functional system as a whole. This principle may be illustrated more clearly by an analysis of a mental function that has been the subject of considerable study. For this purpose we may choose writing, for we have made a special study of this function in the past (Luria, 1950).

Before a person can write what is dictated to him, he must first acoustically analyze the sound composition. This analysis consists of differentiating each separate, discrete element or sound from the continuous sound flow, determining their actual phonemic signs, and comparing these sounds with other sounds of speech in accordance with these signs. Acoustic analysis and synthesis, which occupy the whole of the initial period of learning how to write, have been shown by special investigations (Nazarova, 1952, and others) to involve the very close participation of articulation. The sound composition of the work is later "recoded" into the visual images of letters, which can be written down. Every sound of speech identified with the aid of hearing and articulation is firmly associated with a definite visual image of a letter, or "grapheme," which may be written in various ways (as a capital or small letter, simply or elaborately). The recoding of each phoneme into the visual scheme of a grapheme must be accomplished with due regard to its topological properties and to the spatial arrangement of its elements. This act is preparatory for the third stage in the process of writing—the recoding of the outlines of the visual letters into a kinesthetic system of successive movements required to write them. In the writing of the various letters, a complex kinetic "melody," requiring a definite organization of motor acts in space and in time, a smooth flow of movement, etc., is created. The relative importance of these factors does not remain constant throughout the various stages of development of the motor skill. In the first stages, the writer's attention is concentrated on the sound analysis of the word and, sometimes, on the search for the required grapheme. When the skill to write has been acquired but not yet automatized, these factors fade into the background and are called upon only for a particularly complicated word.

When writing has become automatized, it is converted into smooth, kinetic stereotypes.

To meet the needs of our argument, the analysis of the psychological aspect of writing has been considerably simplified. Many factors, such as the variations in phonemes depending on their position in a word and the maintenance of the required sequence of sounds in a word and of words in a phrase, have not been dwelled upon. This account will suffice to show how complex the process of writing is and how dependent it is on a varied concatenation of links.

The complexity of the composite function of writing is matched by the complexity of its graded (or systematic) localization. It follows that the act of writing cannot by any means be regarded as the result of the activity of any one "center;" its performance requires a complete system of interconnected but highly differentiated cortical zones.

The performance of the act of writing is conditional on the integrity of the primary and, in particular, of the secondary fields of the auditory cortex of the left temporal region, which together with the inferior portion of the postcentral (kinesthetic) and premotor portions of the cortex takes part in the phonematic analysis and integration of speech. Another essential requirement is integrity of the visual-kinesthetic areas of the cortex, without which recoding of the phonematic structure into a system of graphemes, with maintenance of the topological characteristics and spatial coordinates, is impossible. Integrity of the kinesthetic and motor (postcentral and premotor) portions of the cortex is also essential for normal writing activity, i.e., for the recoding of graphic schemes into smooth kinetic "melodies" of motor acts. As shall be indicated subsequently, the proper performance of higher mental functions is impossible without the integrity of the whole brain, including its frontal regions.

It can therefore be stated with justification that normal writing can be carried out only if a highly complex group of cortical zones remains intact. This complex comprises practically the whole brain and yet forms a highly differentiated system, each component of which performs a specific function.

Meanwhile, it must be remembered that the complex constellation of zones concerned in the act of writing may vary at different stages of formation of the skill. Moreover, it may vary with different languages. For instance, special investigations (Luria, 1947, 1960) have shown that phonetic writing in Russian or German has a very different structure from hieroglyphic writing in Chinese and even from mixed (containing both phonetic and conventional components) writing in French. There is every reason to suppose that writing in these languages is based on different constellations of cerebral zones.

It is evident that writing can be disordered by circumscribed lesions of widely different areas of the cerebral cortex, but in every case the disorder in writing will show qualitative peculiarities depending on which link is destroyed and which primary defects are responsible for the disorder of the whole functional system.

If the lesion is situated in the cortical territory of the auditory analyzer, systematized reception of the sound flow will be impossible. Complex sound combinations will be perceived as inarticulate noises and closely similar phonemes will be confused. A patient with such a lesion, although retaining smooth motor skills and the ability to form graphemes, will not be able to formulate a clear "program" necessary for the writing of words.

Closely similar but (as shall be enumerated) essentially different results ensue from a lesion of the cortical divisions of the kinesthetic analyzer. Such lesions prevent normal participation of articulation in the process of analysis of the sounds of speech. In these conditions, very typical writing defects will develop.

A completely different form of writing defect is seen with lesions of the parieto-occipital divisions of the cortex, i.e., areas directly concerned with visual-spatial analysis and synthesis of external stimuli. In these cases the perception of the sound composition of speech remains intact, but its recoding into visual-spatial schemes (graphemes) is impossible. The topological scheme of the letters and the spatial arrangement of their elements are disturbed.

Finally, with lesions situated within the cortical divisions of the motor analyzer, it is the kinetic organization of the acts that suffers most. The writing defect in such cases will therefore take the form of loss of the required order of the elements to be written, disturbance of the smoothness of the necessary movements, increased inertia of the nervous pathways once formed, difficulty in switching from one motor element to another, etc. The discussion of writing disturbances in the presence of local brain lesions will be continued subsequently (Part III, Section 9).

All that has been said regarding the graded localization and systematic pathology of the writing process has general relevance and leads to fundamental conclusions. The first of these, which has already been stated, is that a complex functional system may be disordered by lesions situated in the most widely separated areas of the cortex but that each disorder has its own specific character. In each case the "proper" function* of the affected cortical area is primarily upset, so that this particular link of the functional system cannot perform normally. The secondary (or systematic) consequence of this disturbance is the collapse of the functional system as a whole. Finally, functional adaptations take place in the pathologically changed system and lead to compensation of the defect by calling into play the intact links of the cortical apparatus. An important fact in our opinion is that the secondary and tertiary changes in a functional system resulting

* In this instance the term "function" is used in the first of its meanings that was given (Part I, Section 1B): the activity peculiar to that particular area of the cerebral apparatus.

from lesions in different locations show variations in character that make it possible to judge the nature of the primary disturbance. Consequently, *for every local lesion functional systems develop specific defects and undergo specific adaptations*. Analysis of this specific character of the disturbance of the higher cortical functions accompanying local brain lesions enables identification of the primary defect underlying the disturbance. In this way the main purpose of the clinical-psychological investigation is accomplished.

Our understanding of disturbances of the higher mental functions in the presence of circumscribed brain lesions leads to the second conclusion, which is of fundamental importance to questions of technique. We must recognize the need, not merely to state that a symptom is present, but also to qualify it or define its structure. In other words, in order to know the cerebral location of the corresponding function it is not sufficient to merely state that a particular function is lost (as was frequently done by classical neurologists), for this leads to mistaken attempts to localize the lost function directly in the affected area of the brain and inevitably gives a wrong idea of the actual mechanism of the particular symptom. The symptom can be correctly understood only by *qualitative analysis, by the study of the structure of the disturbance, and ultimately, by the identification of the factor or primary defect responsible for the development of the observed phenomenon*. This is the only way by which the true mechanism of a disturbance can be discovered. Symptoms that at first glance appear to be identical turn out, when examined more closely, to be the result of completely different pathological factors. Distinguishing between the external manifestation of a defect and its qualitative structure, i.e., to identify the primary defect and its secondary (systematic) consequences, is an essential condition of the topical analysis of disturbances arising from local brain lesions. This is the only approach that can provide for topical evaluation of the lesion, which, in practice, is so important.*

• • •

After analysis of the defect underlying the symptom and of its secondary (systematic) consequences, we come to the last principle, which is equally

* An approach to disturbances of functions which is not based on the assessment of symptoms as the result of a local lesion but which considers the observed disturbances to be the result of dissociation of brain systems, has recently been revived in neurology. This approach is reflected most clearly in a recently published investigation by Geschwind (1965).

At first glance it might appear that such an approach would be radically opposed to that adopted in this book. However, such an objection does not withstand careful analysis.

There is no doubt that dissociation between the functions of individual brain formations may give rise to significant disturbances of higher cortical functions, which are always constructed on a basis of the combined activity of cortical areas and discrete brain formations belonging to different systems. However, such dissociation can arise not only in lesions of the conducting systems of the brain (the importance of important when analyzing disturbance of the higher mental functions by circumscribed brain lesions.

The classical neurologists noticed the fact, so paradoxical at first glance, that *a lesion of a single, circumscribed area of the cerebral cortex often leads to the development, not of an isolated symptom, but of a group of disturbances, apparently far removed from each other.* They usually singled out the most obvious feature, which they regarded as the basic symptom, and considered the rest to be accessory symptoms. However, with the accumulation of more data, it became apparent that the presence of a group of symptoms with a lesion of a circumscribed area of the cerebral cortex is the rule and not the exception. Moreover, this rule militates against the views that the cerebral cortex contains a number of isolated centers and that the different cortical regions are equipotential. If, as we assume, the complex mental processes are functional systems, the development of a group of disturbances from a lesion of a circumscribed area of the cerebral cortex is inevitable.

It is known that different higher mental functions (or, more precisely, functional systems) have common links, or components, in their mechanism. For instance, writing, like the pronunciation of words, has as one of its components the reception of the acoustic elements of speech. Operations involving spatial relationships or calculation, externally very different functions, also possess a common link—simultaneous spatial analysis and synthesis. There are myriad other such examples. The primary disturbance of sound analysis and synthesis occurring with a cortical lesion of the left temporal lobe invariably causes a disturbance of the ability not only to write, but also to memorize words, retain a long series of spoken sounds, etc. without, however, affecting functions such as calculation or spatial perception. In contrast, a cortical lesion of the left parieto-occipital region invariably causes poor execution of spatial operations and of calculation (as well as of several other functions of no immediate concern here) but not of the perception of the sound composition of words or of the attendant functions of writing, pronunciation of words, etc.

Thus, the presence of a primary defect, interfering with the proper function of a given part of the brain, inevitably leads to disturbances of a group of functional systems, i.e., to the appearance of a symptom-complex, or syndrome, composed of externally heterogeneous but, in fact, internally interconnected symptoms.

The analysis of such syndromes and the discovery of the common links at

---

which must not be underestimated), but also in lesions of secondary or tertiary areas of the cortex, which themselves must be regarded as structures responsible for integrating the work of the various brain systems. The primary aim of the present book is to analyze disturbances which arise in lesions of these areas; the symptoms that are the result of lesions of the conducting tracts of the brain still await special neuropsychological investigation.

the basis of their component symptoms are essential parts of the psychological investigation of the disturbances arising from local brain lesions. By analysis of the whole syndrome, a more reliable estimate can be given of the probable location of the lesion than would be possible from the isolation of a single symptom. The qualitative analysis of the syndrome as a whole is therefore an essential step in the clinical analysis of disturbances of higher cortical functions from local brain lesions.

By defining the syndrome as a whole and establishing the links uniting groups of functional systems we are brought face to face with well-known tenets in modern psychology. Writers such as Spearman (1932) and Thurstone (1947), whose psychometric investigations revealed the mutual connection between individual mental processes, concluded that particular groups of functions are based on common factors and will therefore show a high degree of correlation with changes in certain specific functions and an absence of correlation with changes in others. Research such as this led to the creation of a system of psychological investigation known as "factor analysis," embodying accurate mathematical methods for determining common and special factors.* Syndrome analysis, concerned with the factual pathology of higher mental functions, can be regarded as a legitimate variant of factor analysis, the only difference being that syndrome analysis is directed toward the investigation of the organization of mental processes in a single subject.

• • •

The foregoing remarks require additional clarification in one important respect. The basic factor concerned in different disturbances is not necessarily a primary defect of the "proper function" of the affected area of the brain, nor does it necessarily lead to the total loss of this function. In many cases the function is merely depressed, and this is demonstrated by local disturbances in the neurodynamics of a particular function. Finally, in many cases of generalized brain pathology this factor has no particular topical character; it may take the form of the general pathological changes in neurodynamics studied extensively by Pavlov's school (Ivanov-Smolenskii, 1949; etc.).

In all these cases, various disturbances may appear: a weakening or inadequate mobility of nervous processes, a weakening of internal inhibition, or a pathologically increased external inhibition of processes that have already developed. These may be manifested equally in several different analyzers and may thus lose their local selectivity. *The most important fact,* however, *is that a generalized disturbance in the dynamics of the nervous processes must make its effect felt primarily on those forms of cortical activity with the most complex organization.* We may therefore suppose that in these cases it is the

*The method of "factor analysis" of psychological factors has recently been applied by B. M. Teplov and his associates to the study of symptoms mainly related to the physiological aspects of nervous process (Nebylitsyn, 1960; etc.).

higher level of organization of the mental processes that suffers most and that a depression of various forms of mental activity occurs, a phenomenon that attracted the attention of many eminent neuropathologists, starting with Baillarger (1865) and Jackson (1884) and ending with Head (1926) and Ombredane (1951). The discovery of the physiological mechanisms of this depression of psychophysiological processes will undoubtedly be one of the most important advances in neurological knowledge.

• • •

We have formulated some general principles to guide us in our subsequent examination of our case material. In our opinion, they are well-grounded and have proved their practical validity over a long period of time in the topical diagnosis of local brain lesions.

It only remains for us to mention one more group of conditions that must be satisfied when disturbances of higher cortical functions resulting from local brain lesions are studied. It is a subject for further research rather than conclusions based on past experience, namely, the need for a neurodynamic characterization of the disturbances that are to be studied.

We know that the disturbance of a function arising as a result of a pathological change in the state of a definite area of the brain (or of the brain as a whole) frequently does not lead to loss of the function but merely to the appearance of symptoms of depression or of excitation of the activity of the particular area.

This was a point repeatedly made by classical neurologists, who constantly reiterated that an action which cannot be performed voluntarily can in some cases take place if it is incorporated in a well-automated system (Jackson). This fact can be illustrated by the case, well-known in the neurological literature and described by Gowers, when a patient, unable to utter the word "No" of her own accord, exclaimed after several unsuccessful attempts: "No, doctor, I cannot say 'no'! . . ."

The physiological nature of this temporary inhibition of a function, if that function has to be performed as an independent action under voluntary control, deserves the closest attention in order to elucidate its basic mechanisms. It is only recently that substantial progress has been made in this direction and that the process of "blocking" of functions in local brain lesions and its restoration by "deblocking" have been subjected to special and close analysis (Weigl, 1963).

This pathological state of the brain (or of its individual areas), as has been pointed out, manifests itself by significant changes in the dynamics of the higher nervous processes, leading to a weakening of these processes, to a disturbance of the most complex forms of internal inhibition, to an imbalance of the nervous processes, to increased pathological inertia, to a diminution of the integrated forms of activity (often termed a "narrowing of the range" of a particular function), to a lessening of the aftereffect, etc. This neurodynamic characterization of pathological cortical activity became possible only with the introduction of modern methods of studying higher nervous activity, and the further development of these methods is the most urgent task in the investigation of the pathology of higher cortical functions.

The completion of this task must entail the work of a whole generation of research workers. It is for this reason that the present book, which is more a review of past research than an account of work in progress at the moment, deals inadequately with the neurodynamics of pathological changes in the cortical processes arising from local brain lesions and emphasizes that this is a matter for further research.

II

DISTURBANCES OF THE HIGHER CORTICAL FUNCTIONS IN THE PRESENCE OF LOCAL BRAIN LESIONS

1. Some Functional Investigative Problems

A. PRINCIPAL FORMS OF DISTURBANCE OF THE HIGHER CORTICAL FUNCTIONS RESULTING FROM LOCAL BRAIN LESIONS

In classical neurology, the syndromes of disturbances of the higher cortical functions accompanying local brain lesions were subdivided into three main independent groups: agnosia, apraxia, and aphasia. To these were added the more specialized disorders of alexia, agraphia, acalculia, amusia, etc.

There are clinical grounds for differentiating the basic syndromes of agnosia, apraxia, and aphasia. When disturbances of the higher cortical functions associated with circumscribed brain lesions are investigated, the emphasis is frequently on perceptual, motor, or speech disorders. Nowadays, however, this approach to the pathology of the higher cortical functions resulting from local brain lesions meets with both factual and theoretical objections. The classification of the syndromes of agnosia, apraxia, and aphasia as clearly demarcated, independent symptom-complexes was based on the belief that these disorders develop independently both of disturbances of more elementary functions and of each other.

Classical neurologists, distinguishing between disturbances of the higher and the more elementary functions, defined agnosia as a disturbance in the perception of the nature of sensation with the preservation of the ability to experience sensation and apraxia as a disorder of skilled action with the elementary motor functions remaining intact. In defining aphasia as "speech asymbolia," a concept formulated by Finkelburg (1870) and Kussmaul (1885), speech was also so distinguished and speech disorders were looked upon as independent of more elementary defects.

Agnosia, apraxia, and aphasia finally came to be understood as disorders of higher "symbolic" activity, in sharp contradistinction to disturbances of a more elementary type. Meanwhile, another tendency appeared in the classical approach to the agnosias, apraxias, and aphasias: These disorders were frequently represented as being independent of each other. These views had a theoretical basis in contemporary psychology, according to which the complex motor, perceptual, and speech processes are higher symbolic functions to be distinguished from the sensorimotor level of activity.

As time went on, however, data accumulated that conflicted with these viewpoints. Clinical evidence appeared suggesting that the agnosias may be based on more elementary sensory defects and the apraxias on more elementary motor defects. Cases were reported that showed that even in speech disorders there can be disturbances of the sensory and motor components of speech activity. More recently, this tendency to bridge the gap between the relatively elementary and complex disturbances and to make a more physiological analysis of the mechanisms underlying the complex symbolic disorders has gained momentum. As a result of a series of investigations (e.g., Bay, 1950, 1957*a*; Denny-Brown, 1951, 1958; Zangwill, 1951; Teuber, 1955, 1959, 1960*a*, etc.; Ajuriaguerra and Hécaen, 1960), convincing evidence was obtained of the importance of changes in the relatively elementary sensory and motor processes in agnostic, apractic, and aphasic disorders.

Meanwhile, clinical practice yielded more and more factual data indicating that the agnosias, apraxias, and aphasias could no longer be regarded as independent, isolated disturbances. Observations showed that disturbances in visual spatial orientation (spatial agnosia), well known in clinical practice, are, as a rule, accompanied by well-defined motor disturbances; since the necessary spatial afferent control is lacking, movement becomes apractic in character. A close relationship was established between astereognosis and a disturbance in fine and precisely organized palpatory movements. Finally, reports appeared that optic-gnostic disorders were frequently accompanied by marked disturbances in eye movement, sometimes so severe that it was difficult to determine whether a gnostic or a practic defect was responsible for the disorder. Findings such as these prevented many workers from making hard and fast distinctions between the agnosias and apraxias. Neurologists began to employ the term "apractognosia" to reflect the unity of sensory and motor defects, and with the increasing wealth of clinical experience, the use of this word became the rule rather than the exception. The view that the agnosias, apraxias, and aphasias are sharply demarcated from the more elementary disorders also met with serious theoretical objections.

As mentioned (Part I, Section 1B and C), according to the modern theories of physiology and psychology propounded by Sechenov and Pavlov, sensory processes are the result of the work of analyzers and the higher perceptual processes are not dissociated from their elementary components. It is clear from the Pavlovian concept of reflex analysis that it serves no useful purpose to describe disturbances of higher cortical functions in subjective terms, such as "disturbance of perception" or "disturbance of the integrity of vision." They may have been excellent descriptive terms in Munk's time, but they did obstruct progress in physiological analysis. At present, therefore, progressive minds in neurophysiological research, while accepting the qualitative specificity of the more complex forms of analyticosynthetic activity, regard as their most urgent task the study of the elementary components of these forms.

Modern psychology, too, has decisively rejected the once dominant view that sensory and motor processes are isolated functions that are sharply demarcated from each other.

As stated, according to the reflex concept, sensations and perceptions constitute selective, systematized reflection of the external world and have both sensory (afferent) and motor (efferent) components. Sechenov himself, by including the active "probing" movements of the eyes among the processes of visual perception, called attention to the reflex, afferent-efferent nature of this act. Further investigation extended this principle to the cutaneokinesthetic and even to the acoustic fields of perception, demonstrating that motor components are involved in each of these "sensory" processes. In recent decades neuroanatomists have discovered and described the motor apparatuses belonging to the receptors and the efferent fibers contained in the nervous apparatus of every analyzer (Part I, Section 2D). Modern views on the organization of the sensory processes have thereby been formulated on a sound morphological footing. The second important problem in modern neurophysiology, therefore, is the relationship between complex sensory and motor disorders, on the one hand, and between practic and gnostic afferent disturbances, on the other.

These important considerations also compel re-examination of the classical concept of the apraxias and the directing of our main attention to the afferent bases of disturbances of complex voluntary movements.

The science of psychology long ago divested itself of the notion that voluntary movements are undetermined, free-willed acts with no afferent basis. Considerable influence was exerted on this change of viewpoint by the materialistic philosophy and by the findings of physiological research. The findings of Krasnogorskii (1911) and of Konorskii and Miller (1936) were used by Pavlov when, for the first time, he included the processes of analysis and synthesis of kinesthetic stimuli in his study of the physiological basis of voluntary movement and thus created the concept of the "motor analyzer." In this manner he extended the application of the principles used in the examination of all afferent zones of the cerebral cortex (cutaneokinesthetic, visual, auditory) to the motor cortex and made voluntary movement accessible to objective physiological study. In his investigation of motor acts, Bernshtein (1926, 1935, 1947, etc.) defined the afferent basis of voluntary movement and established the role of returning afferent impulses in their regulation. Nevertheless, there is still an urgent need for the study of the afferent basis of disturbances of the higher forms of movement and activity. Modern scientific theories of the reflex structure of sensory and motor processes thus emphasize the interdependence of these processes and justify the consideration of gnostic and practic disorders as mutually related phenomena.

The analysis of speech processes and of their disturbances by circumscribed brain lesions must be similarly modified. Attempts have recently been made to interpret sensory aphasia as a disturbance of acoustic gnosis (approximating it to the patterns of the acoustic agnosias) and motor aphasia as a special form of apraxia. This tendency to seek more elementary motor disorders in motor-speech defects has recently been strengthened by the work of Bay (1950, 1957*b*), who attempted to distinguish paretic, dystonic, and dyspractic components in motor aphasias.

Despite the considerable progress that has been made in the investigation of the sensory and motor components of speech, complex speech disorders are still often interpreted as a completely independent sphere comprised of disturbances of some form of symbolic activity or of specific speech "images" and their transmission. Many clinical descriptions of aphasic symptoms are given without proper analysis, and the classifications of these disturbances are based either on hypothetical schemes, in which patterns of "conduction" or "transcortical" aphasia (usually unconfirmed by clinicopsychological investigation) are identified, or on purely linguistic descriptions of "nominal," "syntactical," and "semantic" aphasias, which do not reflect the true richness of the clinical syndromes and bear no relationship to their underlying physiological mechanisms.

This interpretation of speech disorders proved unproductive and introduced great, and ultimately unsurmountable, difficulties into the study of the aphasias. An urgent need for a new approach to the aphasias has thus been created. Their study should be brought more into line with the analysis of agnosia and apraxia, on the one hand, and with the identification of the more elementary changes in cerebral activity leading to these complex disturbances, on the other.

Speech is the result of a highly complex integration of nervous processes instigated by the combined activities of different parts of the brain. In the narrow meaning of the term, speech processes involve complex systems of sensorimotor coordinations with their own specific organization. The perception of speech is based on the analysis and synthesis of elements in the flow of sound by the combined work of the auditory and kinesthetic analyzers. The pronunciation of words is accomplished by a complex system of coordinated articulatory movements, formed on the basis of previous experience; the afferent basis of this process is the work of the same kinesthetic and auditory analyzers that are involved in the perception of speech. The processes involved in writing are no less complex in character; as has been discussed, they are based on the combined work of the auditory, visual, and motor analyzers. Obviously, therefore, these disturbances cannot be properly analyzed unless the study of the pathology of the speech act includes the study of the special forms of sensory and motor disorders.

Because of the foregoing explanations, agnosias, apraxias, and aphasias cannot be considered isolated phenomena and the long-held view that these forms of disturbance constitute the entire pathology of the higher cortical functions caused by local brain lesions can no longer be accepted. Besides the arguments that have been presented, we must be struck by the fact that disturbances of the higher cortical processes accompanying circumscribed brain lesions are incomparably complex in form. To interpret the whole range of observed facts by these basic (and often ill-defined) concepts would be to eliminate much of the infinite variety of these disorders from consideration. This matter will often be returned to in the course of this account.

This book is concerned with disturbances of the higher cortical functions arising from local brain lesions and with the analysis of the underlying mechanisms of these disturbances. This implies that *the primary object is to analyze what is contributed by a particular analyzer to the structure of each functional system and what disturbances of the higher cortical functions arise as a result of a lesion of one of the responsible cortical divisions.*

With this task in mind, the plan of the subsequent account can be appreciated. Relatively localized lesions of those zones of the cerebral cortex that are the cortical divisions of a particular analyzer will be the initial object for study. The changes in the relatively elementary forms of analytic-synthetic activity directly resulting from these lesions and the disturbances of the higher cortical functions based upon them will then be examined. Following this, the complex speech disorders developing as a secondary (systematic) result of these localized brain lesions will be described. At the same time, the factors underlying the whole complex of disturbances arising from local brain lesions will be analyzed and identified. This means that, by starting with the analysis of topographically localized brain lesions, we shall try, wherever possible, to ascertain the psychophysiological mechanisms of the disturbances of the higher cortical functions.

• • •

Analysis of a disturbance of higher cortical functions, identification of the elementary functional components, and examination of the connection between the afferent and efferent aspects of cortical activity are not the only methods of investigation of our chosen problem. When studying the psychophysiological basis of the disturbances to be described, the specifically human types of organization of the higher cortical processes, in whose formation and disturbance speech plays a most important part, must be constantly borne in mind.

It has been advanced (Part I, Section 1C) that the higher mental functions of man are functional systems, social in origin and mediate in structure. This primarily means that no single complex form of human mental activity can take place without the direct or indirect participation of speech and that the connections of the second signal system play a decisive role in the formation of these activities.

By adopting this point of view, the usual notion of speech as one of the special forms of mental activity must be modified slightly and, besides speech processes being understood by the narrow meaning of the term, the general speech organization of mental processes must be distinguished. The speech organization of mental processes is revealed by the complex pattern of integration of their functional properties and is based upon the principle of nervous activity that was advanced with the introduction of the concept of the second signal system. Because of speech, abstraction and generalization of direct stimuli received from the outside world is made possible; speech can thus encompass relationships and associations between objects and events extending far beyond the limits of direct sensory perception. Because of speech, our perception acquires a selective systematic character. Finally, because of speech, higher nervous activity in man acquired that property that enabled Pavlov (*Complete Collected Works*, Vol. 3, p. 577) to describe the second signal system as the "higher regulator of human behavior." Speech activity, in this wide sense of the term, extends far beyond the bounds of the processes that may be observed during verbal communication between people.

Naturally, therefore, the speech organization of mental processes must be considered the activity of the brain as a whole, i.e., based on the combined work of the whole complex of analyzers. We are still only at the beginning of the investigation of the cerebral mechanisms responsible for this specifically human form of organization of cortical processes. At present, we can only postulate that the extreme complexity of the structure of the human cerebral cortex, with the development of overlapping zones of the cortical endings of the individual analyzers and with the intensive development of the upper layers of the cortex, is associated phylogenetically with the introduction of this new principle of nervous activity.

Because of its exceptional complexity, the speech organization of the higher cortical functions is very easily deranged by any local or general brain lesion. We shall inevitably encounter manifestations of these disturbances when we investigate phenomena lying far beyond the limits of the aphasias. When studying the symptoms of a disturbance of the sensory or motor (gnostic or practic) processes accompanying a local brain lesion, we must, therefore, carefully analyze the manner in which the relationship between the two signal systems changes and note which aspects of the speech organization of mental processes are thereby affected.

First, therefore, it is necessary to study disturbances of the higher cortical functions in the closest relationship with more elementary sensorimotor defects. Second, it is no less important to investigate the changes taking place in their speech organization. It is only by satisfying both of these conditions that disturbances of the higher cortical functions resulting from local brain lesions can be properly analyzed.

The study of the disturbance of the speech organization of mental processes accompanying local brain lesions is only in its infancy, whereas the pathophysiological investigation of general organic and functional disorders of cerebral processes has made considerable progress and rests on a broad factual basis. Thus, the problem with which we are concerned here has attracted far less study.

The investigation of how the speech organization of mental processes is disordered by local brain lesions and of how the different aspects of this organization are affected unequally by lesions of different parts of the brain is presently only in its initial stages. For this reason the reader must interpret the subsequent analysis as merely the first attempt in this new and inadequately explored field.

B. THE PROBLEM OF THE DOMINANT HEMISPHERE

Ever since the classical investigations of Broca (1861*a* and *b*) and Wernicke (1874) it has been known that, despite their morphological symmetry, the two cerebral hemispheres are not equal in functional importance. In right-handed persons the left hemisphere is predominantly concerned with speech functions and is dominant in this respect, whereas the right hemisphere does not carry such important (primarily speech) functions and may therefore be designated as subordinate.

For this reason, most investigations have been concerned with the study of the disturbances of higher cortical functions arising from lesions of the left (dominant) hemisphere, whereas the symptomatology of lesions of the right (subordinate) hemisphere has, until very recently, not received adequate attention.

Various workers have shown that in right-handed persons, a lesion of certain definite areas of the frontotemporal-parietal divisions of the left hemisphere causes a disturbance of speech whereas a lesion of symmetrically opposite areas of the right hemisphere does not produce symptoms of this nature. This fact has led many writers to distinguish speech areas in the cerebral cortex (Fig. 23). In periodic investigations (Luria, 1947, etc.) of large numbers of patients with gunshot wounds of different parts of the brain, speech disturbances were observed in the period soon after injury when wide areas of the left hemisphere were affected, but the speech defects remained permanent only when the lesion affected much more highly localized areas of the brain, usually corresponding to the aforementioned speech areas (Fig. 24).

Nevertheless, the dominance of one hemisphere in relation to speech functions proved not to be so absolute as was supposed, and research showed that the degree of dominance varied considerably from subject to subject and from function to function. Jackson (1869) originally suggested that speech results from the combined work of both hemispheres, with the left, or dominant, hemisphere associated with the most complex forms of voluntary speech and the right hemisphere responsible for the more elementary functions of automatized speech. Many workers have returned to the concept that both

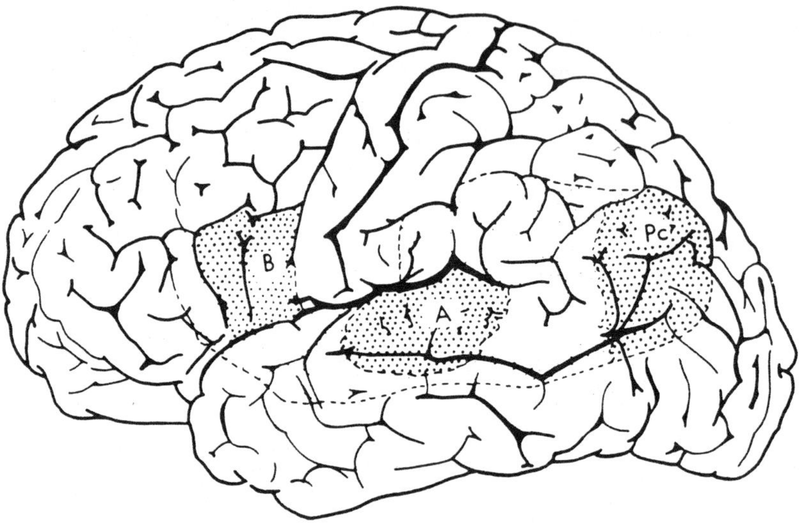

FIGURE 23 Speech zones of the cortex. (*A*) Wernicke's area; (*B*) Broca's area; (*Pc*) area of visual images of words. (*From Déjerine, 1914.*)

hemispheres participate jointly in the performance of complex mental functions (including speech); in Soviet psychology this trend has been developed by Anan'ev (1960). We also consider that the higher mental functions, including speech, result from the combined activity of both cerebral hemispheres, with each making its own, though not equal, contribution. The parts played by the two hemispheres in the organization of higher mental functions, including that of speech, is a matter for future research.

Although the role of the subordinate (right) hemisphere in the higher cortical functions cannot yet be defined, the clinical observations of many writers (Chester, 1936; Luria, 1947; Humphrey and Zangwill, 1952; Goodglass and Quadfasel, 1954; Ettlinger, Jackson, and Zangwill, 1955; Subirana, 1958; Ajuriaguerra and Hécaen, 1960; Zangwill, 1960; etc.) have convincingly shown that in left-handed persons lesions of the subordinate (left) hemisphere also lead to definite disturbances of speech and its related perceptual processes. Correspondingly, with lesions of the dominant hemisphere, speech (as well as its related functions) is disturbed to a different degree in different subjects and may redevelop unequally being restored comparatively satisfactorily in some and hardly at all in others. These findings cannot entirely be explained by the severity of the lesion (the size of the focus, the presence of complicating factors, etc.). It is evident that the degree of dominance of one hemisphere in relation to lateralized processes such as speech varies considerably from case to case, and this factor introduces a considerable element of diversity into the local pathology of higher cortical functions. This may also account for the fact that circumscribed lesions in the same location may produce symptoms of unequal severity in different individuals. Some important observations have been made

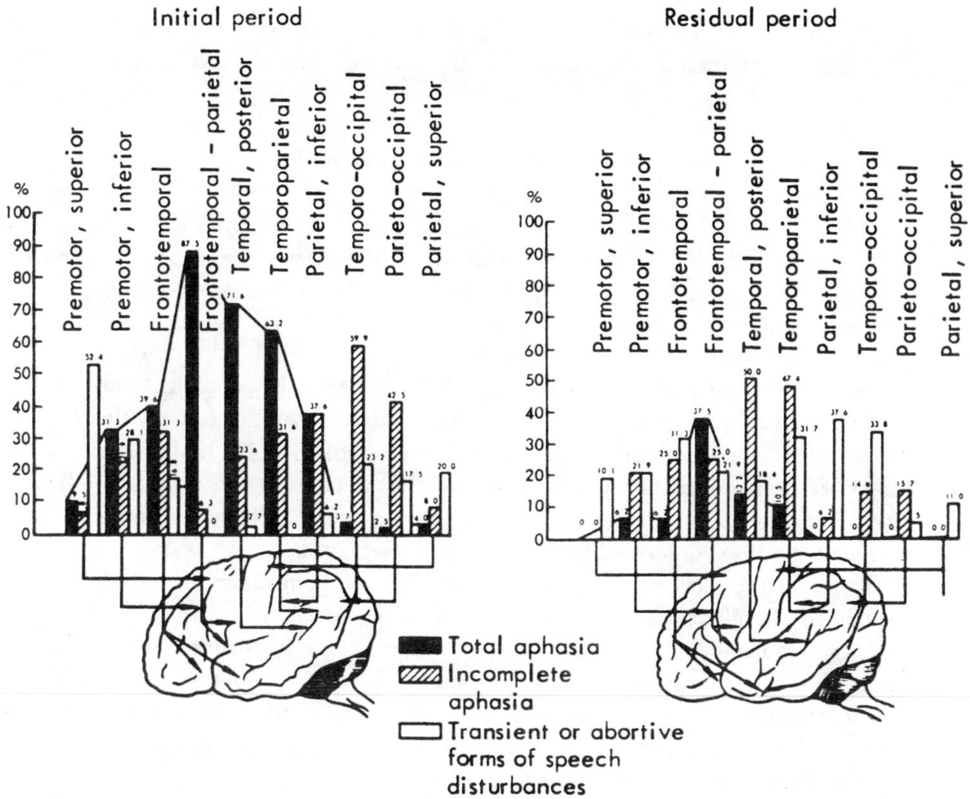

FIGURE 24 Distribution of speech disturbances from gunshot wounds of different parts of the brain in the initial and residual periods after trauma, in approximately 800 patients. The diagrams show the percentage of cases with a gunshot wound of a particular area of the left hemisphere that resulted in speech disorders of different degrees of severity. (*After Luria, 1947.*)

indicating that a lesion destroying the speech areas of the left hemisphere need not be followed by any detectable symptoms (for example, if the lesion develops in early childhood or if it progresses very slowly). We may also add that absolute dominance of one hemisphere in respect to all mental functions is evidently far rarer than has been supposed and that many persons show only partial or unequal dominance of the hemisphere in respect to different functions. For example, a person may be "right-handed" in respect to speech yet have a functionally dominant left eye. Methods of detecting general and partial dominance of a hemisphere will be discussed subsequently (Part III, Section 2).

Recent observations (Zangwill, 1960; Hécaen and Angelergues, 1962; Milner, Branch, and Rasmussen, 1964), for instance, show that whereas in the great majority of right-handed people speech processes are firmly linked with the function of the left hemisphere, in left-handed persons the connection between speech functions and the right hemisphere alone is expressed to a much lower degree. The observations of Milner, Branch, and Rasmussen, obtained by injection of sodium amytal into the external carotid artery (Wada's test, 1949), showed, for instance, that speech functions are connected with the right hemisphere in only 20% of left-handed and ambidextrous persons, whereas in 64% they remain dependent on the left hemisphere. It is only in those left-handed and ambidextrous subjects, in whom a lesion of the left hemisphere was present in early childhood, that in 67% of cases speech processes are linked with the right hemisphere; even in this group, however, in 22% of cases the left hemisphere continues to play an essential role in speech activity.

The conclusions regarding dominance of one (usually the left) hemisphere have usually been drawn from observations only on disturbances of speech, arising as a rule in right-handed subjects with lesions of the left hemisphere. These observations have been supplemented by certain indirect features indicating predominance of the function of the right (or left) hand and the right (or left) eye. Suitable methods of determining this dominance will be described below (Part III, Section 2).

However, the data on the dominant role of one hemisphere in relation to speech, the hand, and the eye have proved to be very contradictory. The impression has been obtained either than these methods are insufficiently reliable or that the dominance of one hemisphere (usually the left) is only relative in character, and that in some cases dominance for one feature (e.g., speech) does not coincide with dominance of the same hemisphere for another feature (e.g., the hand or eye).

There is an urgent need for additional features to be discovered which would make it possible to determine sufficiently reliably both the dominance and the degree of dominance of one hemisphere and also to decide whether this dominance is general or is functionally specific.

An important step toward the solution of this problem was taken by the Japanese neurologist Wada (1949), who suggested the first objective test for the reliable determination of the degree of hemispheric dominance for speech. This test involved injecting sodium amytal into the left or right carotid artery, supplying blood to the corresponding hemisphere. The appearance of transient aphasia after the injection of sodium amytal indicated that this hemisphere was dominant with respect to speech.

Observations, which I shall discuss again below (Part III, Section 2) have shown that injection of sodium amytal into the left carotid artery of right-handed subjects causes a disturbance of speech for 3–5 min, whereas its injection into the right carotid artery causes no disorders of this kind but often produces totally different symptoms: affective changes, disorders of the body schema, and sometimes a disturbance of direct spatial orientation—symptoms of a lesion of the nondominant hemisphere. Right-handed people with latent left-handedness (born left-handed), repressed left-handedness, or ambidexterity will give a correspondingly less definitive picture; the disorders arising will be less clear-cut and transient in character.

The use of Wada's method to detect hemispheric dominance, however reliable it may be, has important limitations: it is a surgical operation which must be carefully performed and supervised and which is attended by a certain risk.

That is why it is still extremely necessary to find other methods for the diagnosis of hemispheric dominance that can be used in any situation, yet be just as reliable.

One such method has been suggested by Kimura (1963, 1967). It has gained wide acceptance as the "dichotic listening test" and it is performed as follows: By means of a stereophonic tape recorder two different series of simple words or sounds are presented to the subject, one to his right ear, the other to his left. He is told that although the course of the two auditory pathways is bilateral, the pathway from one hemisphere to the contralateral ear is dominant. The subject who has a dominant left hemisphere will therefore recall many more words directed to his right ear than to his left ear. This phenomenon has been called the "right ear effect," and it is widely used for the diagnosis of hemispheric dominance.

The "right ear effect" has been found to be observed clearly only if dominance of the left hemisphere is total, and if incomplete (as is often the case in ambidextrous subjects) words presented to the right ear are recalled with equal probability. Dominance of the right hemisphere gives the opposite effect, so that the subject pays greater attention to words presented to the left ear and recalls them with greater probability.

It has also been found that during dichotic presentation of nonverbal stimuli (sounds or melodies) a "left ear effect" is observed, indicating that the right (nondominant for speech) hemisphere may play the leading role in the analysis of nonverbal acoustic information.

Another characteristic is that the "right ear effect" by no means coincides with dominance of the right hand, and in some clearly right-handed individuals the right ear effect may be indistinct or even totally absent. These findings again emphasize the fact that in reality there is no such thing as global dominance of the hemispheres affecting all analyzers equally, but instead there is differential dominance of the hemispheres with respect to modality-specific and materially-specific (verbal-nonverbal) signals.

Further, an indistinct right ear effect, or its total absence, may be frequently observed in right-handed subjects who were left-handed at birth or, in other words, in subjects with genetically determined left-handedness. This is an important fact in connection with the elucidation of the mechanisms of hemispheric dominance for speech.

The use of this method on patients with local brain lesions has yielded important facts. Patients with lesions of the dominant left hemisphere have been found to exhibit not only a contralateral, but also a bilateral effect. In other words, the volume of words recalled by both the right and the left ear is considerably reduced. But in patients with lesions of the right hemisphere the effect of a narrowing of the range of recalled words is found only in the contralateral (left) ear.

This fact is very similar to the well-known clinical phenomena in which patients with lesions of the dominant (left) hemisphere have difficulty in performing complex types of praxis not only with the right hand, but with both hands. It shows that the influence of the dominant hemisphere is directed not only to the contralateral side, but that it also has a general organizing character, reflected equally on the functions of both sides of the body. The data just described can take us an important step further toward the solution of the problem of the genesis of hemispheric dominance, on the one hand, and the problem of differences in the manifestation of a pathological focus located in each of the two hemispheres in children. In both these situations fresh light is shed on the problem of pediatric neuropsychology, a branch of the subject which had been totally neglected until recently.

The view that both cerebral hemispheres are equipotential in infancy and that up to a certain moment of time dominance of one hemisphere is not exhibited in children is widely quoted in the literature (Zangwill, 1960).

However, experiments by Simernitskaya and her colleagues have shown that a "right ear effect" can be clearly observed in children also; however, it is seen in children in a less definite form, with wider scatter of its indices. What is particularly interesting is that in children of 6–8 years a "negative right ear effect" can be seen much more often than in adults: in other words, the range of recall of words presented to the left ear is greater than to the right. The frequency with which this phenomenon is found decreases with age: in children of 6–8 years a "negative right ear effect" is observed more often than in children of 10–12 years. In adults it is found in about 5% of cases.

These facts suggest that dominance of the left hemisphere for speech is not inborn, but it is something which develops gradually, being present in rudimentary form early in life and only gradually assuming a more definite character. Meanwhile, they also suggest that the nondominant (right) hemisphere can play a much more important role in children than in adults, and that in the early period of the child's development the right hemisphere exerts a much greater influence on the course of speech processes than in older children and in adults. This can evidently be explained by the fact that the psychological structure of speech activity changes during development, and in the early stages of the child's development the direct sensory component of speech plays a much more important role than in the adult. I shall turn again to certain aspects of this problem below when I discuss interaction between the hemispheres in the performance of psychological processes (Part II, Section 7).

Equally important facts indicating profound changes in the cerebral organization of psychological functions during the child's development have been obtained by analysis of the effects of a local lesion of one hemisphere at successive stages of childhood.

As was stated above, in adults a pathological focus in the left (dominant) hemisphere can be bilateral in its manifestations, i.e., it can impair receptor or motor functions bilaterally, whereas a focus in the right (nondominant) hemisphere has only a partial, contralateral effect (observed only in the left ear or left hand, contralateral to the focus).

Results obtained by Simernitskaya and her colleagues have shown that the character of the effect produced by a focus in one hemisphere may be totally different in children and in adults. Dichotic listening tests on children with lesions of the left and right hemispheres have yielded the following results.

As a rule, the influence of a focus in the left hemisphere has been found to extend only contralaterally, i.e., it reduces the right ear effect without lowering the productivity of the ipsilateral left ear; conversely, a focus in the right hemisphere very often gives a bilateral effect, i.e., it leads to a change in the volume of trace imprinting from signals directed to both the left and the right ear.

This finding shows that the mechanisms lying at the basis of hemispheric dominance in children are different from those in adults, and that the bilateral effect characteristic of lesions of the dominant hemisphere arises in children with pathological foci not in the left, but in the right hemisphere.

However, bilateral changes in dichotic perception observable in children with lesions of the right hemisphere characteristically differ qualitatively from the corresponding bilateral effect in adults with lesions of the left hemisphere. The difference is that in adult patients bilateral changes of dichotic perception are uniform in character whereas in children they are divergent: disturbances of perception of verbal stimuli by the left ear are combined, not with a decrease, but with a reciprocal increase in the range of perception of identical information reaching the ipsilateral, right ear.

This observation shows clearly that the organization of brain activity in childhood differs from that of adults, since in childhood a disturbance of functions arising through a lesion of the left hemisphere is very likely to prove compensatable by activation of the opposite, right hemisphere.

Evidence in support of this hypothesis is given by many clinical observations which show that disorders of speech function (aphasia) and disturbances of forms of gnosis, praxis, and intellectual activity connected with speech due to a lesion of the left hemisphere run a much milder course in children than in adults and are compensated incomparably more easily (evidently through the implication of the opposite, right hemisphere in the function), and that these defects are manifested for much shorter periods, and sometimes not at all.

The hypothesis of the more important role of the right hemisphere in children than in adults is also supported by the clinical observations of Simernitskaya et al. who showed that the symptoms due to a lesion of the right hemisphere, which I have already mentioned and will turn to again (Part II, Section 7) as spatial agnosia, unawareness of the left side, disturbance of drawing, and apraxia of dressing, evidently connected with disturbance of the body schema, are manifested much more clearly in childhood than the symptoms of a lesion of the left hemisphere mentioned above, and that they are much more enduring in character.

All these observations open up fresh prospects for research aimed at analyzing changes in interhemispheric relations during their development of the child. These investigations will mark a new stage in neuropsychology, and without doubt they will be undertaken by future generations of scientists.

I shall describe here only facts that have been obtained in the last few years by the dichotic listening test and I shall only briefly mention a very productive method of investigation of hemispheric dominance, that of the study of differences in the perception and analysis of visual information addressed to the right or left visual field. Such investigations, using a tachistoscopic method of visual stimulation of one side of the visual field, have recently been carried out by many investigators. They have shown that signals addressed to the right visual field are perceived faster by subjects with dominance of the left hemisphere than signals addressed to the left half of the visual field; that components of speech codes (letters, words) are distinguished much more clearly by the right visual field, whereas nonverbal stimuli (nonsense figures, faces) are better perceived by the left visual field.

These investigations have led to significant progress toward a more precise definition of the true function of the left and right hemispheres and of the contribution which each of them makes to complex forms of psychological activity. I shall turn again to the appropriate data below.

As already stated, the degree of dominance of the hemispheres varies not only from subject to subject, but also from function to function. Whereas speech processes, as a rule, show a marked degree of lateralization and depend on the dominant hemisphere, there are many functions with a much smaller degree of lateralization.

As shall be discussed again, the processes of visual perception are apparently associated to a much smaller degree with one dominant hemisphere, and the most marked and permanent gnostic disorders arise from bilateral lesions of corresponding parts of the cortex (Part II, Section 3C).

Similar findings have been observed in impairment of the selective organization of voluntary activity resulting from a lesion of the frontal regions of the brain (Part II, Section 5C-G). All these findings suggest that the different mental functions vary in their degree of lateralization.

It is easy to see that the relative importance of the dominant hemisphere to the performance of different functions is an important factor that, in conjunction with the differences in the degree of dominance of one hemisphere in different persons, greatly complicates the investigation of the pathology of the higher cortical functions in the presence of local brain lesions. Nor must it be forgotten that the right hemisphere *is* dominant with respect to certain mental processes. There is evidence that such processes include those concerned with music and the awareness of a personal disability. The unequal participation of the two hemispheres in the performance of complex forms of mental activity is not limited, however, to what has been described. Research during the past decade (Anan'ev, 1959, 1960; etc.) has shown that, as a rule, many functions require the participation of both hemispheres but that, because one hand plays a dominant and the other a subsidiary role, the nature of the participation of the left and right hemispheres in these functions is profoundly different. This fact has been demonstrated most clearly by Teuber and his co-workers (Semmes, Weinstein, Ghent, and Teuber, 1960). During their study of the disturbances of tactile sensation after gunshot wounds of the right and left hemispheres, these workers observed that even with respect to functions as remote from speech as tactile sensation the character of the functional organization of the two hemispheres is different. Whereas in the left (dominant) hemisphere, the sensory functions are very highly differentiated, in the right (subordinate) hemisphere they are represented more diffusely. Therefore, a lesion confined to the sensorimotor areas of the left hemisphere leads to a disturbance of sensation in the opposite hand, whereas wounds outside these areas are not followed by sensory disorders. On the other hand, wounds of the right hemisphere may cause sensory defects even if not situated within the sensorimotor area; these wounds frequently cause disturbances in the ipsilateral hand as well.

The conception that the two hemispheres, although morphologically identical in structure, are not identical in their degree of functional differentiation, not only in regard to speech but also to sensory (and, possibly, motor) functions, has only recently found expression in the literature. Further research in this direction may yield important results.

It is easy to see that our lack of knowledge concerning the degree of dominance of the hemispheres in different persons and with respect to different functions is a great handicap in the clinical investigation of patients with local brain lesions. For this reason, some important problems can be solved only tentatively at the present time. These include, in particular, the problem of the disturbances of higher cortical functions arising from lesions of the right hemisphere and, more important still, the problem of the part played by the right hemisphere in the compensation for defects caused by lesions of the left hemisphere. In this book we shall deliberately bypass all of these problems, in the confidence that they can and will be solved when sufficient factual information has been accumulated.

C. GENERAL CEREBRAL COMPONENTS IN CASES OF LOCAL BRAIN LESIONS

Let us consider the last factor that considerably complicates the topical analysis of disturbances of the higher cortical functions, namely, the effect of general cerebral abnormalities on the disturbance of those functions affected by various circumscribed lesions of the brain. General cerebral abnormalities are prominent in cases of gunshot wounds of the brain, particularly in the early stages after injury, when, as Smirnov (1947) showed, perifocal phenomena, changes in the circulation of the blood and cerebrospinal fluid, and contrecoup effects may be especially well marked. Very few pathological conditions, for example certain depressed fractures of the skull and residual states after gunshot wounds of the skull (tangential and perforating), will give rise to purely local manifestations.

General cerebral manifestations are particularly prominent with vascular disorders and tumors of the brain. For example, vascular disorders leading to hemorrhage or thrombosis are usually associated with circulatory changes that (especially in elderly patients) cause impaired nutrition and arteriosclerotic changes of the brain, as have often been described in the literature. However, the hemorrhage or the thrombosis itself may lead to additional manifestations extending far beyond the limits of local disturbance. Hemorrhage from a relatively large artery (or thrombosis of such a vessel) usually involves a large area of the brain receiving its blood supply from that vessel. To these may be added manifestations of local reflex disturbances of vascular activity. In this way, the changes that develop spread far beyond the actual limits of the underlying pathological focus.

Equally prominent are the general cerebral components in cases of cerebral tumor. As a rule, every tumor, especially if large, is accompanied by hypertension and dislocation, which, in turn, lead to changes in the circulation of the cerebrospinal fluid in the form of interference with the outflow of the fluid and of internal or external hydrocephalus. A cerebral tumor also has a significant effect on the blood supply and vascular system, causing mechanical and reflexive changes in the vessels that lead to disturbance of the normal nutrition of the brain tissue beyond the area of the lesion. If we also consider that in cases of rapidly expanding and extensively disintegrating cerebral tumors the local injury is augmented by a general cerebral toxic factor, we may begin to appreciate the complexity of the topical analysis of the effects of a cerebral tumor. The relative importance of the local and general factors must obviously differ in extracerebral tumors (e.g., arachnoid endotheliomas), in relatively slow-growing and localized tumors (e.g., astrocytomas and oligodendrogliomas), and in malignant, rapidly growing tumors (e.g., medulloblastomas and spongioblastoma multiforme); growth of the tumor not only destroys the nerve cells but is also accompanied by marked toxic effects (Smirnov, 1951).

The relationship between general and local cerebral components may vary significantly in a patient with a brain tumor during growth of the tumor, with disturbance of the compensating mechanisms occurring at a given moment. It may also change considerably in the postoperative period, when cerebral edema and swelling may develop. Special psychological investigations (Spirin, 1951) have shown the variability of these manifestations of edema and swelling during the days immediately after operation and their correlation with the disturbances of higher cortical functions.

Finally, the relationship between local and general cerebral components does not remain constant from day to day or even from hour to hour. Every clinician knows that an increase in intracranial pressure, resulting from any of a whole series of possible factors, may produce an exacerbation of the patient's general condition, with aggravation of the symptoms of increased pressure, lasting for periods of hours or days. During such periods the patient can only be studied after measures have been adopted for lowering the intracranial pressure. Clinicians also know how easily the functions become fatigued in such patients and, consequently, how variable are the results of investigation.

The presence of general cerebral components in practically every case of local brain lesion greatly complicates the evaluation of the local symptomatology (Rapoport, 1936–1941, 1948, 1957) but does not make it impossible. General cerebral factors cause pathological changes in the dynamics of nervous processes, disturb the relationship between excitation and inhibition, alter the mobility of the nervous processes, and induce signs of a pathological inertia of these processes. All these disturbances lead to changes in mental activity, mainly in the complex forms of mental processes. In these cases, however, neurodynamic disturbances are apparent in not one but many systems, a feature that distinguishes them from local neurodynamic defects. It is only in the severest cases that the general cerebral manifestations mask the local symptoms to such an extent that the local diagnosis cannot be established.

In evaluating disturbances of the higher mental functions, special attention should be given to the influence exerted on the course of cortical processes by pathological changes in the deep portions of the brain, notably by lesions of the brain stem and diencephalon. Besides the phenomena that have been described, these lesions cause special disturbances of the functions of the activating reticular formation, as a result of which the tone of the cortex is markedly modified and the patient's general condition may be affected. These factors may also lead to a considerable disturbance of cortical functioning and may hamper the diagnosis of a local lesion.

Finally, in many cases such factors as perifocal inflammation, increased intracranial pressure, and dislocation may so extend the scope of the disturbances caused by the primary focus that the investigator may be confronted with regional, rather than a local, symptomatology, including several disturbances caused by the pathological process in areas of the brain adjacent to the lesion (Rapoport, 1936–1941, etc.).

Another important component of the general clinical picture is the influence exerted by the primary local lesion on remote parts of the brain. This remote influence may induce, for example, secondary symptoms from malfunctioning of the frontal lobes (or "pseudofrontal" symptoms); such secondary symptoms may appear in association with lesions situated, in particular, in the posterior cranial fossa or the occipital regions and create considerable difficulty in topical diagnosis (Konovalov, 1954, 1957, 1960). However, it must be realized that in some cases general cerebral factors do not mask but actually exacerbate the symptoms of local lesions, so that these become apparent only when, for instance, the intracranial pressure is raised.

For these reasons, the study of the various disturbances of the higher cortical functions accompanying local brain lesions is rendered highly complex. It would be wrong, however, to suppose that such an investigation is thereby impossible or that the role of the local lesion in the disturbance of the higher mental processes cannot be defined. Experience shows that, despite all these complications, the psychological investigation of the higher cortical functions has a role in the topical diagnosis of brain lesions and that it is a method that can be used for these purposes in neurological and neurosurgical practice.

In the subsequent account, these complicating factors will be deliberately ignored. Giving a somewhat abbreviated general account of the clinical findings, we shall mainly dwell on findings illustrative of the relationship between symptoms and local lesions of the cerebral cortex. The account is rather schematic, for our purpose is to describe the changes in the higher mental processes arising as a result of local brain lesions.

2. *Disturbances of Higher Cortical Functions with Lesions of the Temporal Region*

The temporal region of the cerebral cortex is complex in structure and in functional organization. It includes divisions acting as the cortical nuclear zone of the auditory analyzer (Areas 41, 42, and 22), the extranuclear zones of the auditory portion of the cortex (Area 21), and the formations of the inferior and basal divisions unconnected with the functions of auditory analysis and integration (Area 20). In addition, the temporal region also includes, in its medial surface, those formations belonging to the archipallium and the transitional portion of the cortex constituting part of the limbic system; these formations are associated with apparatuses closely involved in the regulation of afferent processes and form a specialized structure of the cerebral cortex. Finally, the temporal zones bordering the parietal and occipital regions (the posterior portions of Areas 22 and 37), as well as the wholly specialized areas formed by the structures of the pole of the temporal lobe, constitute other divisions.

Since the aim of this book is the examination of only the higher mental functions and their disturbances in the presence of local brain lesions, we shall not analyze the symptoms arising from lesions of the divisions of the temporal region as a whole (Rapoport, 1948, etc.) but shall confine our attention to those disturbances associated with lesions of the auditory divisions of the temporal portion of the cortex.

Naturally, the symptoms arising from left temporal lesions will be considered first. This will enable us to lead up to the problems of impairment of the acoustic aspect of speech and immediately introduces the most complex and fundamental problems of those speech defects vitally involved in disturbances of the higher cortical functions.

A. HISTORICAL SURVEY

The history of the study of the disturbances arising from lesions of the temporal region of the cerebral hemispheres largely consists of the analysis of defects accompanying lesions of the *left* temporal region; comparatively little attempt has been made to study the symptomatology of lesions of the right (subordinate) temporal region, and this region will hardly concern us in our analysis. The history of the clinical study of the syndromes associated with a lesion of the left temporal region will be briefly surveyed. These syndromes are of considerable interest from the point of view of their underlying nature.

As previously mentioned, the first detailed account of disturbances arising from a lesion of the cortex of the left temporal lobe was given by Wernicke (1874), 13 years after Broca's discovery. Wernicke stated that a lesion of the posterior third of the first temporal gyrus of the left hemisphere leads to a disturbance of speech comprehension, in which speech is perceived as inarticulate noise. The patient's own ability to communicate by language is likewise disturbed; he cannot repeat words addressed to him, he cannot name objects, and he cannot write from dictation. His speech contains paraphrases and is sometimes converted into a word salad. In these cases, however, the receptive (or "impressive," as they are frequently termed) disturbances of speech remain dominant, a finding that led Wernicke to describe this whole syndrome as sensory aphasia.

Although the pattern of the sensory speech disturbances described by Wernicke has remained, without any great modification, an accepted clinical representation, it always proved difficult to explain. Two opposing interpretations exist. Wernicke himself, when comparing his description with previous approaches to aphasia as an intellectual or symbolic disorder (Finkelburg, 1870), expressed the opinion that sensory aphasia is an auditory disturbance in which the sensory images of speech (which he designated by the somewhat unusual term "Wortbegriff") are disturbed, in contrast to Broca's aphasia, in which the motor images are impaired.

In an attempt to decipher the mechanisms of these disturbances, he later suggested that auditory fibers corresponding to the part of the tone scale (b_1–g_2) within which audible speech takes place, referred to by Bezold as the "speech part of the tone scale," terminate in the posterior third of the first temporal gyrus. Sensory aphasia thus began to be interpreted as partial deafness or, more accurately, deafness to the speech zone of the tone scale.

However, Wernicke's hypothesis of the partial, auditory character of sensory aphasia met with criticism on both factual and theoretical grounds. Flechsig (1900) showed the invalidity of the claim that auditory fibers of the speech spectrum terminate in the posterior third of the first temporal gyrus. Subsequent investigations revealed that all fibers of the auditory tract terminate in Heschl's transverse gyrus and not in the convex cortical portions of the temporal lobe; this finding itself was sufficient to invalidate Wernicke's interpretation.

Moreover, several workers (Frankfurter and Thiele, 1912; Bonvicini, 1929; Katz, 1930; etc.) showed that in patients with sensory aphasia auditory perception of the speech zone of the tone scale is preserved and that, in general, these patients have no constant impairment in tonal hearing. In other words, the speech disturbances arising in sensory aphasia proved so complex and varied that the contention that they are nothing more than a defect in elementary hearing began to be doubted.

For this reason, not long after the publication of Wernicke's article, sensory aphasia began to be interpreted not as a specialized, auditory disorder, but as a more general, symbolic or intellectual defect. These views, intrinsically akin to those of Finkelburg in Germany and Jackson in England, were formulated most clearly by the French neurologist Marie (1906), who claimed that one with sensory aphasia hears but does not understand what is said, or, in other words, that sensory aphasia is not a disorder of hearing as such but a disorder of the intellect (or of "intellectual analysis"). It is easy to see that this attempt to seek the source of sensory aphasia in intellectual defects divorced speech from its sensory components and came dangerously close to those overtly idealistic doctrines in which the intellect is regarded as a phenomenon independent of its sensory basis.

Marie's view of the intellectual nature of sensory aphasic defects proved no more satisfactory to investigators, however, than Wernicke's hypothesis of the loss of the speech zone of the tone scale. Neurologists were becoming more and more convinced that the disturbance in speech comprehension in sensory aphasia is primarily a disturbance of the hearing of speech and that it is not by accident that such patients say that in their condition the sounds of speech become inarticulate noises, like the rustling of leaves. With increasing frequency suggestions were made in the literature that the basis of sensory aphasia is a disturbance of "discriminative hearing" (Henschen, 1920-1922); Schuster and Taterka, 1926; etc.) and that one with sensory aphasia may display a peculiar form of "sound-unawareness" ("*Nicht-Beachtung der Sprache*": Pick, 1931).

Meanwhile, attempts were being made to give a different interpretation of the functions of the convex divisions of the temporal portion of the cortex, especially of its superior portions. By limiting the primary (projection) auditory zones to the area of Heschl's transverse gyri (Area 41 and perhaps Area 42), some workers suggested that the cortex of the superior temporal gyrus (Area 22) be regarded as a "psychosensory" zone (Campbell, 1905), i.e., as a zone responsible for discriminative hearing.

Nevertheless, the scientific interpretation both of this discriminative hearing and of the functions of the secondary auditory fields remained obscure for a long time. Further scientific progress was necessary before the nature of discriminative hearing and of the functions of the cortical apparatuses responsible for it could be adequately explained. Progress here was achieved mainly through advances in the neurophysiology of the auditory analyzer, on the one hand, and in knowledge of the structure of spoken language (phonology), on the other.

B. THE AUDITORY ANALYZER AND THE STRUCTURE OF THE AUDITORY CORTEX

The principal reason why classical research into sensory aphasia failed to surmount the difficulties just described was that the investigators had no adequate scientific theory of sensory processes in general and of auditory processes in particular to work with.

According to the receptor theory of sensation, accepted at that time, any afferent excitation (including excitation traveling along the auditory nerve) is received passively by the cortex; only when it reaches the cortex does it undergo "mental conversion," i.e., transformation from a sensation into an idea and, hence, into a complex sensory image. As a result of this concept, these workers drew a hard and fast line between the elementary sensory zones (receiving only afferent excitation from the periphery) and the psychic or psychosensory zones (transforming them in accordance with psychological laws). Guided by this theory, they attempted to interpret the phenomena of sensory aphasia as hearing disorders and to seek their causes either in a diminution of the sharpness of hearing, in a defect in perceiving certain frequencies of the tone scale, or, again, in a lesion of those areas of the cortex regarded as the depot of auditory images or ideas. With any other interpretation, analysis of hearing defects would necessarily lead to the conclusion that the patient was suffering from mental, or intellectual, disorders.

The understanding of sensory (especially auditory) processes underwent a radical change as a result of the introduction of Pavlov's *reflex theory of sensation* and concept of *analyzers*. The foundations of this theory were laid by Sechenov and the theory was further developed by several Soviet physiologists, notably Gershuni (1945, 1965), Leont'ev (1959), and Sokolov (1958). According to this theory, sensation is always an active reflex process associated with the selection of the essential (signal) components of stimuli and the inhibition of the nonessential, subsidiary components. It always incorporates effector mechanisms leading to the tuning of the peripheral receptor apparatus and responsible for carrying out the selective reactions to determine the signal components of the stimulus. It envisages a continuous process of increased excitability in respect to some components of the stimulus and of decreased excitability in respect to others (Granit, 1955; Sokolov, 1958; Gershuni, 1965; Hernandez-Peon, 1955). In other words, *sensation incorporates the process of analysis and synthesis of signals while they are still in the first stages of arrival.* These concepts, so fundamentally opposed to the previous hypothesis of dualism (the passivity of the first physiological and the activity of the subsequent psychological stages of perception), constitute the principal distinguishing feature of the Pavlovian view of the sensory organs as analyzers. According to this view, from the very beginning the sensory cortical divisions participate in the analysis and integration of complex, not elementary, signals. The units of any sensory process (including hearing) are not only acts of reception of individual signals, measurable in terms of thresholds of sensation, but also acts of complex analysis and integration of signals, measurable in units of comparison and discrimination.* The sensory divisions of the cortex are the

*A similar position is propounded by the modern probability theory of perception. According to this theory, every perception is the result of a process of selection from a series of possible alternatives (Bruner, 1957; Sokolov, 1960; etc.).

apparatuses responsible for this analysis, and indications of a lesion of these apparatuses are to be found, not so much in a lowering of the acuity of the sensations, as in a disturbance of the analytic-synthetic function. In a lesion of the sensory divisions of the cortex, the thresholds of sensation may, under certain conditions, remain normal (and sometimes, as when there is a pathological increase in the excitability of the cortex, they may actually be lowered) whereas the disturbances of the higher forms of analytic-synthetic activity of the analyzer and the related selectivity in the receptor processes become predominant. It follows, therefore, that these may serve as adequate indicators of the pathological changes in the corresponding divisions of the cerebral cortex.

It is only very recently that new evidence of the role played by the temporal zones of the cortex in the detection of very short sounds has been obtained; these facts (Baru, Gershuni, and Tonkonogii, 1964; Gershuni, 1965; Karaseva, 1967) suggest that the auditory cortex has other important functions, for it prolongs excitation evoked by very short stimuli, thus rendering them amenable to analysis. This function of the auditory cortex, not previously described, explains the fact that an animal with a lesion of that area can no longer differentiate short sounds although it can still differentiate long sounds.

This explains why, when investigating the results of extirpation of the sensory cortex from animals, Pavlov and his co-workers (Babkin, 1910; Kudrin, 1910; Kryzhanovskii, 1909; Él'yasson, 1908; etc.) were able to discover not merely a disturbance of previously formed reflexes to single sound stimuli, but something more important: a disturbance of the relatively complex ability to differentiate between single and complex signals and an incapacity to form new conditioned reflexes in response to complex sound stimuli. Similar findings have recently been obtained by American workers (Butler, Diamond, and Neff, 1957; Goldberg, Diamond, and Neff, 1957), who observed that destruction of the auditory divisions of the cortex in cats severely limits the ability of the animals to differentiate between sound groups although they can still discriminate between simple changes in pitch.

These findings demonstrate that those workers who tried to discover the basis of sensory aphasia in a defect in perceiving certain parts of the tone scale were mistaken, for they failed to make use of those indicators that could actually reflect the pathological state of the auditory cortex. It is not so much the indices of the sharpness of hearing as the more complex forms of differential auditory analysis that reflect the pathology of the auditory divisions of the cortex.

With the development of scientific knowledge, it was not only the concept of the nature of auditory sensation that changed. Information on the structure of the auditory divisions of the cerebral cortex has increased significantly so that, in addition to the theory of the reflex nature of auditory analysis, there is now a firmer basis for understanding the symptoms arising from lesions of this region.

Investigations of the fine structure of the cerebral cortex and of the conducting pathways showed that the principal primary (projection) auditory zone of the cortex (or the central part of the cortical nucleus of the auditory analyzer) consists of the transverse gyri of Heschl (Area 41 and part of Area 42) and that auditory fibers from both ears are represented in the transverse gyri of both hemispheres. These central, or projection, fields of the cortical nuclei of the auditory analyzer are distinguished by the typical coniocortical structure of the receptor zones and by the marked predominance of the fourth afferent layer of cells. The investigations of Pfeiffer (1936) and Bremer and Dow (1939) showed that these fields have the typical somatotopic structure of the primary fields. Fibers carrying impulses from high frequencies of the tone scale are projected in their medial divisions and corresponding fibers from the low frequencies are projected in their lateral divisions.

The areas of the superior temporal gyrus belonging to the secondary fields of the cortical ending of the auditory analyzer possess significantly different morphological properties from the primary fields in that the second and third (association) layers of cells predominate. The fibers arriving in these areas arise from the nuclei of the thalamus and communicate only indirectly with the periphery; they belong to the internal portion of the vertical connections transmitting impulses that have already been analyzed and integrated. No information regarding the somatotopic character of the projections of this region is available. The more recent investigations of Bremer (1952) and others have shown that stimulation of the peripheral auditory receptor may also induce potentials from these secondary fields; however, more intensive stimulation is necessary and the effect possesses none of those somatotopic signs that are found if the potentials are recorded from areas situated in the primary auditory zone.

Certain anatomical and neuronographic discoveries made during the subsequent study of the secondary divisions of the auditory region in animals and man proved to be of the utmost significance. It was shown that the secondary auditory zones possess much wider systematic connections than the primary ones, enabling them to work in conjunction with adjacent regions of the cortex. By tracing the anatomical connections of the temporal region, Blinkov (1955) showed that the temporal region possesses powerfully developed associative links with the inferior divisions of the premotor (Broca's) area and that these links actually terminate in the posterior third of the first temporal gyrus (Fig. 25).

Similar results were obtained from neuronographic investigations. Whereas direct stimulation of the primary divisions of the auditory cortex does not produce potentials that spread far over the brain, stimulation of the secondary zones (Areas 22 and 21) gives rise to potentials that may be traced to the inferior segments of the premotor and frontal portions of the cortex (Areas 44, 46, and 10). In this way, conditions are created for the auditory and motor analyzers, especially those parts of the latter concerned with the innervation of the vocal organs, to work together. All these findings provide further evidence that *the secondary divisions of the auditory cortex are responsible for analysis and integration, acting as the "combination center" of the auditory analyzer, but carry out this work in close conjunction with those areas of the inferior segments of the frontal region considered to be the cortical endings of the motor analyzer, having special speech functions in man.*

Thus, we see that *the secondary divisions of the auditory cortex*, which have always been looked upon as auditory psychosensory zones, may be interpreted physiologically as *secondary fields of the nuclear zone of the auditory analyzer*, responsible for the *analysis and integration of sound signals and that these processes are carried out by the combined activity of the several cortical zones taking part in speech activity.*

C. LANGUAGE SOUNDS AND THE HEARING OF SPEECH

While modern knowledge of the structure and function of the sensory zones of the cortex indicates the correct ways to analyze their pathological states, advances in linguistics have resulted in a much greater understanding of the formations that are actually disordered by lesions of these zones.

What are the sounds of speech? What exactly do we mean by a disturbance of discriminative hearing of speech, such as may arise from a lesion of the temporal divisions of the cerebral cortex?

The sounds of speech cannot be regarded as simple or complex groups of tones or noises that are distinguishable merely with the aid of sufficiently acute hearing. Modern linguistics tells us that the articulated sounds of speech differ radically from sounds not related to speech. Two features characterize the sounds of human speech: In their origin and structure they are always organized in a definite objective language system, and, consequently, they are special, generalized sounds. Physiologically they are always complex and are produced with the aid of the phonation-articulation apparatus, without which they can be neither pronounced nor perceived.

Physically, the sounds of speech consist of a series of tones (vowels) and other sounds (consonants). The tones may merge with each other without interruption (as was shown, for example, by Hellwag's well-known triangle); this is also true of the other sounds. Therefore, it is often physically difficult to draw a line between the vowels "u-o-a-e-i" or between the consonants "p" and "b," "s" and "z," etc. However, for the sounds of speech to perform their function as carriers of precise meaning, they had to be discrete, i.e., to be clearly distinguishable from each other. If "u" would merge imperceptibly with "o" and "o" with "a" and "a" with "e," the words "put," "pot," "pat," and "pet" would be indistinguishable from each other. A similarly

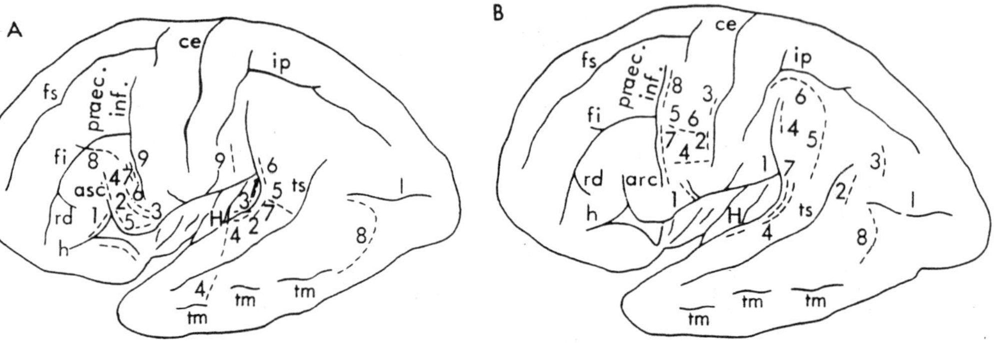

FIGURE 25 Connections between the temporal and inferior frontal regions. Diagrams of the points of communication between individual bundles of fibers composing the fasciculus arcuatus. Connections of each bundle of fibers with the cortex are denoted by identical numbers on the surface of corresponding parts of the brain: (*a*) Connections between the temporal lobe and inferofrontal gyrus; (*b*) connections between the temporal lobe and anterocentral gyrus. (*From Blinkov, 1955.*)

clear distinction must be maintained between the voiced "b" and the unvoiced "p" (e.g., to distinguish "bet" from "pet"), the voiced "d" and the unvoiced "t" (e.g., to distinguish "do" from "to"), etc.

Because of the discreteness of the sounds of speech, in every language certain sound signs acquire the property of allowing for differentiation of meaning while others remain unimportant, i.e., not able to change the meaning of a word. In modern linguistics the former are known as phonemic, and the sounds of different meaning made distinct by these signs are called "phonemes"; the others are known as "variants." Modern linguistics, or, more accurately, that subdivision of linguistics called "phonology" (developed by Troubezkoi [1939], Jakobson and Halle [1956], etc.), has established that every language possesses its own rigid phonemic system with certain sound signs standing out as distinguishing between meaning (phonemic). The whole sound structure of the language is determined by the system of opposites, in which a difference in a single phonemic sign changes the meaning of the pronounced word. In Russian, for example, phonemic signs are voice or voiceless ("dom"-"tom," "balka"-"palka"), softness or hardness ("pyl"-"pyl'," "byl"-"byl'"), and the presence or absence of stress ("zámok" – "zamók"). Signs of phonemic significance in other languages, such as the length of the sound in German ("Satt" – "Saat," "Stadt" – "Staat"), the fricative in English ("vine" – "wine"), and the openness of the vowels in French ("le"-"les"-"laid"), have no such significance in Russian. Thus, the fundamental feature of the speech process is the selection of *distinguishing, phonemic signs* from the flow of sound during both the pronunciation and the perception of speech sounds. *Differentiation of the sounds of speech is accomplished by identification and amplification of these distinctive*

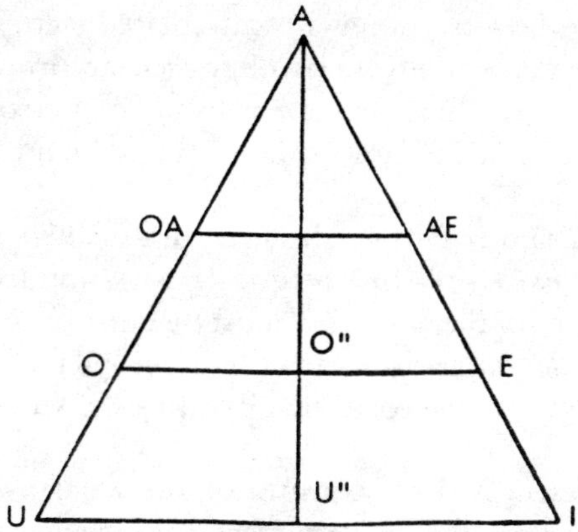

Hellwag's triangle

signs and separation of them from the unimportant, fortuitous signs that are of no phonemic significance.

The development of the ability to perceive spoken sounds and to hear speech requires the closest participation of the articulatory apparatus and assumes its final character only in the process of active articulatory experience. The first years of development of speech are taken up with this acquisition of the ability to hear speech, with the participation of articulation. This process of auditory-articulatory analysis is at first manifest and overt in character. As electromyographic studies have shown (Sokolov, 1959; Novikova, 1955; etc.), it recedes into the background only gradually, so that when or shortly before the child begins to attend school the hearing of speech ceases to require the actual participation of articulation. However, if the child is told a word with a complicated sound or, still more, asked to write it, the articulatory apparatus will again be brought into visible use to aid in the perception and recognition of the precise sound structure of the word.

The articulation of the sounds of speech, like the process of perception of these sounds by ear, thus obeys the laws of analysis and integration, or, what amounts to the same thing, the laws of differentiation and identification of the essential (phonemic) and inhibition of the unessential signs, the only difference being that the distinctive, phonemic signs on which the speech sounds are based are themselves determined by the language system. Their character is complex, generalized, and social in its origin.

It is clear, therefore, that the perception of speech by hearing requires not merely delicate, but also systematized, hearing. When this selection of the essential, phonemic signs is no longer possible, phonemic hearing is disturbed. This is why the boundary between hearing speech and understanding it loses its sharp distinction. A person ignorant of a foreign language not only does not understand it, but does not even hear it, i.e., he does not distinguish from the flow of sounds the articulated elements of the language and does not systematize the sounds of speech according to its laws. The unfamiliar language is thus perceived by that person as a stream of unarticulated sounds, not only impossible to understand, but inaccessible for accurate auditory analysis.

All that has been said regarding the structure of the sounds of a language and regarding the hearing of speech is of decisive importance to the understanding of the nature of the work that must be done by *the secondary divisions of the auditory cortex of the left hemisphere,* those divisions that, as has been stated, are closely associated with the cortical apparatuses of kinesthetic (articulatory) analysis.

The work of these divisions consists of the *analysis and integration of the sound flow by identification of the phonemic signs of the objective system of the language.* This work must be carried out with the very close participation of articulatory acts, which, like the singing activity of the vocal cords for the hearing of music, constitute the efferent link for the perception of the sounds of speech. It consists of differentiating the significant, phonemic signs of the spoken sounds, inhibiting the unessential, nonphonemic signs, and comparing the perceived sound complexes on this phonemic basis. It refracts the newly arriving sounds through a system of dynamic stereotypes formed while the language was being learned and thus carries out its task on the basis of objective, historically established systems of connections. This deciphering of sound signals in accordance with historically established codes of spoken speech and the organization of auditory experience into new systems constitute the basic activity of the speech areas of the auditory cortex.

Investigations by L. A. Chistovich and co-workers have recently given a clear insight into the physiological basis of the process of perception of the sounds of speech and the role of articulatory impulses in it. According to these investigations the assessment of the sounds of speech can take place at two different levels, by two correspondingly different mechanisms.

The direct perception of the sounds of speech, a very rapid process, takes place, according to all the evidence, with the closest participation of the auditory cortex; it consists essentially of the acoustic identification of the most informative feature, and it is the basis for the simplest forms of imitation of sounds perceived. By contrast, the more complex process of qualification of a speech sound takes place at a higher level. It requires the identification of additional articulatory features of the sound and the participation of special "articular commands"; it is a much slower process, for it includes the classification of speech sounds into categories, and it evidently requires the close participation of kinesthetic areas of the cortex and also, perhaps, other and still more complex systems.

A lesion of these cortical divisions, therefore, must cause, not the simple loss of acuity of hearing, but the disintegration of the whole complex structure of analytic-synthetic activity underlying the process of the systematization of speech experience. It will be from this standpoint that lesions of the auditory cortex of the left hemisphere causing auditory agnosia and sensory aphasia will be considered.

D. DISTURBANCES OF HIGHER CORTICAL FUNCTIONS WITH LESIONS OF THE CORTICAL NUCLEUS OF THE AUDITORY ANALYZER. ACOUSTIC AGNOSIA AND SENSORY APHASIA

After these remarks on the working of the auditory analyzer, the structure of the secondary divisions of the auditory cortex, and the distinctive qualities of word hearing, we can go on to describe the basic defect arising from a lesion of the superior divisions of the left temporal region and to analyze the syndrome of sensory aphasia, the typical result of such lesions. Our purpose will be to discover the *fundamental defect* resulting from a lesion of the secondary divisions of the auditory cortex and to deduce from this the group of disturbances systematically dependent on the fundamental defect. *We shall naturally seek this fundamental defect in a disturbance of the complex forms of auditory analysis and integration, in particular in a disturbance of phonemic hearing.* As shall be explained, this disturbance lies at the root of the whole syndrome of sensory aphasia.

Investigation of patients with a lesion of the posterior third of the first temporal gyrus of the left hemisphere and with sensory aphasia* shows that, as a rule, they have no permanent hearing disturbances in the sphere of sounds not concerned with speech. Conditioned reactions to individual tones can be formed in these patients quickly enough and are stable enough once they have been produced. The problem of changes in the dynamics of the hearing function caused by lesions of the auditory cortex, as expressed by changes in auditory adaptation, in the stability of orienting reflexes to sound stimuli, etc., remains unsolved and awaits special investigation.

No sooner, however, do we proceed to investigate relatively fine differentiation between sounds in these patients than we discover considerable defects, notably in those cases in which these sounds formed parts of whole complexes. Korst and Fantalova (1959), for instance, found that patients with lesions of the temporal lobes began to have difficulty in identifying like sounds, which they looked upon as different, with the result that the ability to differentiate between sounds became impaired. It was also found (Traugott, 1947; Kaidanova, 1954; Babenkova, 1954; Kabelyanskaya, 1957; Shmidt and

*As stated, in discussing this syndrome we shall always have in mind right-handed individuals, for a similar syndrome arises in left-handed persons with a lesion of the corresponding divisions of the right hemisphere.

Sukhovaskaya, 1954) that the difficulty in sound discrimination was especially conspicuous when the patients were presented with complexes consisting of the same components but in a different order. An interesting fact that emerged from these investigations was that the difficulties were confined to the sphere of hearing; no obvious defects could be found in these patients with respect to visual differentiation (including differentiation between complex groups of colors). This situation is appropriately illustrated in Fig. 26. These diagrams also show that this acoustic disturbance is not so conspicuous in patients with a lesion of the inferior divisions of the left temporal region and with the syndrome of "transcortical" aphasia as it is in those with lesions of the superior divisions and that it is therefore manifestly focal in character.

The observations of Semernitskaya (1945) on the ability of patients of this group to reproduce rhythmic patterns were similar. As a rule, such patients have considerable difficulty in repeating rhythmic taps executed relatively quickly (e.g., ″ ″ ″ or ‴ ‴ ‴ or ″∪∪∪″∪∪∪ ∪∪∪″∪∪∪″). These patients state that they cannot discern the rhythmic pattern by ear and therefore cannot repeat it. A patient with a lesion of the temporal region *can* reproduce a rhythmic pattern if it is executed slowly, when it can be counted out.

Patients whose functions of auditory analysis and integration are disturbed can perceive (and reproduce) single rhythmic groups but are frequently unable to repeat this rhythmic pattern over and over again (as a series). They complain that they are given far too many taps to be able to identify their pattern. All of these difficulties point to a serious defect of auditory analysis accompanying a lesion of a superior division of the left temporal region.*

Very recently Gershuni and his co-workers have described a significant increase in the threshold of perception of short sounds in patients with lesions of the temporal cortex. Characteristically this type of disturbance was found in patients with lesions either of the left or of the right temporal cortex, and in every case it was manifested particularly clearly in the ear opposite to the pathological focus (Baru, Gershuni, and Tonkonogii, 1964). This fact is illustrated in Fig. 27.

The same fact has been confirmed by Karaseva (1968) in a larger series of cases.

Examination of the *word hearing* of these patients reveals much more marked disorders of auditory analysis and integration. In the severest cases, the patient cannot distinguish clearly between single sounds of speech or repeat them (e.g., pronouncing "u" as "o" or "o" as "u" or "a" and repeating "t" as "k" or "s" as "sh," "zh," or "z"). Only if the oral image is reinforced by visual perception can the patient repeat the desired sounds. In less severe cases,

*Disturbances in the analysis of complex rhythmic patterns may also arise from lesions of the symmetrically opposite areas of the right temporal region but then they do not constitute part of the syndrome of sensory aphasia.

disturbances in the differentiation between speech sounds arise when the patient is presented with two similar sounds, differing only in a single sign (oppositional or correlating phonemes). These patients easily repeat pairs of widely differing sounds (e.g., "r" and "m" and "d" and "s") but cannot correctly reproduce pairs of sounds such as "d-t" and "t-d," "b-p" and "p-b," and "z-s" and "s-z," which they repeat in the form of the preceding sound ("t-t," "d-d," etc.). Sometimes the patients state that there is some difference between these sounds, but they cannot pinpoint exactly what it is.

Similar results may be obtained by asking the patient to write these sounds or by carrying out an experiment involving differential movements in response to closely similar sounds (for example, asking the patient to lift a hand in

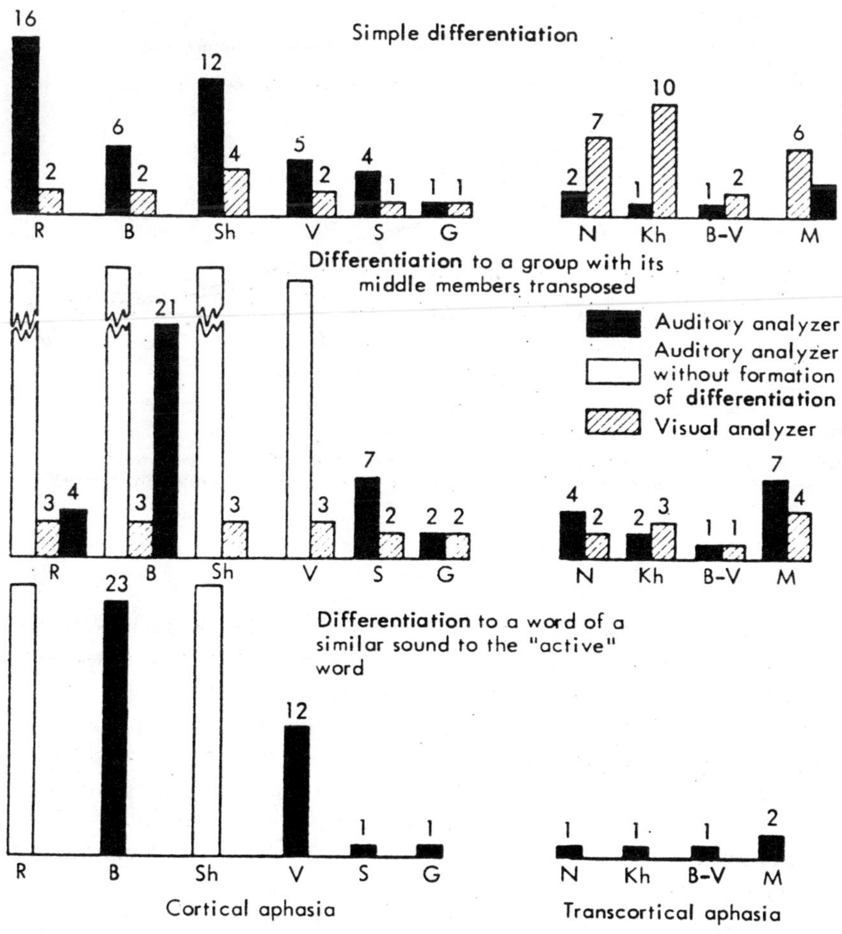

FIGURE 26 Disturbance of sound differentiation in patients with lesions of the left temporal region. The letters denote the initial of the patient's surname; the numbers denote the number of combinations after which stable differentiation was obtained. (*After Kabenyanskaya, 1957.*)

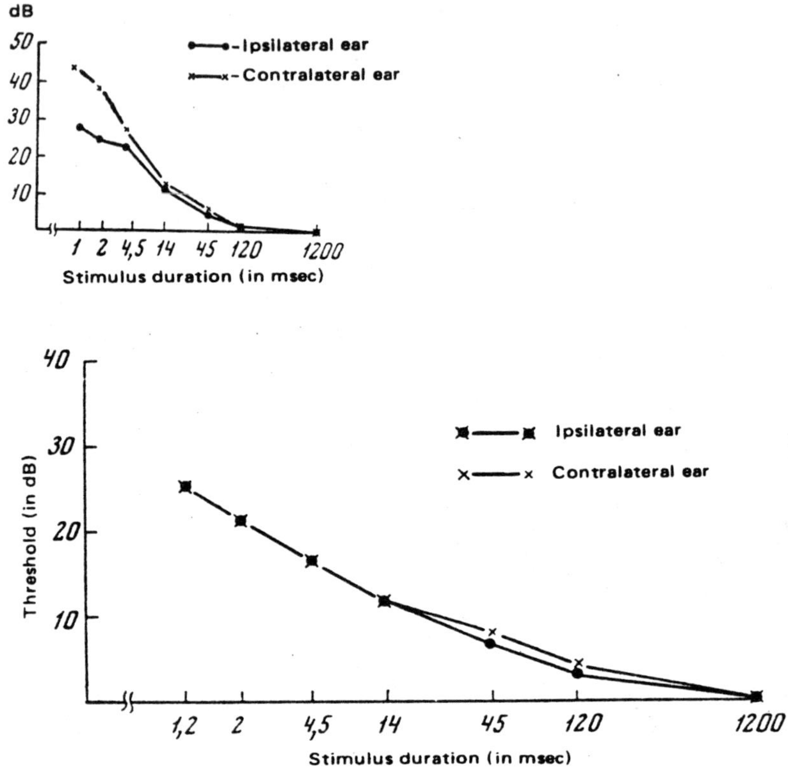

FIGURE 27 Changes in threshold of perception of short sounds in patients with temporal lesions (after Karaseva): above, normal subjects; below, patient with lesion (tumor) of right temporal region.

response to the sound "b" and not to move it in response to the sound "p"). In such examinations patients of this group display an obvious disturbance of sound differentiation; sometimes it is sufficient to alter the delivery of the sounds (for example, to pronounce "b" with a low and "p" with a high overtone) for the phonemic sign (voice) to lose its differential significance.

It follows, therefore, that a lesion of the secondary divisions of the auditory cortex of the left hemisphere results in a disturbance in the ability to decipher the phonemic code, on which the process of analysis and integration of the sounds of speech is based.

Figure 27 summarizes the results of the examination of phonemic hearing (by presentation of similar, correlating phonemes) in over 800 patients with gunshot wounds of the brain. This diagram shows that a disturbance

Characteristically disturbances of verbal (phonemic) hearing arising in lesions of the left temporal lobe are not necessarily accompanied by a disturbance of musical hearing. As several workers have described, the discrimination of tonal relationships and musical hearing may remain intact in patients with lesions of the left temporal lobe but may be severely affected in some patients with lesions of the right temporal lobe (Feuchtwanger, 1930; Ustvedt, 1937; Ombrédane, 1945; Luria, Tsvetkova, and Futer, 1966) and in patients with lesions of the temporal pole.

Hence, the *disturbance of discriminative hearing*, which can now be interpreted as a *disturbance in the analytic-synthetic activity of the auditory cortex* (in the form of a disturbance of the differential system of speech sounds), may be regarded as the *fundamental symptom of a lesion of the superior temporal region of the left hemisphere*, and *the resulting acoustic agnosia may be regarded as the fundamental source of speech disturbance*. The group of defects constituting the syndrome of temporal acoustic aphasia arises entirely as a result of disturbances of phonemic hearing.

These disturbances may be divided into two closely related groups: disturbances of the phonetic aspect of speech and disturbances of its

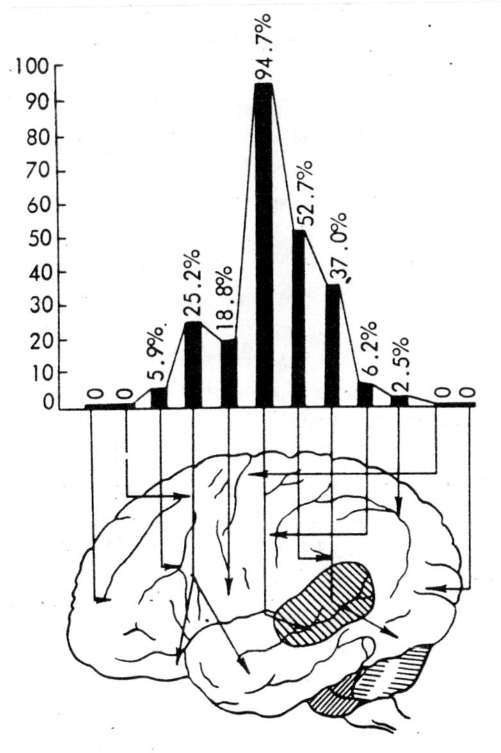

FIGURE 28 Percentage of over 800 patients with gunshot wounds of the brain who displayed derangement of phonemic hearing. (*From Luria, 1947*.)

conceptual aspect. There are other symptoms of the phonetic disturbance of speech in sensory aphasia than difficulty in discriminating between perceived sounds of speech, e.g., difficulty in pronouncing sounds and difficulty in analyzing the sound composition of speech and writing.

Although he shows no primary disturbance of articulation and can easily reproduce any position of the mouth presented to him visually or on the basis of kinesthetic analysis, a patient with temporal aphasia experiences considerable difficulty in pronouncing a word that he has heard. The word "kolos" (ear of corn), for example, sounds to him like "golos," "kholos," or "goros." Although he usually manages to retain the general melodic pattern of this word, he is unable to repeat it without distorting its sound composition. This type of distortion of the sound composition of a word, usually called "literal paraphasia," is a typical symptom of disturbed phonemic hearing in temporal aphasia. Another somewhat neglected fact must also be mentioned, namely, that in patients with a lesion of the cortical divisions of the auditory analyzer, disturbances of the motor aspect of speech may also be present.

The forms of literal paraphasia just described are not the only speech disturbances occurring in temporal aphasia. Frequently, such patients substitute for defective words other groups of sounds, firmly established in the past and belonging to the same conceptual sphere. Therefore, besides pronouncing a desired word in a distorted manner, patients of this group sometimes replace it by another word of similar sound and sometimes of similar meaning ("verbal paraphasia"). For instance, instead of the word "kolos" he may say "kolkhoz" (a collective farm). Often a patient, guessing the meaning of the word but not being able to formulate it, substitutes a descriptive term ("you know, flour is made from it" or "you find them in the fields").

A disturbance of active (repetitive or original) speech is typical of the acoustic agnostic disorders of the type that has been described. Active speech is associated with preservation of the primary kinesthetic basis of articulation. In the mildest cases of temporal aphasia this disturbance may appear as nothing more than difficulty in finding necessary words and occasional mistakes in pronouncing them; in more severe cases the patient's speech may become unintelligible and may come to resemble the word salad mentioned by workers investigating sensory aphasia.

Nevertheless, these disturbances of the phonetic aspect of speech, although characteristic of temporal aphasia, are not always apparent. The ability to produce habitual words, which do not require special sound analysis for their pronunciation and which had been transformed long ago into est. blished speech-motor stereotypes, may not be disturbed. For instance, such patients can easily pronounce words such as "well, of course" or "that is to say," although they cannot produce words not so well established.

The *disintegration of the sound structure of speech* is particularly conspicuous in all types of *externally controlled analysis of the sound structure of speech*, such as lies at the basis of writing. It is well known that the highly automatized speech of the adult ceases, in some cases, to rest on the auditory analysis of speech and begins to be pronounced on the basis of well-established kinesthetic epigrams. For writing, however, it is essential to have fully preserved, precise phonemic hearing. If phonemic hearing is disturbed, the patient has great difficulty in stating the number of sounds (or letters) comprising a given word, the order of the sounds (or letters), etc. Similar difficulties arise in attempts to synthesize a whole word from a given series of sounds presented separately (for example, "m," "i," "s," "t"). The identification of isolated sounds from a sound-complex, their differentiation from similarly sounding phonemes, and the maintenance of their proper order are difficult for a patient with a lesion of the superior temporal region, and only relatively few succeed in overcoming this problem.

It was stated that a disturbance in the analysis and synthesis of the sound composition of speech inevitably leads to disintegration of the ability to write, one of the most serious and frequent manifestations of a lesion of the left temporal region.

As a rule, patients with a lesion of this part of the cortex can copy a text correctly, write habitual words based on established kinesthetic epigrams, and write symbols (such as USSR and USA) that have become converted into established optic ideograms. However, they cannot write from dictation or their own composition. In the most severe cases, any form of free writing or writing from dictation becomes impossible; and the patient is able to form only random and inappropriate assortments of letters. In milder cases, the patient makes mistakes with words requiring special sound analysis. Substitution of oppositional phonemes (e.g., the Russian words "sobor" and "zapor" for "zabor," "okules" for "ogurets"), inability to articulate individual phonemes from a stream of consonants, and transposition (anticipation, postposition, and perseveration) of sounds are, therefore, the signs by which a patient with a disturbance of the functions of sound analysis and synthesis may be readily distinguished. Examples of impaired writing in such patients are given in Fig. 29.

Closely similar in nature is the disturbance of the reading ability that is found in these patients. As stated, they have no difficulty recognizing familiar ideograms, for the latter have become firmly entrenched from previous speech experience (their surname, the town where they live, etc.). If they have had considerable reading experience, they may even be able to look at newspapers and understand the general meaning of what is written; however, they cannot make out individual letters, syllables, or less familiar words. The discrepancy between the continued ability to recognize familiar words and the profound disturbance of true reading ability is one of the most characteristic features of the reading of these patients.

The disturbance in the phonetic aspect of speech in temporal (acoustic)

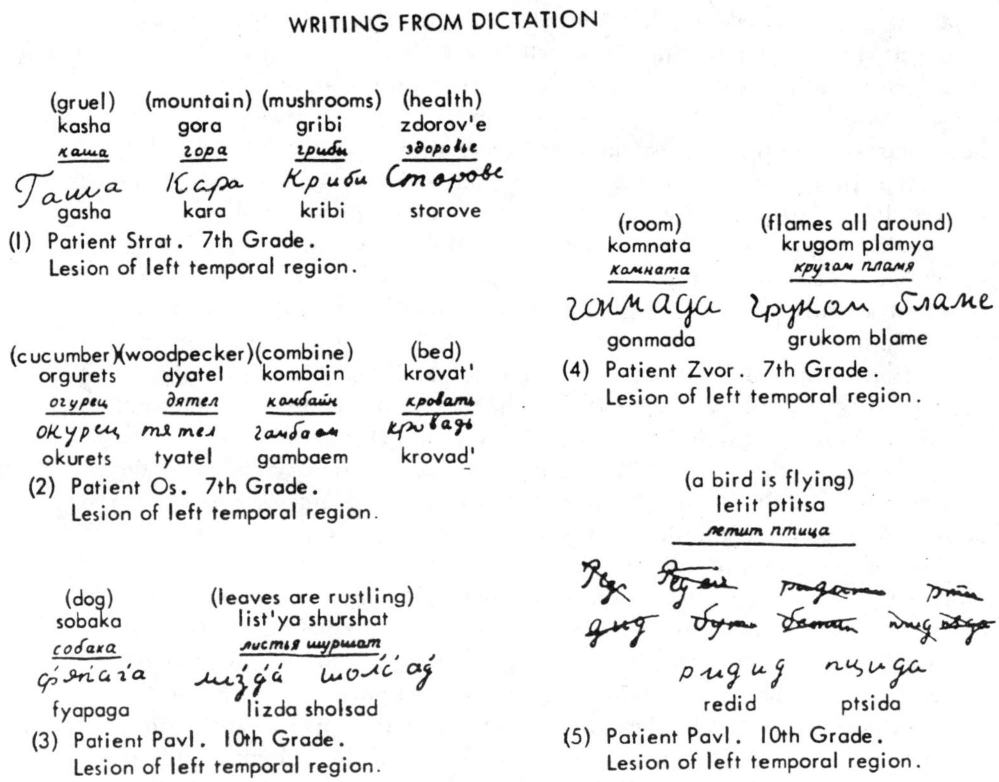

FIGURE 29 Examples of impaired writing in temporal (acoustic) aphasia. [In addition to the translation, the transliterated spelling of each dictated and written word has been provided: note that all the examples show substitution of the letter pairs k–g, z–s, d–t, b–p, r–l.] *(From Luria, 1947.)*

aphasia is closely related to the disturbance in its conceptual structure. The phoneme, the primary differentiation of which is disturbed in these cases, is a unity of sound and meaning, and phonemic hearing is sense-discriminating hearing. It is quite natural, therefore, that when the sound (phonemic) structure of speech is disordered, the system of word meaning based on this structure must also be disordered.

This disturbance in the conceptual aspect of speech is clearly manifested in the well-known syndrome of sensory aphasia, so termed because of the disturbance in the comprehension of the meaning of words. If the word "kolos" sounds like something between "golos," "goroz," "kholost," etc., with only the rhythm of the word being grasped, its meaning, or, more precisely, *its objective attribute is lost*. The word "kolos" becomes a meaningless collection of sounds, or it retains only a vague and undifferentiated meaning of something to do with a field, to farming ("kolos"-"kolkhoz"), to foodstuffs, etc. Often, only diffuse conceptual associations of the original meaning of the word remain, arising from the individual fragments of the sound complex. It is sometimes difficult to suggest what conceptual associations may arise in a patient whose speech has lost not only its sound composition, but also its precise objective attribute (Bein, 1957).

Although in severe cases of sensory aphasia this disintegration of the conceptual structure of speech is almost complete, in milder forms it becomes obvious only as a result of especially sensitive tests. One such test, as shall be described (Part III, Section 8C) is that based on retention of the meaning of several spoken words. If a patient with a not very apparent form of sensory aphasia, who can still understand the meaning of the words "eyes," "nose," and "ear," is asked repeatedly to point to the parts of the face so named, it will very soon become clear that the meaning of these words is beginning to go astray and that their objective attribute is being lost; the patient helplessly repeats "nos . . . [Russian for "nose"] nosh . . . nozh . . . nos . . . " and begins to point to parts of the face that have only just been named.

It is natural that this type of disturbance will be particularly obvious when a word denoting an object is spoken in the absence of the object itself. The difficulty can be largely overcome if the presentation of the word is accompanied by pointing out of the named object, for limitation of the choice of alternatives helps the patient to fix the meaning of the word. This is one method that is used in the rehabilitation of patients with sensory aphasia (Kogan, 1961).

Investigators have always observed some degree of irregularity in the manifestations of the disturbance of the conceptual aspect of speech in temporal aphasia. It should be remembered that such impairment is basically closely related to the disintegration of the phonemic structure of speech. The nature of this irregularity requires further, detailed study.

It has always been maintained that the ability to pronounce words denoting objects and their qualities (nouns and to some extent adjectives) is more severely affected than that of words denoting actions or relationships (the latter function to be treated fully in Part II, Section 4F). This is revealed in the typical speech of one with sensory aphasia, which is almost completely without substantives and consists mainly of auxiliary words (conjunctions, prepositions, adverbs, and interjections) that are joined together to form expressions with unity of intonation and melody. Because of this, the speech of a person with sensory aphasia may remain to some extent comprehensible although it is almost totally without objective words.

Irregularity is also revealed by the deterioration of the objective words themselves, with both their active use and understanding of them more difficult. The general, wide meaning of words, i.e., the system of associations and relationships built upon them, is far better preserved despite its diffuseness than the concrete, objective attribute of words. For this reason a patient with sensory aphasia often appreciates only the general implications of a given word and can neither differentiate it nor, still less, understand its concrete significance. This phenomenon stands out clearly in the form of a multitude of "paragnosias" (imprecise or incorrect understanding of the meaning of a word) and "verbal paraphasias" (replacement of the proper word with another from a closely related conceptual sphere) (Bein, 1947, 1957).

At present it is difficult to explain this phenomenon, although there is good reason to suppose that a defect in the system of phoneme selection is invariably accompanied by disturbed selectivity throughout the entire conceptual structure of speech. It was this character of the disturbances of the conceptual aspect of speech in sensory aphasia that led Jakobson and Halle (1956) to formulate the hypothesis that there are forms of aphasia in which the "code" system of the language is much more severely deranged than the system of its "context," so that compensatory attempts are largely confined to these context associations. While such a distinction is highly probable, its psychophysiological basis requires further, careful study.

The disturbance of the understanding of word meaning (alienation of word meaning) observed in patients with left temporal lesions is not always the result of disintegration of phonemic hearing, whereby the sounds of a word becomes indistinct and loses its stability.

In clinical medicine forms of this condition are known in which a disturbance of the understanding of word meaning arises despite the relative integrity of phonemic hearing. In such cases (which were described in the older literature under the name of "transcortical sensory aphasia") the patient continues to distinguish similar phonemes relatively well, and sometimes he can even write, but he begins to give the wrong meaning to words he hears. There is reason to suppose that in these cases, which some writers have described as "associative auditory agnosia," the disturbance of formation of word meaning takes place at a different stage from that described above. The mechanisms of these "relatively rare" forms of sensory aphasia are not yet clearly understood, and an explanation of the reasons why they arise is still awaited.

Closely related to these disturbances of the conceptual aspect of speech in temporal aphasia are the changes affecting *speech memory*, the latter type of disorder constituting an essential part of this syndrome. It would be wrong to regard speech memory as the retention of isolated word epigrams and the process of memorizing as the simple ecphoria of these isolated, latent pictures. To a greater or lesser degree memorizing is always the adoption of selective systems of word associations, while reproduction is the process of analysis of these systems with the selection of the associations to be used and the simultaneous inhibition of those that are not required.

Can it be assumed that the process of memorizing and reproducing words remains intact when the structure of the phonemic and conceptual aspects of speech is itself disturbed? Observations in cases of temporal aphasia have shown that a lesion of the systems of the superior temporal region leads to an obvious disturbance of the memorization and reproduction of words. In other words, a disturbance of sensory speech is always accompanied by manifestations of *speech amnesia.*

The phenomenon just described can be observed in word repetition experiments. As shall be explained more fully, sometimes a patient with a relatively mild form of temporal aphasia has only to be presented with one or two words, or a pause of 3 to 5 seconds introduced, and difficulties will arise in the repetition of the given word, which is replaced by paraphrases. Difficulties in memorizing and reproducing words are seen still more clearly when the patient is asked to repeat a series of words or an entire phrase.

An analysis of these disturbances, comparing sensory aphasia with the condition known as "conduction aphasia," is dealt with specially below (Part II, Section 2E).

Obvious disturbances of word memory associated with the diffuseness of the phonemic and conceptual structure of speech are also evident during experiments concerned with the naming of objects.

The naming of an object (or the designation of an object by a certain conventional group of sounds, forming a word) is a much more complex phenomenon than the simple association of the visual appearance of an object with a conventional acoustic complex. It involves the abstraction of the known identification features of the object and the choice, from a large number of alternatives, of the name by which the object can be designated. Naturally, therefore, the naming of an object may be affected under different conditions, when any one stage of this complex process is disturbed.

Lesions of the left temporal cortex, causing a disturbance of phonemic hearing, naturally impair the process of identification of the acoustic complex which designates the given object and, as a result, the required acoustic engram begins to be confused easily with other engrams sharing a certain common component. A disturbance of simple differentiation of audioverbal complexes, which arises as an inevitable result of sensory aphasia, causes words or groups of sounds similar in their acoustic composition to be no longer clearly distinguished, so that a person who normally could easily find the required name can no longer do so. Irrelevant acoustic complexes, which under normal conditions would have a very small chance of appearing during the perception of that particular object or the appearance of a given pattern, now appear just as probably as the appropriate words; the number of different acoustic complexes springing up in such a patient may often be so great that he is quite unable to pick out the required name, and the selectivity of the process of word finding is lost. These numerous searches and paraphasias (sometimes "literal," when instead of the necessary word similar sounds are uttered; sometimes "verbal," when the required word is replaced by another of similar meaning) become the objective features of the disturbance of audioverbal selectivity that result from a disturbance of the differential activity of the audioverbal cortex.

A characteristic feature of this disturbance, which can justifiably be called "amnestic aphasia," and which arises on the basis of a sensory (acoustico-gnostic) defect, is the fact that prompting the patient does not revive the necessary selective acoustico-verbal traces and cannot therefore help him to find the word he requires. Such a patient, when trying to name an object shown to him, makes helpless attempts to select the required sound from the whole range of possible acoustic complexes.

Psycholinguistic investigations of the probability that different acoustic complexes arise in such cases have not yet been specially undertaken, nor have there been any special studies of the physiological nature of this defect since the earlier work of Sapir (1929, 1934) and of Gal'perin and Golubova (1933).

• • •

The syndrome of the disturbance of higher cortical functions accompanying lesions of the auditory divisions of the cortex of the left temporal lobe has been described. As mentioned, this syndrome is based on a disorder of those aspects of the working of the cortical divisions of the auditory analyzer that are responsible for the analysis and synthesis of the sounds of speech, under the controlling influence of the phonemic structure of language. This disorder results in a collapse of the phonemic structure of speech, together with a conceptual disturbance composed of extinction of the meanings of words and loss of their objective attributes. The disorder of the phonemic pattern of speech also leads to marked impairment of the word memory, brought to light both in the naming of objects and in the course of spontaneous speech; as stated, attempts to activate these latent pictures of the required words by prompting are useless in such cases.

Another characteristic feature of sensory (acoustic) aphasia is the fact that all functions not related to the defect of sound analysis and synthesis are usually preserved. A patient with a lesion of the temporal systems continues to correctly perform tasks requiring the visual analysis of images; he has a sound idea of the spatial arrangement of lines, and he successfully accomplishes the operations of spatial praxis. Frequently, all of these functions are so well preserved that the patient may actually use them to compensate for his defect. Assistance from kinesthetic and visual-spatial analysis and synthesis may therefore be used for rehabilitation of patients in this group.*

E. DISTURBANCES OF HIGHER CORTICAL FUNCTIONS WITH LESIONS OF THE MIDDLE SEGMENTS OF THE TEMPORAL REGION. ACOUSTIC-MNESTIC APHASIA

We have so far analyzed disturbances of the higher cortical functions associated with a lesion of that part of the superior divisions of the

*The present author has previously outlined rehabilitative methods based on the use of residual systems (Luria, 1947, 1948).

left temporal region composed of the secondary fields of the cortical nucleus of the auditory analyzer. What disturbances may arise from lesions of the middle segments of the convex portion of the left temporal lobe, i.e., those segments not directly related to the cortical nucleus of the auditory analyzer and conventionally called its "extranuclear" divisions?

While this question is of great practical importance because of the high incidence of lesions of this region (tumors and abscesses of the temporal region frequently affect these segments), the answer is highly complex. Its complexity is due to the fact that far less is known about the direct functions of this cortical region than of the others and to the fact that the disturbances associated with lesions situated here are much less clearly defined clinically than those elsewhere.

Since the temporal region of the cortex possesses close connections both with the auditory and visual divisions of the cortex and with the mediobasal segments directly related to the nonspecific, tone-controlling mechanisms and affective processes, its role in the performance of the higher cortical functions is evidently very complex. The disturbances of the higher cortical processes (especially speech) arising from lesions of these segments is accordingly of great interest.

The middle segments of the convex part of the temporal region (of the dominant hemisphere), corresponding to Areas 21 and 37, differ in their structure and connections from the aforementioned formations. Like the secondary fields of the nuclear zone of the auditory analyzer, these parts receive fibers from the thalamic nuclei not directly communicating with the periphery and thus are among the structurally more complex zones of the cerebral cortex.

They are particularly well developed in man and are composed of relatively new formations of the cerebral cortex. They possess two essential features. Firstly, a part of these segments is closely connected with the cortical formations belonging to the system of another (the visual) analyzer and may be regarded as the overlapping zone of the cortical endings of these two analyzers. Secondly, these formations retain their connections with more primitive structures, namely, the limbic lobe and the basal segments of the temporal portion of the cortex together with the hippocampus and amygdaloid body, the region most closely concerned with regulation of cortical tone and of the affective processes. Campbell (1905) referred to the superior divisions of the temporal region as "acoustic-psychic," preferring to call the remainder of the convex divisions simply the "temporal cortex," without any additional qualification.

Animal experiments in which the temporal region was extirpated gave complex and inconsistent results. They showed that this region of the cortex is, in fact, related to both the auditory and the visual analyzers and to the formations regulating the general cerebral tone and closely associated with the emotional aspect of animal behavior.

The clinical picture arising from lesions of the middle segments of the temporal region is also very complex and varied. Besides symptoms related to the auditory and visual spheres (the development of complex auditory and visual hallucinations), tumors of the temporal region cause marked mental disorders (the dreamy states originally described by Jackson [1931-1932, Vol. 1]) and emotional changes; these disturbances are especially pronounced when the pathological process has spread to the deep portions of the temporal region and has begun to affect the hippocampal region and the amygdaloid body (Part II, Section 2G). Several writers (Grünthal, 1947; Scoville *et al.*, 1953; Milner, 1956; etc.) have described distinct disturbances of the direct fixation of traces, associated, from all evidence, with changes in the state of the cortex temporal lobe and with pathological processes or reactions in the deep divisions.

Important results were obtained by Penfield and Roberts (1959) following stimulation of the convex surface of the temporal region. They observed the complex hallucinations, memory images, and changes in the state of consciousness. On the basis of these findings, these authors attributed mnestic functions to the cortical portion of the temporal lobe and distinguished, besides the auditory ("sensory") region of the cortex, the "interpretative" region of the cortex, to which, following Jackson, they ascribed functions "more complex than the simple functions of perception."

The importance of these symptoms is enhanced by the fact that many of the pathological processes associated with intracranial tumors and abscesses in this region have a direct effect on these particular segments of the temporal cortex.

For the time being we shall leave aside the interpretation of the effects of lesions situated in the middle segments of the temporal region of the left hemisphere. They should probably be regarded as the result of the perifocal influence of the pathological process on the region of the superior temporal gyrus. It is likewise possible that we are dealing with a disturbance of the general state of cortical excitability, as a result of the action of the pathological process on the connections between the temporal region and the occipital and mediobasal formations. Notwithstanding the variety of possible interpretations, the nature of the disturbances of the higher mental functions (especially speech) arising from lesions of this region is sufficiently well defined. Different writers give different descriptions of these disturbances; some designate them as manifestations of "transcortical sensory aphasia" while others call them "amnestic aphasia" or "acoustico-mnestic aphasia." None of these terms reflects the clinical picture of the disturbances with sufficient precision.

The main difference between this form of aphasia and the acoustic-gnostic speech disturbances that have been described is that in these cases phonemic hearing is completely or partially preserved, and when there is any impairment it is only after suitable "loading." These patients have no difficulty in repeating closely related (oppositional) phonemes without confusing them; confusion arises only if the problem is made more complicated. They easily understand words and exhibit no clear evidence of alienation of word meaning. They easily repeat individual words, without altering their sound composition and without giving any literal paraphasias. They often correctly write individual words from dictation, making mistakes only when the words are unfamiliar or complex in sound composition.

These patients exhibit marked disturbances when they attempt to remember words given to them orally. Although they can retain single words well, they have great difficulty in retaining and repeating series of (three or four) words. Usually the patient reproduces only one or two words but cannot repeat the whole series. Sometimes he begins to replace the required words by perseverations of words previously given. A similar but even more marked defect arises when the patient is presented with a series of a few short phrases (like "the house is burning, the moon is shining, the broom is sweeping"). As a rule, the patient forgets the last phrase or confuses the phrases.

These patients also have considerable *difficulty in reproducing words or word series under more complicated conditions.* Nothing more is needed than to separate the reproduction of the word series from its presentation by an interval of 5 to 10 seconds and to fill this interval with unrelated speech activity, for example, by asking the patient questions. Tests have shown that in these cases the traces of the given word series easily disappear, and the patient is unable to recall them.

Finally, the disturbance of the ability to retain word series is revealed by the fact that, although retaining the essential elements of the series, the patient *cannot reproduce them in the proper order* but constantly changes their sequence of presentation. Sometimes the correct order of a series cannot be reproduced after as many as ten or fifteen repetitions of four or five words. This disturbance of the order of verbal traces is evidence of weakness of the tracer function of the cortex in this region. This phenomenon is often accompanied by a marked disturbance in the mobility of the auditory processes of speech, for after a few correct repetitions of a series of words, such patients have difficulty in repeating the same words in a different order and continue to mechanically repeat the words in their previously established order.

It is characteristic that the traces of visually presented series of signs (e.g., geometrical figures) are retained much better than traces of word signals presented orally.

A series of curves taken from tests on a patient with acoustic-mnestic aphasia is given in Fig. 30 (Luria, Klimkovskii, and Sokolov, 1966). These results show that the process of memorizing of sounds, whether words or numbers, presented by ear is severely affected in these cases, whereas the memorizing of the same material if presented visually remains intact. Similar results were obtained in a comparative investigation of the retention of verbal and kinesthetic series (Luria and Rapoport, 1962).

The instability of retention of a series of words presented orally is particularly acute in these patients. It is this finding that has led to the application of the term "amnestic aphasia" to describe this group of disorders as a whole. Even if word amnesia appears to be absent, it can easily be brought to light by suggesting to the patient that he name not a single object, but a group of two or three. In these cases the patient will name one object correctly but will be unable to name the second or third, and he usually perseverates the word previously given. Characteristically, that an incorrect word was given is not usually perceived by the patient, thus demonstrating that the disturbance present is one affecting direct word meaning. As in the group of disturbances previously described, prompting usually does not help the patient.

The significant narrowing of the range of word operations available to the patient and the inhibitory effect of one word on another are clear indications of the pathological state of the cortex in the temporal region.

Similar disorders of the amnestic-aphasic type also appear in the active speech of these patients. While animation of intonation and melody is preserved, their speech usually abounds in the same seeking for words as in the experiments involving the naming of objects. As in that type of experiment, the active speech of the patients of this group contains paraphasias. Usually, however, these are verbal rather than literal in character.

The foregoing account shows the highly distinctive character of the disturbance of higher cortical activity arising from lesions of the extra-auditory divisions of the left temporal region and its complex relationship to the symptoms described in the preceding section. It must be added that the writing of the patients of this group may remain relatively unaffected, signs of a disorder being discovered only if the conditions are made more complicated (for example, by widening the range of words to be written).

The acoustic-mnestic disturbances arising in this group of cases differ from those observed in frank sensory aphasia by the fact that they do not include a gross disintegration of the sound structure of speech (phonemic substitutions, difficulty in sound analysis of words, writing disorders, etc.). Nevertheless, several symptoms are common to both groups. If the range of the word material is broadened, amnestic symptoms are joined by marked manifestations of sensory aphasia in the form of extinction of meaning; as a rule, prompting does not assist with the ecphoria of the required word.

The physiological basis of the disturbances described above was incompletely understood until recently, when an attempt was made (Luria, Klimkovskii, and Sokolov, 1966) to describe the conditions that impair the retention and recall of series of acoustic and audioverbal traces in the patients of this group.

These observations show that at least two mechanisms may lie at the basis of these disturbances. In some cases the mechanism may be increased proactive and retroactive inhibition of weakened audioverbal traces. As a result of this factor, although the patient can easily remember individual sounds or words, he cannot recall a series of sounds or words, because the individual elements of the series easily inhibit each other. In many cases this has the result that the repetition of a series of 3, 4, or 5 words starts

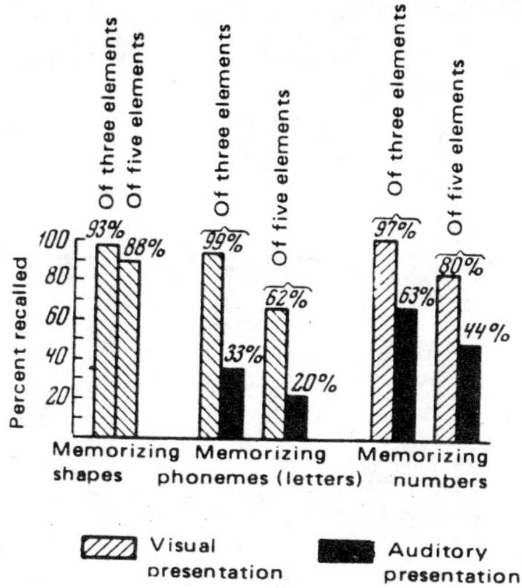

FIGURE 30 Difference in memorizing series of sounds, words, and numbers shown or dictated to a patient with acoustic-mnestic aphasia (after Klimkovskii, Luria, and Sokolov).

with repetition of the last word, all the others being retroactively inhibited and impossible to recall; characteristically this takes place only during the repetition of audioverbal series and not during the recall of visually presented material. This fact is illustrated in Fig. 31.

Another characteristic feature of the patients of this group is the clear manifestations of reminiscence which they exhibit; after a short pause the effect of proactive and retroactive inhibition becomes so reduced that the patient can repeat material which he could not recall directly.

In another group of cases the retention and correct recall of an audioverbal series are prevented by a mechanism of "equalization of trace intensity." Whereas under normal conditions the trace of a stimulus just presented is much stronger than traces of previous stimuli and, consequently, the probability of its recall is much greater, in this pathological state of the temporal cortex the strength of recent and previous traces, or of important and unimportant traces, may become equal and, consequently, the required trace is less likely to be recalled. In such cases even a short pause between presentation and recall of the audioverbal series is sufficient for the traces of the recently presented series to become equal in intensity to those of past series, and their selective ecphoria is impaired. The phenomena of paraphasia (the recall of irrelevant traces with the same or

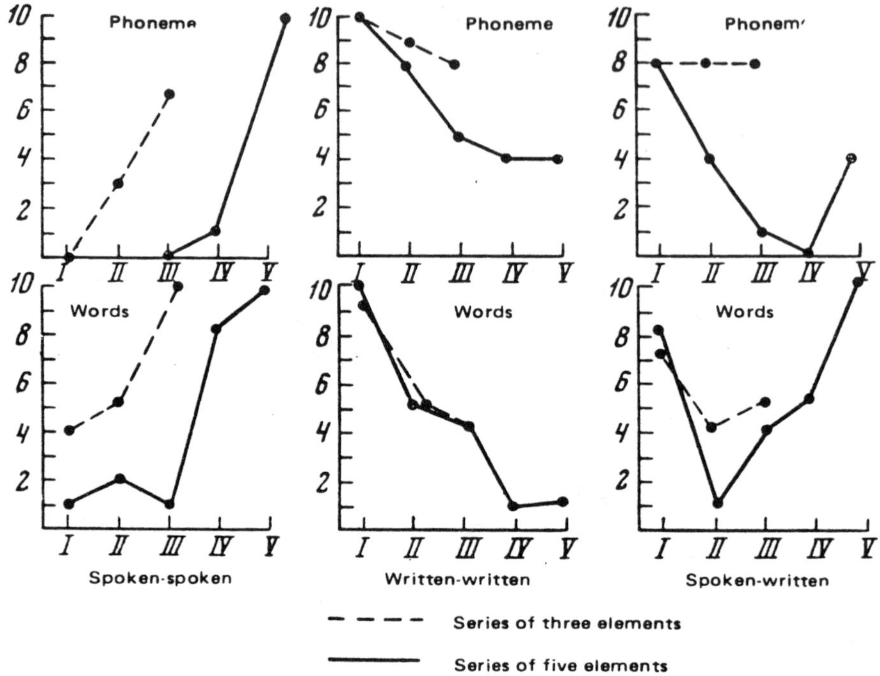

FIGURE 31 Phenomena of retroactive inhibition during recall of audioverbal and visual series by patient with acoustic-mnestic aphasia (after Luria, Sokolov, and Klimkovskii). When sounds or words are dictated, the patient recalls and recites the last word of the series; if they are presented in writing, he recalls the first elements of the series in writing. Tests with dictation and recall in writing give intermediate results.

almost the same probability as the required trace) observed in such cases (Luria, Sokolov, and Klimkovskii, 1967) make this explanation a very likely one.

These facts provide an approach to the physiological analysis of some forms of "conduction aphasia" and show them to be an attenuated form of acoustic-mnestic disturbances (Luria, 1962, unpublished work; Luria and Rapoport, 1962; Tonkonogii, 1964; Luria, Sokolov, and Klimkovskii, 1967; Klimkovskii, 1966).

. . .

The phenomena encountered in the presence of lesions of the extra-auditory divisions of the left temporal region have been described. However, the analysis of the pathophysiological mechanisms underlying these phenomena is a matter for future consideration. There can be no doubt that some of these phenomena—the difficulty in retaining the sequence of a series of elements presented orally, the marked narrowing of the range of sound (especially word) stimuli that is capable of being retained, the inhibiting effect of one word upon another, and, finally, the clear evidence of auditory-verbal perseverations—indicate a significant change in the neurodynamics within the cortical divisions of the auditory analyzer; the nature of the impairment is a decrease in the strength of the nervous processes and a disturbance in their mobility. However, it is only by a careful psychophysiological investigation of these phenomena that the nature of the mechanisms underlying these disturbances can be established.

Our account of the pathological changes accompanying lesions of the extra-auditory divisions of the left temporal region would be incomplete without mentioning one very characteristic symptom of lesions of the temporo-occipital portion of the left hemisphere. This relates to the *extinction of word meaning*, whose psychological characteristics differ considerably from those encompassed by the syndrome of sensory (acoustic-gnostic) aphasia.

Patients with a lesion in this region may not experience much difficulty in differentiating between similar sounds, readily carry out tasks involving the phonemic analysis and synthesis of words, write quite difficult words accurately, and recognize and correct any word that is incorrectly pronounced. However, while they may pronounce words faultlessly, they frequently cannot remember their meaning. This type of extinction of word meaning, i.e., a profound amnesia of word meaning, presents a pattern quite different from that observed in lesions of the cortical nucleus of the auditory analyzer. The mechanisms responsible for these phenomena are not yet known, but on the basis of certain findings it seems likely that they are concerned not so much with a disturbance of the phonemic structure of speech, as with a disintegration of auditory-visual synthesis and of the connections between visual images and their word names; such synthesis and connections are conditions essential for maintaining the normal structure of speech. This hypothesis has been confirmed by experiments (conducted by Blinkov and the present author) in which patients have been asked to make drawings; while they can readily copy drawings shown to them (even difficult ones), they cannot reproduce what they have drawn when the drawings are removed. Although words apparently retain their direct significance, they do not bring to mind the precise visual image that usually arises in a normal subject or in a patient with a lesion of the superior divisions of the temporal region. Examples of such disturbances are given in Fig. 32.

A possible mechanism for them may be a disturbance of the combined working of the cortical portions of the temporal (hearing, speech) and occipital (visual) regions. The fact that the patient can copy drawings indicates that visual analysis and synthesis as such are preserved; the preservation of the phonemic aspect of speech indicates the normal working of the cortical divisions of the auditory analyzer. The inability to produce the corresponding visual images through the speech system and the great instability of the visual images suggest that processes that can be carried out only by the combined work of both regions are disturbed. These considerations do not, of course, constitute an adequate explanation of this symptom, and the analysis of the defects arising from a lesion of the border zones responsible for the combined working of two analyzers (in this case, auditory and visual) must be a subject for future research.

F. DISTURBANCES OF INTELLECTUAL PROCESSES WITH TEMPORAL LESIONS

We have confined our attention so far to the analysis of acoustic-gnostic and speech disturbances arising from lesions of the systems of the left temporal region. The question, however, arises: Are the intellectual processes of these patients preserved, and, if not, what is the exact nature of the derangement?

This question is particularly important because, as mentioned, certain workers believe that the whole of sensory aphasia is the result of primary intellectual disorders and regard the functional defects as essentially an abnormality of the intellect or as a partial dementia. Marie (1906), notably, held this view.

What are the features of the intellectual processes in patients with temporal aphasia? Much factual evidence has recently been gathered on this problem, and part of the question can now be answered. Observations made in recent decades (Luria, 1940*a*; Bein, 1947; Ombredane, 1951; etc.) are in disagreement with Marie's hypothesis; they reveal that the intellectual processes of patients with temporal aphasia are not affected to the same extent and in the same manner as he suggested. Analysis of the manner in which the conceptual structure of speech is disturbed in temporal aphasia revealed a distinctive inequality in the conceptual defects (Part II, Section 2D). As pointed out, the direct significance (or objective attribute) of speech is affected to a far greater degree in such patients than is its generalizing function.

Many observations suggest that the ability to grasp the general meaning of words and sensitivity to their conceptual sphere may remain relatively intact in these patients, although certain definite changes are found. This is shown by the fact that with lesions of this type prepositions and conjunctions are better preserved, and these connecting words, as stated, continue to constitute a large proportion of the speech of the sensory aphasic.

Ordinarily, the "rule" in any brain lesion is that the most complex formations, those last to develop (primarily the abstract forms of intellectual activity), are most severely affected, but this obviously does not apply in cases of sensory aphasia. During a careful study of the paraphasias of patients with temporal aphasia, Bein (1957) found that conceptual substitutions (verbal paraphasias) frequently have a very abstract basis; the groundlessness

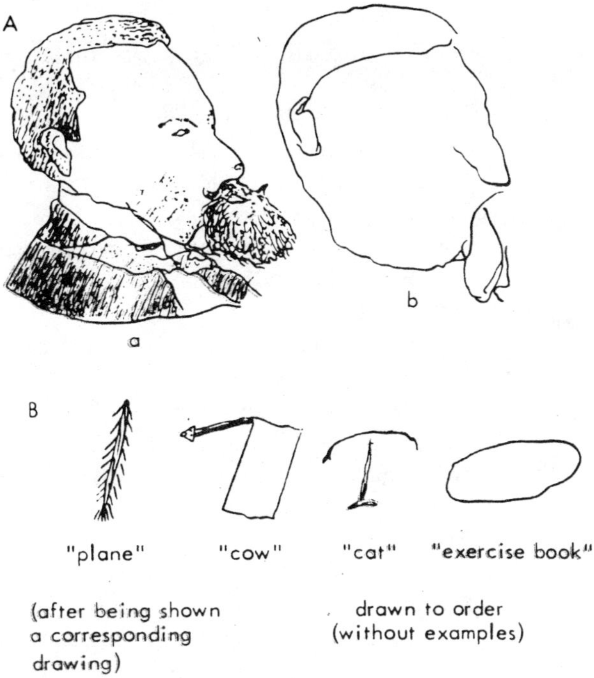

FIGURE 32 Drawings by patients with wounds of the temporo-occipital region of the cortex. (*A*) Patient M. (*a*) Portrait copies from life. (*b*) Portrait drawn from memory. (*B*) Patient R. Drawings of objects to a spoken order. (*After Blinkov and Luria.*)

intellectual activity was thereby confirmed.

Further convincing evidence that patients with sensory aphasia can still carry out operations involving abstract intellectual activity (classification of objects, type relationships of the "genus-species" form, etc.) was obtained by Isserlin (1929–1932, 1936), Lotmar (1919, 1935), Kuenburg (1923), and, in particular, Ombredane (1951). From these investigations (and also from the observations of Bein, 1957, and Luria, 1947) it became clear that a patient with sensory aphasia can grasp the meaning of abstract ideas, such as "development," "cause," and "limitation," and can understand the proper meaning of metaphors. He can carry out transfer operations and can even detect relationships of analogy, although naturally within the limits imposed by the degree of preservation of the function of understanding the direct meanings of the words he uses. Contrary to Goldstein's (1948) opinion, we believe that within certain limits a patient with temporal aphasia retains the ability to classify and possesses the function of abstract orientation which the disciples of the noetic school considered to be defective in all aphasics.

The preservation of the ability to understand abstract relationships is also revealed when the investigation of speech operations is left for what is called the investigation of "nonverbal intellect." The findings demonstrate that a patient with acoustic agnosia and sensory aphasia can successfully carry out operations involving geometrical relationships, mentally transform the spatial relationships of elements, make spatial analogies, etc. As Ombredane (1951) has shown, such patients can also perform operations with series of pictures, although they frequently make mistakes when deciding on the order of presentation of a subject in pictorial form.

Finally, clinical evidence discloses that the ability to perform basic arithmetical operations is potentially preserved even in severe cases of temporal aphasia, provided that they are performed in a written form and are not dependent on the preservation of verbal traces (as in the case of mental arithmetic).*

These observations show that several of the fundamental operations of abstract intellectual activity may be largely preserved in lesions of the left temporal region. However, the patient with a disturbance of the phonemic and conceptual structure of the speech processes always experiences *considerable difficulty* notwithstanding the adequate preservation of the ability to engage in certain forms of abstract intellectual activity, when he attempts to carry out *systematic, successive operations with relationships requiring the constant participation of speech associations as mediators*. In such circumstances the ability to discriminate between relationships becomes manifestly inadequate and the patient's intellectual operations begin to suffer.

The intellectual defects of a patient with temporal aphasia become apparent in nonspeech operations in which an essential part of the process entails the use of systems of speech associations retained in the memory. For instance, a patient who could still sort out a series of pictures telling a story, provided he was allowed to mix them up himself, found the process very difficult if he was not allowed to touch the pictures and was asked to put them in the proper order as indicated by the appropriate numbers (Ombredane, 1951). These patients experience similar difficulties with series of geometrical operations. The defects were found to be particularly serious when such patients attempted to do mental arithmetical calculations. They had no difficulty in grasping numerical relationships but, although usually preserving the general plan of the necessary actions, they became helpless when given problems requiring a series of successive operations with some of the results to be kept in mind. An attempt to assist the process by allowing them to speak out loud was unsuccessful, and without the support of a well-established and differentiated system of word associations it was seriously impaired.

It should be noted that the operations of discursive intellectual activity, which are wholly dependent on speech, for example, the solution of logical problems as in Burt's tests on the establishment of multiple relationships (Part III, Section 8E), remained completely beyond these patients' ability. They

*Among our patients was a bookkeeper with a severe form of sensory aphasia who could still draw up the annual balance sheet in spite of severe disturbances of speech and although he was unable to remember the names of his subordinates and used to refer to them incorrectly.

could not perform these operations because of difficulties associated with the constant alienation of word meanings, the instability of word values, and the impossibility of retaining traces of word associations and sequence.

Hence, the unique feature of disturbances of the intellectual processes accompanying a lesion of the temporal systems with manifestations of acoustic aphasia is that, although able to directly recognize relationships (visual-spatial or logical equally well), these patients are *incapable of performing discursive operations necessitating the participation of a system of differentiated verbal associations with well-established traces.* The attempt to enlist the aid of speaking aloud impairs rather than improves the process, making it quite impossible to carry out the required task. The defect may be partially compensated for only by means of visual aids, in substitution for the deranged verbal traces. Only in these conditions can the patients cope with relatively simple intellectual operations. The preservation of the general plan of the presented task, together with the impossibility of accomplishing it by means of a series of successive operations, constitute the distinctive feature of the intellectual disturbance in patients with temporal aphasia, distinguishing it from the forms of intellectual impairment accompanying other lesions of the brain, especially lesions of the frontal divisions, which we shall consider below.

How can this peculiar preservation of the direct comprehension of spatial and, in particular, of logical relationships in patients with such severe disturbances of speech be explained? There can be no doubt that the system of abstract logical relationships grew and took shape on the basis of speech. Can this system remain intact in speech disorders?

In our attempt to interpret this fact we should not fall into the error typical of the idealistic doctrine of the Würzburg school, according to which intellectual activity is quite distinct from speech and is a primary and independent function. We must therefore make one point in our argument clearer.

The speech disturbances arising from lesions of the temporal region do not destroy speech completely. They damage only the phonemic structure of speech and, consequently, the processes requiring the constant participation of the differentiated system of words, with their precise objective attribute. We may gather from this that as a result of lesions of the temporal systems speech is not completely destroyed and that some types of operations involving ideas may remain relatively intact.

On the other hand, we know that it is only in the earliest stages that the systems of associations based on speech are dependent on the fully developed system of spoken speech, with its kinesthetic impulses passing to the cerebral cortex and constituting the basal component of the second signal system. During their subsequent development, however, they become more firmly established and gradually begin to lose their dependence on this kinesthetic support. This fact has been studied in detail in the psychological investigations of Vygotskii (1934, 1956) and Gal'perin (1959), in special experiments by A. N. Sokolov (1959), and in electrophysiological investigations by Novikova

(1955) and Bassin and Bein (1957). These investigations showed that when intellectual operations are sufficiently established they begin to be performed without the visible aid of speech kinesthesia and, in all probability, become to some extent independent of the fully developed processes of articulated speech, which the subject calls upon for aid only when performing complex discursive operations.

Cases of temporal acoustic aphasia provide another example of the relative preservation of some processes of understanding of abstract relationships when the fully developed forms of discursive intellectual speech activity are disordered. These cases present a great many hitherto unstudied problems, such as the characteristics of internal speech in patients with lesions of the temporal systems and the participation of external speech support in the performance of various intellectual operations, and it cannot be doubted that a determined analysis of these problems will shed considerable light on this relatively unexplored field.

I have described the disturbances of audioverbal processes and of the forms of psychological activity connected with them that are found in patients with lesions of the lateral zones of the left temporal region.

Unfortunately we still know very little about the functions of the right temporal region and of the disturbances resulting from its lesions.

Clinical observations as a rule reveal no appreciable disturbances of verbal hearing or of speech processes in these cases. Symptoms of speech disorders, almost imperceptible in form, become apparent in patients with such lesions only if features of left-handedness are well marked, and for that reason lesions of the right temporal lobe in right-handed persons as a rule are symptom free.

Some workers have noted that patients with lesions of the right temporal region may be unaware of the left side in the acoustic or visual field, that massive lesions of the right temporal lobe may give rise to phenomena of hyperamusia or, sometimes, disturbances of musical hearing (Part II, Section 2D) and, finally, that symptoms of disturbances arising in lesions of the right temporal region (imprecise evaluation of time, sometimes disturbances of recognition of pictures) are superposed on a background of disinhibitedness and impulsiveness, characteristic features of syndromes resulting from lesions of the nondominant right hemisphere. All that can be said at present is that the symptomatology of disturbances of higher cortical functions in lesions of the right temporal lobe still awaits detailed investigation.

G. DISTURBANCE OF PSYCHOLOGICAL PROCESSES IN LESIONS OF THE MEDIAL ZONES OF THE TEMPORAL REGIONS

So far we have described disturbances of higher psychological functions found in patients with lesions of the lateral zones of the temporal region (in particular, of the dominant, left hemisphere).

The lateral zones of the left temporal region belong to the central part of the auditory analyzer, and they play an important role in the processing of auditory (and audioverbal) information. Naturally, therefore, my attention was drawn initially to the description of disturbances exhibited in such cases in complex forms of analysis and synthesis of the sounds of speech and of speech processes taking place with their participation.

However, not all parts of the temporal region belong to cortical zones of the auditory analyzer. There are large portions of the temporal lobe which belong to completely different systems and which, as regards both their origin and their functional characteristics, must be given special attention.

In 1937, Klüver and Bucy originally described a unique combination of disturbances arising as the result of bilateral removal of the temporal region in monkeys. After this operation the animals showed distinct changes in visual perception, marked behavioral changes (associated with sudden attacks of rage), and certain memory disturbances, which at that time were insufficiently well understood. In the same year, Papez (1937) put forward the suggestion that the medial zones of the temporal region are very closely related to the central mechanisms of the emotions.

The descriptions given by Klüver, Bucy, and Papez prompted intensive research in the following years, with the result that an extensive literature began to appear in the 1940's and 1950's. The number of publications on the subject is now very large.

As a result of these investigations, attention was concentrated on the medial zones of the temporal region, which had hitherto attracted comparatively little interest; they belonged to the formations of the archicortex and paleocortex, and are components of the limbic region, which had not yet been adequately studied at that time. This region, previously included in the olfactory system, as much careful research subsequently showed, is in fact quite different in its origin, structure, connections, and functions.

As the now classical investigations of Filimonov (1949) showed originally, this region, partly belonging to the archicortex and partly to the paleocortex, exists even in animals which have no olfactory function (dolphins), and it differs completely from the neocortex in its cytoarchitectonic structure. Subsequent investigations showed that the limbic system and, in particular, the region of the hippocampus which forms part of it, has very close connections with the nonspecific nuclei of the thalamus and hypothalamic region and with the brain-stem reticular formation (McLean, 1955, 1959; Nauta, 1955, 1958; Pribram and Kruger, 1954; Pribram and Weiskrantz, 1957; Adey, 1958), and that these connections are responsible for the circulation of excitation around a circuit including the hippocampus, the nuclei of the thalamus and septum, and the mamillary bodies, which later came to be known in the literature as the "hippocampal circle" or "circle of Papez" (Fig. 33). The existence of this circle, which ensures a very close connection between the medial zones of the temporal region and the autonomic formations of the hypothalamus and nonspecific nuclei of the reticular formation, was also demonstrated by the observation that stimulation of the hippocampus evoked discharges in the anterior and dorsomedial nuclei of the thalamus (Adey, 1958; Green and Adey, 1956; Green, 1964), and that stimulation of the nuclei of the reticular formation evoked changes in hippocampal electrical activity.

These facts provided solid arguments for regarding the medial zones of the temporal region (especially the hippocampus) as a system which participates not so much in the analysis and synthesis of exteroceptive (predominantly acoustic) stimuli as in the regulation of the state of activity of the cerebral cortex as a whole. These suggestions are confirmed both by electrophysiological findings obtained by the use of microelectrode techniques (see above Part I, Section 2F) and also by observations on animals.

Numerous experiments by Pribram and co-workers (1954, 1957), McLean (1955, 1959), Olds (1958), and many others have shown that bilateral extirpation of the hippocampus causes substantial changes in an animal's behavior. Changes in the animal's needs or in its affective life are combined with changes in its state of wakefulness or with disturbances of its memory. The animals in these experiments developed noticeable changes in their inclinations and had sudden attacks of rage (as described previously by Klüver and Bucy); skills learned previously disappeared, and the animals were unable to acquire new ones. More recent experiments have shown that this region plays an essential role also in the mechanism

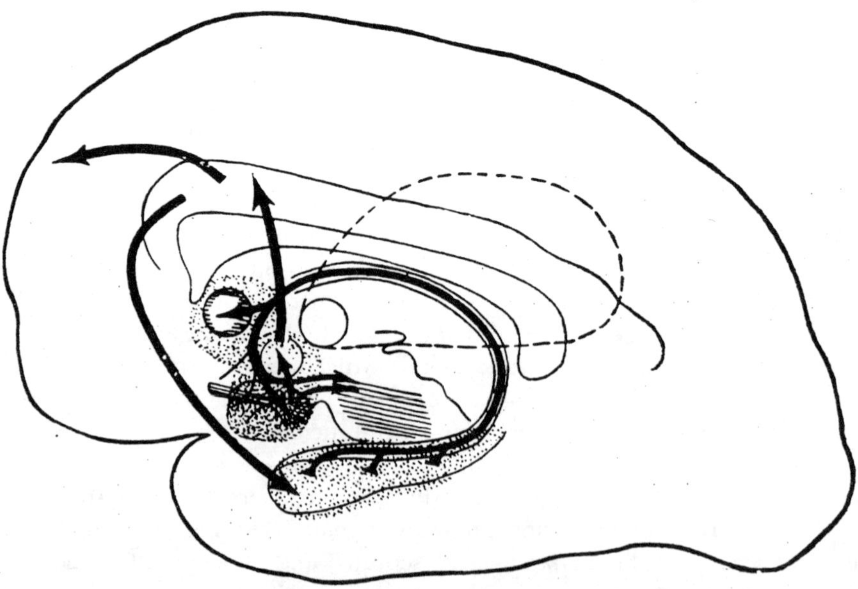

FIGURE 33 Scheme of the hippocampal circle (the circle of Papez).

of the orienting reflex, and for this reason the appearance of an orienting reflex evokes discharges in the hippocampal region (Adey, 1958; McAdam, 1962), whereas destruction of the hippocampus leads to marked changes in the orienting reaction (Grastyan, 1959).

It can accordingly be concluded that the medial zones of the temporal lobe belong to a system which regulates the state of activity of the animal and its emotions and that they play an important role in processes responsible for the preservation and activation of traces of impressions from the outside world. These suggestions were confirmed by clinical observations on patients with "temporal epilepsy" and with disturbances arising as a result of lesions of the deep zones and the medial formations.

Observations on patients with temporal epilepsy (Penfield and Ericson, 1941; Penfield and Jasper, 1954; Alajouanine, 1961; Bragina, 1965) have shown that stimulation of the medial temporal zones give rise not so much to audioverbal disorders and auditory hallucinations but rather to general affective changes and special states of consciousness. The aura of such epileptic fits frequently consists of accentuation of the sense of taste and emotional changes, disturbances of autonomic processes, and general motor excitation. These facts are all added evidence of the role of the medial formations of the brain in the regulation of the general tone of brain activity.

Similar results indicating the role of the medial temporal zones in the regulation of states of wakefulness were obtained in observations on stationary changes in behavior which arise following the destruction of this region by a pathological process or resection.

Observations made by various workers and generalized by Bragina (1965) showed that deep tumors affecting the medial zones of the temporal region and adjacent formations are manifested primarily as changes in the waking state and emotional sphere of the patient. Such patients very often show fluctuations of their state of consciousness, sometimes falling into a state of drowsiness: they are no longer sure of their bearings and they start to experience vague emotionally colored sensations, assuming the form of general alarm or anxiety, sometimes accompanied by visual or auditory hallucinations, but more often with the character of general confusion. Frequently these pathological foci evoke characteristic motor disorders which assume the character of stupor or of generalized restless movements (Bragina, 1965).

The changes observed in patients with lesions of the medial temporal zones and adjacent formations are reflected particularly clearly in the *patient's general memory.* It is in the patients of this group that we find an impairment of direct trace retention, which in the less severe cases leads to a fluctuating state of consciousness, but in patients with massive lesions of this region causes profound disturbances of imprinting with a picture resembling Korsakov's syndrome.

At the beginning of the century, Bekhterev (1900) drew attention to the fact that bilateral lesions of the anteromedial temporal zones can lead to severe disturbances of memory reminiscent in many respects of Korsakov's syndrome: similar observations were made later by Gilyarovskii (1912) and by Grünthal, who described a profound disturbance of memory in patients with lesions of the mammillary bodies (1939) and, later still, in bilateral lesions of the hippocampal cortex (1947). Finally, a few years later, Scoville (1954), and Milner (1957), and Penfield and Milner (1958) described similar disturbances of memory caused by bilateral resection of the hippocampal region. Similar observations also were made by Walker (1957), Baldwin (1956), and others after unilateral temporal lobectomy.

A profound disturbance of states of consciousness and of direct trace imprinting can be observed both during the sequelae of acute trauma (accompanied by diencephalic lesions) and in patients with deep tumors in the temporal region (Shmar'yan, 1949).

A very distinctive picture was observed in a systematic neuropsychological investigation of these cases by Popova (1964) under the author's direction. Patients with massive lesions of the medial temporal zones, although sometimes showing definite changes in the emotional state (alarm, depression, anxiety), as a rule exhibited marked changes of consciousness. In the milder cases these changes consisted of instability and fluctuation of general tone, so that when they were given problems to solve sometimes they succeeded, but sometimes they did not. In patients with more massive lesions cortical tone was so reduced that the patients easily passed into a level of consciousness marked by drowsiness, and their orientation in their surroundings became distinctly unstable.

Disturbances of these patients' direct memory are particularly clear. Traces from external environmental influences are imprinted insufficiently firmly in these patients, and sometimes they disappear after only a short time; if the lesion is not confined to the medial temporal zones but also affects the diencephalon, these defects may be manifested particularly clearly. Such patients have a confused notion of time, they can be seriously wrong in their estimate of the time of day, they cannot say whether they have eaten a meal or not; they do not clearly recognize the physician treating them, and sometimes if the person examining them is absent from the ward for 10 or 15 minutes, they greet him on his return as someone they do not know or they declare that it was several days since he was last with them.

Such patients can correctly repeat a series of words presented to them without any transpositions or inaccuracies such as are characteristic of patients with lesions of the lateral zones of the left temporal region; if, however, they are requested to repeat the same series of words after an interval of 3 or 4 minutes, not only can not they do so, but often they cannot even remember that they have just taken part in a test. A similar situation arises in tests of relating the theme of stories. Having correctly related the meaning of a fragment immediately after it was read to them, ten minutes later they do not even recall that a story was read to them, and even after prompting their recollection of the theme is very vague (Popova, 1964). Sometimes these defects of trace retention are accompanied by confabulations. The patient's attitude, however, is that he cannot be sure that these confabulations correspond to the forgotten theme.

Because of the instability of preservation of direct traces, the patients of this group have noticeable difficulty in Konorski's test, in which the subject has to decide whether two stimuli, applied at intervals of 1.5–2 min, are similar or different; in such tests these patients give many more incorrect answers than patients with lesions elsewhere in the brain.

Another feature of this group of patients (in whom a lesion of the medial zones of the left temporal region spread to diencephalic formations) was the instability of their fixed set phenomena; the illusion obtained during testing by Uznadze's method disappeared after a pause of only 5–7 sec (Filippycheva and Konovalov, unpublished investigation).

If we add to this the fact that the disturbances described above are superposed upon distinct autonomic changes, clearly the pattern of disturbances arising in lesions of the medial temporal zones and adjacent formations becomes sufficiently well defined.

The above facts show how functions of the medial temporal zones differ from those of the lateral temporal zones, and they emphasize how different in character are the disturbances of psychological processes which accompany these lesions.

3. *Disturbances of Higher Cortical Functions with Lesions of the Occipital and Occipitoparietal Regions*

In our account of the symptomatology of lesions of the temporal region we described pathological changes in hearing and in the complex forms of its organization through speech. When we turn to the subject of lesions of the occipital and occipitoparietal regions, we move to a different group of disturbances of the analytic-synthetic activity of the brain.

As long ago as 1878, when discussing the "elements of thought," Sechenov (see Sechenov, 1947) suggested that the whole system comprising the complex forms of activity of the human sense organs may be divided into two large categories. Whereas the complexes of *sound signals* arriving from the external environment are *integrated into successive series*, the complexes of *visual and tactile stimuli* are combined into definite groups that reflect systems of *simultaneous* spatial influences. According to Sechenov, the combination of individual stimuli into successive series is the principle guiding auditory (and to some extent, motor) analysis and synthesis, whereas the combination of individual stimuli into simultaneous groups is the principle guiding visual and tactile analysis and synthesis. The central apparatus of visual and tactile analysis is encompassed in the occipital and parietal areas of the cerebral cortex.

The disturbances affecting simultaneous synthesis arising in association with lesions of these areas of the brain may take different forms. Whereas in lesions of the occipital areas of the cortex, representing the cortical termination of the visual analyzer, we may expect to find disturbances of highly specialized (visual) forms of analysis and synthesis, in lesions of the parietal areas, i.e., of the cortical termination of the cutaneokinesthetic analyzer, the disturbances are confined to the tactile sphere; finally, in lesions of those cortical regions forming part of the overlapping zone of the central ends of the visual and tactile analyzers and responsible for the most complex forms of joint activity of these analyzers, the defects of simultaneous synthesis may acquire a particularly complex character and lead to intricate forms of disturbance of spatial perception.

The disturbance of simultaneous synthesis associated with lesions of the occipital and occipitoparietal cortical divisions may be seen to affect processes differing in complexity. In some cases it may be nothing more than a disturbance of sensory syntheses, manifested by defects of visual or olfactory perception and partially compensated for by the connections of the second signal system which are still preserved. Examples of such disorders are the visual and tactile agnosias arising from lesions of the occipital or parietal areas. In more complicated cases these disturbances may mainly be apparent in the more complex mnestic processes and may alter the basis of the symbolic forms of activity, especially of speech activity, which require simultaneous spatial synthesis for their execution. In these cases the lesions lead to more complex, secondary disturbances, clinically known as "semantic aphasia," "acalculia," and other forms of impairment of complex perceptual operations.

This group of disturbances will now be considered, starting with the relatively simple forms. Those changes in the higher cortical functions that have been more closely studied from the clinical point of view, and which may help in the interpretation of the functional pathology of these cerebral areas, will receive primary attention.

A. HISTORICAL SURVEY

The study of disturbances of visual processes arising from lesions of the occipital regions of the brain began with the clinical analysis of the phenomena of total or partial central blindness and of visual agnosia. This branch of neurology then became associated with a cycle of investigations on disturbances of the more complex forms of perceptual activity arising from lesions of closely situated regions. The two groups of investigations are closely associated in the history of science, and they must therefore be described together.

In 1855 the Italian neurologist Panizza reported an important finding: Permanent blindness developed in individuals with a lesion of the occipital region. He called this condition "central blindness." This discovery of central blindness was later augmented by observations that animals with such lesions retained sight but lost the more complex forms of visual perception. In the latter half of the last century, Munk (1881) observed that destruction of the occipital divisions of the cerebral hemispheres of the dog leads to a characteristic phenomenon: The dog retains its ability to see and to avoid objects but it ceases to "recognize" them. The idea that pathological changes of perception are possible in a form in which the animal retains its elementary visual functions yet cannot recognize objects was later applied to clinical medicine, where it prompted the appearance of an extensive literature on the question of defects of visual and tactile perception in man arising from circumscribed lesions of the occipital and parietal regions of the brain.

Somewhat earlier, Jackson (1876) had postulated the existence of distinctive clinical "imperception," phenomena in which the patient's sensory processes are apparently preserved although the ability to recognize objects is not. Freud (1891) reached a similar conclusion a little later, and applied the name "agnosia" to these phenomena, by which he meant a disturbance of the optical perception of an object although all the elementary processes of visual sensation are preserved. Similar accounts of "mental blindness" were given by Charcot (1886–1887), Lissauer (1889), and others. The patients observed by these writers also retained their vision, apparently without loss of acuity, but could not recognize objects presented to them. Sometimes these patients could describe the individual parts, even quite small ones, of objects and could reproduce their outline accurately, yet they were quite unable to recognize the objects as a whole. Although these writers described the clinical facts fully, they found great difficulty in explaining them.

Some, like Munk, went no further than to state that "the animal can see but cannot recognize," although, as Pavlov repeatedly pointed out later, this does not pave the way for further investigation. Others, following Finkelburg (1870), attempted to explain imperception not by a disturbance of vision, but by a disturbance of the complex symbolic function, the "Facultas signatrix" of Kant, and interpreted the disturbance of recognition of objects as a special form of "asymbolia." Finally, a third group, continuing the traditions of associative psychology, believed that these phenomena, subsequently named "agnosia," are manifestations of a disturbance of the "visual images of memory" or a disturbance of the secondary analysis of intact visual perceptions. These authors assumed that the material basis of this defect was a disturbance of the associative connections between the visual region of the cortex and a hypothetical "center of ideas," which they localized in Flechsig's great posterior associative center. This position was subsequently accepted by writers such as Broadbent (1872), Kussmaul (1885), Lichtheim (1885), Charcot (1886–1887), and others without further analysis.

The view of agnosia as a disorder of memory or of ideas or a defect of some form of symbolic function, and not as a true disturbance of vision, persisted for a long time in the neurological and psychopathological literature. The classical writings of Lissauer (1889) included descriptions of two different forms of visual agnosia; in one the patient ceases to differentiate and integrate the components of the visual image of an object, and in the other he continues to see the object clearly but cannot recognize it. These forms were described as "apperceptive" and "associative" mental blindness, respectively.

The arbitrary gap between elementary sensory processes and the higher forms of perception, lying at the root of most of the classical studies of agnosia, soon came to be regarded as unsatisfactory, and at the beginning of the present century there were requests for more accurate studies of the state of the sensory processes in patients with optic agnosia. Attempts were made to discover changes caused by the pathological process and to fill the artificial gap separating the pathology of the "elementary" and "higher" cortical functions.

The first attempts to abandon the concept of agnosia as a disorder of recognition quite unconnected with vision were made by Monakow (1914) and his pupil Stauffenberg (1914, 1918). Both of these workers claimed that the disorder of cognitive activity in the visual agnosias must be interpreted as a disorganization of visual processes of different complexity or as the result of pathological changes in the visual divisions of the cerebral cortex that disturb the "subsequent process of synthetic vision."

These investigations laid the foundations for a whole series of investigations aimed at studying optic agnosia in terms of disturbances of visual activity per se. With exceptional thoroughness, various clinical forms of visual disturbance were described (Poppelreuter, 1917–1918; Holmes, 1919; Gelb and Goldstein, 1920; Pötzl, 1928; Kleist, 1934; Lange, 1936; Denny-Brown and co-workers [Denny-Brown, Meyer, and Horenstein, 1952, etc.]; Zangwill and co-workers [Paterson and Zangwill, 1944, 1945; Ettlinger, Warrington, and Zangwill, 1957; etc.]; Bay, 1950; Hécaen and Ajuriaguerra, 1956, etc.). In an attempt to explain the findings, Pötzl (1928) made various suppositions regarding the physiological phenomena arising in pathological states of the cortex of the occipital and occipitoparietal regions. Some of the other workers cited (Holmes, Zangwill, etc.) claimed the existence of changes in "visual attention." A third group of workers (Teuber, 1959; Semmes *et al.*, 1960), while accepting the idea of the presence of a disturbance of integrative processes, emphasized the narrowing of the range of simultaneously perceived signals as the principal sign of a pathological state of the brain. Denny-Brown and co-workers (1952) suggested that the inability to combine perceived elements into a unified whole be called a disturbance of "amorphosynthesis."

These attempts to draw nearer to a physiological analysis of the relatively more elementary sensory phenomena lying at the root of the agnosias reflect what must be regarded as the most progressive tendencies in modern neurology. Admittedly, some writers detract from the value of their analysis by limiting it to the schemes put forward by Gestalt psychologists, who believe that a change in the relationship of figure and background is the basis of the pathology of perception (Gelb and Goldstein, 1920); others (Stein and Weizsäcker, 1927, and, more recently, Bay 1950), on the other hand, attempt to reduce complex amnestic defects to a disturbance of the excitability of individual points of the retina or to the manifestations of the instability of the optic function ("*Funktionswandel*"). There can be no doubt, however, that the pathophysiological analysis of the agnosias will yield facts that will put this subject on a firm scientific basis.

The history of the study of the optic agnosias is thus the history of the description of the distinctive features of different forms of disturbed visual perception and the history of attempts to make a pathophysiological analysis of the mechanisms lying at the root of these changes. What are the neurophysiological mechanisms which may help us to understand these phenomena? This is a question of crucial importance and we shall now examine it.

B. THE VISUAL ANALYZER AND THE STRUCTURE OF THE VISUAL CORTEX

The main obstacle in the way of a correct understanding of the cerebral mechanisms of optic perception and of the physiological analysis of the phenomena of optic agnosia has been the *receptor theory of sensation and perception*, which dominated the psychological and neurological thought of the nineteenth and early twentieth centuries.

As stated, this theory postulated that sensation is a passive process resulting from the stimulation of the organs of the senses by external agents. Excitation from the retina is directed to the receptor centers of the cerebral cortex, where it acquires the character of sensations; only then are these sensations combined into perceptions, which in turn are analyzed and converted into the more complex units of perceptual activity. The first stages of this complex process were regarded as elementary and passive physiological operations and the last stages were regarded as complex and active mental forms of activity. This theory inevitably led to the postulated gap between the elementary and higher forms of perceptual activity to which we have referred.

A different approach to many of these phenomena is provided by the reflex conception of perception, originated by Sechenov and developed experimentally by Pavlov. In more recent psychophysiological investigations (Granit, 1955; Sokolov, 1958; etc.) this theory has also been applied to the study of human perception. According to the reflex theory, sensation and perception are active processes distinguished by a degree of selectivity and incorporating efferent (motor) components. The physiological mechanisms of this selective analysis and synthesis of stimuli were studied by Pavlov and his collaborators, who laid the foundations for the understanding of the physiology of the analyzers. The analyzers were considered responsible for the discrimination of "signal" (essential to the organism) signs and for the rejection of unessential signs. This made up the core of the reflex theory of perception.

From the point of view of the reflex theory many of the mechanisms of perception began to take on different significance. Sechenov declared that every act of visual perception incorporates both centripetal (afferent) and centrifugal (efferent) mechanisms. When it perceives objects in the external environment, the eye actively "senses" them, and these sensing movements are incorporated, along with the proprioceptive signals from the oculomotor muscles, as elements of visual perception. Sechenov's discovery was the starting point of a large series of investigations that yielded a rich harvest, especially during recent years, when technological advances have made it possible to record the electrophysiological phenomena taking place in the various parts of the visual analyzer from the retina to the visual cortex. Recordings showed that the processes taking place in the various parts of the optic pathways are not unidirectional (centripetal) but bidirectional (centripetal-centrifugal or afferent-efferent) in nature and that, along with the discharges recorded in the optic nerve and the higher, central portions of the visual analyzer, changes may also be detected in the retina during stimulation of the central portions of the optic apparatus. These facts, reflecting well-known psychological phenomena (for example, the increase in visual acuity due to active fixation of attention or due to the subject's orientation), were studied physiologically by Granit (1955), who described changes in the retinal potentials occurring under the influence of central stimulation, and by Sokolov (1958, 1959), who examined the role of orienting reactions in perception and in the complex forms of selective sensory processes that are possible only in the presence of cortical dominance. These investigations demonstrated the selective character of the processes of perception taking place with the participation of the system of two-directional (afferent-efferent) connections and provided the factual basis for the reflex theory of sensation.

What is the apparatus responsible for the complex analytico-synthetic processes lying at the root of the visual-tactile forms of perception? What do we know of its structural and functional characteristics? How are we to envisage the disturbances of perceptual activity developing from lesions of this apparatus?

We shall first describe as briefly as possible what is known about the structure of the visual analyzer, especially of its cortical divisions.

• • •

To fully describe the structure of the visual portions of the cerebral cortex, situated in the occipital region, would be to duplicate much that has already been said in the description of the structure of the cortical divisions of the auditory analyzer. Therefore, the relevant facts will be summarized on the basis of the most general features.

In contrast to the other peripheral receptors, the retina is a highly complex nervous structure, considered by some writers to be a part of the cerebral cortex which has moved toward the outer surface of the body. In a series of inner layers of the retina there are groups of neurons, some of which receive excitation arising in the light-sensitive cells of the outer layer, and transmit it in the form of isolated or combined impulses along the fibers of the optic nerve to the central nervous formations. Other groups of neurons receive efferent impulses arriving from the central formations, and act as apparatuses for effecting the central regulation of the excitability of individual points of the retina.

This apparatus, highly complex in structure, is shown schematically in Fig. 34. The presence of elements providing for both the centripetal and the centrifugal organization of impulses demonstrates the reflex, afferent-efferent structural principle of this peripheral part of the visual analyzer. Hence, the retina is an apparatus that not only receives specific stimuli from the outside, but also is regulated by direct influences from central impulses that modify the excitability of individual receptor elements and thus break up or unify the structure of excitation.

The impulses of excitation arising in the retina are transmitted along the optic fibers, partially decussating in the chiasma, to the central subcortical and cortical nervous apparatuses, i.e., to the lateral geniculate body and nuclei of the thalamus and thence to the visual portions of the occipital region of the cerebral cortex. Until recently it was believed that the fibers of the optic nerve, the optic tract, and that part of the optic pathway that passes within the white matter of the cerebral hemispheres and is called the "optic radiation" are wholly centripetal and afferent. However, Polyak (1957), Shkol'nik-Yarros (1958), and others have shown that all these parts of the optic pathway also contain a considerable number of centripetal afferent fibers and that the central apparatus of vision is thus reflex in character in the full meaning of this word.

The scheme developed by Shkol'nik-Yarros (Fig. 35) shows that most fibers passing from the retina relay in the nuclei of the lateral geniculate body pass to that part of

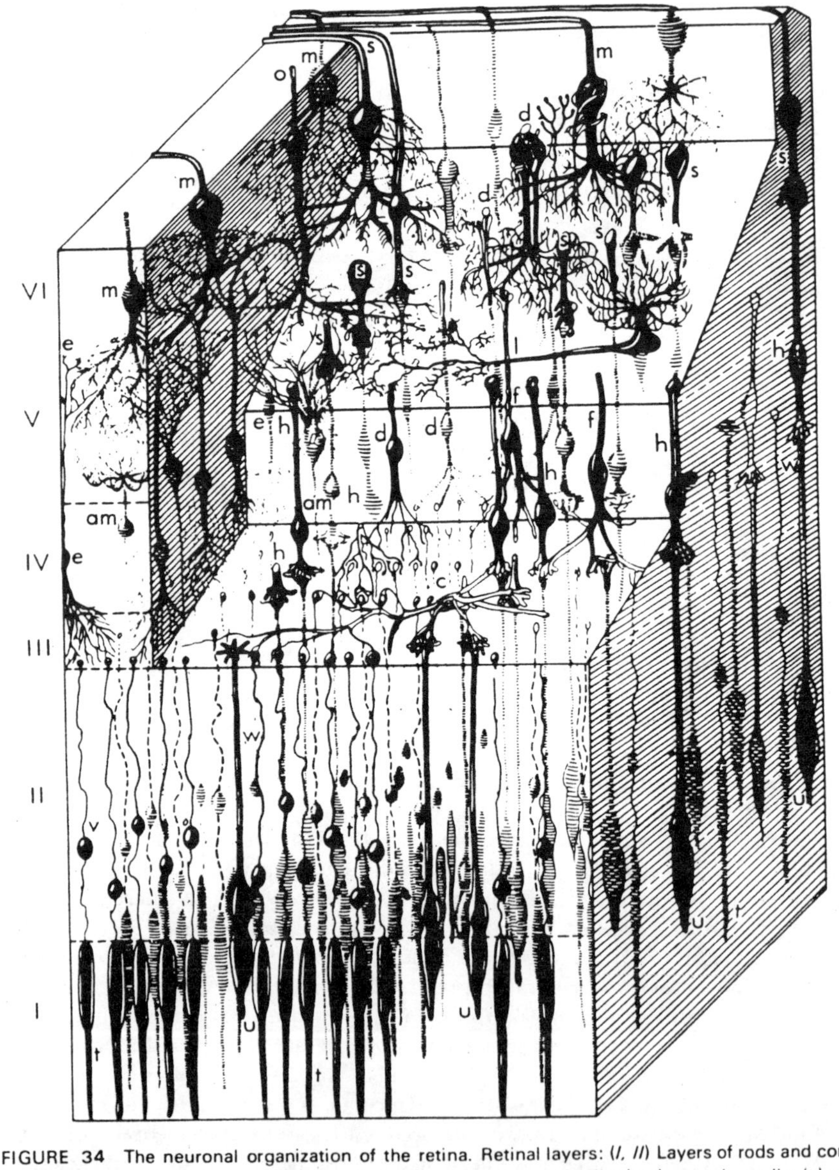

FIGURE 34 The neuronal organization of the retina. Retinal layers: (*I, II*) Layers of rods and cones: (*III–V*) layers of bipolar cells; (*VI*) layer of ganglion cells. Types of cells: (*am*) amacrine cells; (*c*) outer horizontal cells; (*l*) inner horizontal cells; (*d–h*) bipolar cells; (*m–s*) ganglionic cells; (*t–u*) receptive parts of cones and rods. (*From Krieg, 1942.*)

the occipital portion of the cortex situated at the pole of the occipital region and then run along its medial surface. This area (Area 17) can justifiably be regarded as

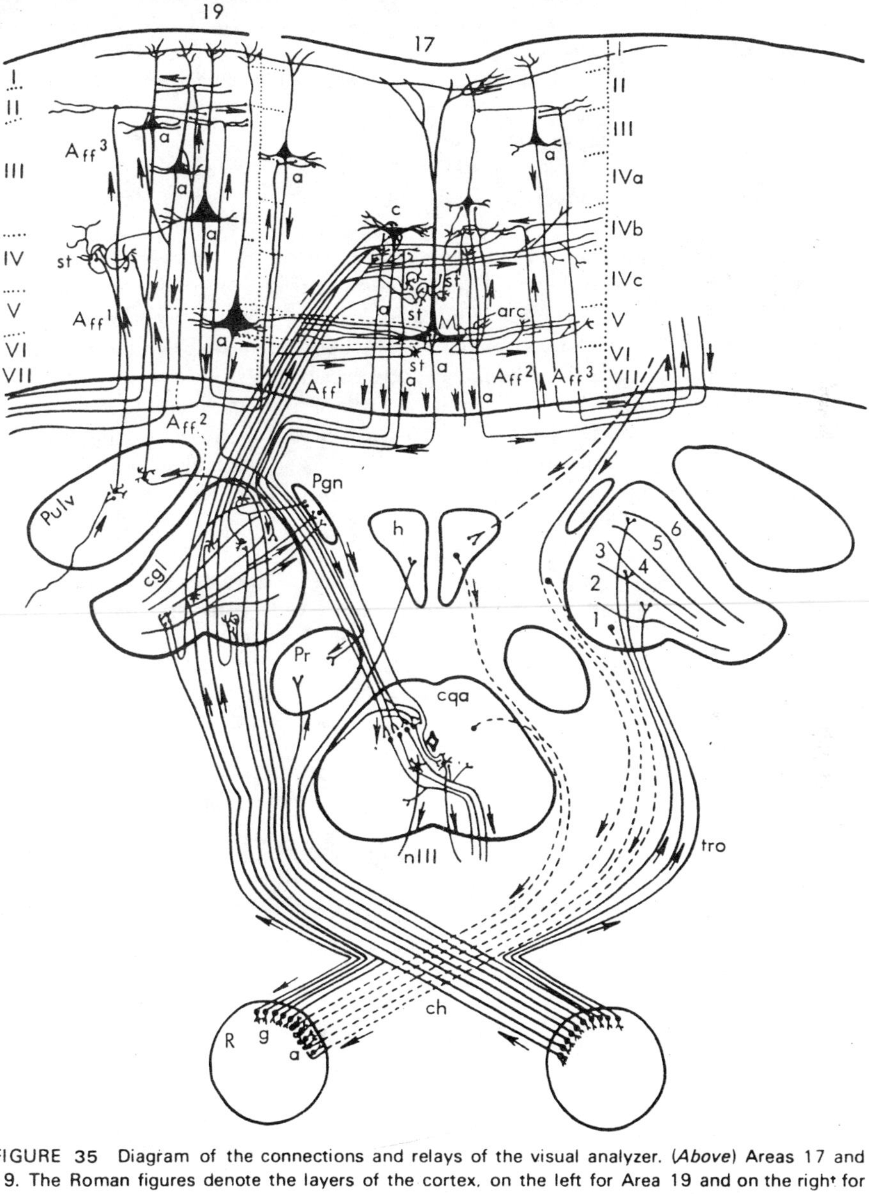

FIGURE 35 Diagram of the connections and relays of the visual analyzer. (*Above*) Areas 17 and 19. The Roman figures denote the layers of the cortex, on the left for Area 19 and on the right for Area 17. Area 18, situated between Areas 17 and 19, is not designated on the scheme. (*Middle*) Subcortical formations. (*Below*) Retina. Centripetal (continuous lines) and centrifugal (broken lines) connections of the retina are shown. (*Pulv*) Pulvinar; (*cgl*) lateral geniculate body; (*Pgn*) pregeniculate nucleus; (*h*) hypothalamus; (*Pr*) pretectal nucleus; (*cqa*) anterior corpora quadragemina; (*nIII*) oculomotor nerve; (*ch*) chiasma; (*R*) retina; (*g*) ganglionic cells of retina; (*a*) amacrine cells of retina; (*tro*) optic tract. The arrows denote the direction of transmission of excitation. (*Composed from personal observations and data from the literature [Minkowski, Le Gros Clark, Polyak, Cajal, Novokhatskii, Chow, etc.] by Shkol'nik-Yarros, 1958.*)

the primary field of the cortical nucleus of the visual analyzer. A few afferent fibers, after relaying in the lateral geniculate body and passing to the secondary (ventral and posterior) nuclei of the thalamus, reach the divisions of the occipital cortex (Areas 18 and 19), which may be called the "wide visual sphere" (Pötzl, 1928) or the secondary fields of the cortical nucleus of the visual analyzer (Part I, Section 2).

All of the fields of the visual portion of the cortex that have been referred to give rise to both afferent fibers, directed toward the subcortical optic nuclei and thence to the retina, and associative fibers, passing from Area 17 to Areas 18 and 19 and vice versa. Together they constitute the reflex apparatus of the visual cortex, responsible for the complex acts of visual perception and, therefore, whose pathology is of interest to us.

The topical organization of the visual cortex itself is just as important as the afferent-efferent structure of the conducting system of the optic perception. Since the time of Brouwer (1917–1932, summarized in 1936) it has been known that the fibers leaving the retina are arranged in strict order, so that definite parts of the lateral geniculate body and of the projection areas of the visual portion of the cortex correspond to definite areas of the retina (Fig. 36). For this reason, stimulation of the corresponding points of the visual cortex causes photopsia in definite parts of the visual field while destruction of these parts leads to a strictly defined inactivation of the corresponding (contralateral) parts of the visual field, with the development of hemianopsia or scotoma. These phenomena were investigated in detail by Teuber (1960).

Next to the central or projection area of the cortical nucleus of the visual analyzer lie the secondary visual fields, or the fields of the wide visual sphere (Areas 18 and 19). They differ in their cytoarchitectonic structure from Area 17 in that their fourth afferent layer of cells becomes narrowed and is overshadowed by the more highly

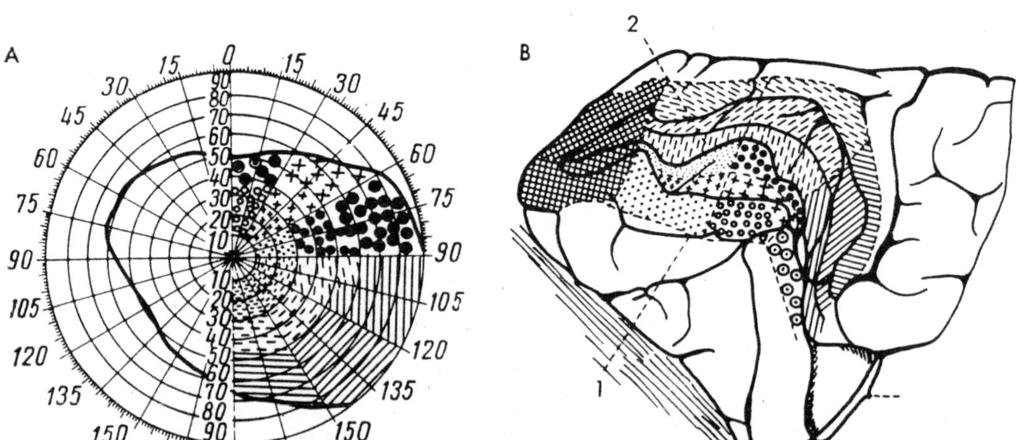

FIGURE 36 Projection of the retina on the cortex showing the correlation between areas of the visual zone of the cortex (Area 17) and areas of the visual field. (*a*) Visual field; (*b*) visual zone of the cortex. (*1*) Lower lip of calcarine fissure; (*2*) upper lip of calcarine fissure. (*After Holmes, 1938.*)

developed, mainly associative, complex of the second and third layer. As is also the case in the secondary auditory portion of the cortex, fibers pass to Areas 18 and 19 from nuclei of the thalamus having no direct connection with periphery, carrying impulses that have already received preliminary analysis in the subjacent subcortical formations (Polyak, 1957; etc.). These zones (like Area 22 of the temporal cortex) thus also belong to the group of secondary cortical zones.

Neuronographic investigations conducted on animals by von Bonin, Garol, and McCulloch (1942) and others have shown that this architectonic structure of the secondary fields of the occipital region is associated with particular physiological properties. It is clear from Fig. 37 that with stimulation of the projection areas of the visual portion of the cortex (Area 17) the spread of excitation is limited to that particular field whereas the effect of stimulation of Area 18 is much more widely felt, with possible detection in adjacent or more distant parts of the same hemisphere and even in the opposite hemisphere. If we are to believe the findings of these workers, local stimulation of Area 19 leads to an equally extensive (although opposite in sign) inhibitory effect.

Similar results were obtained in man with stimulation of the occipital region of the cortex of patients on the operating table. Investigations started by Hoff and Pötzl (1930) and extended by Penfield (1941, 1954, etc.) showed that stimulation of the projection areas of the occipital region is followed only by the development of elementary visual sensations (colored rings, fog, tongues of flame, etc.) while stimulation of the secondary divisions of the occipital cortex leads to more complex and significant visual hallucinations, with the reanimation of visual images formed by the patient in the past. Figure 38 shows points of the cortex whose stimulation has produced visual hallucinations. The belief that the work of individual areas of the visual cortex differs in its complexity is confirmed by the results of these experiments.

The role of the occipital portion of the cortex in the analysis and synthesis of visual stimuli was investigated in detail by Pavlov and his collaborators

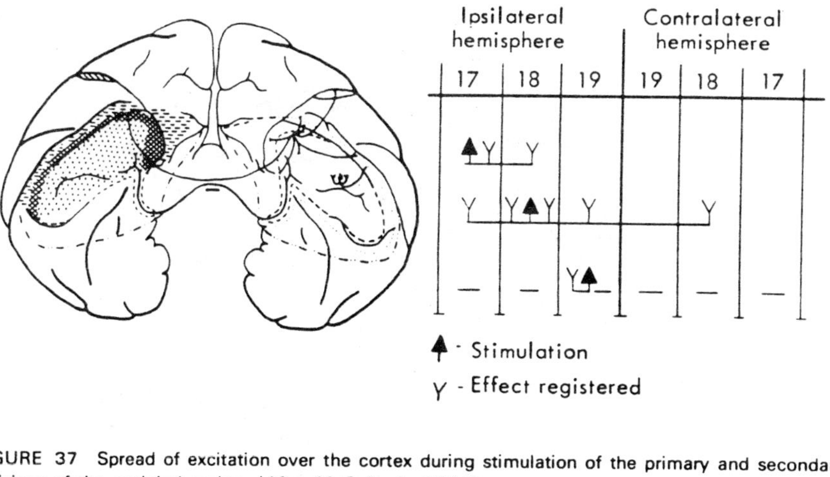

FIGURE 37 Spread of excitation over the cortex during stimulation of the primary and secondary divisions of the occipital region. (*After McCulloch, 1944.*)

in dogs, by Lashley (1930–1942) in rats, and by Klüver (1927, 1937, 1941) in monkeys. These workers showed that, although at lower evolutionary levels the elementary forms of visual analysis and synthesis can still be carried out by the subcortical formations, even in rodents extirpation of the occipital portion of the cortex, while it permits gross recognition of light, makes the discrimination of shapes quite impossible. Still more serious disturbances of visual analysis and synthesis are found after extirpation of these cortical areas in primates. The most significant fact, however, as Pavlov and his school demonstrated, is that extirpation of the occipital portion of the cortex in the dog leads not so much to a decrease in visual acuity as to a disturbance of the more complex forms of analysis and synthesis of visual signals. Research conducted by this school showed that conditioned reflexes can be formed in a dog after extirpation of the occipital region only in response to simple visual cues and that more complex forms of differentiation based on the discrimination between more detailed visual cues (shape, color, etc.) cannot be achieved; the reactions to these visual signals lose their selective character. This disturbance in selectivity is the feature that, according to Pavlov's theory, reflects the functional state of the visual portion of the cortex.

Similar findings in monkeys were obtained more recently by American workers (Chow, 1952; Mishkin, 1954; Mishkin and Pribram, 1954; Orbach and Fantz, 1958; etc.). They showed that extirpation of those parts of the cortex that constitute the homologous secondary fields of the cortical nucleus of the visual analyzer is followed by a marked disturbance in the development of complex visual differentiation, although the more elementary visual functions remain relatively preserved.

These experimental findings obtained in animals are of undoubted interest and contribute to the understanding of the general principles governing the

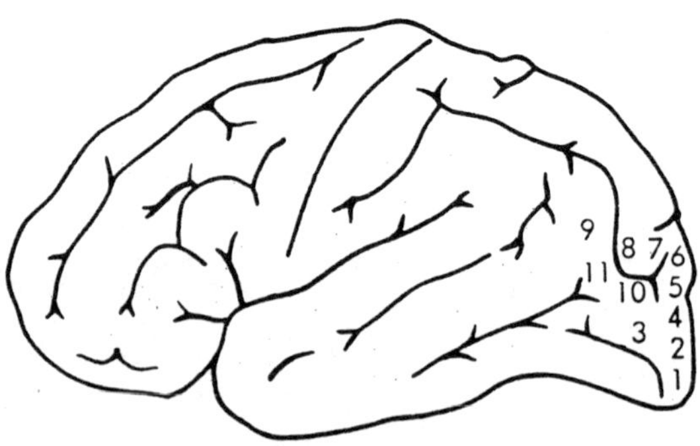

FIGURE 38 Diagram showing points of the occipital region whose stimulation causes visual hallucinations. Stimulation of Area 17: (*1*) "Illuminated balls"; (*2*) "colored light"; (*3*) "white light"; (*4*) "blue disk"; (*5*) "flame"; (*6*) "blue fog." Stimulation of Areas 18 and 19: (*7*) "faces, sounds coming from the side below"; (*8*) "a man coming from the side"; (*9*) "faces"; (*10*) "wild animals"; (*11*) "faces and butterflies." (*After Hoff and Pötzl, 1930, and others.*)

work of the visual cortex. However, the most valuable findings are those pertaining to the functional changes occurring in man as a result of lesions of the occipital region of the cerebral cortex.

C. DISTURBED OBJECT PERCEPTION WITH LESIONS OF THE VISUAL CORTEX AND CONCURRENT AGNOSIA

The complexity of the process of visual perception of objects and of the representation of objects is well known. Numerous investigations over a period of years, summarized in the recent survey by Bruner (1957), have shown that the apparent simplicity and directness of visual perception of an actual object or of its representation is often imaginary, for no sooner are the conditions of visual perception made slightly more difficult (for example, by making the relationship between object and background more complex or by presenting rapidly flashing shapes) than the true complexity of this process is at once fully apparent. It is in such cases that it becomes clear that the final recognition of objects, and of their representations in particular, is the result of complex perceptual activity, beginning with the identification of one particular sign of an object and the creation of a "perceptual hypothesis" and continuing with the selection of a particular sign from a series of alternatives; during the latter activity the important signs are brought to the foreground and are integrated, while the subsidiary, unimportant signs are inhibited.

Hence, investigation of visual perception under special conditions shows that it possesses a complex structure similar to that of tactile perception, whereby the hand successively and selectively palpates a series of signs and then gradually integrates them into a single, simultaneous entity (Kotlyarova, 1948; Anan'ev, 1959). Genetic investigations (Piaget, 1935; Zaporozhets, 1960; Zinchenko, 1958; etc.) have shown that the development of visual perception in the child passes through corresponding stages. Initially the hand feels the whole object and the eye examines it and only in the later stages do more abbreviated and refined forms of perception prevail. If the conditions of visual perception are made more complex, the process of orientation to the individual signs of a perceived object and, especially, of the representation of an object again reverts to the unshortened form and the examination is transformed into prolonged scanning of the object by the moving eye. Figure 39 shows the recorded eye movements during an examination of a photograph.

All of these results indicate that visual perception of an object or of its representation is a complex, active process, consisting of the identification of individual signs of the object or likeness, the integration of these signs into groups, and, finally, the selection of their meaning from a series of alternatives. This is a complicated reflex process requiring the participation of sensory and motor apparatuses, particularly the apparatus of eye movement (responsible for performing orienting and exploratory activity). It thus becomes clear why lesions of the occipital areas of the cerebral cortex lead to dissimilar, and sometimes highly complex, forms of disturbance of visual perception.

A few of these forms will be considered for a closer view of the psychophysiological aspect of the visual act.

A lesion of the primary area of the visual cortex (Area 17) is not followed by the specific disturbances of complex visual perception that have been discussed. Total destruction of the visual projection cortex of both hemispheres causes central blindness; the same degree of destruction limited to one hemisphere leads, as stated, to a unilateral (contralateral) loss of the field of vision (hemianopsia); a partial lesion of this area on one side leads to a localized manifestation of central blindness (scotoma). Nevertheless, the remaining, intact visual zone continues to function, as Gelb and Goldstein (1920) and Teuber (1960*a*) showed, and compensates successfully for the defect caused by constriction of the visual field. The recording made of the eye movements of a patient whose field of vision was constricted by

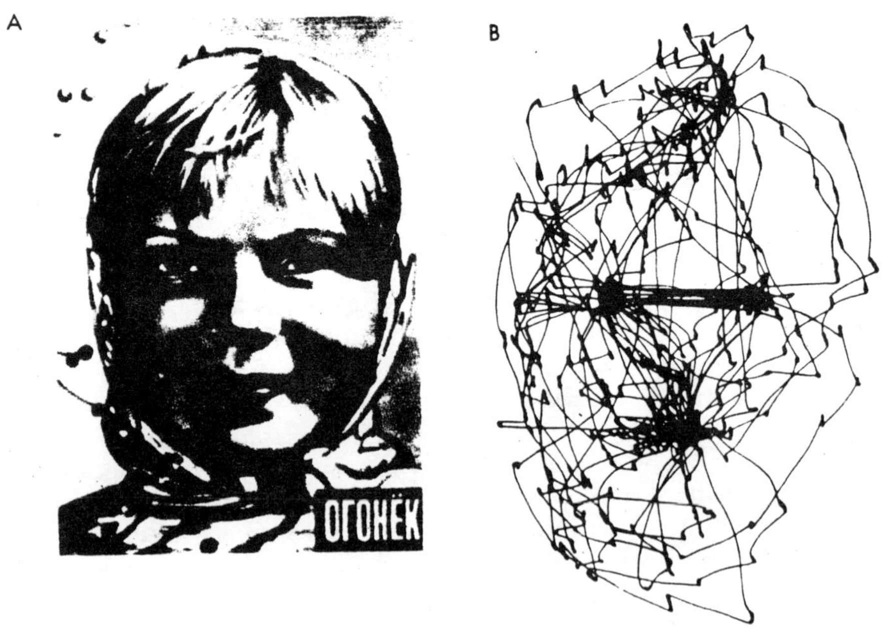

FIGURE 39 Eye movements during examination of a photograph by a normal subject. (*A*) Photograph given to subject for examination. (*B*) Recording of the eye movements during the examination of the photograph. (*After Yarbus, 1961.*)

opticochiasmal arachnoiditis to a narrow cone with an angle of only 6 to 8° is shown in Fig. 40. Similar compensatory eye movements apparently take place with lesions of the projection divisions of the occipital cortex accompanied by hemianopsia. In all of these cases the visual synthesis of integrated likenesses can still be achieved, and only during the early stages of the lesion (resulting from trauma or hemorrhage) is it possible to observe the gradual transition from total central blindness through indistinct intermediate stages to functionally perfect vision. With such lesions, however, the disturbance of vision does not assume the character of optic agnosia but takes the form of either a blurring of vision, which completely recedes after a short period (Pötzl, 1928), or of a partial loss of the field of vision.

It is quite a different matter if the lesion extends beyond the limits of the primary visual cortical fields. Investigations (Holmes and Horrax, 1919; Hoff, 1930; Brain, 1941; Paterson and Zangwill, 1944; Denny-Brown et al., 1952; Hécaen and Ajuriaguerra, 1956; etc.) have shown that unilateral lesions of the wide visual sphere, extending beyond the limits of the occipital pole and sometimes involving the parieto-occipital divisions of the cortex as well (especially if situated in the right hemisphere), may lead to phenomena outwardly similar to those just described yet essentially very different from them. In these cases, one of which has been described by us (Luria and Skorodumova, 1950), hemianopsia also occurs; it differs, however, in that one (usually the left) side of the field of vision is lost to the patient, the eye movements evidently play no part in compensating for the defect, and the hemianopsia becomes "fixed" in character. The patient suffers from that

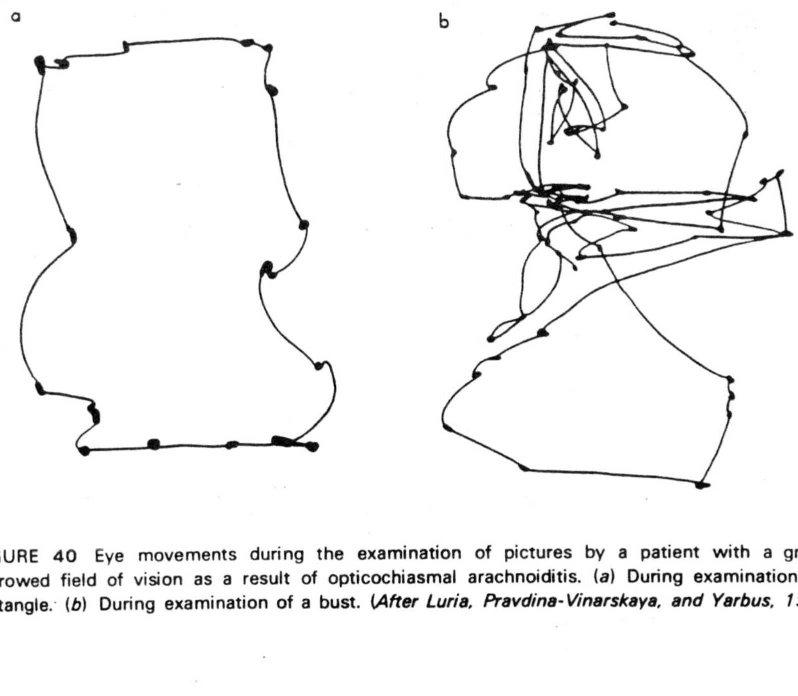

FIGURE 40 Eye movements during the examination of pictures by a patient with a grossly narrowed field of vision as a result of opticochiasmal arachnoiditis. (*a*) During examination of a rectangle. (*b*) During examination of a bust. (*After Luria, Pravdina-Vinarskaya, and Yarbus, 1961.*)

"unilateral spatial agnosia" (Ajuriaguerra and Hécaen, 1960) interpreted by some writers as a disturbance of visual attention and by others as a primary, unilateral disintegration of the visual process. An example of such a loss of the left half of the field of vision as revealed by the drawing of pictures is given in Fig. 41.

If the circumscribed lesion does not extend beyond the limits of the wide visual sphere (Areas 18 and 19) but involves both hemispheres or their connections, the disturbance of visual perception may become more severe and, at the same time, the nature of its structure may change. In such cases, known since the time of Willbrandt (1887) and Lissauer (1889) as cases of "optic agnosia," the patient appears to have no marked defect of visual acuity; nevertheless, his visual perception of objects and, in particular, of their representation is grossly impaired.

In the most extensive lesions of this region, a patient with the "classical" form of optic agnosia, which Lissauer (1889) described as "apperceptive mental blindness," cannot recognize by sight even the simplest objects and, in particular, pictures of simple objects (although he can recognize them by touch). In less severe cases he can recognize objects that are of simple structure or familiar but cannot correctly interpret more complicated objects, whose recognition calls for the identification and integration of a number of their more important signs. It is a significant fact that such a patient will usually pick out one particular sign and then go on to make logical guesses. He will try to decipher the meaning of the picture or object by a method based on

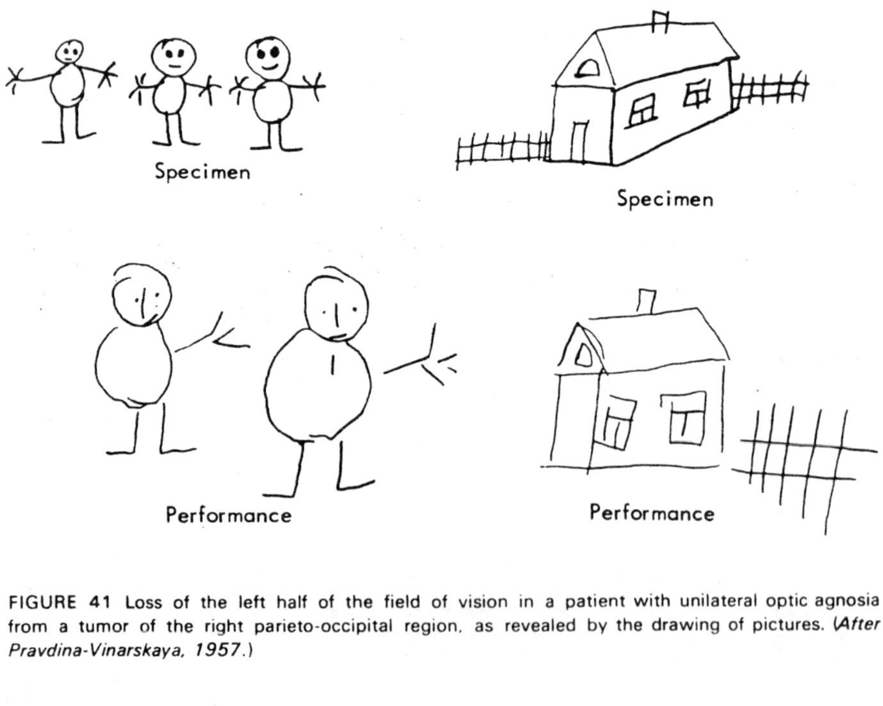

FIGURE 41 Loss of the left half of the field of vision in a patient with unilateral optic agnosia from a tumor of the right parieto-occipital region, as revealed by the drawing of pictures. (*After Pravdina-Vinarskaya, 1957.*)

verbal logic but frequently will reach wrong conclusions owing to the fact that it corresponds to the object under examination in only one respect. As examples, after a prolonged attempt a patient may tentatively call a picture of a pair of spectacles a bicycle ("a circle, then another circle, and some sort of crossbar . . . it must be a bicycle? . . . ") or may interpret a picture of a cock with bright colored feathers as "a fire, of course" (the feathers are tongues of flame); the picture of a sofa with two cushions becomes "an automobile, of course" (the cushions are headlamps), and a key is "something metallic and long . . . it must be a knife or spoon . . . ."

Sometimes during regression of this syndrome (for example, after removal of a tumor of the occipital region) these gross disturbances gradually disappear. And sometimes the patient who at first could not even distinguish between a line drawing and a written word begins to correctly identify drawings as the postoperative edema of the occipital regions of the brain subsides (Fig. 42).

In less marked cases these defects of visual perception of pictures may become apparent only when conditions are made more complicated, e.g., if unnecessary lines are drawn across the outline drawing of an object or if the pictures are presented in quick succession. An example of this type of disturbance is shown in Fig. 43.

Although the manifestations of optic agnosia were described long ago, insufficient attention has been paid to the study of their nature and we can do no more than suggest their psychological features and physiological mechanisms.

One fact stands out clearly in every case so far described: The structure of the visual act is incomplete. The patient identifies a particular sign from a complex object or picture or sometimes he may manage to pick out a second

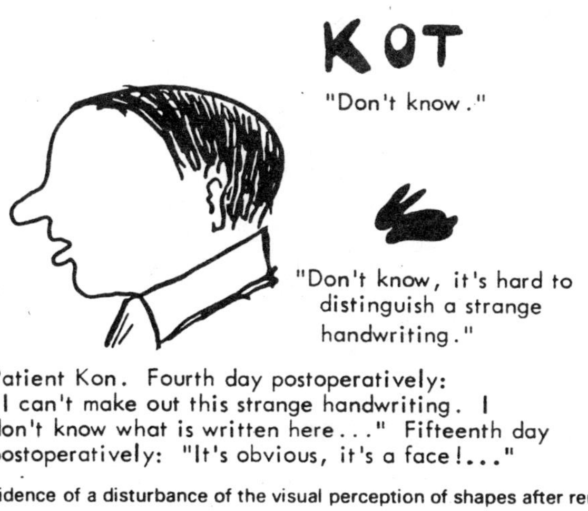
KOT
"Don't know."
"Don't know, it's hard to distinguish a strange handwriting."
Patient Kon. Fourth day postoperatively: "I can't make out this strange handwriting. I don't know what is written here..." Fifteenth day postoperatively: "It's obvious, it's a face!..."

FIGURE 42 Subsidence of a disturbance of the visual perception of shapes after removal of a tumor from the occipital region of the brain as revealed by the patient's growing ability to identify this drawing.

sign, but he cannot synthesize these signs visually and cannot convert them into the components of an integral whole.

Characteristically, the system of speech associations by means of which the patient attempts to compensate for his defect remains intact, and the process of visual analysis is converted into a series of spoken attempts to decipher the meaning of perceived signs and to integrate them into a whole visual image. Conclusions regarding the meaning of the picture as a whole, which patients with optic agnosia usually reach on the basis of individual signs of an object, thus frequently prove to be wrong or excessively general. For example, when attempting to identify the picture of a monkey, such a patient will say "eyes . . . mouth . . . of course, it's an animal!" If shown the picture of a telephone he may say "a dial . . . numbers . . . of course, it's a watch or some sort of machine!"

Evidence in support of this view was published by Birenbaum (1948). Patients with optic agnosia were shown partly uncovered pictures. It was found that these patients interpreted these incomplete pictures just as successfully as they did the complete pictures (of which they recognized only a

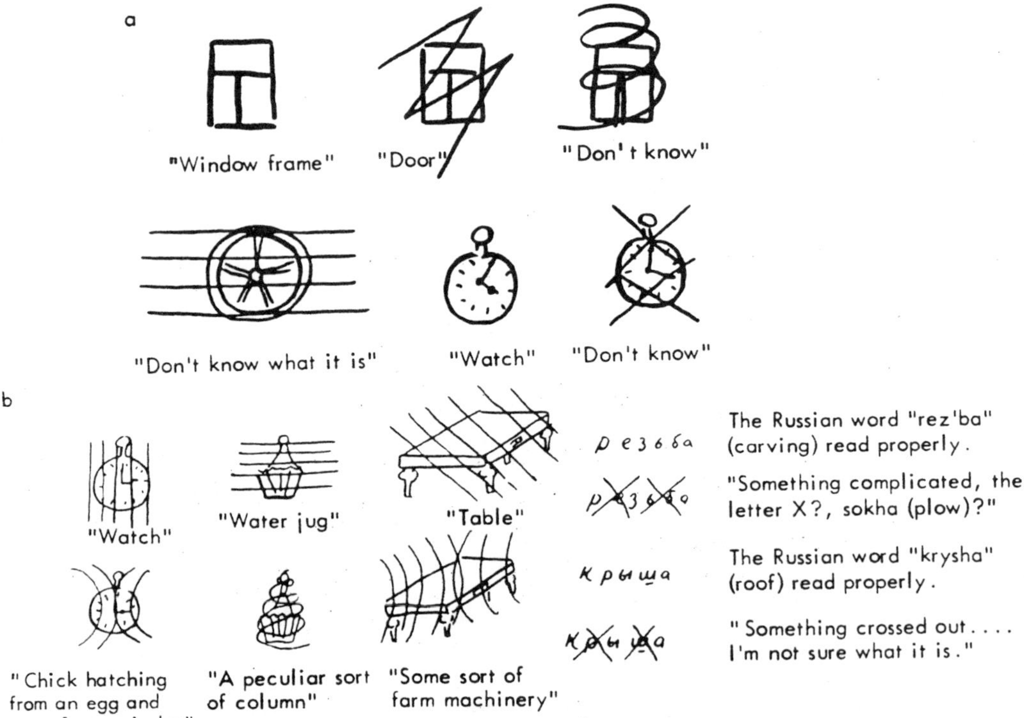

FIGURE 43 Disturbance of the perception of crossed-out figures in a patient with optic agnosia. (*a*) Patient Kon. Extracerebral tumor of occipital region. (*b*) Patient Eng. Deep area of softening in the left parieto-occipital region.

particular group of details) whereas normal subjects were much less successful in this regard.

Similar findings, indicating that the basic defect in optic agnosia is, in fact, a disturbance of the ability to synthesize isolated visual signs into an integral whole, may also be obtained by watching these patients draw. Examples of how a patient with optic agnosia draws an elephant and a man are given in Fig. 44. Although such patients draw the individual parts of the object reasonably well, they cannot integrate these parts into a complete drawing. The drawing of an elephant becomes a "graphic narration" of its details.

The foregoing observations suggest that the form of optic agnosia we have described is based neither on a disturbance of "memory images" (as postulated by Charcot, 1886–1887) nor on a disturbance of the symbolic function (Finkelburg, 1870, and subsequent writers). Rather, they suggest that optic agnosia is a complex visual disturbance of the synthesis of isolated elements of visual perception, and of the integration of these elements into simultaneously

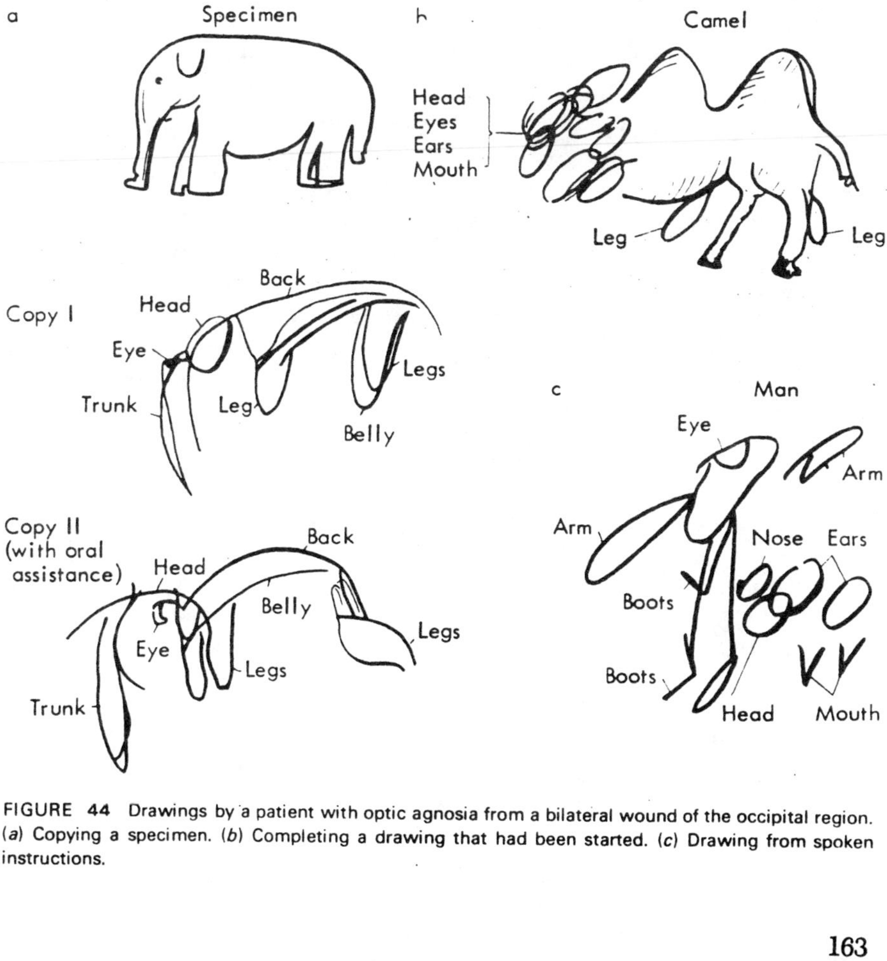

FIGURE 44 Drawings by a patient with optic agnosia from a bilateral wound of the occipital region. (*a*) Copying a specimen. (*b*) Completing a drawing that had been started. (*c*) Drawing from spoken instructions.

perceived groups, the basic processes in the normal recognition of whole pictures. We therefore feel that the suggestion made by Denny-Brown and co-workers (1952) that certain forms of agnosia are based on the pathological manifestation of amorphosynthesis (i.e., the integration of single signs into a whole structure) is most probably correct and may be applied not only to cases of tactile agnosia, where this phenomenon is especially marked (as shall be discussed in Section 3D of this part), but also to disturbance of optic gnosis.

We still know too little about the physiological mechanisms of optic agnosia. There can be no doubt, however, that a careful pathophysiological study of patients with this disorder will reveal a number of sensory disorders (rapid fatigue from visual reception, impaired visual adaptation, raising of thresholds, etc.) that probably become more pronounced when challenged by more complex forms of visual perception. This is suggested by the findings of Stein and Weiszäcker (1927), Bay (1950), Denny-Brown and co-workers (1952), and others.

Additional findings, of great importance to our understanding of the optic agnosias, may be obtained by studying patients without such obvious symptoms of disturbance of objective perception but in whom such a disturbance can be demonstrated by rather different means. In 1909, Balint described a case of bilateral lesions of the occipitoparietal systems that affords us an unusual and clear example. The patient showed no signs of marked object agnosia and readily distinguished between objects and pictures representing them. The significant feature of this case, however, was that the patient could perceive only one object at a time, regardless of its size. When the field of vision contained two objects (for example, a needle and the flame of a candle) the patient could see only one of them; if he looked at the needle, the flame of the candle in the background disappeared and vice versa. The narrowing of the field of vision in this case was thus expressed not in units of space but by the number of simultaneously perceived objects. This disturbance was also accompanied by another associated symptom, namely, gross ataxia of gaze. The patient was unable to transfer his gaze smoothly from one object to another, and if an object was pointed out to him he soon lost it because of the ataxic wandering of his gaze. Because of this phenomenon, Balint called the whole syndrome a "mental disturbance of gaze" ("*Seelenlähmung des Schauens*"). Similar cases were subsequently reported by Holmes (1919), Hécaen and Ajuriaguerra (1952), Luria (1959*a* [Eng.]), and Luria, Pravdina-Vinarskaya, and Yarbus (1961).

In all such patients a special variant of disturbed integration of elements into groups may be observed. These cases introduce certain mechanisms of disturbance of visual perception associated with lesions of the occipital and occipitoparietal regions of the brain whose full significance will probably not be discovered until further investigations have been made. For this reason we shall discuss them in rather more detail.

The phenomenon of "simultaneous agnosia" has been studied for many years. Janet originally described this disturbance in the case of a Polish officer who sustained a bilateral wound of the parietal region; the officer's visual perception and visual imagery were severely limited, so that he was able to picture or recall only one visual object at a time. When he analyzed this case at one of his "Clinical Wednesdays," Pavlov (1949) put forward the suggestion that the cerebral cortex, weakened as the result of the pathological condition, was incapable of dealing simultaneously with two stimuli so that one excited point has an inhibitory effect on the other, making it apparently "insignificant." We ourselves have observed similar phenomena in two cases of bilateral lesions of the parieto-occipital region and we have made some progress in the psychophysiological analysis of the symptoms observed (Luria, 1959*a* [Eng.]; Luria, Pravdina-Vinarskaya, and Yarbus, 1961).

The first patient whom we studied was one with a bilateral perforating wound of the occipitoparietal region. Unlike patients with optic agnosia, he could recognize individual objects. For practical purposes, however, he led the life of a blind man. This was because, like Janet's and Balint's patients, he could perceive only one object at a time (a figure or letter), except for the very rare instances when he could recognize a group of elements psychologically suggesting a single visual structure (for example, familiar words). As in the patients described by Janet and Balint, our patient's visual synthesis of individual signs into an integral structure was deranged. These defects were especially marked when the perception of pictures telling a story or of a printed text was investigated; on these occasions it became obvious that the patient's ability to scan the elements of an integral whole in an organized manner was severely disturbed and that the signs of amorphosynthesis that had been absent during the perception of single pictures had appeared. Meanwhile this patient exhibited the same symptom of optic ataxia as did the patient described by Balint. He could not place a dot in the center of a circle or draw a line around a shape; when his gaze was directed toward the point of the pencil, the shape he had been looking at disappeared and he could not carry out the optic coordination of his movement. For the same reason he could not write and keep to the line or draw complex shapes (Fig. 45).

When a patient was given a small dose (from 0.05 to 0.1 g) of caffeine solution, in order to stimulate the intact nervous elements of the occipital portion of the cortex, there characteristically was a temporary diminution of the severity of these defects; for 30 to 40 minutes the patient was able to perceive two objects simultaneously and to perform actions requiring visual-motor coordination. This effect is illustrated in Fig. 46. Pavlov's postulate of weakened functioning of the inhibited cortical cells of the occiput as the basis for this defect appears to conform to the facts (Luria, 1959*a* [Eng.]).

Similar findings were observed in the other patient who developed an analogous syndrome after a bilateral vascular lesion of the parieto-occipital portion of the cortex (Luria, Pravdina-Vinarskaya, and Yarbus, 1961). In this patient we observed a disturbance of coordinated ocular movements, which together with concurrent agnosia and optic ataxia constituted the essence of the syndrome. As in the preceding patient, perception was grossly constricted, so that he could comprehend only one object at a time and was quite incapable of performing tasks requiring visual-motor coordination (Fig. 47). The defects of visual perception were characteristically accompanied by disturbances of eye-fixation movements, and when we recorded these movements while the patient examined a simple geometrical figure or a portrait we obtained results very different from those seen in normal subjects or patients with disturbances of the peripheral section of the visual analyzer. The corresponding tracings are shown in Fig. 48. These demonstrate that the phenomenon of simultaneous agnosia in this patient was, in fact, accompanied by a profound disturbance of the motor apparatus of vision, an apparatus responsible for visual perception.

The fact that the narrowing of visual perception down to a single element is always accompanied by a disturbance of the visual analysis and synthesis of complex objects leads to important conclusions regarding the mechanism of complex visual perception.

The normal process of perception of a complex visual object involves the isolation of items carrying the maximal useful information and the comparison of these items with each other. For this process to be successful, visual perception must have at least two active receptor points, one of which (macular) receives the necessary information, whereas the other (peripheral) gives information about the presence of other components of the visual field and evokes an orienting reflex, consisting of a shift of fixation, so that the object in question falls into the central (macular) area of vision.

In patients with the "constriction" of visual perception down to a single element, described above, this mechanism disintegrates, the organized shift of fixation becomes impossible, and adequate perception of complex visual objects is disturbed.

In the course of the last few years I have seen different degrees of this defect, always occurring in patients with bilateral lesions of the occipital region and disturbing the optical behavior of these patients to a varied degree.

The basic mechanisms of this disturbance are not yet known. Their investigation is still only in its infancy. We can cite only the work of Kok (1958), who discovered obvious disturbances in the differentiation of visual complexes with lesions of the parieto-occipital systems, and the preliminary observations of Sorkina and Khomskaya (1960). The latter reported that the systems of visual differentiation of color formed in patients with occipitoparietal lesions remained relatively stable as long as the patients were required to discriminate between elements of the same system (from a pair of stimuli) but that they quickly disintegrated when the patients were asked to discriminate among several (two or three) pairs of visual signals.

There is no doubt, however, that further research will shed light on the neurodynamic principles governing opticognostic disorders and on the roles of constricted visual perception and disturbed visual synthesis in the different forms of optic agnosia. It is evident that disturbances of visual traces and the pathological change in the mobility of the visual analyzer are essentially involved in opticognostic disorders.

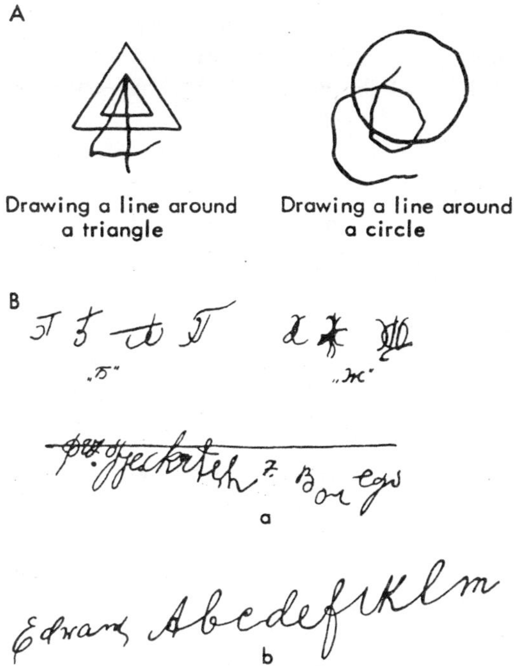

FIGURE 45 Signs of visual-motor ataxia in a patient (Patient V) with a bilateral wound of the parieto-occipital region. (*A*) Drawing around a shape. (*B*) Writing: (*a*) with the eyes open; (*b*) with the eyes shut.

The pathological manifestations seen in other, more specialized forms of optic agnosia have received even less study. They include agnosia to color and agnosia to symbols (letters and numbers), which sometimes accompany the forms of object and simultaneous agnosia that have been described and sometimes exist independently of them. These disturbances have often been described in the literature (Pötzl, 1928; Lange, 1936; Ajuriaguerra and Hécaen, 1960; etc.), and we shall not consider them further.

. . .

Our description of the syndromes of optic agnosia would be incomplete without mention of another form, whose mechanisms remain unexplained but which must differ essentially from those described.

During the early stages in the study of optic agnosia a form called "associative mental blindness" was described (Lissauer, 1889). Patients with this type of disturbance have no difficulty in visually perceiving objects or pictures of objects. The essential defect in this condition is difficulty in recognizing the nature of the objects and pictures.

This disturbance is especially conspicuous in those with lesions of the subordinate (usually the right) hemisphere. They are particularly typified by a peculiar "agnosia for faces," which has been described by Pötzl and Hoff (1937), Hécaen and Ajuriaguerra (1952), Chlenov and Bein (1958), and others. The faces of persons to whom he is speaking can be distinguished perfectly well by such a patient, but his perception of them loses its sense of familiarity. The ability to accurately copy a drawing remains intact, but such a patient is unable to reproduce an object or picture from memory. An example is given in Fig. 49.

These disturbances of recognition without apparent specific sensory defects are encountered fairly frequently, and the study of the mechanisms responsible for their production must accordingly be regarded as one of the most important and urgent aspects of the psychophysiological investigation of these lesions of the human brain.

D. DISTURBED TACTILE PERCEPTION AND TACTILE AGNOSIA

We will leave the analysis of opticognostic disorders in order to examine very briefly the closely related disturbances of tactile synthesis, which have been called "tactile agnosia" or "astereognosis." These disturbances may arise from lesions of the parietal areas of the cerebral cortex, areas constituting the cortical portion of the cutaneokinesthetic analyzer, and they have much in common with the phenomena of optic agnosia.

Whereas in normal visual perception, as has been pointed out, the process of synthesis of elements into an integral picture takes place rapidly and comprehensively, the corresponding process in tactile perception, involving the palpation of objects, is comparatively extended. The successive stages of tactile perception can therefore be examined.

Tactile perception per se has been considered in detail (Katz, 1925; Kotlyarova, 1948; Anan'ev, 1959; Zinchenko, 1959; etc.), and its modification

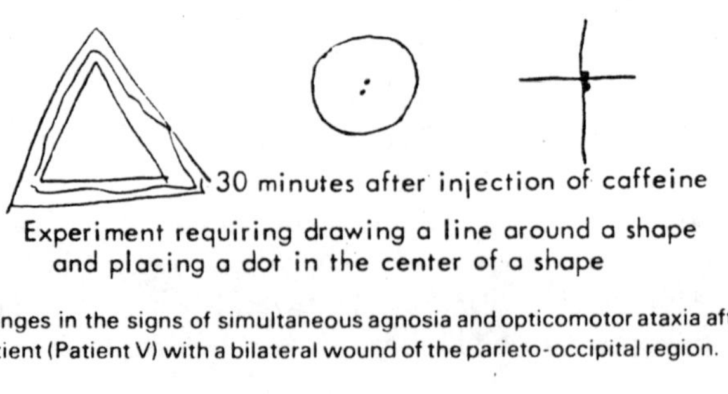

FIGURE 46 Changes in the signs of simultaneous agnosia and opticomotor ataxia after administration of caffeine to a patient (Patient V) with a bilateral wound of the parieto-occipital region.

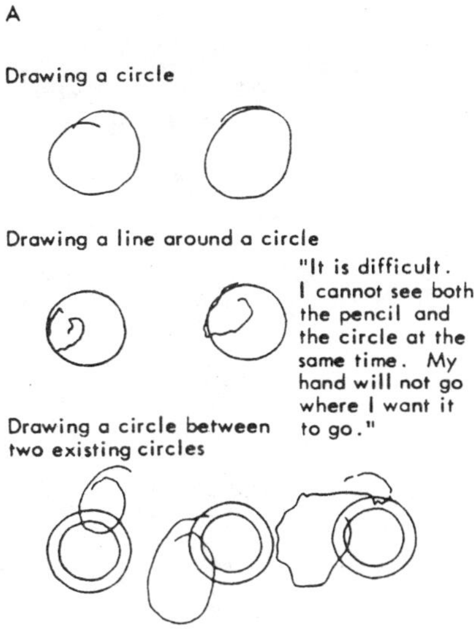

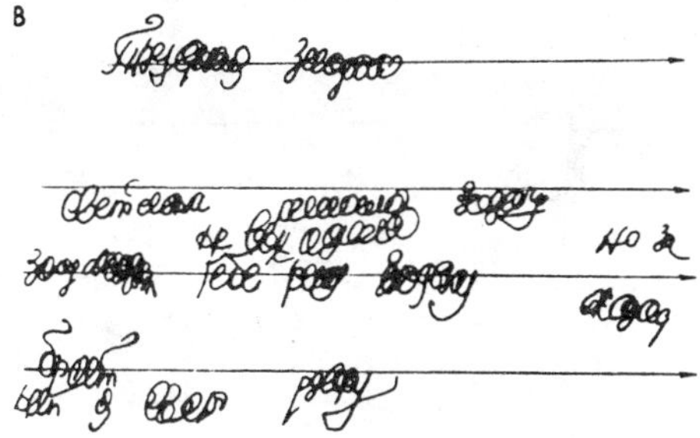

FIGURE 47 Disturbance of visual-motor coordination in a patient (Patient R) with a bilateral vascular lesion of the occipital region. (*A*) Drawing shapes and drawing a line around them. (*B*) Writing.

by pathological processes has also received much attention (summarized by Chlenov, 1934, and others). Nevertheless, the psychophysiological analysis of these disorders, having much in common with what has been described in connection with the pathology of visual perception, still awaits special investigation. It is only recently that investigations have been published to show that the phenomena of astereognosis may be based on disturbances of general forms of spatial synthesis (Teuber, 1965; Semmes, 1965).

We know that a lesion of the posterior central gyrus, a formation considered to be the cortical nucleus of the cutaneokinesthetic analyzer, leads to disturbed cutaneous sensation on the contralateral half of the body. Because of the work of Head (1920), we also know that a lesion of these cortical areas causes the most persistent disturbances of complex epicritic sensation, which may at best be restored only in the very last stages of resolution of the pathological process.

However, there have been frequent clinical reports (starting with that of Wernicke, 1894) of disturbances accompanying lesions of the secondary fields of the postcentral, tactile region of the brain in which the elementary forms of pain and tactile sensation apparently remained intact and the complex forms of discriminatory sensation were principally affected. Among these disturbances were instances in which the patient responded to discrete touch quite well but could not recognize a shape or cipher drawn on his skin, could not localize the place of touch with sufficient clarity, and could not determine the direction of a stroke. Such patients frequently exhibited disturbances in the complex forms of deep muscle sensation and developed manifestations of astereognosis. They could not recognize an object by touch, although they could easily do so by sight.

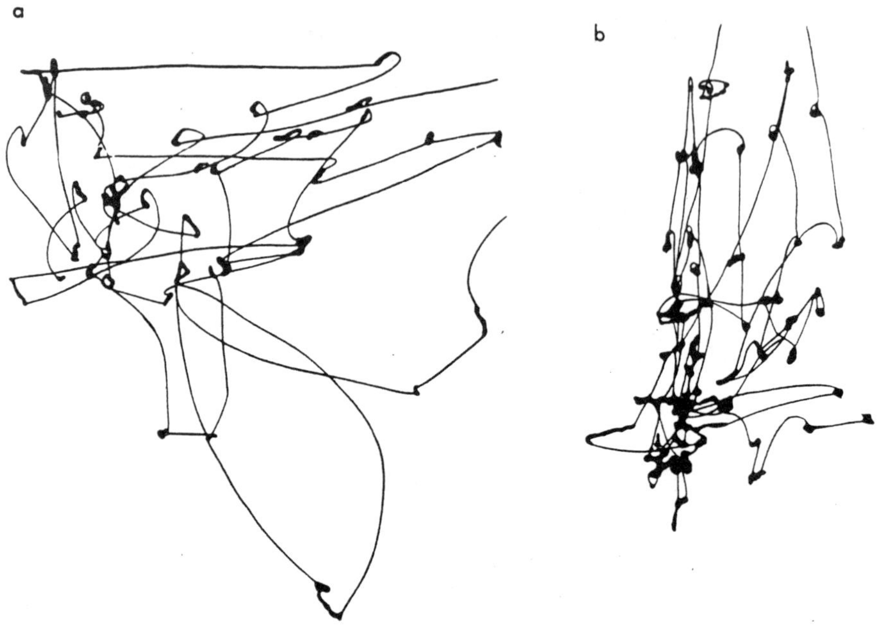

FIGURE 48 Eye movements of a patient (Patient R) with simultaneous agnosis and optic ataxia during examination of pictures. (*A*) When examining a rectangle. (*B*) When examining a face. *(After Luria, Pradina-Vinarskaya, and Yarbus, 1961.)*

At first glance these phenomena appear to be the negation of optic agnosia, but closer inspection shows that they have many features in common. Just as for optic agnosia, many workers investigating astereognosis tended to approach it as a symbolic rather than as a sensory disorder, pointing out that the elementary sensory functions remain generally preserved. Such disturbances have been called "tactical asymbolia" (Wernicke, 1894), "parietal tactile agnosia" (Nielsen, 1946), etc. On the other hand, another group of workers considered these phenomena to be the result of more elementary sensory disorders. Déjerine (1914) believed that they are a special form of sensory disturbance developing as the problems presented to the patient become increasingly difficult. Bay (1944) suggested that tactile agnosia is based on a complex group of elementary sensory disorders manifested as changes in threshold, disturbance in adaptation, etc. Interesting results relating to the dynamic analysis of the sensory disturbance from lesions of the parietal cortical region subsequently obtained by Korst and Fantalova (1959).

More recently this search for disturbances of elementary sensory components in cases of tactile agnosia and astereognosis has been rewarded by new and important data. According to these observations, these phenomena can now be regarded as products of disturbances of integrative processes in the tactile sphere, closely related to the defects of synthesis of simultaneous groups encountered in optic agnosia.

Head (1920) showed that a lesion of the parietal region of the cortex leads to inability to perceive two tactile stimuli applied simultaneously to the skin areas corresponding to the site of the brain lesion. Beginning in 1945, the intensive research of Bender and Teuber (Bender, 1952; Bender and Teuber, 1948; Semmes *et al.*, 1960) showed that perception of stimulation applied to affected (contralateral to the pathological focus) areas very quickly ceased. Orienting reflexes produced by stimulation of skin areas contralateral to the focus were quickly extinguished, and the perception of two or several simultaneously applied cutaneous stimuli was disturbed. This constriction of perception is reminiscent of the narrowing of attention so prominent in simultaneous agnosia. In the opinion of several writers (Denny-Brown *et al.*, 1952), it may also lead to a disturbance of the "spatial summation" of excitation and ultimately to the phenomenon of amorphosynthesis with which we are already familiar, although this time we find it in the tactile sphere.

The inability to recognize an object by touch or to distinguish a shape or cipher outlined by someone else on the skin is not, therefore, the result of any symbolic disorder but the manifestation of a disturbance of those sensory syntheses that have been discussed. We have not ourselves investigated disturbances of tactile syntheses; we mention them only because incorporation of this topic into the program of future research may lead to elucidation of some general aspects of the structure of agnostic disorders that have hitherto not been understood.

E. SPATIAL DISORIENTATION AND CONSTRUCTIVE APRACTAGNOSIA

In the previous pages the disturbances of visual and tactile perception arising from lesions of the secondary divisions of the visual and cutaneo-

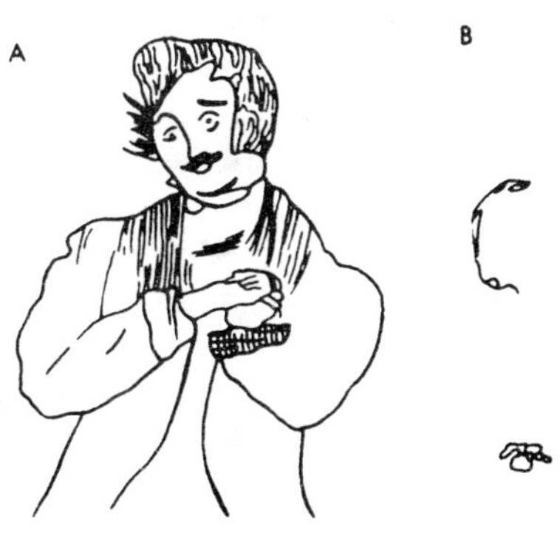

FIGURE 49 Drawings from life and from memory by a patient with agnosia for faces from a bilateral vascular lesion of the occipital region. (*A*) Copy of an existing picture. (*B*) The same picture drawn from memory.

kinesthetic areas of the cerebral cortex have been described. The analysis of these phenomena has led us to recognize a *disturbance in the ability to integrate single stimuli into simultaneous structures or groups* as the common factor responsible for these disorders.

We shall now turn to other phenomena that may arise from lesions of the occipitoparietal cortical divisions and that directly bring up some important problems in the pathology of spatial orientation.

The posterior parts of the inferoparietal region (Area 39), directly continuous with the occipital divisions, constitute one of the newest cortical formations connecting the central apparatuses of the kinesthetic, vestibular, and visual analyzers. They play a dominant part in the integration of all of these various stimuli, and a lesion of these areas is inevitably followed by some degree of disturbance of the more complex forms of visual-spatial synthesis. This type of disturbance leads to a breakdown of spatial orientation and to the phenomena of spatial apraxia collectively known as the "apractognosias"; they have been described fully in the literature.

• • •

The perception of spatial relationships and orientation in space are among the most complex forms of reflection of the outside world. Spiritualistic attempts to depict the perception of space as one of the forms of "*a priori* synthetic judgments" (Kant) or to approach it from the nativistic point of view, in which the reflection of space is considered an inborn form of cognition, could not be farther from the truth.

The perception of space is based on visual orientation toward the objects of the outside world, or, more precisely, on those processes of visual analysis and synthesis that have just been discussed. However, as ontogenetic investigations, notably by workers such as Piaget (1935), have shown, visual orientation in space is only the last and most refined form of spatial perception. These ontogenetic investigations revealed that in the early stages of development, spatial orientation is already implicated in the child's practical activity; this orientation becomes possible at the end of the first year of life, when the combined work of the visual, kinesthetic, and vestibular analyzers is established (Shchelovanov, 1925; Figurin and Denisova, 1949). Only after the establishment of this combined activity, responsible for the processes of inspection, palpation, head orientation, and eye movements, can the complex forms of reflection of spatial relationships develop, which remain unchanged even if the position of the body is altered. This accounts for the great interest shown in cases in which a disturbance of one of these components, for example the vestibular apparatus, leads to obvious changes in spatial orientation as a whole (Beritov, 1959, 1961).

However, the perception of spatial relationships in man is more than the combined activity of the three analyzers just mentioned. An essential feature of human spatial perception is the fact that it is always asymmetrical, manifesting obvious lateralization. In the surrounding space we can distinguish the right and left sides and what lies before, behind, above, and below us; in other words, we perceive space by means of a system of basic geometrical coordinates. However, not all of these geometrical coordinates have the same value. Orientation in space essentially always consists of distinguishing what in external space lies on the right; being related to the dominant right hand, it differs from what lies on the left. These notions of right and left are subsequently designated by words. The subject begins to depend on a complete system of signs for his orientation in space. This system includes a complex group of "local signs," some of which are associated with the activity of the vestibular apparatus, some with muscle sense, and some with vision. Finally, these coordinates usually become defined by words and so become subject to the organizing influence of the language system. Several workers, starting with Lotze (1852) and ending with Schilder (1935), Shemyakin (1940, 1954, 1959), and Korolenok (1946), have given detailed accounts of the complex group of factors lying at the root of orientation in space.

Orientation in space may be disturbed by various factors. The most prominent forms of disturbance of spatial orientation are to be found when the lesion affects those parts of the cerebral cortex responsible for the combined work of all of the aforementioned analyzers. It is for this reason that disturbances in spatial orientation occupy so important a place in the pathology of the occipitoparietal regions of the brain.

• • •

Disturbances in the perception of spatial relationships and in spatial orientation occurring from lesions of the parieto-occipital divisions of the cortex have been described by many workers (Holmes, 1919; Head, 1926; Critchley, 1953; Zangwill and co-workers [Paterson and Zangwill, 1944, 1945; Ettlinger, Warrington, and Zangwill, 1957; etc.] in England. Zucker, 1934; Gerstmann, 1924; Pötzl, 1928; Conrad, 1932; Kleist, 1934; Ranschburg and Schill, 1932; Lange, 1936 and many others in Germany. Krol' (1933) in the Soviet Union. Lhermitte and co-workers [Ajuriaguerra, Mouzon, 1942] and Hécaen and Ajuriaguerra, 1956, and co-workers in France. Bender and Teuber [1947, 1948, etc.] in the United States). In the cases reported, defects in spatial perception were usually combined with defects in spatially organized activity. That is why certain writers have suggested calling this condition "spatial apractognosia."

The phenomena of spatial apractagnosia are by no means always associated with gross disturbances in the visual or tactile ability to identify objects. Even in cases of astereognosis a general disturbance of the "spatial factor" exceeding the limits of tactile defects can be postulated (Semmes, 1965). Only if the pathological focus deranges the normal work of the anterior occipital cortical areas do they mainly affect the visual sphere, and then they are complicated by the presence of optic agnosia; if, on the other hand, the pathological process affects the postcentral cortical areas, these phenomena begin to assume a marked tactile-kinesthetic nature and they are combined with astereognosis. This shows that spatial apractagnosia has several variants, for which further careful study is needed.

Signs of a disturbance of orientation in space are exhibited in the course of their ordinary behavior. Often such patients cannot find the way to their own ward, have lost their sense of direction (they go to the right, for example, when they should go to the left), are unable to carry out the ordinary daily tasks requiring the use of spatial relationships, cannot dress themselves, cannot make the bed, etc.

They experience considerable difficulty in the course of special tests, for example when asked to put the hand in a particular position in space. They confuse vertical with horizontal, frontal, and sagittal directions; they cannot properly arrange matches in the shape of required geometrical figures. These disturbances become especially marked when the patients are confronted with tasks requiring the conscious transfer of certain spatial relationships, for example, when the doctor, sitting opposite the patient, asks him to reproduce the spatial position of his hands by mentally reversing the relationships perceived visually or, similarly, to transfer the relationships between the elements of a figure formed from matches.

Similar difficulties may arise when such patients attempt to copy geometrical figures with asymmetrically arranged elements, especially if these elements are not in their usual positions. Characteristically, in patients with optic-spatial disorders it is not only the phenomena of apractognosia or constructive apraxia type that occur. These patients have difficulty in reproducing letters and show signs of mirror image writing ("optic-spatial agraphia"). Examples of such disturbances are shown in Fig. 50.

However, the disturbances in patients with the syndrome just described extend far beyond the range of orientation in space as perceived by direct vision. *These defects are seen most clearly in relation to spatial ideas*, whose integrity is the fundamental condition for the performance of many operations.

Two tests reveal this defect particularly well. One is associated with estimation of the position of the hands of a clock, the other, with analysis of the coordinates of a map. Both of these operations involve the processes most severely deranged in patients with a lesion of the occipitoparietal areas of the cortex. Both are carried out in an externally symmetrical field, whose analysis, however, requires the use of conventional asymmetrical coordinates. The symmetrically opposite points of a clock face denote 3 and 9, 12 and 6; superimposed upon this basic system of coordinates are conventional systems attaching a different value to externally symmetrical points. If we add that all of these coordinates have values expressed in conventional speech formulas (for example, 10 minutes past 6 and 10 minutes to 6; 20 minutes past 7 and 20 minutes to 7), the complexity of this organization of space in the process of estimating the time from the position of the hands of a clock will become quite obvious. Similar complexities are seen in confrontations with the spatial organization of a map, in which geometrically symmetrical directions (east and west) assume completely different meanings. Both of these operations necessitate the deciphering of a directly perceived, symmetrical space with the use of the entire range of lateralized afferent systems.

Observations show that a disturbance in the comprehension of the spatial relationships on a clock face and on a map, in which symmetrically opposite points are interchanged, is one of the most common symptoms of a lesion of the parieto-occipital divisions of the cortex. Figure 51 shows typical examples of such disorganization.

Patients with this syndrome experience similar difficulties in naming their

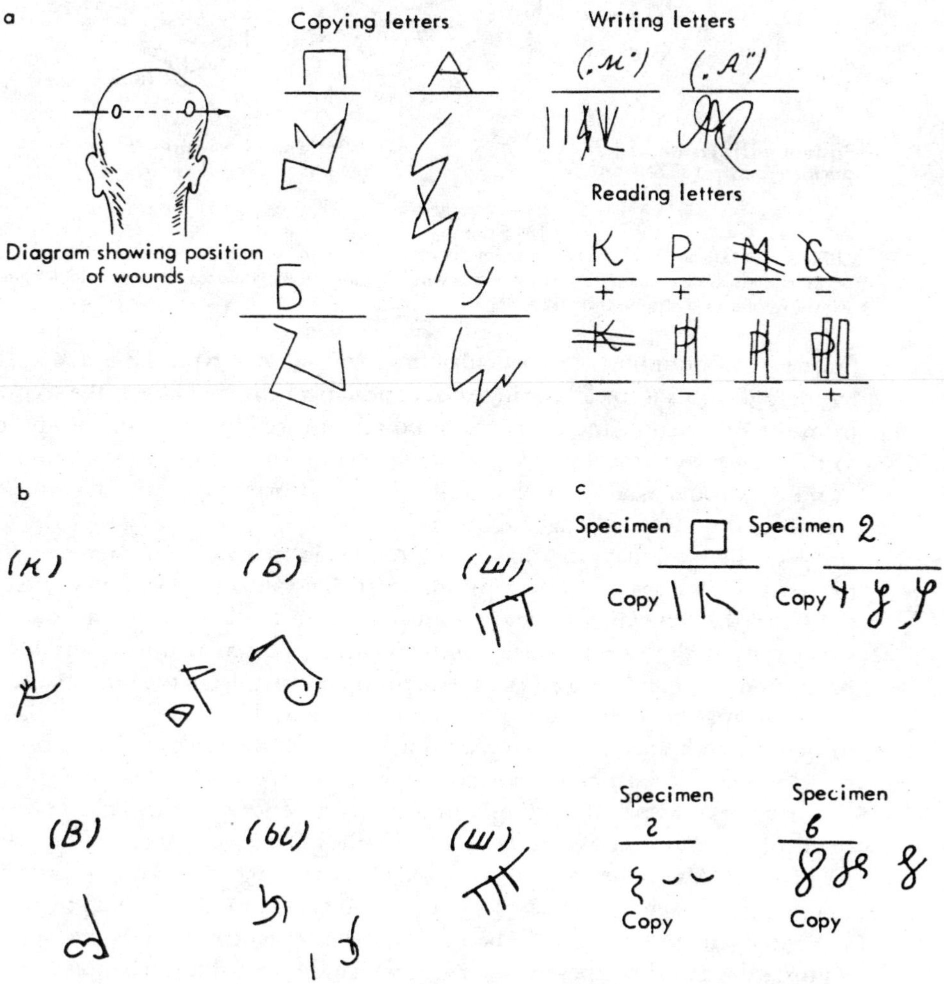

FIGURE 50 Optic-spatial disturbances of writing from dictation and copying in patients with a lesion of the parieto-occipital cortical divisions. (*a*) A patient (Patient Bul.) with a bilateral wound of the occipital region. (*b*) A patient (Patient Erokh.) with a wound of the left parieto-occipital region. (*c*) A patient (Patient M) with a wound of the left parieto-occipital region.

a

b

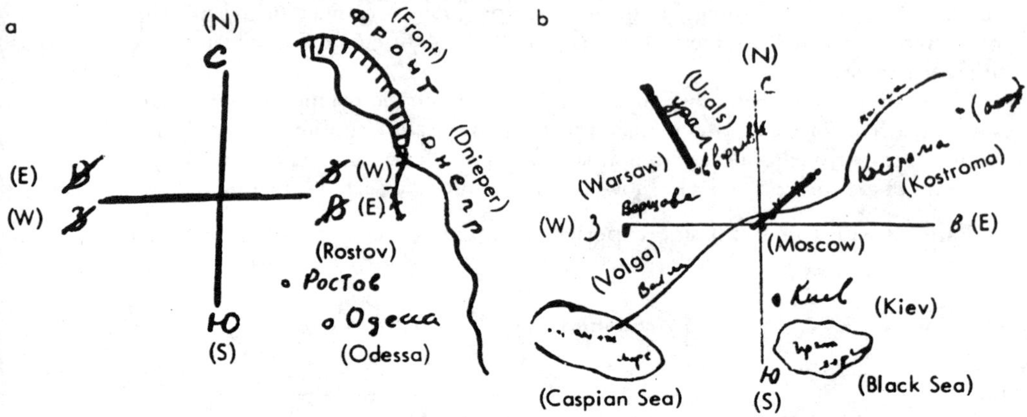

Patient with lesion of left parieto-occipital region

Patient with lesion of right occipital region

FIGURE 51 Disturbance of orientation of points on a map in patients with a lesion of the parieto-occipital cortical divisions. (*a*) A patient with a wound of the left parieto-occipital region. (*b*) A patient with a wound of the right occipital region.

fingers or in pointing to a particular finger by name. A typical mistake made by these patients is to call the index (second) finger the ring finger (the second from the other end), and the corresponding mistake is made when they point to the fingers by name. Symptoms like these comprise such an important part of the syndrome as a whole that, following the work of Gerstmann (1924), it was given the name of "finger agnosia."

All of the symptoms that have been described may be encountered in the presence of lesions of the occipitoparietal divisions of both the dominant (left) and the subordinate (right) hemispheres. In the latter case phenomena such as finger agnosia and the inability to correctly estimate the time from the position of the hands of a clock or to identify countries from their designations on a map may be less marked, a fact indicating that these defects are probably associated with special speech disturbances developing only from lesions of the dominant hemisphere. However, the differences in the character of the disturbances of spatial synthesis produced by lesions of the right and left hemispheres must receive further detailed study. This type of research, started by Hécaen, Ajuriaguerra, and co-workers (1951, 1956, etc.) and by Zangwill and his co-workers (1951, 1957) and others, merits the most serious attention.

Serious attention must also be paid to the phenomena of unilateral spatial agnosia described by these workers, in which the spatial disturbances appear only on one (usually the left) side. These disturbances, usually accompanying lesions of the right hemisphere and proceeding independently of complex speech disorders, must receive special analysis.

A distinctive feature of these disturbances of spatial synthesis, primarily those accompanied by a lesion of the dominant hemisphere, is their association with special speech disorders. We have seen the extent to which the systems of conceptual associations of speech were preserved in patients with optic agnosia and how dominant was their role in attempts to decipher the meaning of an optically perceived object. In spatial apractagnosia there is a completely different state of affairs. Patients with a lesion of the parieto-occipital (or, more accurately, of the parietotemporal-occipital) divisions of the left hemisphere exhibit signs of disturbed spatial synthesis and spatial orientation not only in relation to visual perception and activity, but also in regard to the more complex symbolic forms of activity proceeding at the level of speech processes.

We have in mind the special difficulties in logical-grammatical operations and in arithmetical operations, both of which activities are psychologically closely related to operations involving spatial relationships. (These disorders comprise part of the syndrome of the disturbance of the higher cortical functions arising from lesions of the parieto-occipital divisions of the brain and merit special examination.)

F. DISTURBED LOGICAL-GRAMMATICAL OPERATIONS AND SEMANTIC APHASIA

The view that lesions of the parieto-occipital region of the left hemisphere may lead to a considerable disturbance in speech activity was put forward by clinical neurologists at the beginning of the study of disturbances of the higher cortical functions accompanying local brain lesions. When the study of cortical pathology was still in its infancy, it was observed that lesions of this region may be associated with word amnesia and difficulties in complex logical and grammatical operations. As has been pointed out (Part I, Section 1A), however, the psychological concepts of that period did not lend themselves to more accurate definitions of these disturbances, and writers either reduced the disorders to specialized memory defects or attributed them to a damaged cortical "center" in which complex conceptual functions are localized (Broadbent, 1879); such a damaged center was considered to result in "asymbolia" (Finkelburg, 1880) or "asemia" (Kussmaul, 1885).

Views such as these were held in clinical neurology for many years, and even Head (1926) considered that the disturbances arising from a lesion in this region could be described as "semantic aphasia." Subsequently, the adherents of the noetic school (Bouman and Grünbaum, 1925; van Woerkom, 1925; and especially Goldstein, 1927, 1934, 1948) repeatedly described gross disturbances of speech-regulated intellectual activity in such patients.

The fact that patients with a lesion of the parieto-occipital divisions of the cerebral cortex do, in fact, exhibit serious disturbances of the complex forms of speech activity has been established beyond doubt. As a rule, such patients do not show signs of disturbed articulation or defective phonemic hearing, disturbances which are characteristic of patients with a lesion of the left temporal divisions (Luria, 1940*b*, 1945, 1947, etc.). The extinction of meaning of words that was described in the preceding section and the understanding of both individual words and simple expressions remain reasonably well preserved. Significant disturbances come to light, however, as soon as the more complex forms of speech activity are investigated.

The first and the most prominent symptom observed by many writers (Lotmar, 1919, 1935; Goldstein, 1926*b*, 1948; etc.) is the considerable difficulty in bringing to mind the name of an object. It was this difficulty that led these workers to classify these cases as belonging to the syndrome of "amnestic aphasia." Careful investigation reveals, however, that the disturbance of word memory in these patients is quite different in character from that found in association with temporal lesions, the latter disturbance being based on instability of the sound images of words. Whereas patients with a lesion of the temporal divisions of the cortex are not helped if a story is told to them word by word for they still cannot remember anything of it, it is a different matter with patients of the present group; the latter have only to be told the first sound of a missing word and they will reproduce it rather easily. This suggests that the difficulty these patients have in naming objects is based upon an instability of the sound images of words.

Representatives of the noetic school, previously cited, believed that this special phenomenon hides a far more general defect and that the word amnesia in these patients may be a product of a general intellectual disorder. These ideas were apparently confirmed by various clinical findings.

Head (1926) originally showed that patients who had difficulty in finding the necessary words at the same time experienced considerable difficulty in remembering complex speech constructions. A relatively complicated story that is told to them is converted into a reproduction of isolated and unrelated fragments. They fail to grasp the meaning of the story, for they have considerable difficulty whenever they have to operate with certain logical relationships. Some writers, for example Goldstein and Gelb (1924), feel that the difficulties experienced by these patients are not simply speech defects but are something more, so that a patient with color amnesia, for example, cannot perform "categorical operations." According to these writers, instead of classifying colors into specific groups, such a patient simply recognizes a continuous spectrum of changing hues. Similar disturbances of intellectual operations in such patients were described by Weigl (1927), Conrad (1932), Zucker (1934), and others.

Attempts to regard the disturbances of higher cortical functions accompanying parieto-occipital lesions as the manifestation of general intellectual defects, coupled with psychomorphological notions of a "center for ideas" localized in this region, were not only theoretically faulty, but also contrary to the clinical facts.

Investigations by van Woerkom (1925), Head (1926), Conrad (1932), Zucker (1933), and others revealed facts suggesting that the semantic disturbances observed in this group of patients are completely ungeneralized and that the symptoms are distinctive, being in the nature of those defects of simultaneous synthesis and orientation in space discussed previously.

As shown by these workers and confirmed by some of our own observations (Luria, 1940*a*, 1947, etc.), the patients of this group show adequate preservation of the understanding of individual words (including abstractions). Some investigators (Kogan, 1947) observed a slight narrowing in their range of word meanings. These patients had no difficulty in grasping the meaning of complex ideas such as "causation," "development," "capitalism," and "cooperation"; abstract themes were also quite within their comprehension. Difficulties developed when they were presented with complex logical-grammatical constructions, the understanding of which requires the "co-ordination of details into a common whole" or the "fitting together of details into a single formula" (Head, 1926, pp. 257–262). It is because of these disturbances of certain logical operations and not because of the primary disintegration of some form of abstract orientation that the understanding of certain concepts is significantly impaired.

It is important to note that the disturbance of the understanding of certain speech constructions in these patients has nothing to do with the length of the passages presented to them. Head (1926) originally observed the existence of certain definite speech constructions that are very difficult for the patients of this group to understand, although the units may be very short and sometimes consist of only two or three elements. Among these structures (Luria, 1940*a*, 1945, 1947, 1948; Bubnova, 1946; etc.) are logical-grammatical structures expressing spatial relationships (the prepositions "below" and "above," "before" and "after," etc.; the adverbial clauses "to the right of" and "to the left of"; etc.). Patients with a lesion of the parieto-occipital regions of the brain can understand even quite long phrases that describe a simple event reasonably well, but they have difficulty in carrying out tasks such as drawing a triangle below a circle and a triangle to the right of a cross. They cannot appreciate the difference between the type of verbal constructions represented by "a triangle below a circle" and "a circle below a triangle"; the patients usually draw the corresponding figures in the order in which they are given in the instructions and then, after prolonged trials, exclaim: "I understand 'triangle' and 'circle' but I have no idea how to place them in relation to each other."

The ability to integrate the details into a single whole and to understand that a construction including the same elements may express different relationships between objects is grossly impaired in these patients. A possible means of dealing with this defect in the course of rehabilitative training may be to have the patient make a special study of the meanings of propositions and constructions, with the use of external aids and grammatical rules; growing understanding of them is converted into a series of successive operations (Bubnova, 1946; Luria, 1948). The disturbance of the ability to mentally integrate details into a single whole proves, however, to be fairly permanent. We have noticed in a series of patients studied in great detail that even after many years of training this ability was not regained; although a patient could analyze these constructions "by numbers," he would declare that he could not understand their significance and could not grasp them mentally. I have studied one such case for 30 years, and it has been fully described elsewhere (Luria, 1972).

The disturbances in the understanding of logical-grammatical constructions observed in patients with parieto-occipital lesions are not, however, confined to parts of speech expressing spatial relationships such as those just mentioned. Similar difficulties arise when such patients attempt to understand comparative relationships (for example, the statements in Burt's well-known test that "Kate is lighter than Sonia" and "Sonia is lighter than Kate") or time relationships incorporating a spatial component (for example, "spring before summer" and "winter after autumn"). The difficulty experienced in understanding such constructions is particularly great when three components are compared (for example, "Olga is lighter than Sonia but darker than Kate"). Since it demands some degree of concentration even from a healthy subject, this test proves to be quite beyond the capacity of a patient with a lesion of the parieto-occipital divisions of the brain. Although he can identify the individual elements named in this construction, not even after prolonged work on the problem can he comprehend the system of relationships that it contains. Other grammatical constructions beyond the reach of this group of patients include those with verbs expressing an action transacted from one object to another (for example, "to take to someone" and "to take from someone").

All of these logical-grammatical constructions have one very obvious common factor: All are to some extent verbal expressions of spatial relationships; in some (for example, constructions with the prepositions "below" and "above") this is manifested simply and openly, while in others (for example, comparative or transitional constructions) it is more complex or subtle.

Other logical-grammatical constructions exist in which these spatial relationships are still more masked. By these we mean certain forms of inflected relationships, appearing at a late stage in the history of language. Such constructions include those with an attributive genitive case ("father's brother" or "brother's father," "the dog's master" or "the master's dog"). These constructions, although consisting of two nouns, denote but one object, and sometimes, moreover, this is not even mentioned in the expression (for example, in the term "father's brother," "uncle" is not stated). Before such expressions can be understood, the logical synthesis of the elements into an integral whole is required.

We have proved to our satisfaction, on the basis of a large number of cases (Luria, 1940*a*, 1945, 1947), that patients with a lesion of the parieto-occipital lobes readily perceive the individual components of such expressions but cannot understand the relationships that they denote; after fruitless attempts to grasp the significance, they declare: "Of course, I know what a brother and a father mean, but I cannot imagine what the two are together!"

Frequently, constructions with symmetrically opposite relationships of their component elements (for example, "father's brother" and "brother's father") are perceived by such patients as identical in meaning. Similar difficulties may be observed if a patient in this group is asked to put together two words in which relationships are expressed by means of the passive voice. Such patients, for example, cannot determine which of the following constructions is correct: "the sun is lit by the earth" or "the earth is lit by the sun."

Finally, considerable difficulty is experienced with grammatical constructions in which there is an unfamiliar, inverted position of the elements so that the order of the words is opposite to the order of the action they describe. Besides the types of expression involving the passive voice that have been referred to, the type represented by "Nicky was struck by Peter. Who was the bully?"* should be mentioned in this connection. For this construction to be understood, the relationships must be reversed mentally, but this operation is impossible for the patient with a lesion of the parieto-occipital portion of the cortex. Such patients experience still greater difficulty if they are called upon to understand complex constructions in which the elements bearing certain relationships to each other are some distance apart and separated by other words or clauses, so that the distant elements have to be synthesized before the meaning of the construction becomes clear. This will be discussed in greater detail subsequently (Part III, Section 8E).

We have spent some time on these matters because it is evident that they reveal additional features of the disturbances arising from lesions of the parieto-occipital divisions of the brain. We have no evidence suggesting that lesions of this region are followed by a general disorder of the intellect or by general semantic disorders. Monakow (1914) was essentially right when he labeled "asemia" a generalized disturbance that could arise only from widespread lesions of the whole cerebral cortex and when he maintained that its elements may appear in conjunction with circumscribed brain lesions widely differing in their location.

The "semantic aphasia" that develops in patients with lesions of the parieto-occipital areas of the left hemisphere reveals the considerable difference in the structure and origin of the symptoms. The disturbances in complex speech operations are highly specialized in nature; the internal relationship is maintained by the complex forms of spatial orientation and oriented (or asymmetrical) spatial syntheses are impaired (Part II, Section 3E).

We do not yet know the mechanisms responsible for these disturbances nor have we a sufficiently clear idea of their nature. Most probably, however, they are based on defects of special forms of simultaneous (spatial) syntheses,

*Translator's note: The force of this example is somewhat lost in the translation. The words in Russian are "Nicky," "struck," and "Peter," with the active voice used, but the meaning is disclosed by the fact that "Nicky" is in the accusative case and "Peter" in the nominative. This type of inverted word order is common in Russian.

represented in language and performed with the closest participation of the parieto-occipital cerebral systems. Interpretations of these disturbances as the "inability to combine the details mentally into a single, final whole" (Head, 1926) or the "conversion of a successive survey into an instantaneous over-all picture" (Pötzl, 1928) therefore appear very sensible. Lhermitte, Lévy, and Kyriako (1925) claimed that in patients with a syndrome due to a parieto-occipital lesion there is an insufficiency of spatial schemes. All of these suggestions, though incomplete and descriptive and made from different points of view, would indicate that the disturbances of higher cortical function in patients with a lesion of the parieto-occipital systems of the left hemisphere are associated with defects in the ability to carry out complex spatial synthesis. These perspectives were raised by Sechenov and still provide material for further study.

G. DISTURBANCES OF ARITHMETICAL OPERATIONS AND THE SYNDROME OF ACALCULIA

The disturbances of higher cortical functions from lesions of the parieto-occipital areas of the cerebral cortex are not confined to the system of logical-grammatical operations. They are equally prominent in relation to arithmetical operations, which are closely connected to spatial operations and spatial concepts.

Disturbances of arithmetical operations may be associated with circumscribed lesions of many different parts of the brain; these operations may also be adversely affected by generalized forms of depressed cerebral activity. However, the syndrome of "acalculia," which arises from lesions of the parieto-occipital divisions of the brain (as was clearly demonstrated by Heilbronner, 1910; Peritz, 1918; Head, 1926; Singer and Low, 1933; Lange, 1936; Krapf, 1937; Luria, 1945; Rudenko, 1953; etc.), is so definite in its character that it may be used successfully for the topical diagnosis of these lesions.

Operations involving numbers acquired their abstract character only relatively late in human history; their historical roots lay in geometry, and even now they largely remain spatial in character. Recent investigations (Piaget, 1955, 1956 [Rus.]; Gal'perin, 1959; Menchinskaya, 1955; Davydov, 1957; Nepomnyashchaya, 1958; etc.) have shed light on the complicated ontogenetic path of the formation of the concept of number and of arithmetical operations. They have shown that in the first stages of a child's development the concept of number and arithmetical operations are still based on visual action and require the manipulation of the elements of calculation in an external spatial field; these operations are crystallized only gradually, being first replaced by visual images and then by abstract arithmetical mental operations. However, in the latter stages the concept of number and arithmetical operations retain their spatial components. Long after he has mastered the system of tens and units, a child continues to arrange its elements in the familiar spatial scheme into which the individual numbers fit.

The important role that the spatial factor continues to play in number ideas and in arithmetical operations suggests that the disturbances of spatial synthesis resulting from lesions of the parieto-occipital systems of the brain (as discussed in Part II, Section 3E) must also be accompanied by disturbances of numerical and arithmetical operations. These aspects of numerical operations are discussed more fully elsewhere (Luria, 1945).

Writers who have made a special study of disturbances of the concept of number and of arithmetical operations accompanying lesions of the parieto-occipital divisions of the brain are unanimous in declaring that these disturbances are based on a disorder of definite spatial syntheses or, in their own words, "disturbance of the category of direction in space" or the "factor of asymmetry." According to these writers, with lesions of the parieto-occipital systems of the brain, the reference points in asymmetrical space, which are essential for correct calculation, are lost and arithmetical operations become impossible through the loss of their spatial coordinates.

The disturbances of these spatial syntheses may differ in type, for they depend on the situation and severity of the parieto-occipital lesion. With lesions situated in the occipital region and largely involving the visual system of the cortex, the disturbance of these spatial syntheses may be similar to a disturbance of other visual-spatial processes. Such patients cannot distinguish clearly between numerals with a similar graphic structure; they see them as mirror images when reading and writing letters or numbers. They confuse 6 and 9, and cannot differentiate between 69 and 96, etc. They naturally cannot make out Roman numerals such as IV and VI or IX and XI, and they can deduce the correct value of these outwardly similar compound numbers only by a process of successive analysis involving various accessory, concrete devices. With lesions not extending to the visual region of the cortex, these disturbances of visual perception are not so clear-cut. The disturbances of the system of spatial coordinates are more generalized in character and are manifested at the level of the more complex, more concise, and mainly mnestic operations.

In such patients, impairment of direct orientation in space, the phenomena of finger agnosia and disturbances in logical-grammatical operations accompany arithmetical disorders. The latter are manifested by the *disintegration of the categorical structure of number*. This disturbance appears in the reading and writing of numbers, and it subsequently leads to considerable difficulty in arithmetical operations.

The analysis of compound numbers formed in accordance with the decimal system requires the differentiation of categories occupying different positions in space when written, and even when imagined they retain this spatial organization. It is clear, therefore, that when spatial syntheses are disturbed and oriented (or asymmetrical) spatial ideas have disintegrated, the categorical structure of number is fundamentally upset.

That this is so is apparent from the fact that patients with the most severe form of these disturbances retain direct appreciation of the numerical value of individual numbers (which can be compared with the direct recognition of the meaning or the object categorization of words), yet they can neither write nor read compound numbers. For example, they write 109 as 100 and 9, and 1027 and 1000 and 27; they may write 17 as 71 and read 729 as 7, 2, and 9, without being able to integrate these numbers into a three-figure number. They experience considerable difficulty in understanding the meaning of compound numbers containing several figures, and often fail to take into account the numerical value of each category of figures in the number as a whole, simply taking note of the component figures. For such patients, for example, the number 489 is larger than the number 601 and 1897 is greater than 3002.

Although these defects in the understanding of multifigure numbers are revealed clearly in reading and writing, they are even more conspicuous in the course of special experiments requiring the analysis of the categorical structure of number. As a rule, patients with parieto-occipital lesions cannot point to the figure in a multifigure number representing the tens, hundreds, or units column. They confuse the spatial position of the figures and often refuse to tackle such a comparatively simple problem. These defects are particularly obvious when, in order to overcome the masking effect of the established stereotypes formed previously, the patient is asked to read out a multifigure number whose figures are written vertically. In such instances, even after a full explanation, the patient is unable to analyze the categorical structure of the number.

The disturbance of the ability to discern the categorical structure of a number, by analogy with the accompanying phenomenon of the disturbance of the understanding of the meaning of words and phonemes in speech, is the cause of the profound difficulties in carrying out arithmetical operations, a disturbance that has given this particular syndrome the name "acalculia."

As a rule, patients who cannot identify the categorical structure of number cannot perform even relatively simple arithmetical operations. In severe cases they cannot even manipulate numbers including a tens column, and they can calculate only by counting one by one with the aid of their fingers. In other cases arithmetical operations involving numbers up to ten are still possible but are carried out slowly and evidently depend on other aids. They are quite unable to perform operations with numbers greater than ten. For example, when carrying out arithmetical operations in writing, these patients may omit the stage of transferring from one column to another. We give an example of addition showing this feature:

1
7
+
2
5

If the operation is made more complicated, by arranging the two-figure numbers vertically, the numbers 17 and 25 will be added without regard to their conformity to the "tens" and "units" columns despite detailed explanations (1 + 7 + 2 + 5 = 15; or 1 + 5 = 6, 7 + 2 = 9, total 69; etc.).

The mental addition of two-figure numbers, involving the carrying over of tens, is also difficult for such patients because they cannot make a categorical analysis of the numbers to be added. Even patients whose capacity for mental arithmetic is still apparently unimpaired show defects in the spatial orientation of arithmetical operations; they make mistakes of the type of: 31 − 7 = 22 (30 − 7 = 23, followed by counting off one to the left instead of to the right).

As a rule, long-standing and firmly established speech-motor stereotypes, such as the multiplication table, are preserved in such patients, although less habitual operations than multiplication are disturbed. Division and the manipulation of fractions are also impossible, for they demand a fairly complex system of intermediate links and the ability to perform mathematical operations mentally.

Finally, disturbances in the ability to perform arithmetical operations in patients with parieto-occipital lesions of the brain may be revealed by inability to perform actions associated with the recognition of mathematical signs. If such patients are shown examples in which all the numerical components of the operation are given but the mathematical signs are omitted, the difficulty of the task presented to them will be obvious. When tackling problems such as these, patients with this particular syndrome bridge the gap by using random signs. The precise systems of mathematical coordinates are replaced by a very diffuse notion of "making less" (equally expressible by the signs − or ÷) or of "making bigger" (equally expressible by the signs + or ×). Disintegration of the system of mathematical relationships, in addition to the disintegration of the categorical structure of number, constitutes the picture of true parietal acalculia. Disturbances of counting in local brain lesions (especially in patients with aphasia) have been described in detail by Tsvetkova (1972).

As stated, the disturbances in the concept of number and of mathematical operations accompanying inferoparietal and parieto-occipital lesions are highly significant for the description of this syndrome as a whole. They clearly show how false is the notion of an inferoparietal "center" in which the understanding of number and the arithmetical functions are localized. They indicate that the appreciation of the complex categorical structure of number and the ability to perform arithmetical operations disintegrate primarily as a result of disorders in the complex forms of spatial analysis and synthesis. Such analysis and synthesis constitute one of the important psychophysiological conditions for the formation of many mental functions, including arithmetical operations.

H. DISTURBANCES OF INTELLECTUAL PROCESSES

We have seen that a lesion of the parieto-occipital divisions of the cortex may cause important disturbances in the "synthesis of individual elements into simultaneous groups," as Sechenov (1891) originally pointed out. These disturbances lead to considerable changes in visual perception, in spatial orientation, in the performance of certain logical-grammatical operations, and in calculation functions evidently closely associated with disturbances of the complex forms of spatial analysis and synthesis.

These findings suggest that other types of intellectual processes may also be deranged in these patients (whom we may divide into two groups, depending on the parieto-occipital situation of the lesion). By no means can these disturbances be identified with the disintegration of abstract intellectual activity, as advanced by the followers of the noetic school, for they are far more specialized in nature and are primarily due to impairment of the visual-spatial factor, discussed earlier in this chapter.

It is unfortunate that in clinical medicine there have been only relatively few detailed psychological investigations of the intellectual processes in patients with parieto-occipital lesions of the brain. Many of the investigations that have been made have been concerned with logical-grammatical and arithmetical operations. At present, not much can be said about the disturbances of intellectual activity in patients with occipital lesions of the brain accompanied by the phenomena of optic agnosia; much more is known about these disturbances in patients with lesions of the inferoparietal systems and a syndrome of disturbed spatial synthesis. Analysis of the disturbances of the intellectual processes in the patients reported in the literature shows that the disturbances are associated with the defects that have been described.

The patients in this group* eagerly began to tackle the various problems presented to them, without showing those defects of attention and of the regulating role of spoken instruction that characterize patients with a lesion of the frontal lobes (Part II, Section 5D). They had some difficulty only in

* Besides our personal observations, we also take into account here the investigations made by Zeigarnik and described in her book (1961).

comprehending the instructions, mainly as a result of the aforementioned defects in logical-grammatical operations.

These observations (as well as those of Kok, 1957, 1958, 1960) showed that the patients of this group cope adequately with abstract operations. Concepts such as family and species and cause and effect were comparatively easy for them to grasp, and the performance of operations such as finding the antonym of a given word and choosing a word expressing a family-species or cause-effect relationship met with no special difficulty (ignoring, of course, difficulties arising on account of an amnestic-aphasic defect if one was present). Further observations showed that patients of this group, once they have sorted out the conditions of the problem, can produce a general plan for its solution and that, although they find difficulty in individual logical-grammatical or arithmetical operations, they nevertheless preserve the general scheme of reasoning, which Bruner, Goodnow, and Austin (1956) and Miller, Pribram, and Galanter (1960) call the "general strategy of intellectual activity." It is because of the preservation of the general organization of intellectual activity that these patients respond well to rehabilitative training (Bubnova, 1946; Luria, 1948; etc.).

The principal defects in the intellectual processes of these patients are revealed by their inability to perform the operations necessary for the solution of a given problem if these operations require the identification of visual signs and their spatial organization. Such difficulties may arise, for example, in tests of their "constructive intellect," i.e., when performing tasks with levers, when putting together a Link's cube or Kohs blocks, and so on. These operations involve the analysis of spatial relationships or the assembling of individual elements into an integral whole. As Gadzhiev (1951) reported, when patients with a lesion of the parieto-occipital systems attempt to put a Link's cube together, they not only easily grasp the principles of the task and can formulate them verbally, but also carry out the preparatory actions required by the plan; they have difficulty only in operations needing the direct (visual or mnestic) synthesis of spatial relationships.

The behavior of patients of this group presents similar features when solving arithmetical problems. As our observations and the unpublished data of Nepomnyashohaya and, later, of Tsvetkova showed, these patients produce a correct plan for solving the problem after prolonged analysis of the given conditions but experience great difficulty as soon as they begin concrete arithmetical operations.

Investigations (Luria and Tsvetkova, 1966) have shown that patients with lesions of the parieto-occipital systems of the left hemisphere experience great difficulty with arithmetical problems. The grammatical system of expressions in which the conditions of the problem are formulated are outside their grasp as a logical-grammatical structure to be directly perceived, and this invariably causes them considerable difficulty. The patients of this group try hard to elucidate the meaning of the problem and attentively analyze every sentence composing it. They will ask: "What does 'larger by five kilograms' mean? Why 'five' and 'kilograms?' Where does the 'five' come in?"; they begin to comprehend the meaning expressed by this sentence only after they have learned the meaning of each of these grammatical expressions. Investigations by Bubnova (1946) and later by Tsvetkova (1966) have shown that it is only through the use of special measures, with the exteriorization of the diagnostic features of logical-grammatical structures, that these defects can be overcome and the patient enabled to understand the essential relationships. As soon as this has been done, there is no longer any difficulty in proceeding to the stage of learning the necessary "strategy" of the intellectual act, and the patient only begins to have difficulty in this case when performing the individual operations involved in solving the problem.

Particular interest is attached to the investigation of disturbances of the intellectual operations concerned with abstraction and generalization in these patients conducted by Kok (1957, 1958, 1960). This showed that a system of generalizations may be formed quickly in patients with a well-marked inferoparietal syndrome, based on the abstraction of logical signs; these patients can classify geometrical figures or colors equally easily. However, as soon as the investigation turns to problems in which the patient must identify a more complex sign, including the spatial relationship between elements (for example, one element lying above or below another or movement of one element toward or away from another), stable systems of generalizations cannot be formed.

These findings show that the disturbance of intellectual processes with a lesion of the parieto-occipital divisions of the brain is highly specialized in nature and is not due to a defect of any "symbolic function" or "abstract intellectual activity"; it is evidently more closely related to a disturbance of definite types of spatial syntheses. The investigations of disturbances of higher mental functions in lesions of the parieto-occipital divisions of the cortex are still in their infancy. Psychologists and psychophysiologists are faced with the task of giving a careful and accurate description of the syndromes arising in association with lesions situated in different areas of these divisions of the brain and of studying the factors on which these syndromes are based.

4. *Disturbances of Higher Cortical Functions with Lesions of the Sensorimotor Regions*

So far the disturbances of the higher cortical functions arising from lesions of the cortical divisions of the exteroceptive analyzers have been described. Attention has been directed to this type of disorder in the auditory, visual, and, to some extent, tactile forms of analysis and synthesis of external stimuli and to the changes in the more complex forms of mental activity associated with such local brain defects. Now let us turn to the disturbances of voluntary movement and action observed in the presence of lesions of the sensorimotor divisions of the cerebral cortex, or, in other words, to the study of the pathology of the motor analyzer.

This topic is particularly complex, for the study of voluntary movement, more than any other branch of psychology and physiology, has felt the influence of false, idealistic philosophical concepts. Scientific attempts to tackle this field were slow to begin.

Some of the problems associated with the theory of voluntary movement and the highlights in the study of this function shall be discussed briefly, and the material now available from clinical neurology and psychophysiology will then be described.

A. HISTORICAL SURVEY

Ideas on voluntary movement were for a long time under the direct influence of idealistic philosophy. Whereas sensation and perception were usually regarded as passive states of consciousness arising when stimuli impinged on our sense organs, voluntary movements were regarded, on the contrary, as purely active processes, whereby the conscious mind directed bodily movements.

This idealistic viewpoint was encountered in philosophy, psychology, and physiology, and in all of these fields it was an obstacle to the development of scientific knowledge. In philosophy, it took the form of the well-known doctrine of free will, always the cornerstone of the most extreme idealistic schools of thought. In psychology, it was reflected in the theory of ideomotor acts, which, although it gave a correct subjective description of voluntary movement, regarded them as active phenomena taking place automatically as soon as the corresponding ideas appeared and failed to explain the process scientifically. Ultimately, voluntary movement was considered by subjective psychology to be the result of the influence of a nonmaterial spiritual power (Bergson, 1896) or as the manifestation of a spiritual "fiat" (James, 1890). In physiology, the idealistic conception of voluntary movement was revealed by the suggestion that only those regions of the anterior central gyri which, it was thought, sends "volitional impulses" to the muscles could be regarded as "voluntary motor centers." The origin of these impulses remained unexplained, and the motor area of the cortex was naturally regarded as that part of the brain in which the "spiritual principle enters into the material apparatus of the brain" (Sherrington, 1934; Eccles, 1953).

This idealistic conception of voluntary movement divorced this field from all other fields of scientific knowledge and hindered its materialistic study. A long period of scientific development was necessary before these false ideas could be overthrown and before the study of voluntary movement and the mechanisms responsible for it could be brought within the framework of scientific investigation. The decline of prescientific, idealistic views on voluntary movement was a consequence of the development of the reflex theory and of the radical changes taking place in ideas on the psychophysiological structure of self-regulating voluntary movement and actions.

A century ago, in his *Reflexes of the Brain* (1861), Sechenov formulated the hypothesis that all forms of movements, starting with the most elementary, involuntary and ending with the most complex, voluntary, are determined (or obligatory) movements and that the basic difference between the most complex forms of movement must be sought in the system of stimuli evoking them. Twenty years later, Sechenov again turned to this subject, in his *Physiology of the Nervous Centers* (1881), and propounded his hypothesis more fully, pointing out that with the change to complex forms of mental processes in man "feeling changes to reason and purpose, and movement to action."

This idea of the reflex structure of voluntary movement radically changed the orientation of its concrete investigation. By compelling abandonment of the idea that such movements are "free," undetermined acts, it directed attention to the *afferent* organization of voluntary movement and to the change in the afferent organization accompanying the transition from elementary, unconditioned reflex, or instinctive, movements to "voluntary" movements of animals and to the truly voluntary movements and actions of man.

This concept, which revolutionized the previous concepts on voluntary movement, underlies the hypothesis advanced by Pavlov that the efferent mechanisms of the motor act are merely the final effector links in the chain of its organization. According to this hypothesis, the "voluntary" movements of animals and, in particular, the truly voluntary movements of man are the result of the "integrated activity of the whole cortex" and the individual parts of the cortex perform the function of analysis and synthesis of exteroceptive and proprioceptive stimuli and constitute the various afferent mechanisms of the motor act.

An original position was adopted by Bernshtein (1947), who, following Pavlov, concluded from a series of investigations that voluntary movements cannot, in principle, be controlled by efferent impulses alone. For complex movements (locomotor or purposeful) to be controlled, Bernshtein believes that there must be a constant flow of afferent impulses, not only from external objects that are to be taken into account when the movement is constructed, but also, and primarily, from the subject's own locomotor apparatus, whose every change in the position alters the conditions of movement. That is why the decisive factors in the construction of movement are not so much the effector impulses (which are of a rather purely executive character), as the complex system of afferent impulses that give precision to the composition of the motor act and that ensure that the movements are subjected to a wide system of correction.

Similar views were expressed by Orbeli (1935) and Anokhin (1935, etc.), who showed that de-afferentation of a limb, by making the motor impulses diffuse and incapable of correction, completely abolishes the ability to control movement.

It would be wrong to suppose that the system of afferent impulses determining the motor act is simple in construction and limited to a single group of analyzers. It is easy to see that the conditions determining the structure of a voluntary movement must include visual, auditory, tactile, and in particular, kinesthetic afferent impulses. Each of these afferent systems (whose disturbances have already been examined) is responsible for one aspect of the organization of the motor act; however, the analysis and synthesis of the stimuli on which performance of the movement is based involve the participation of all of these specialized systems. The central apparatus of movement production, or what Pavlov called the "motor analyzer," is therefore the most complex and the most generalized of all the mechanisms for analysis and synthesis, with the aforementioned analyzers constituting its specialized components. Disturbances in the working of the motor analyzer and changes in the course of motor processes may therefore develop from lesions in the most widely separated parts of the brain.

An essential fact is that the system of afferent impulses determining the motor act changes at different levels of ontogenesis and in different conditions for the performance of movement. Many investigations conducted during recent years (cited by Piaget, 1935, and Zaporozhets, 1960) have shown that not only in the various stages of phylogenesis, but that also during the ontogenetic development of the child, the psychological and psychophysiological structure of voluntary movements undergoes considerable change.

In the very earliest stages—during the intra-uterine and early postnatal periods of development—the movements of the fetus and infant are almost entirely determined by interoceptive and proprioceptive controlling influences and are elementary and diffuse in character. Following Coghill (1929) and Anokhin (1935, etc.), we conducted a series of experiments in which we observed that stimulation of the facial skin of a five-month human fetus caused a diffuse wave of excitation. Only those movements evoked by stimulation of the lips and included in the system of the instinctive act of sucking, becoming perfected at that time, bore anything like a precisely organized character (Luria, 1932 [Eng.]). Subsequently these elementary unconditioned-reflex movements begin to be supplemented by new, acquired movements that require the closest participation of the cortical apparatus and that gradually come more and more under the control of the telereceptors. The child's first year is largely taken up by the formation of these more complex movements, voluntary in the wide sense of the term (locomotor and objective); they receive afferent impulses from both the visual and the kinesthetic systems and begin to come under the domination of complex systems of afferent syntheses (Figurin and Denisova, 1949; etc.).

However, the formation of the integrated afferent organization of motor acts may be regarded as only the beginning of the long road to (or as the prehistory of) the development of truly voluntary movements. The formation of truly voluntary movements is intimately related to another factor, the latter playing a decisive role in the structure of this formation. Analysis of this factor will enable us to probe deeply into the nature of the internal mechanisms of voluntary movement and action.

From the initial stages of the child's development (from the second year of life), the system of speech signals is incorporated into the mechanism of construction of the child's actions—initially in the form of an adult's spoken instructions and later in the form of the child's own speech and the communication system based upon it. The participation of speech in the formation of the child's motor acts has been the subject of detailed study in recent years (Kol'tsova, 1958; Luria, 1955, 1956–1958, 1959*b* [Eng.]; Yakovleva, 1958; Tikhomirov, 1958, etc.) and has enabled the essential steps in the development of voluntary movements to be identified and studied. As these investigations (which will be considered again) showed, in the first stages the spoken instruction of the adult can only trigger individual movements but cannot restrain or control them and cannot correct movements of long duration. Only in the subsequent stages can the speech of the adult, and later the speech of the child itself, undertake the task of formulating, at first externally and later internally as well, the dimensions and plan of the motor act, introducing the necessary corrections into the movements, and comparing the result of the movement with its intention. These are the mechanisms that bring about the change from the quasi-voluntary movements of the infant to the truly voluntary movements of the older child and the adult.

The analysis of voluntary movements made during recent decades by physiologists and psychologists and the aforementioned investigations on the formation of voluntary movements are of fundamental importance. They showed that the idealistic view of voluntary movements as the result of purely willed acts obstructed the path to the scientific investigation of these movements and must give way to the idea that *voluntary movements are complex reflex acts* carried out under the influence of a group of afferent systems. These afferent systems, situated at various levels in the brain, include the system of speech signals. The connections formed on the basis of these signals are included in the mechanisms forming the truly voluntary motor act, determining its direction and controlling its course. The planning and organization of the motor act constitute a specific feature of voluntary movement and action proper and of complex, perfected voluntary activity, which will be examined subsequently (Part II, Section 5D).

By replacing the idealistic conception of voluntary movement by the scientific, deterministic analysis of the mechanisms involved, the reflex theory supplies ample ground for rejecting any attempt to approach voluntary movement and action from the standpoint of narrow localization.

By regarding efferent mechanisms as only part of the cerebral organization of motor acts, and redirecting attention to those afferent systems taking part in the construction of the motor act, the reflex theory shows that voluntary movement is the result of the integrated activity of the whole brain and that as the most highly organized activity, it may be impaired by many lesions of the cerebral hemispheres. The great vulnerability of voluntary movements to many, varied lesions of the brain may be attributed to the fact that a lesion of any zone of the cortex comprising part of the complex afferent system involved with organization of voluntary movement must inevitably affect the performance of the movement. That is why the study of the pathological basis of voluntary movements, of defects in their architectonics, and of disturbances of their neurodynamics constitutes so complex a chapter in clinical neurology and psychophysiology.

• • •

The history of the study of disorders in voluntary movement will be reviewed briefly. The study of disturbances of voluntary movement arising from circumscribed brain lesions, known as "apraxia," began much later than the study of disorders of speech and gnosis. The first stage in this study was largely taken up with the description of the special features of these disturbances in psychological terms; the subsequent development of the study of the apraxias was connected with attempts to overcome the concepts of subjective psychology and to analyze the mechanisms lying at the basis of these disturbances.

When Liepmann (1900) first introduced the concept of apraxia, his main purpose was to differentiate this type of motor disorder from the more elementary phenomena of paralysis, ataxia, and disturbances in tone. For this reason he was inclined from the start to include this phenomenon in the group of disturbances of the higher mental functions known since the time of Finkelburg (1870) as "asymbolias" (i.e., disturbances of the symbolic functions of the mind) and to associate it with the disturbances of voluntary movement described by Meynert (1899) as "motor asymbolia."

Following in the footsteps of Freud (1891), who defined agnosia as a disturbance of visual perception in which the elementary visual functions are preserved, Leipmann defined apraxia as the "inability to perform purposeful movement" in the absence of paresis, ataxia, or a disturbance of tone. He regarded it as the result of a lesion of "those parts of the brain which, in the language of psychology, can disturb the domination of the mind over the individual members of the body, even though the latter are undamaged and remain capable of movement" (Liepmann, 1900). Liepmann's description of the "psychological" form of motor disturbance marked an important contribution to the neurological literature. However, his analysis of the pathology of movement was conducted from the standpoint of associative psychology, just as Wernicke, before him, had investigated aphasia and Lissauer agnosia.

According to Liepmann, the voluntary motor act is the result of a mental idea of a movement and of the motor effect that this idea evokes. He therefore believed that it would be possible to distinguish, as the factors responsible for the voluntary movement, *ideas* of the purpose of the action and of the possible ways of performing the action and that these ideas are composed, in turn, of visual and kinesthetic ideas, which ultimately produce the required movement. These ideas are stored in the form of "engrams" or "memory images" in the corresponding (mainly the postcentral, inferoparietal, and parieto-occipital) regions of the cortex and may be reanimated when a general "ideational plan" of movement arises. If the general plan of a movement leads to the retrieval, or ecphoria, of mnestic-associative connections firmly established by previous experience, the movement will be highly automatized in character, the corresponding "ideas" will be stripped of their complex psychological signs, and the act becomes a simplified physiological process.

In Liepmann's opinion, circumscribed brain lesions may disturb several different links of this mechanism of movement construction. In some cases they make the plan of the movement itself impossible, leading to what is called "ideational apraxia," in which the patient cannot create an image of the required movement. In other cases the image of the required movement is present but the connections between this image and the nervous apparatuses responsible for putting it into operation are interrupted. In these cases the patient, even when he knows what movement he must carry out, cannot put it into effect because the engrams that have been laid down by his previous motor experience cannot be revived. As a result, there emerges that form of apraxia that Liepmann called "motor apraxia." Liepmann subdivided this disorder into "ideokinetic" apraxia (disturbance of voluntary movements resulting from the dissociation of the purpose of the movement from the corresponding innervation) and "limb-kinetic" apraxia ("Gliedkinetische Apraxie"), by which he meant disturbance of special schemes of movements of the hand, or of the articulatory apparatus, etc. laid down in previous experience. The more the focus encroaches on the posterior (parietal and parieto-occipital) portions of the brain, the more the motor disturbances approximate the ideational form of apraxia; when they involve the postcentral region, limb-kinetic apraxia develops. This state of affairs is illustrated in Fig. 52.

This theory of apraxia which Liepmann developed in a series of published reports (1900, 1905, 1913, 1920) and which was supported by neurologists such as Kleist (1907, 1911) and Pick (1905), was the first attempt to analyze disturbances of the higher motor functions and to differentiate their various forms. Liepmann's clinical investigations were so thorough that many of his descriptions of the apraxias retain their interest even today.

Despite Liepmann's valuable contribution to the clinical understanding of apraxia in general and of its forms, his theory immediately came up against several serious theoretical and practical difficulties. These were due primarily to the basic psychological standpoints from which Liepmann regarded voluntary movement, i.e., as the result of subjective ideas or volitional impulses. Because of this point of view, Liepmann in effect continued the psychomorphological tradition. He directly compared the "nonspatial psychological concepts" with the "spatial pattern of the brain." Discussions of this sort inevitably closed the door to the scientific analysis of the phenomena and also, which is particularly important, wrongly placed the apraxias (both ideational and ideokinetic) in a class apart from the more elementary forms of disturbances of the afferent systems lying at the basis of the construction of every movement. Soon after Liepmann published his theories, Monakow (1914) therefore came out with a strong criticism against them and urged that the apraxias be approached from the strictly physiological point of view. He regarded apraxia as a pathology of automatized movements resulting from a disturbance by the brain lesion of "the excitability of certain areas of the cortex, leading to interference with the course of certain reflex arcs and to elimination of certain reflex components" (1914, p. 96). Monakow refrained from making the sharp division between the apraxias and the more elementary disorders that Liepmann had made and looked for forms of motor disorders that would bridge the gap between apraxia and paresis, on the one hand, and sensory disturbances, on the other. He accordingly recognized the existence of various forms of "motor" and "sensory" apraxias and distinguished them from the "gnostic" apraxias.

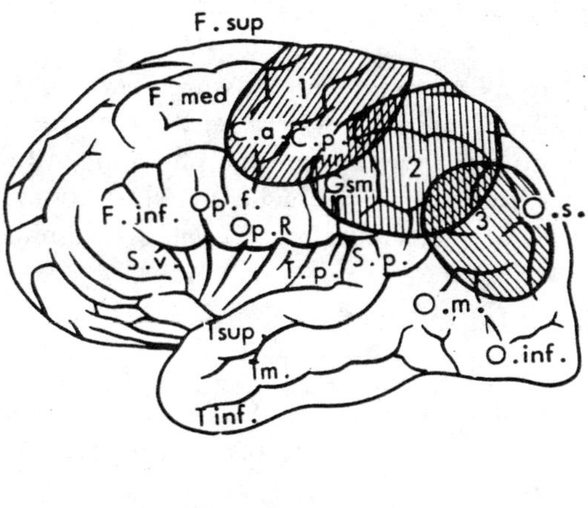

FIGURE 52 Localization of the apraxias according to Liepmann (1900, etc.). (*1*) A lesion of this area causes limb-kinetic apraxia. (*2*) A lesion of this area causes ideokinetic apraxia. (*3*) A lesion of this area causes ideational apraxia.

Monakow's views were developed further by his pupil Brun (1921) and to some extent by Sittig (1931), who carried the analysis of disturbances of voluntary movements of varying degrees of automatism associated with local brain lesions a significant step further.

The difficulties that beset Liepmann were also of a practical nature. Regarding the apraxias as disturbances in the ideas of movement and associating them mainly with foci in the posterior divisions of the brain led, in fact, to the limitation of the concept of apraxia, which no longer included all the rich and varied forms of movement disturbances described by clinicians. Later on, Liepmann himself was forced to recognize the possibility that ideational apraxia could exist in association with circumscribed lesions in the frontal region. Additional findings pertaining to the role of lesions lying outside the parietal divisions of the brain in the development of apraxia were reported by Pick (1905, etc.), who described "perseveratory apraxia," by Kleist (1907), who described "apraxia of the sequence of action," and, later, by Denny-Brown (1958), who distinguished between frontal and parietal forms of apraxia. A crisis developed in the study of apraxia, which called for a radical re-examination of the original subjective psychological concepts, for release from the bonds of psychomorphological doctrine, and for considerable extension of the physiological analysis of the cerebral mechanisms of voluntary movement. This reorientation characterized the last period in the study of disorders of voluntary movement. Investigation was now concerned with bridging the gap between the elementary and the complex disorders of motor function and with giving a more reliable analysis of the neurodynamic mechanisms underlying motor disturbances arising from brain lesions.

The investigations started by Wilson (1908) and continued by Head (1920), Pötzl (1937), and others demonstrated the role of the integration of kinesthetic impulses in the construction and realization of movements. Their findings were re-examined by Schilder (1935), who analyzed the role of the "body image" in movement construction, and by Mayer-Gross (1935), who undertook a special investigation of the components responsible for the disturbance of automatized movements arising in apraxia. Finally, Critchley (1953) and, in particular, Denny-Brown and co-workers (1952, 1958) made detailed studies of the physiological conditions underlying apraxia.

These studies, whose purpose it is to bridge the gap between the pathology of comparatively elementary and that of complex forms of motor activity and to concentrate on the physiological analysis of the disturbances fundamentally concerned in apraxia, are still in their early stages. Nevertheless, they indicate clearly enough the future direction for the study of disturbances of voluntary movements accompanying local brain lesions.

The way in which the study of apraxia developed in classical neurology has been outlined very briefly. We shall now turn to considerations on the structure of the cortical divisions of the motor analyzer and on the physiology of the voluntary motor act. Following this, pathology of the higher motor functions resulting from circumscribed lesions of the cerebral cortex will be examined.

B. THE MOTOR ANALYZER AND THE STRUCTURE OF THE SENSORIMOTOR REGION

As a result of the general revision of ideas regarding the structure of motor processes, considerable modifications have recently been introduced into the description of the cerebral mechanisms of voluntary movements. The starting point for this revision was the reflex theory of voluntary movement, which has already been considered. The introduction of the reflex theory necessitated an entirely different approach to the cerebral mechanisms of the motor act.

Only rather recently has there been general acceptance of the view that the cortical apparatus of voluntary movements is localized in the motor area of the cortex, or Brodmann's Area 4, and in the corresponding extrapyramidal subcortical motor ganglia. Ever since the historic investigations of Betz (1874), who discovered the giant pyramidal cells in the fifth layer of this zone, the view has been held that the postcentral region is the sensory projection area and that the anterior central gyrus is the motor apparatus of the cerebral cortex, regulating voluntary movements and directing its impulses along the efferent pyramidal tract to the anterior horns of the spinal cord.

The reflex theory of movement, formulated by Pavlov and his pupils (Krasnogorskii, 1911; Konorski and Miller, 1936; Skipin, 1947, 1956, 1958) and developed by Orbeli (1935), Anokhin (1935), and Bernshtein (1947), compelled modification of this concept.

The view that the efferent motor impulses are only the final stage in the preparation of the motor act by the brain and that a fundamental role in this process is played by the system of afferent syntheses forming these motor impulses led to the replacement of the concept of cortical motor centers by the much wider concept of cortical divisions of the motor analyzer. According to this new idea, the cortical divisions of the motor analyzer embrace a large group of cortical zones and its activity is responsible for the various preparatory processes of the motor act. Some of these organize voluntary movements in the system of external spatial coordinates, another group analyzes the impulses arriving from the muscles and joints, and a third group implements the regulating influence of speech connections, an important component of the organization of voluntary movement. Some authors (Bernshtein, 1947; Luria, 1957) believe that all of these regions of the brain must be considered components of the cortical part of the motor analyzer in the broad meaning of the term. As shall be discussed more fully, each region contributes to the organization of the motor act, each being responsible for one particular aspect of the production of the movement.

However, in addition to the broad concept of the cortical divisions of the motor analyzer, there are perfectly legitimate grounds, in connection with the differentiation of the cortical nucleus of the motor analyzer, for a narrower concept of these divisions. The feature of the cortical nucleus of the motor analyzer distinguishing it from the corresponding divisions of the other analyzers is that it is related not to one, but to *two zones of the cerebral cortex, usually designated as the postcentral and precentral regions. These two regions work in close cooperation with one another* and, together, form a single functional apparatus, the *sensorimotor region of the cortex.*

This distinctive feature of the cortical apparatus of the motor analyzer has its basis in structural, dynamic, and genetic factors. The structural and dynamic basis for the identification of the sensorimotor region as the cortical nucleus of the motor analyzer is the very fact that the motor act is a complex functional system. Before a voluntary movement can be carried out, the visual, vestibular, or acoustic impulses must first be recoded into a definite system of kinesthetic signals. This system forms a three-dimensional grid, enabling the efferent signals to be correctly directed to the appropriate muscle groups and at the same time dynamically altering the direction of these signals in accordance with the position of the muscles and joints in space. Without this kinesthetic basis, no movement can be performed. This is demonstrated by the well-known experiments in which de-afferentation of a limb (at any level of the afferent apparatus) causes disappearance of the precision and differentiation of the motor impulses. This kinesthetic basis of movement is the responsibility of the postcentral divisions of the cortical nucleus of the motor analyzer, which recode exteroceptive signals into kinesthetic constellations and integrate impulses into *simultaneous groups*, as discussed previously (Part II, Section 3C).

Nevertheless, kinesthetic integration is only one aspect of the cortical organization of voluntary movements. Every voluntary movement is a *series of successive innervations* rather than a single spatially organized motor act. This can be observed for practically every movement, but it stands out particularly clearly in every complex motor skill, which consists of a series of successively changing innervations; this series of innervations comprises a single kinetic melody. As many writers have shown (Lashley, 1937; Luria, 1957; etc.), this kinetic melody cannot be composed by the same cerebral apparatus that is responsible for the spatial organization of motor impulses. All the evidence indicates that it requires a special cerebral mechanism, which brings about the inhibition of the motor impulse once it has appeared and integrates the successive impulses into a single motor stereotype that has developed over a period of time. There are many grounds for localizing this aspect of the efferent integration of the motor act in the anterior divisions of the cortical nucleus of the motor analyzer, especially in the premotor region (Part II, Section 4E).

The complex character of the cortical nucleus of the motor analyzer, responsible for both the kinesthetic and the kinetic organization of movements, is revealed by genetic, anatomical, and neurophysiological data. Phylogenetic investigations (Brodmann, 1909; Polyakov, 1938–1948; Kukuev, 1940; Khachaturyan, 1949; etc.) have shown that in the early stages of phylogenesis the sensorimotor region constituted a morphologically unified system; only comparatively recently did it differentiate into sensory and motor zones. However, after the structural unity of the sensorimotor region had given way to the morphological separation into two regions, these regions continued to be functionally united, as revealed by both morphological and physiological signs.

As was discussed (Part I, Section 2C), when excitation reaches the postcentral portion of the cortex it is relayed to the precentral portion of the motor cortex, either through transcortical connections or through the ventrolateral nucleus of the thalamus, which is the subcortical integrative apparatus of the motor system. Another fact bearing on this discussion is that in both the postcentral and the precentral region of the cerebral cortex there are both afferent and efferent groups of fibers, affording further proof of the structural and functional unity of the two parts of the cortical nucleus of the motor analyzer. If to these facts is added the important discovery made by Lassek (1954) that, contrary to previous ideas, only a comparatively small part of the fibers of the pyramidal tract arise in the giant Betz cells of the anterior central gyrus and that a large proportion of them originate in the postcentral and premotor divisions of the cortex, the unity of these divisions of the sensorimotor cortex will be still more apparent.

Because of these facts, a fresh interpretation has to be given to the function of the anterior central gyrus, long regarded as the motor center of the cerebral cortex. The giant pyramidal cells of Betz are without doubt apparatuses generating efferent motor impulses and components of the "anterior horns of the brain" (Bernshtein, 1947). However, their neurophysiological role is not simply that of directing the impulses generated therein toward the muscles at the periphery; it also includes the reception of the many different dynamic influences arising in other afferent divisions of the sensorimotor portion of the cortex. The higher in the evolutionary scale the animal stands, the more complex the system of afferent impulses received by the Betz cells. That is why, as von Bonin (1943) has pointed out, evolution is accompanied by an increase in the size of the Betz cells and by a reduction in their number per cubic millimeter of gray matter and, therefore, in an increase in the ratio between the total mass of the gray matter and the mass of the bodies of the Betz cells (Table 1).

Table 1

Phylogenetic Development of the Cortical Structures of the Anterior Central Gyrus *(After von Bonin, 1943)*

	Diameter of Betz cells (in μ)	*Number of Betz cells per cubic millimeter gray matter*	*Ratio of mass of gray matter to mass of Betz cell bodies*
Lower monkeys	3, 7	31	52
Higher monkeys	—	—	113
Man	6, 1	12	233

It may be concluded from the foregoing facts that the cortical nucleus of the motor analyzer is, in fact, the sensorimotor portion of the cortex, morphologically differentiated but behaving as a functional unit. This conclusion has been confirmed by a number of physiological observations.

The neuronographic investigations of McCulloch (1943) showed that excitation caused by application of a stimulus to the postcentral portion of the cortex spreads to the precentral portion, i.e., the impulses arising from this stimulation may be followed to Area 4. Conversely, if a stimulus is applied to the precentral cortical divisions, the excitation spreads to the postcentral divisions, and its effect may be traced to the entire group of fields composing this region (Fig. 53).

That is why, as Penfield and Rasmussen (1950) showed, stimulation of the sensory divisions of the postcentral region may give rise not only to a sensory, but also to a motor effect (Fig. 54). Therefore, there is every reason to suppose that the "motor center" of the cortex, in the narrow meaning of the term, is a complex formation consisting of two regions (postcentral and precentral), both participating in a combined operation but each, as will be demonstrated, having its own specific function.

The organization of the two zones composing the cortical nucleus of the motor analyzer has much in common with what has already been elucidated in regard to the cortical structure of other analyzers. The central (or primary) field of each of these components comprises the projection areas of the cerebral cortex. The projection areas of the postcentral portions (Area 3) contain the terminations of fibers coming from the periphery and carrying impulses

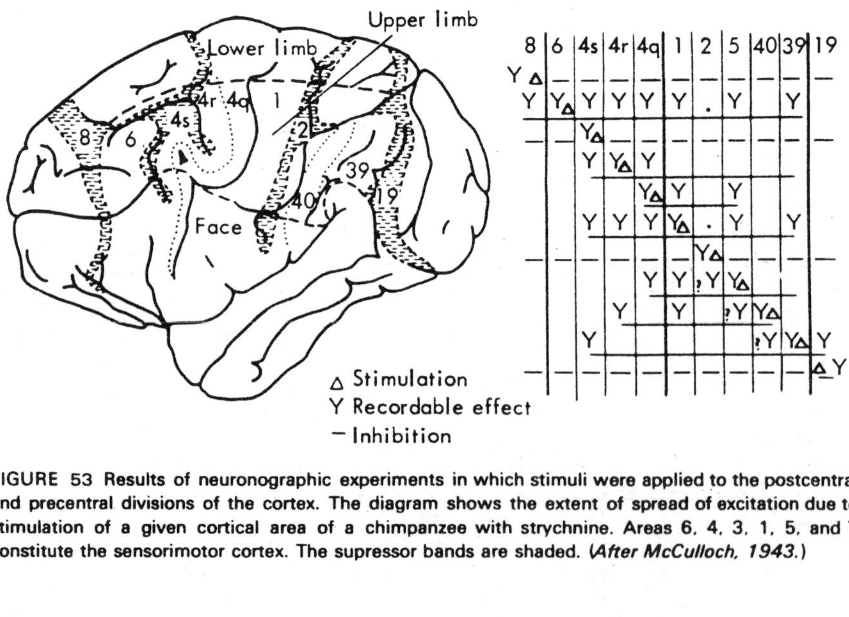

FIGURE 53 Results of neuronographic experiments in which stimuli were applied to the postcentral and precentral divisions of the cortex. The diagram shows the extent of spread of excitation due to stimulation of a given cortical area of a chimpanzee with strychnine. Areas 6, 4, 3, 1, 5, and 7 constitute the sensorimotor cortex. The supressor bands are shaded. (*After McCulloch, 1943.*)

from one of the receptor zones, while fibers whose course lies in the pyramidal tract, passing to the motor neurons of the spinal cord, originate in the projection area of the precentral region (Area 4). The projections of the fibers in these parts of the cortex characteristically possess distinct somatotopic features, for the lower limbs are represented in the contralateral upper sensorimotor portion, while the upper limbs and face are represented in the middle and lower portions of this region. The most characteristic feature (which cannot be seen as clearly in the cortical divisions of the other analyzers) is that, as mentioned (Part I, Section 2B), the projection of the corresponding divisions of the peripheral sensorimotor apparatus is represented in these sensorimotor cortical divisions in accordance with a *functional and not a geometrical principle.* The greater the functional importance of a given organ, the richer its system of connections, the greater its role in the system of voluntary movements, and the larger the area occupied by its projection in the cerebral cortex. Turning

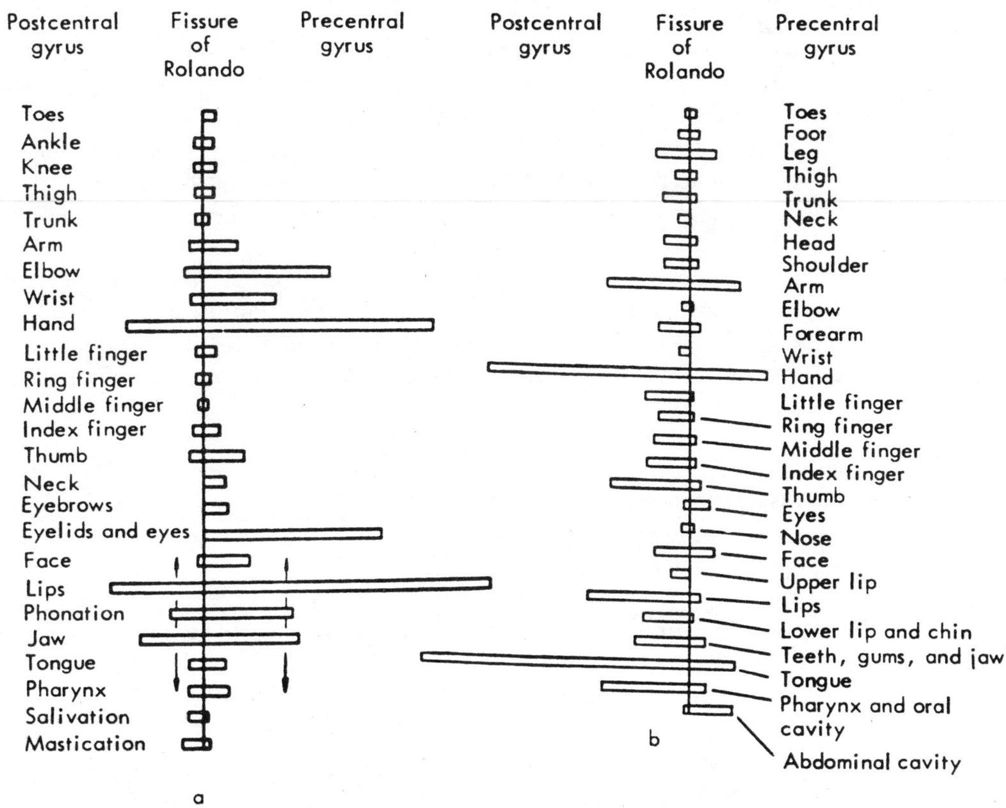

FIGURE 54 Motor and sensory reactions during stimulation of the precentral and postcentral divisions of the cortex. (*a*) Representation of the motor processes in the cerebral cortex. (*b*) Representation of the sensory processes in the cerebral cortex. The length of the columns indicates the relative number of motor and sensory reactions caused by stimulation of the points situated anteriorly or posteriorly to the fissure of Rolando. (*After Penfield and Rasmussen, 1950.*)

back to Fig. 10, the results of Penfield's experiments may be seen, in which he stimulated various areas of the sensorimotor cortex and obtained sensory or motor responses in the corresponding parts of the body. It is easy to see what a large area is covered by the cortical projections of the upper limb and of the organs of speech compared with the projection area of the trunk, thighs, and legs.

The primary (projection) fields of the cortical nucleus of the motor analyzer are in juxtaposition to the secondary fields: Areas 2, 1, 5, and 7 of the postcentral gyrus and Areas 6 and 8 of the premotor region. The latter are similar in nature to the secondary fields of the nuclear zone of other analyzers. As repeatedly mentioned, they play an important part in the integration of individual stimuli into "groups" (in the postcentral region) and "series" (in the premotor region).

The whole of the apparatus responsible for the cortical analysis and integration of voluntary movements is superimposed on the apparatus of the subcortical motor ganglia, which in man are not important in their own right but provide only what have been called the "background components of the motor act" (Bernshtein, 1947; etc.). We shall not concern ourselves in any great detail with the symptomatology of lesions of these formations.

Analysis of the cortical organization of voluntary movements and of their disturbances discloses two groups of movements that are especially interesting in connection with the pathology of higher mental functions, namely, movements of the hand, incorporated in various forms of voluntary action, and movements of the oral apparatus, constituting the basis of speech. In turn, the role of the "afferent" (postcentral) and "efferent"* (premotor) cortical divisions in the organization of these movements and the forms of disturbance associated with lesions of these parts of the brain will be examined.

C. DISTURBANCES OF THE AFFERENT BASIS OF VOLUNTARY MOVEMENT. AFFERENT (KINESTHETIC) APRAXIA

Disorders in voluntary movements arising from lesions of the motor area of the cortex (Area 4, the zone of giant pyramidal cells) or of its tracts is a familiar condition in neurology. The loss of precise movements, the diminished power of movement (pareses), and, finally, if the pathological condition is severe in degree, the motor paralyses have often been described in the literature and are among the best known cortical symptoms.

*The term "efferent" is used here and subsequently in a conventional and by no means precise sense. As will be clear from the subsequent account, it is also used to describe a unique form of afferent innervation of the motor act, the reason being that this afferent system is completely specialized in character.

Much less is known about the motor disturbances resulting from a lesion of the postcentral divisions of the cerebral cortex, especially of those fields belonging to the postcentral part of the cortical nucleus of the motor analyzer (Areas 3, 1, 2, 5, and, to some extent, 7). The postcentral cortical region is usually regarded as the sensory cortical region, whose function, from the clinical point of view, is completely separate from that of the motor portion of the cortex. In the analysis of lesions of this region, attention has therefore been concentrated on sensory disorders.

Nevertheless, the postcentral portion of the cortex must not be regarded solely as a sensory center. Embryogenetically, it develops as part of a single sensorimotor region, becoming an independent unit only in relatively late stages. Further, it is closely connected by association fibers to the motor fields, working with the latter in close cooperation. The anatomical and physiological evidence for this statement has previously been given (Part I, Sections 2B and C). However, the most significant evidence of the participation of the postcentral divisions in the regulation of motor acts has been obtained during clinical observations of patients with local lesions of this region.

Foerster (1936) was one of the first neurologists to make a careful study of motor disturbances arising from lesions of the postcentral divisions of the sensorimotor region. When examining a patient with a localized lesion of Areas 3, 1, and 2, he found not only sensory disturbances in the contralateral limb, but also gross motor defects. In the most severe cases, these resembled pareses, the only difference being that the potential power of the muscles was preserved. Nevertheless, the required movement could not be performed, for the corresponding motor impulse had lost its selectivity and, being unable to find the right destination, produced a diffuse contraction of both agonists and antagonists. Foerster called this phenomenon "afferent paresis." In less severe cases, the required movement was performed but was not sufficiently differentiated. It lost its clearly defined topological pattern and ceased to bear any resemblance to the required objective act, so that the clear difference that is present, for example, in the movements of a person holding a needle or carrying a large object disappeared. Foerster called this undifferentiated complex of hand movements "spade-hand movements." Similar phenomena are observed if such a patient is asked to reproduce various finger positions. Instead of the required movements, the patient gives undifferentiated, quasi-athetoid movements. The manner in which motor analysis is affected by lesions of these divisions of the cortical nucleus of the motor analyzer is illustrated in Fig. 55.

Similar disturbances arise from lesions of neighboring divisions of the parietal region situated posteriorly to those we have been considering (Area 5). As Foerster observed, the performance of differentiated movements without the support of visual control is frequently impossible. These clinical observations become somewhat more comprehensible after electromyographic recording of voluntary movements in patients with lesions of this region. In

Fig. 56 the results of such a recording in a patient with a meningioma of the postcentral region, made in our laboratory by Zambran (unpublished investigation), is presented. These experiments show that with a lesion of this region the motor impulses do, in fact, lose their selectivity and pass to both agonists and antagonists at the same time. When the tumor was removed, this diffusion of impulses gradually disappeared.

The severest of such movement disturbances may be called "afferent kinestatic ataxia"; for less complex cases an appropriate name would be "afferent" or "kinesthetic apraxia." As has been stated these disturbances result from a lesion of the posterior divisions of the cortical nucleus of the motor analyzer. A lesion of this region leads to a disorganization of spatial integration or to disturbance of those "kinesthetic schemes" of movement, upon which the construction of the motor act is based (Head, 1920; Denny-Brown, 1958).

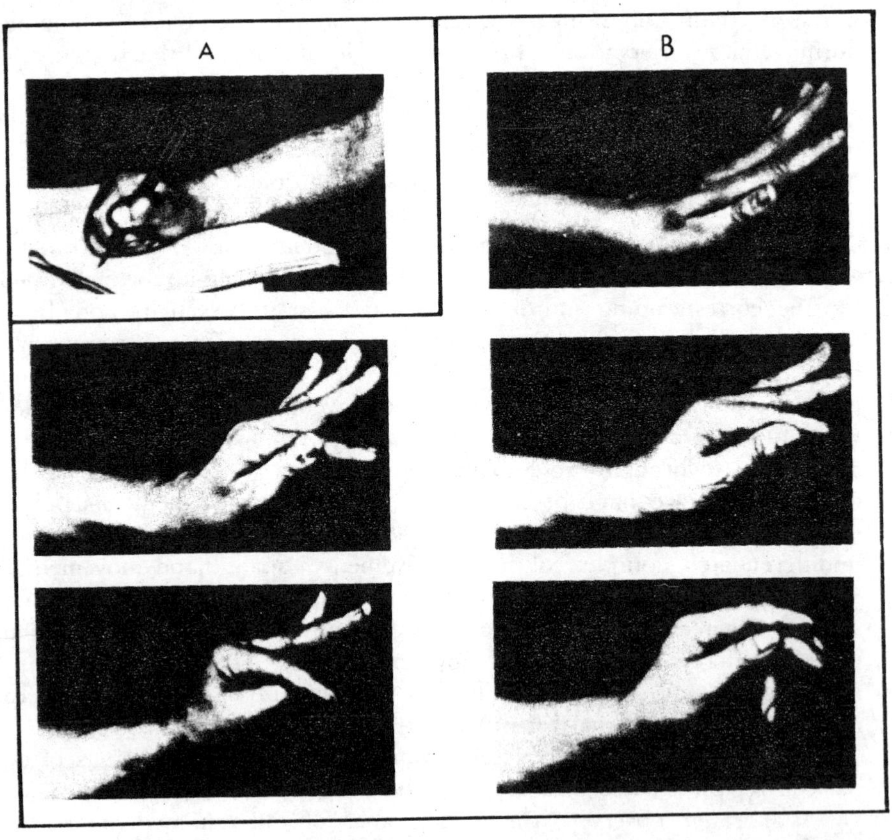

FIGURE 55 Disturbances of differentiated hand movements resulting from a lesion of the postcentral region. (*A*) Disturbance of fine writing movements. (*B*) Static ataxia in a lesion of the postcentral region. (*After Foerster, 1936.*)

All of the intermediate stages between the phenomena of kinesthetic paresis and kinesthetic ataxias and those of the more complex forms of kinesthetic apraxia are not yet known. It is possible that the variety of the disturbances observed clinically is due to different severity, the different extent, or even the different sites of the lesions. There is no doubt, however, that a more detailed study of the neurodynamic disturbances in the analysis and integration of kinesthetic impulses, of the grouping of these impulses, of their shifting to new systems at the appropriate time, etc. will help to elucidate the nature of these complex disorders.

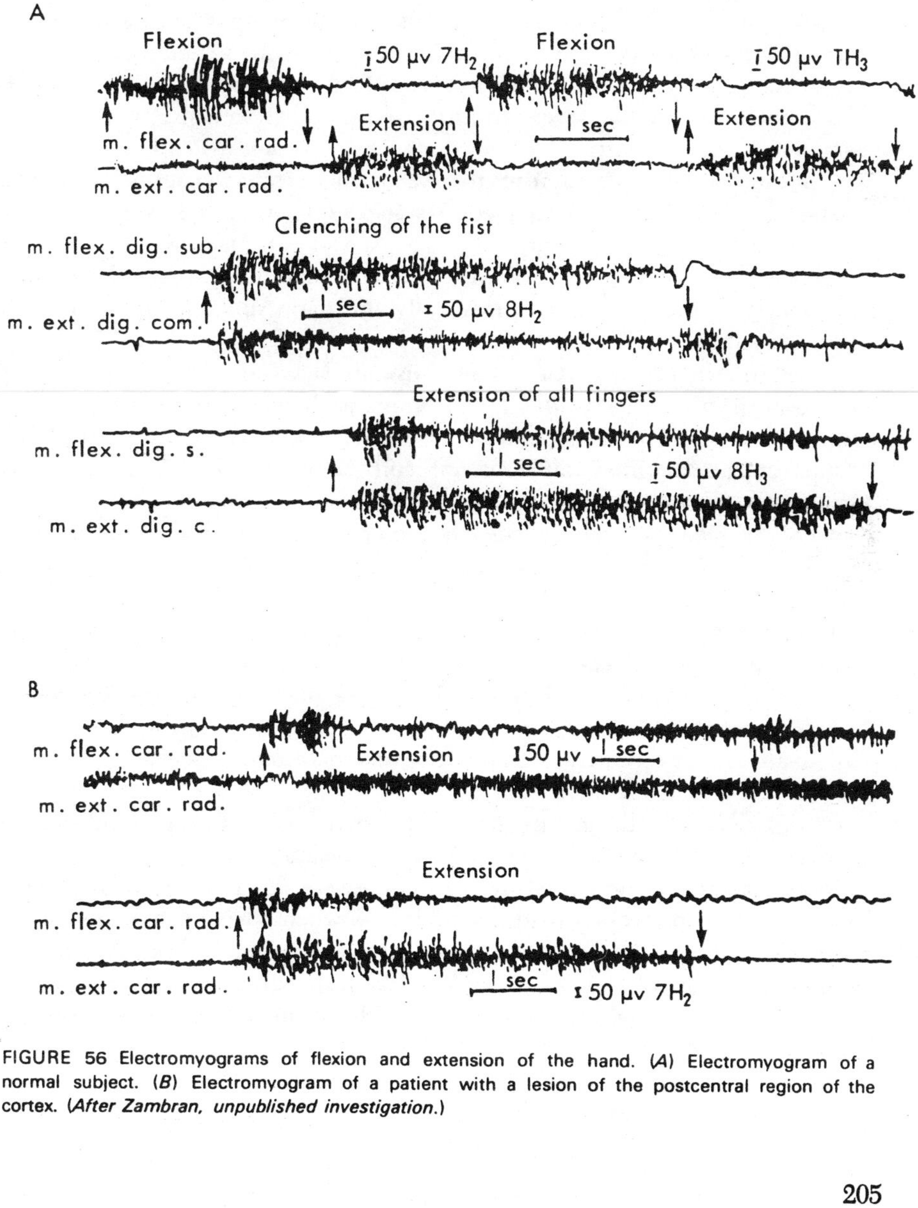

FIGURE 56 Electromyograms of flexion and extension of the hand. (*A*) Electromyogram of a normal subject. (*B*) Electromyogram of a patient with a lesion of the postcentral region of the cortex. (*After Zambran, unpublished investigation.*)

Kinesthetic apraxia is one of the forms of disturbance of voluntary movements resembling the relatively more elementary forms of movement disorder. It is based on an impairment in the cortical analysis of motor impulses and in the kinesthetic integration of movements. Although the disturbances occurring in this type of apraxia affect muscle systems organized in space, kinesthetic apraxia differs essentially from the visual-motor disturbances of orientation in space described previously (Part II, Section 3E). In this form of apraxia, the visual organization of external spatial coordinates (up, down, right, left) may remain intact; what is affected is primarily the ability to select the required kinesthetic impulses for bringing about the movement.

A patient with kinesthetic apraxia, in contrast to a patient with spatial apractagnosia, can control the direction of his movements perfectly well. He does not hold a knife or spoon in the wrong position (for example, upside down), as does the latter; he does not turn to the left instead of to the right, etc. However, when he attempts to take an object, to fasten a button, or to tie a shoelace, he cannot make the required selection of movements. He will spend a long time seeking the required positions and eventually will carry out the movement with the other, sound hand. This inability to make the required movement selection is characteristically the main difficulty present in this form of apraxia.

The kinesthetic form of apraxia usually develops from lesions of the postcentral divisions of the left (dominant) hemisphere and is exhibited most clearly in the contralateral upper limb (where it frequently is complicated by paresis); sometimes, however, difficulty may also be experienced in the ipsilateral upper limb. In lesions of the left postcentral region, therefore, analysis of the movements of the left hand may also reveal signs of kinesthetic apraxia. When the presence of afferent paresis in the right hand makes fine movement impossible and thereby masks the possible manifestations of kinesthetic apraxia, the investigation of the motor functions of the left upper limb may help with the topical diagnosis. However, many cases have been described in which kinesthetic apraxia developed in one hand only. These cases, which have been studied physiologically by Liepmann (1905, 1920) and, more recently, by Denny-Brown (1958) and Hécaen and co-workers (1956), are of particular interest.

Kinesthetic apraxia giving rise to disturbances of objective and imitative movements is particularly prominent in instances in which the patient's movements are unsupported by vision. The reproduction of actions by such patients is therefore particularly impaired when the object is not present (for example, if asked to show how tea is poured into a cup). Hence, the kinesthetic basis of the organization of action is an essential component of symbolic actions, and a disturbance in such actions is regarded in neurology as an apraxic entity.

From what has been said, the importance of detailed study of disturbances in the analysis and integration of kinesthetic impulses in this type of apraxia is evident. Much knowledge of the kinesthetic basis of movement can be obtained by clinical investigation, for example by repeating the system of upper limb movements recorded at different angles (which is easily done by means of a kinematometer), transferring the system of movements to the other hand, forming conditioned motor reactions on a kinesthetic basis, etc. Details of clinical methods of investigation of the kinesthesias will be given subsequently (Part III, Section 3B).

• • •

A disturbance of kinesthetic analysis and integration of movements may sometimes not be generalized but may mainly be manifested in relation to one zone or system. Besides apraxias of the hand, oral apraxia in which the kinesthetic basis of speech movements is disturbed can be distinguished. Its structure is similar to that of kinesthetic apraxia. This type of oral apraxia is clearly revealed by tests involving the repetition of indicated movements of the lips and tongue (for example, puffing out one cheek or putting the tongue between the lips and teeth) or by tests in which the required movements are to be performed by command. These tests are very difficult for such patients, for the necessary neural connections cannot be immediately established; consequently, the ensuing movements are imprecise and diffuse. Sometimes these diffuse movements are substituted for by the reproduction of stereotypes, formed previously, or by motor perseverations. Partial compensation for these defects is possible only with the aid of additional visual afferent impulses. In these cases the patient discovers the necessary movements only in a roundabout manner.

The kinesthetic form of apraxia differs from Liepmann's ideational apraxia and is closer to the "limb-kinetic" apraxia described some time ago by Kleist and referred to by Liepmann as one form of "ideokinetic" apraxia. The difference is based only on the fact that kinesthetic apraxia is distinguished by a causal, dynamic sign, and, therefore, only those forms of apraxia based on the disturbance of kinesthetic analysis and integration can be so designated. These disturbances may develop either independently or as a component of more complex forms of apraxia.

D. DISTURBANCES OF THE KINESTHETIC BASIS OF SPEECH. AFFERENT (KINESTHETIC) MOTOR APHASIA

Examination of the kinesthetic forms of apraxia and of the disturbance of oral praxis leads directly to one of the most complex problems—that of motor aphasia and of its underlying physiological mechanisms.

Motor aphasia, which has always been defined as a disturbance, despite preservation of elementary oral movements, of the ability to articulate words and to use speech, has always been one of the most complex problems in neurology. The reasons why a patient who apparently has the power of articulation cannot speak have not been discovered. It is, therefore, of the greatest importance to analyze motor aphasia and to identify those components of impaired speech leading to various types of difficulty in the articulation of words. In this section this problem will be examined. Analysis of the various factors responsible for the disturbance of the motor aspect of speech will be attempted, with a view to differentiating the possible types of motor aphasia.

The study of motor aphasia began much earlier than the study of the agnosias and apraxias. It passed through the same stages and encountered the same difficulties as those noted in the preceding historical surveys. As stated, Broca first described the syndrome of motor aphasia a century ago and localized the underlying lesion in the inferior zone of the third frontal gyrus of the left hemisphere. This discovery laid the foundation for a new era in the study of the localization of functions in the cerebral cortex.

In his description of motor aphasia, Broca attempted to draw a line between this condition and two sharply contrasting disorders: intellectual impairment ("alogia") and a disturbance of the motor function of the organs of speech ("mechanical alalia"). Nevertheless, Broca did not believe that motor aphasia presents a single picture. On the basis of his distinction between two forms of disturbance of active speech, he recognized "verbal amnesia," in which the patient's ability to find the required words is lost on account of the "loss of memory for words," and "aphemia" or "true motor aphasia," in which the basis of the defect is a disturbance of the "ability to articulate" or, the "ability to produce coordinated motor acts, at the same time intellectual and muscular, constituting articulated speech." According to Broca's description, the patient with "aphemia" retains the relationships between thoughts and words extremely well but has lost the ability to express these relationships by the coordinated movements that have been formed and consolidated during long practice. He loses the "special type of memory—not memory for words, but memory for the movements essential for the articulation of words." Broca localized this "memory for the motor images of words" at the base of the third frontal gyrus of the left hemisphere. Subsequently, this area of the brain came to be regarded as the "center for motor speech" or "Broca's center."

It would not have been possible in Broca's time, because of lack of knowledge of the fine structure of and the physiological laws governing the working of the cerebral cortex, to give a more precise clinical description of motor aphasia. Nevertheless, it was quite obvious that the psychomorphological system of concepts from which this theory was drawn was inadequate. Tendencies like sharply demarcating disorders of memory for articulatory movements from other motor disorders and localizing the motor images of words in a circumscribed area of the inferior frontal gyrus at once encountered theoretical and practical difficulties and soon became a hindrance to further scientific development.

The limitation of Broca's concept was that it necessitated drawing a sharp distinction between disturbances of the motor images of words and all other sensory and motor disorders and required that this psychological phenomenon be localized within a narrow region of the brain. This naturally closed the door both to the more accurate description of the clinical forms of these disturbances and to the further study of the psychophysiological mechanisms underlying this condition. From the practical point of view, the defect of this concept was that, by fixing attention on the base of the third frontal gyrus as the center of the motor images of speech, it detracted from the wealth of clinical factors, ignored many findings outside its compass, and thus was unable to analyze the components of motor aphasia. The contradictions of Broca's theory are at once apparent from his first examination of a patient's brain (Fig. 57). As Pierre Marie originally pointed out, the lesion observed in this patient extended far beyond the borders of the base of the third frontal gyrus, affecting the lower divisions of the postcentral and part of the upper divisions of the temporal region.

Further investigations showed that, besides cases of motor aphasia in which the lesion was actually situated in Broca's area, there were others in which Broca's area remained completely uninvolved, although the clinical picture showed well-defined motor aphasic disorders. In the latter cases the lesion was situated entirely in the lower part of the postcentral region. One such patient was investigated by Nissl von Meyendorff (1930). These findings called for a reappraisal of ideas concerning motor aphasia and for revision of Broca's theories.

Fundamental misgivings were expressed about Broca's principal hypothesis, i.e., any case of motor aphasia must be due to a lesion of the third frontal gyrus. Investigators were doubtful about the claim that all aphasias are based on a disturbance of the motor images of words quite independent of sensory components and unassociated with more elementary neurological defects.

Two factors influenced the subsequent development of the study of motor aphasia: the accumulating knowledge of the structure and function of the sensory regions of the cerebral cortex and the newly expressed theory of the apraxias. As a result of these two factors, suggestions were made that the phenomena of motor aphasia (or, at least, those of some types) may be classed among the apraxias and that forms of speech apraxia may exist in which the focus lies not in the anterior, motor region but in the posterior, kinesthetic regions of the cortex.

The idea of motor aphasia as an apraxia was put forward by Liepmann (1913), who believed that motor aphasia may be regarded as a variant of limb-kinetic apraxia. He claimed that motor aphasia (or, at least, some of its forms) is based on a disturbance

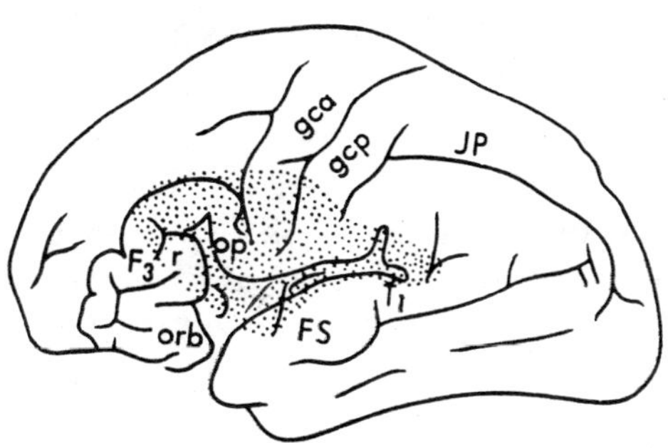

FIGURE 57 Scheme of the brain lesion in Broca's first patient with motor aphasia. The region of softening is shown by punctate shading. (*After Broca, 1861a.*)

of the kinesthetic engrams forming the framework of every motor act. Very similar suggestions (although formulated from completely different, grossly psychomorphological standpoints) were made by Kleist (1907, 1934). A competent defense of the view that motor aphasia may be regarded as "amnesia verbalis kinesthetica" was put up by Nissl von Meyendorff (1930), who not only gave a detailed analysis of the kinesthetic afferent systems lying at the root of articulated speech, but also showed that motor aphasia may develop as a result of a lesion situated in the Rolandic area and involving the inferior portions of the postcentral kinesthetic region of the cortex.

Recently, fresh suggestions have been made to supplement those discussed above, and a new approach to the problem of motor aphasia must consequently be made.

Although, as has been mentioned, from the very beginning the classical theories on aphasia made a sharp distinction between motor aphasia and the more elementary sensory and motor disorders, the tendency in recent decades to approach the apraxias from the physiological point of view has led to a bridging of the postulated gap between elementary sensory and motor defects and disturbances of the motor aspect of speech. The fundamental question then arose: Are particular sensory or motor defects of a more elementary nature at the basis of these disturbances of the motor organization of the act of speech?

This question was answered in the affirmative by Alajouanine, Ombredane, and their collaborators (Alajouanine, Ombredane, and Durant, 1939; Alajouanine and Mozziconacci, 1947; Alajouanine, 1956) by Bay (1952, 1957*a* and *b*), who pointed out that varied and fine disturbances of the motor aspect of speech, in the forms of pareses, dystonias, and dyspraxias, may be observed in patients with motor aphasia, and also by Leonhardt (1962, 1964), who in some of his writings expressed the thought that lesions of the postcentral zones of the cortex in fact play an important role in the origin of the disorders of motor aphasia. This attempt to make a structural analysis of disturbances of motor aphasia and to bring investigations of motor aphasia more into line with the general neurological study of the pathology of motor function must be regarded as a giant step forward, opening the way to further scientific study of this complex phenomenon.

This tendency to bring the analysis of motor aphasia closer to the analysis of other motor disorders, and thus include motor aphasia among the apraxias, is undoubtedly one of the progressive tendencies in modern neurology. It facilitates the study of the physiological mechanisms of the motor disturbances of speech in the light of the knowledge of the structure and pathology of function of the cortical divisions of the motor analyzer, which have been discussed at some length.

Nevertheless, from the latter point of view the tendency to consider all forms of motor aphasia as disturbances of the "amnesia verbalis kinesthetica" type can hardly be considered correct. The problem raised by modern ideas on the structure of the cortical divisions of the motor analyzer is evidently far more complex. It may be defined as the *identification of the various basic components of motor aphasia* and the description of those forms of motor-speech disorder accompanying lesions of both the posterior and anterior divisions of the cortical end of the motor analyzer. Keeping this task in mind, the disturbances arising from lesions of the inferior divisions of the postcentral region of the left hemisphere will first be described. The possibilities that the entity of motor aphasia is based upon various factors and that the analysis of the disturbances of speech from lesions of the postcentral and premotor divisions of the speech zone is helpful in the identification of the individual components of the motor aspect of speech will be taken into account.

Lesions of the inferior divisions of the postcentral region of the left hemisphere (adjacent to the operculum Rolandi) do not lead to motor aphasia as an isolated phenomenon. As a rule, the disturbance appears as a series of apraxic disorders in the working of the oral apparatus, which have already been described. These defects are reflected particularly clearly in the most complex forms of movement of speech apparatus composing the system of speech articulation. In many cases these defects of articulation, constituting the chief symptom of this form of motor aphasia, may be interpreted as the result of a disturbance of the kinesthetic (afferent) organization of motor acts.

A patient with such a disturbance is unable to articulate sounds or words quickly and without concentration. The innervation of articulatory actions has lost its usual selectivity, and as a result the patient cannot immediately assume the correct positions of tongue and lips.

This disturbance is distinguished from dysarthria by the fact that sometimes the required sounds are pronounced clearly enough, the patient showing none of that slurring and monotony of speech characteristic of bulbar or pseudobulbar dysarthria. As a rule, such a patient does not exhibit the dysphonic disorders of speech usually produced by bilateral lesions of this region. The principal defect that can be found in disturbances of the kinesthetic basis of speech consists of *substitutions for individual articulations*. In gross afferent motor aphasia these substitutions are very prominent; the patient may confuse the posterior palatals and the explosives "k," "kh," and "t," which are very different in regard to articulation. With less severe lesions, substitutions in articulation take place only within the range of particular "articulatory oppositions" so that sounds similar in articulation (for example, prepalatolinguals or labials) begin to be confused. It follows, therefore, that substitution of similar articulemes, such as the prepalatolinguals "l" for "n" or "d" or the labials "b" for "m" or "p," are the most typical mistakes in the speech of a patient with afferent motor aphasia.

There are different degrees of speech impairment in kinesthetic motor aphasia. Usually some habitual expressions, well-established kinesthetic stereotypes, remain relatively intact, whereas less firmly established and more highly differentiated forms of speech articulation are more seriously affected. Particularly disordered in these patients are forms of speech requiring precise repetition of a definite system of articulemes and, consequently, depending on a constant mental control over each articulation. That is why apparently paradoxical descriptions of these particular forms of motor aphasia may be encountered in which the repetition of words or phrases (demanding the conscious discrimination between complex groups of sounds and articulations) are reported to be no less and sometimes actually more severely affected than more arbitrary forms of speech activity that do not require the special analysis of particular articulemes. It is possible that many of the phenomena of what is called "conduction aphasia," in which repetitive speech is particularly severely disordered, may be explained not by disturbances of the "categorical situation," as Goldstein attempted to do, but by the inadequacy of the kinesthetic afferent supply of the speech act. The fact that in afferent motor aphasia speaking aloud may be much more severely affected than reading by the patient to himself is explained by the nature of the principal defect—disturbance of the ability to analyze and integrate the kinesthetic signals that comprise the basis of speech.

The disturbances in articulation that have been described are evident in patients of this group even when they attempt to pronounce individual sounds and words. A characteristic feature of this form of motor aphasia is that its most prominent manifestation is difficulty in finding the required articulemes, whereas difficulty in transferring from one articulation to another and disturbances of the motor aspect of speech from pathological inertia of existing movements may be less conspicuous and may sometimes be overcome relatively easily by retraining. Another characteristic feature is the fact that, although such patients have difficulty in articulating individual sounds, they may be able to pronounce whole phrases rather easily. These two features of afferent (kinesthetic) motor aphasia distinguish it fundamentally from the premotor (kinetic) form of motor aphasia, in which difficulties arise involving inhibition of a preceding speech movement with transition to the next movement or where difficulties in transition from a word to a whole sentence become particularly evident (Part II, Section 4F).

It would be wrong, however, to infer that the disturbances found in the kinesthetic form of motor aphasia are limited to difficulties of external articulation.

In recent investigations by Vinarskaya (1969), fresh attempts were made to show that speech articulation (in its external and internal forms) is a means of refining sounds and of placing them in a given category. These investigations showed that whereas the direct imitation of the sounds of speech which, according to Chistovich's views, can take place even in the absence of generalization of sounds (Kozhevnikov and Chistovich, 1965), may remain intact in some patients with lesions of the postcentral zones, the more complex level of analysis of speech sounds and their categorization is invariably impaired in disturbances of the kinesthetic basis of speech. That is why patients with the afferent form of motor aphasia are unable not only to pronounce a required sound of speech precisely, but often also to differentiate clearly between pairs of phonemes (for example, "d" and "n," or "l" and "t"), whether presented to them in spoken or written form. As a rule, writing and, in certain conditions, reading and the understanding of words and phrases are also seriously deranged in patients of this group.

In the early stages of learning how to write, articulatory movements play an active part in the analysis of the sound composition of words. We drew attention to the experiments of Nazarova (1952) in which it was shown that when articulation was not permitted the number of mistakes in writing made by pupils in the first and second grades was increased 5 to 6 times. Since there is active participation of articulation in writing, it may be concluded that the disturbance of the system of articulemes from lesions of the post-central cortical divisions may make writing difficult or even impossible.

Clinical observation has shown that the severest forms of kinesthetic motor aphasia, especially if occurring in patients in whom the ability to write has not been firmly established, may be associated with total loss of the writing skill or, at least, with its marked derangement. Such patients sometimes cannot even identify individual sounds. They write the wrong sounds and make characteristic articulatory substitutions. These mistakes can be prevented if the patient is allowed to pronounce the required word aloud and, at the same time, to have the aid of a visual oral image of the particular word (for example, by looking at his mouth in a mirror). The principal writing mistake made by patients of this group is the use of incorrect articulemes. For example, they may write the Russian word "parna" for "parta," "khadat" for "khalat," "snot" or "slon" for "stol," etc., confusing the similar homorganic articulemes "l," "n," "d," and "t" (Fig. 58). However, with the aid of a visual oral image they may write correctly (Fig. 59).

The writing disorders just described usually appear in severe cases of kinesthetic motor aphasia. However, in cases in which writing ability is apparently still intact, visible disturbances of writing may develop during special "refined" tests, e.g., if the patient is requested to write words that, on account of the complexity of their sound composition, require special articulatory analysis (the Russian words "korablekrushenie" [shipwreck], "paravozostroenie" [shipbuilding], etc.). The defects in writing are particularly obvious if the patient is forbidden to say the word aloud and if the only aid permitted is internal articulation (by requesting the patient to write the required word with his mouth open or with his tongue gripped between his teeth). Under such conditions writing is disturbed, although in normal conditions it is intact (Fig. 60). Our findings concur with those of Blinkov (1948), who showed that writing is deranged in patients with a lesion of the postcentral region of the cortex when external articulation is precluded (Fig. 61).

The disturbances in the ability to read in these patients are closely

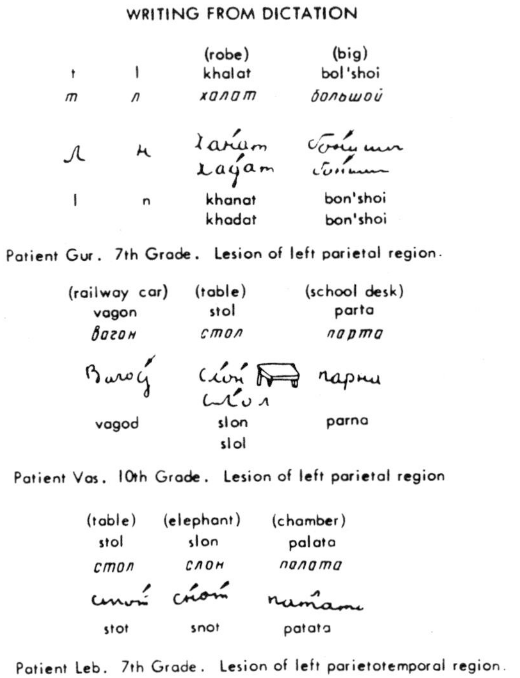

FIGURE 58 Impaired writing ability in afferent motor aphasia.

similar in character to the disturbances in speech. The ability to read firmly established words, especially to oneself, is relatively well preserved, but the ability to read aloud words with a complex sound composition, requiring for their analysis articulation, is diminished because substitution of articulemes creates difficulty in understanding what is written. They cannot pronounce written letters or syllables properly, and they therefore cannot understand the meaning of written words. Because of the articulatory substitutions, these patients usually find it more difficult to read aloud than to read to themselves. Evidently the direct recognition of firmly established visual images of words is of secondary importance in this activity. Impairment in the ability to articulate leads to distortion in the pronunciation of words, so that the understanding of speech is severely impaired.

There is no doubt that the careful study of disturbances of the higher level of phonemic analysis and synthesis, which requires the closest participation of the kinesthetic zones of the cortex, will provide us with new data on the structure of speech processes and may perhaps necessitate a substantial revision of our present views of the physiological basis of speech.

• • •

Some of the characteristic features of the defects in articulated speech occurring in one form of motor aphasia and the closely related disturbances of the kinesthetic basis of the motor act developing from lesions of the inferior divisions of the postcentral region of the left hemisphere have been

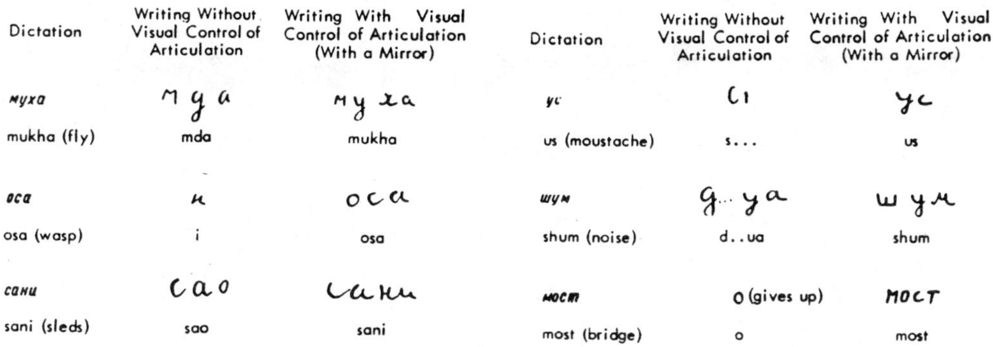

FIGURE 59 Changes in the writing of a patient with afferent motor aphasia who was aided by visual analysis of the oral image.

described. In the face of these findings it seems that these speech defects may be brought more into line with the apraxic disorders observed in the presence of these lesions and that the type of motor aphasia that has been described may be regarded as a special form of disturbance of complex voluntary movements.

As has been stated, articulatory disturbances of this type may occur in isolation in the presence of circumscribed lesions of the inferior divisions of the postcentral portion of the cortex of the left hemisphere. However, impairment of the kinesthetic basis of speech articulation may also be a component of the more generalized syndrome of motor aphasia. By analysis of the kinesthetic basis of the speech act, a special form of motor aphasia may be distinguished and one of the important components of any syndrome involving a motor disorder of the act of speech may be defined.

E. DISTURBANCES OF MOTOR FUNCTIONS WITH LESIONS OF THE PREMOTOR REGION

The organization of voluntary movements is not confined to the mechanisms of kinesthetic afferent innervation, whose disturbances have just been described. As has been mentioned, every complex voluntary movement, especially every complex motor skill, consists of a chain of successive motor acts. A dynamic stereotype, with its organization based on time, is thereby produced. In automatized motor skills, this series may take the form of smooth kinetic melodies.

The organization of a complex motor act involves more than the participation of the postcentral divisions of the cerebral cortex. An important part in this organization of motor activity is played by premotor divisions of the cortex, the secondary fields of the cortical nucleus of the motor analyzer.

The contribution made by these cortical divisions to the motor act will

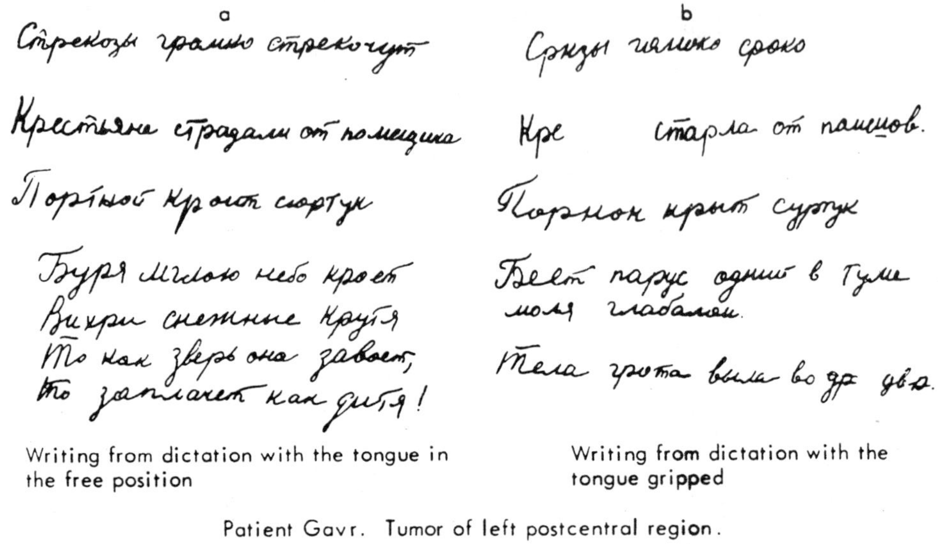

FIGURE 60 Changes in the writing of a patient with a lesion of the postcentral divisions of the cortex after exclusion of external articulation. (*a*) Three simple phrases and a few lines of a poem are written free of error. (*b*) The same phrases, but incomplete and badly jumbled.

now be considered, and the changes in voluntary movements arising from lesions of the premotor divisions of the brain will be examined.

• • •

The investigation of the functions of the premotor zone of the cortex began much later than that of the precentral and postcentral divisions of the cortex, and, indeed, it may be considered to be an achievement of the present generation.

At the beginning of this century the motor region of the cortex was regarded as a single entity, bounded by the limits of the anterior central gyrus. It was not until 1905 that Campbell distinguished the special "intermediate motor zone," which Brodmann later subdivided (1909) into Areas 6 (premotor) and 8 (oculomotor). More recently still were the functions of these areas described in detail and were observations made on the results of lesions affecting them; this was the work in particular of Foerster (1936) and Fulton (1937, 1943, 1949), who stimulated considerable research at that period. The results of these investigations will be briefly examined.

The premotor zone of the cerebral cortex is a part of the cortical motor region, being distinguished from Area 4 only by the absence of the giant pyramidal cells of Betz. Basically, Area 6 retains the same cytoarchitectonic structure as Area 4, a structure characteristic of the whole motor cortex. Distinctive features of the structure of Area 6 are the predominance of the components of the third (association) layer of cells and the large number of axodendritic connections. The premotor portion of the cortex may therefore be classed as one of the secondary, projection-association divisions of the cortex (Polyakov, 1956, 1959).

Genetically, the premotor zone and the motor zone together form a single entity. The premotor zone first appears as a separate formation in the carnivores (Kukuev, 1940), and it is distinguished by a particularly intensive rate of evolutionary development. Whereas in the lower monkeys (lemurs) it occupies a much smaller area (21 mm²) than Area 4 (80 mm²), in man the relationship is reversed; in the latter Area 6 extends over 2418 mm² whereas Area 4 comprises 739 mm². According to Glezer's (1955) calculations, the premotor region in man accounts for over 80% of the whole precentral cortical region. A similar high rate of development of the premotor zone may also be observed during ontogenesis. While the neuronal apparatuses of Area 4 have attained full development in a child approximately 4 years of age, Area 6 continues to develop and reaches full maturity only in a 7-year-old child. At this time the premotor region of the cortex also greatly exceeds the motor region in area.

The connections of the premotor region are also much more abundant than those of Area 4. Besides the numerous connections with other cortical regions, Area 6 is directly connected with the subcortical nuclei and the nuclei of the pons. It receives projections from the secondary, "internal" (Rose, 1950) nuclei of the thalamus and is in very close communication with the structures of the reticular formation. These rich connections of the premotor region with the other portions of the brain have been confirmed by neuronography. As McCulloch (1943) has shown, the effect of stimulation of Area 4 spreads only to neighboring regions, whereas stimulation of Area 6 has a much more widespread effect, with signs of excitation noted in Areas 8, 4, 1, 5, and 39 (Fig. 53).

Finally, it should be noted that the premotor divisions of the cortex are very closely connected with the part of the motor zone known as Area 45. McCulloch's (1943) investigations showed that this part of the cortex, directly bordering the premotor zone (some authors, in fact, regard it as part of the premotor zone), possesses special depressor functions. Stimulation of this area leads to depression of

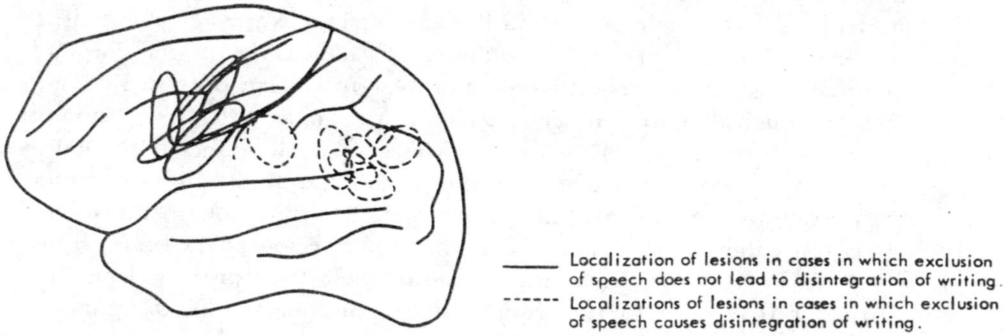

FIGURE 61 Localization of lesions in cases in which the exclusion of external articulation leads to impaired writing. (*After Blinkov, 1948.*)

the activity of the neighboring parts of the cortex and to inhibition of movement previously begun. As shall be shown, the proximity of the premotor zone to these structures of the motor portion of the cortex explains many of its functions.

Because of anatomical and physiological evidence that the premotor region is directly related to the motor portion of the cortex and that its functions are of great complexity, there are grounds for regarding this region as the *secondary field of the cortical nucleus of the motor analyzer*.

This suggestion is confirmed by the changes observed in the motor functions of animals and man after stimulation or destruction of the premotor region of the cortex.

The experiments of Fulton (1935, etc.), Wyss and Obrador (1937), and many other workers showed that stimulation of the premotor portion of the cortex (or, more precisely, of that part of it designated as $6a\beta$) leads, after a long latent period, to the appearance of complex integrated movements, including rotation of the eyes, head, and whole trunk, followed by a movement of the upper limb resembling a grasping action. The epileptiform fits caused by stimulation of the premotor region, described clinically as "adversive," have the same complex character.

The most informative data pertaining to the role of the premotor divisions of the brain in the organization of movement have been obtained from observation of animals after extirpation of these divisions and of patients with lesions localized in the premotor region. After extirpating the premotor cortex in monkeys, Fulton (1943, etc.) and his collaborators found no signs of loss of individual movements. In other words, according to these findings, the premotor region exhibits no signs of somatotopic projection. The temporary disorders of movement that develop disappear relatively quickly. However, as other studies of Fulton (1935, 1937, etc.) have shown, extirpation of the premotor region in monkeys leads to the appearance of a complex group of symptoms, clearly divisible into two components: Firstly, the monkey's movements lost their precise, differentiated character, and skilled movements were noticeably disturbed. Secondly, elements of compulsive movement and motor perseveration stood out clearly (in the form of compulsive grasping, frequent repetition of a movement once carried out, etc.), although they were never observed in the animal after extirpation of the motor area proper of the cortex (Area 4). As will be shown, these two signs—disturbance of skilled movements and the appearance of motor perseveration—are also typical of the changes developing in the motor sphere in patients with lesions of the premotor region of the brain. If the lesion spreads to the subcortical divisions, these signs are augmented by gross disturbances of tone, grasping reflexes, and marked inertia of motor activity.

The disturbances of movement resulting from a lesion of the premotor portion of the cortex are especially prominent in man. Foerster (1936), Kleist (1934), and, later, Shmidt (1942) noted that a lesion of the premotor divisions of the cortex in man does not lead to loss of movements and does not cause permanent paresis. In such cases, however, movement becomes undifferentiated and clumsy; skilled movements of complex composition disintegrate, and each element of the movement begins to require a special effort of will (Foerster, 1936). Sometimes elements of compulsive movements are also observed, and these are regarded by some writers as the revival of primitive automatisms. They are particularly conspicuous in cases in which the pathological process has spread to the basal subcortical ganglia. If to this is added the autonomic disturbances and pathological reflexes (Rossolimo's, Bekhterev-Mendel, and, sometimes, grasping reflexes), the neurological syndrome of a lesion of the premotor zone becomes sufficiently well defined. Disturbances of complex motor actions are the most permanent signs associated with lesions of the premotor portion of the cortex. Although certain neurologists (Walshe, 1935) doubt that the signs, are, in fact, related to the premotor divisions of the cortex and attempt to revert to the old view of the motor portion of the cortex as a single entity, the clinical reality of the facts that have been described is clear enough.

While there has been no doubt about the existence of disturbances of fine movements with lesions of the premotor zone, analysis of the details of these disturbances and of their distinction from other forms of motor disorder remained neglected as a subject for research for a long time. It is only during the last 15 years that these aspects have been given special scrutiny (Luria, 1943, 1945, 1948, etc.; Shkol'nik-Yarros, 1945, etc.). These investigations have shown that disturbances of movement arising from lesions of the premotor zone differ essentially both from disturbances resulting from a lesion of the primary motor zone of the cortex and from those associated with lesions of the postcentral regions, the symptomatology of which has been described. In contrast to lesions of Area 4, with lesions of the premotor portion of the cortex, the ability to perform relatively simple, isolated movements is preserved. The strength of the movements is also preserved in these cases. The basic difference between premotor disturbances and the disturbances of movement accompanying lesions of the posterior portions of the cortical nucleus of the motor analyzer is the fact that the disturbances of movement with lesions of the premotor region are not included in the syndrome of the sensory disorders usually found in the presence of a lesion of the postcentral region. Estimation of the position of a limb in space, like cutaneous sensation, usually remains unimpaired. The sensory disturbances that do occur are quite different and much more complex in character: While retaining deep (muscle and joint) and cutaneous sensation in relation to the individual elements of movement, such a patient shows a considerable defect when evaluating acts composed of a series of individual movements and he loses the kinetic schemes that provide the afferent organization of series of movements.* This defect in kinesthetic synthesis arising from lesions of the premotor portion of the cortex leads to the disintegration of the kinetic structure of motor acts, the central symptom of a disturbance of movement from lesions of this region.

In the aforementioned investigations the movements of patients with lesions of the premotor zone exhibited none of that disturbance of the accurate direction of individual motor impulses forming the principal symptom of lesions of the postcentral regions. A patient with a premotor lesion has no difficulty in reproducing isolated positions of the hand, even relatively complicated ones (for example, keeping the hand in space with the index and little fingers extended). As a rule, the topological scheme of movement remains intact in such cases.

Significant disturbances arise when the patient passes from isolated motor acts to a system of movements incorporating both "principal" and "background" components (Bernshtein, 1947) or to a series of movements of the same type, together forming a single skilled movement or kinetic melody. The earliest symptom of slowly progressive lesions of the premotor divisions of the brain (for example, in slowly expanding meningiomas of this region) is usually the *disintegration of complex skilled movements*. The patients begin to notice that they can no longer carry out habitual operations with skill and smoothness, especially operations requiring the use of both hands. The left hand ceases to carry out automatically its auxiliary ("background") functions; as a result of this defect the swift and smooth interchange of movements in complex skilled operations is disturbed. Typists, for example, lose their facility and celerity of movement and begin to tap out the text with one finger, moving the finger from one key to the other by a conscious effort every time. Musicians can no longer play with the necessary "style" and lose their playing technique. Handwriting begins to change; the letters forming whole words begin to be written separately, and, subsequently, every stroke forming a grapheme requires a separate effort of will. The learning of new operational sequences and complex skilled movements is naturally all but impossible in patients with such lesions. Hence, *disintegration of the dynamics of the motor act and of complex skilled movements constitutes the central symptom of a motor disturbance arising from lesions of the premotor zone of the brain.*

The disturbances of voluntary movement in the presence of lesions of the premotor systems become particularly prominent in special tests requiring the formation of new skilled movements, especially in cases in which the premotor defect is not masked by pareses. Such tests will be described

*The term "kinetic schemes" will subsequently imply schemes providing for the performance of a time sequence of movements, with replacement of successive acts, forming the basis of a kinetic melody.

subsequently (Part III, Section 3B). Cases of this type include, for example, circumscribed lesions of the premotor zone resulting from depressed fractures of the skull with hemorrhages in the premotor region or from extracerebral tumors of this region not extending to the motor zone and not affecting the subcortical ganglia. As a rule, the disorders arise both in the contralateral hand and, to a lesser degree, in the ipsilateral hand. This is usually so with lesions of the premotor region of the dominant hemisphere. This probably implies not merely that connections are present between the premotor zone and structures on the same side, but also that a lesion of this region disturbs the functional organization of any motor act that is a component of complex skilled movements.

Depending on the situation of the lesion within the premotor region, motor defects may be revealed either in movements of the hand or in oral praxis. In each case, however, they are similar in nature and take the form of a disturbance of the *kinetic organization of the motor act*, which has been described.

In the severest cases (especially if the lesion implicates the subcortical systems) this disturbance of the kinetic structure of movement may take the form of a change in the normal relationship between the principal and the background components of the movement. Whereas a normal subject will easily raise his hand in response to a signal to which he is conditioned and immediately lower it again or will press a rubber bulb and then immediately relax the muscles of his hand, these background components of the movement may disappear in a patient with a lesion of the premotor systems. The patient keeps his hand raised or keeps squeezing the bulb, and an additional command must be given before the original position is resumed.

One of the basic motor defects in patients of this type is this disturbance in the automatic inhibition of a movement already in process. If the lesion involves the subcortical extrapyramidal apparatuses, the disturbances in the kinetic organization of movement become apparent even by simple tests. They may also be observed, however, in cases of lesions confined to the premotor divisions of the cortex, more frequently in more complex movements. Such movements include, for example, a complex action in which the hand is thrust forward while, at the same time, the fist is clenched and then the fingers are made into a "ring" (this test is described in Part III, Section 3B). As he carries out one component of this complex movement (for example, thrusting the hand forward), the patient cannot concurrently place his hand in the required position, and he has to perform the two components in succession. Once he has carried out the movement, the patient cannot alternate from one movement to another; he continues, for example, to thrust his hand forward time and time again without changing the ring position of the fingers at all. The extent of the disturbance of the ability to smoothly change from one movement to another is directly related to the severity of the premotor lesion. It is seen to a lesser degree in patients with postcentral lesions, who do not find the inhibition of a movement once it has been carried out as difficult as the assumption of a required pose.

Lesions of the premotor cortical divisions of both hemispheres that are extensions of pathological parasagittal processes (for example, tumors in the region of the longitudinal fissure) may cause similar disturbances, especially in the performance of concurrent movements of both hands. This syndrome was described by Faller (1948). When a patient with a lesion of the premotor divisions is asked, for example, to change the positions of both hands at the same time and with both positions different (e.g., to make a fist with one and to extend the other with the palm up), he will have real trouble with the task. This test of reciprocal coordination was proposed some time ago by Ozeretskii (1930). It will be described in detail subsequently (Part III, Section 3B).

As a rule, smooth and simultaneous positioning of both hands proves impossible for such patients. They either perform the elements of the combined movement in succession or omit one hand from the combined movements (usually the hand contralateral to the side of the lesion). The disturbance of smooth sequence in motor acts leads to a disintegration of complex skilled movements, the principal symptom of a lesion of the premotor divisions of the cortex. Tests of the performance of rhythmic movements, which in recent years have become established as part of the clinical investigation of the motor sphere, may also clearly reveal a disturbance of kinetic organization of the motor act that is produced by lesions of the premotor cortical zone. In these tests the placing of the hand in different positions is not required. In their purest form they aim at identifying the rhythmic organization of movement. Among them may be mentioned, for example, the task of tapping out rhythms of varying degrees of complexity, for instance simple rhythmic groups like " " " or '" '" '" or accented groups like " ∪ ∪ ∪ " ∪ ∪ ∪ or ∪ ∪ ∪ " ∪∪∪". Patients with a lesion of the postcentral regions of the cortex are able to cope with these tasks relatively easily, but a lesion of the premotor cortex gives rise to considerable difficulty in their performance. Frequently such patients cannot combine the individual taps into kinetic melodies, cannot change from one kinetic pattern of rhythm to another, and, in particular, cannot make a rapid and smooth transition in the timing of the accented taps of the rhythmic group. As a rule, the required skilled movement is not executed, the gradually formed motor stereotype becomes inert, and the transition from one established rhythmic pattern to another or any shift in the position of the accented tap becomes impossible. Examples of these disturbances in the performance of tapping tests by patients with lesions of the premotor systems are given in Fig. 62. Similar results have been obtained and studied by Semernitskaya (1945) and Shkol'nik-Yarros (1945). These tests will be described in detail subsequently (Part III, Section 4C).

As the work of Simernitskaya and Bunatyan (1966) has shown, superficial lesions (arachnoidendotheliomas) of the premotor area lead to symptoms of deautomation of motor rhythms, whereas the intracerebral tumors in this area also give rise to additional compulsive movements, which the patient is unable to control.

The disturbance of the kinetic organization of the motor act associated with a lesion of the premotor divisions of the cortex is also brought clearly to light by graphic tests, in which the patient has to alternately draw various elements of a pattern. An example of such tests, which will be described in detail subsequently (Part III, Section 3B), is the drawing of a pattern like ПΛПΛПΛ without lifting the hand from the paper. When asked to draw this pattern, the patient with a lesion of the premotor systems begins to draw each stroke separately or to develop a simple motor stereotype consisting of the repetition of a single element. A firmly established skill in drawing with smooth transition from one element to another cannot be achieved (Fig. 63).

It is easy to see that in all of these cases it is not so much the differential composition or topological scheme that is affected, as the *kinetic organization of the movement.* Hence, the main difficulty experienced by a patient with a lesion of the premotor cortical divisions is not so much in controlling the flow of differentiated impulses to individual muscle groups, as in integrating the impulses in time, an essential for the formation of a smooth kinetic melody.

From the foregoing we are justified in regarding the premotor zone of the cortex as an apparatus responsible for integrating complex series of movements taking place over a period of time.

If the lesion is not confined to the premotor zone of the cortex but extends deeper into the brain, involving the connections between the premotor region and the basal motor ganglia, the aforementioned symptoms are supplemented by changes in tone and by gross *perseverations*, taking the form of the "liberation of primary automatisms." An example of this marked inertia is *forced grasping*, which, according to Fulton (1935, 1937, etc.), is one of the principal symptoms to occur in monkeys after extirpation of the premotor region. In man this symptom appears only with extensive lesions of the premotor region, such lesions disturbing the normal relationships with the basal motor ganglia. Usually the motor perseverations in patients with premotor lesions takes the form of *continuation of a voluntary movement once it has started.* The inability to stop an action once it has began does not disturb the patient's intentions; he does not substitute another action for the required one, although he may inhibit the motor components of the latter action. For example, when the patient draws a circle or a triangle, he continues drawing the same figure time and time again, or when he writes a word (or number), he continues to write the component letters (or numerals) over and over again. Characteristically, these phenomena are aggravated at the period

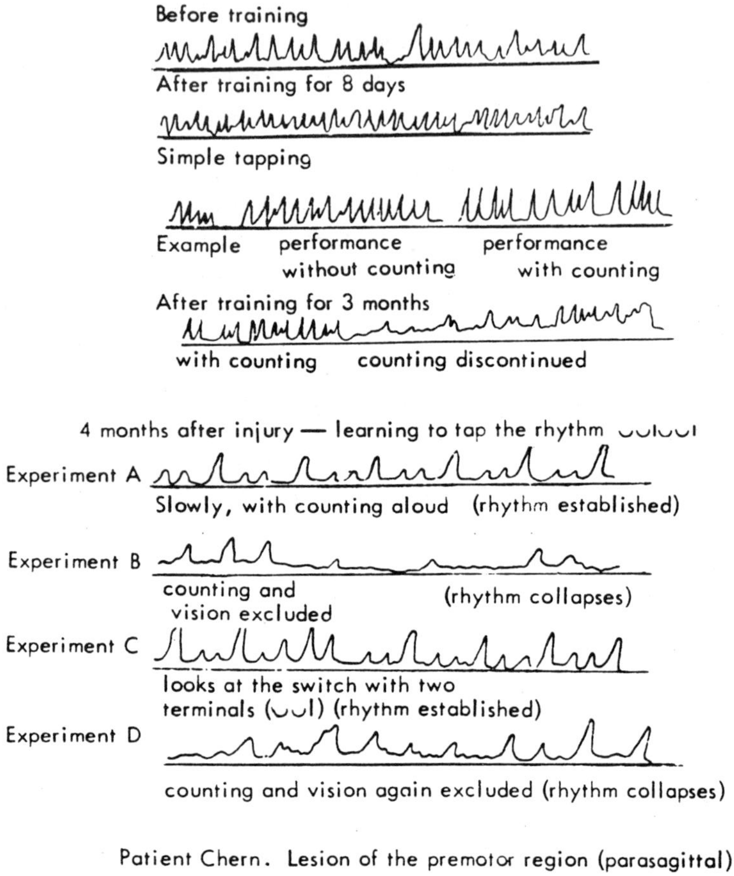

FIGURE 62 Disturbance in the ability to execute rhythmic tapping ("∪∪∪ and ∪∪") in a patient with the premotor syndrome. (*After Luria, 1943, and Shkol'nik-Yarros, 1945.*)

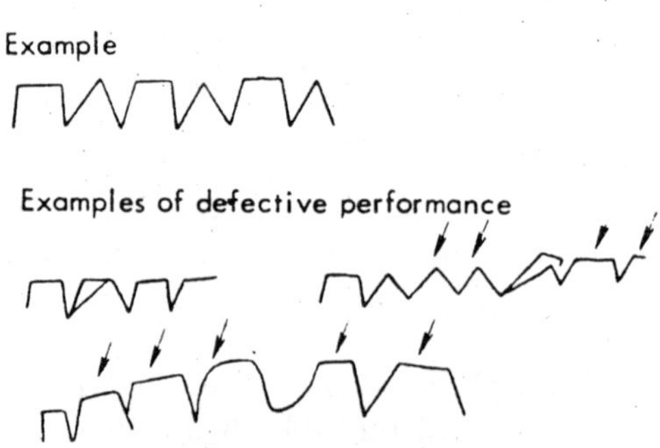

FIGURE 63 Performance of graphic tests requiring alternation by a patient (Patient P) with the premotor syndrome and a lesion of the left premotor region.

of maximal spread of the pathological process in the premotor region of the brain and they gradually disappear as the functioning of this region recovers. In Figs. 64, 65, and 66 are two examples of these compulsive movements taking place during drawing and writing. In the first patient these movements developed after a hemorrhage into the premotor region; in the second patient after a massive injury to the posterior frontal region associated with a deep cyst; in the third they followed the removal of an arachnoid endothelioma of the same region. The perseverations persisted while local edema of the brain was present and gradually disappeared as the edema subsided.

The stability of the symptoms of pathological inertia in the motor analyzer in conjunction with deep-seated lesions of the premotor region and white matter of the brain is so marked that, as the investigations of Spirin (1951) showed, the symptoms can be used to gauge the patient's condition. In certain cases these manifestations of the pathological inertia of the nervous processes also spread to the sensory sphere. As has been observed in similar cases, long after a patient had ceased to make chewing movements he declared that it seemed to him that these movements had continued until he began to speak. Electromyographic investigations in such cases have shown that volleys of impulses recorded in muscles of the upper limb did, in fact, continue long after the movement had ceased. In Fig. 67, taken from a report of Grindel' and Filippycheva (1959), are examples of electromyographic and mechanographic evidence of a static focus of excitation in those portions of the motor analyzer associated with a pathological process of the premotor region of the brain.

These data clearly suggest that a lesion of the premotor systems may lead to definite changes in motor processes of quite a different character from motor disturbances resulting from lesions of the postcentral regions of the brain.

• • •

Certain conclusions may be drawn from the foregoing regarding the functional importance of the premotor region in the organization of voluntary movement in man. This organization is a complex process that depends on the two zones comprising the cortical divisions of the motor analyzer.

The postcentral divisions of the sensorimotor region are responsible for the topological organization of motor impulses, directing them to definite groups of muscles and giving precision to the composition of the motor act. The premotor divisions of the cortex are apparently primarily responsible for the kinetic organization of movement, ensuring the inhibition of movements once they have started, the transfer from one movement to another, and the conversion of individual motor acts into a smoothly and consecutively organized skilled movement.

Investigation of the functions of the premotor zone is still in its early stages, and the phenomena resulting from lesions of the premotor portion of

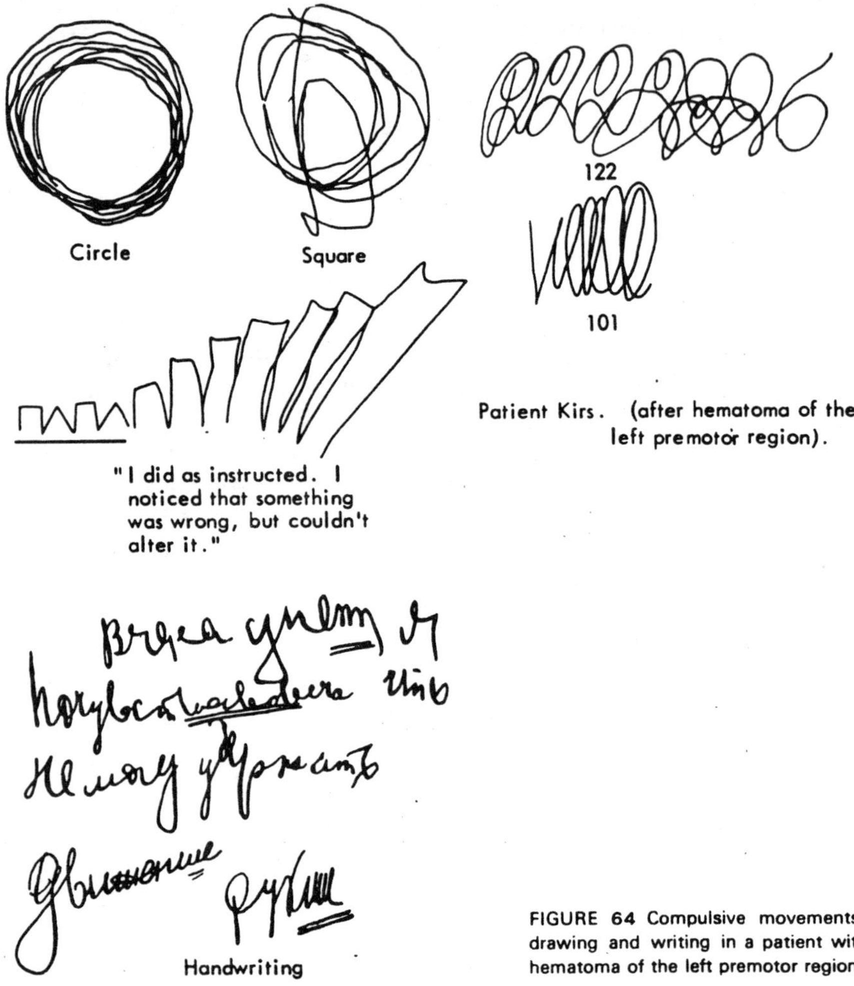

FIGURE 64 Compulsive movements in drawing and writing in a patient with a hematoma of the left premotor region.

the cortex and of the closely connected subcortical extrapyramidal system require further detailed analysis. There is no doubt that such investigations will shed light on the specialized, differential mechanisms responsible for the central organization of movement and will thereby bring us closer to the understanding of the structure of human motor activity.

F. DISTURBANCES OF THE KINETIC STRUCTURE OF SPEECH EFFERENT (KINETIC) MOTOR APHASIA

The disturbances in the kinetic organization of movement and the manifestations of pathological inertia in the motor analyzer, which have just been

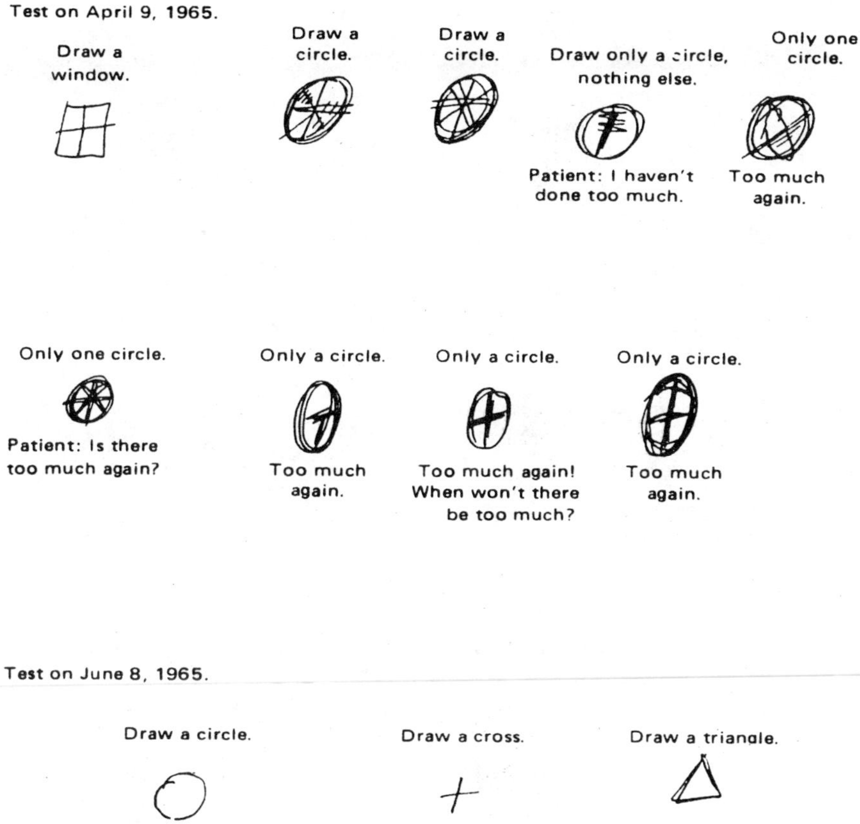

FIGURE 65 Compulsive movements during performance of graphic tests by a patient with an injury to the posterior frontal zones of the brain.

described. In the face of these findings it seems that these speech defects may be brought more into line with the apraxic disorders observed in the examined, lead directly to the analysis of the specific mechanisms of one form of impaired expressive (motor) speech. They play an important role in the overall picture of motor aphasia, and they may be observed in a pure form in patients with a lesion of the inferior divisions of the left premotor cortical zone.

As yet, these disturbances have not received the attention they deserve, and more often than not have not been distinguished from the general aspects of motor aphasia. Motor aphasia has usually been described as a single entity without analysis of the different forms that the disturbance of the motor aspect of speech may assume with lesions of different parts of the brain.

By distinguishing between the two components essential for the perform-

a

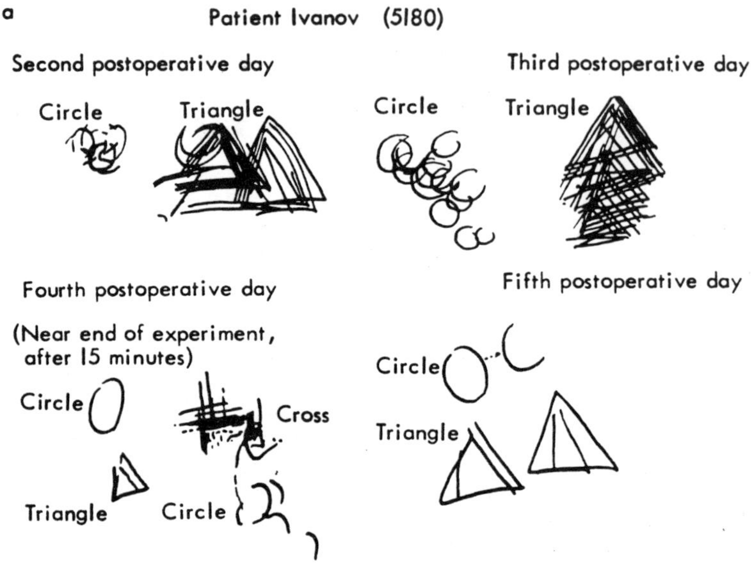
Patient Ivanov (5180)
Second postoperative day
Circle
Triangle
Third postoperative day
Circle
Triangle
Fourth postoperative day
(Near end of experiment, after 15 minutes)
Circle
Cross
Triangle
Circle
Fifth postoperative day
Circle
Triangle

b

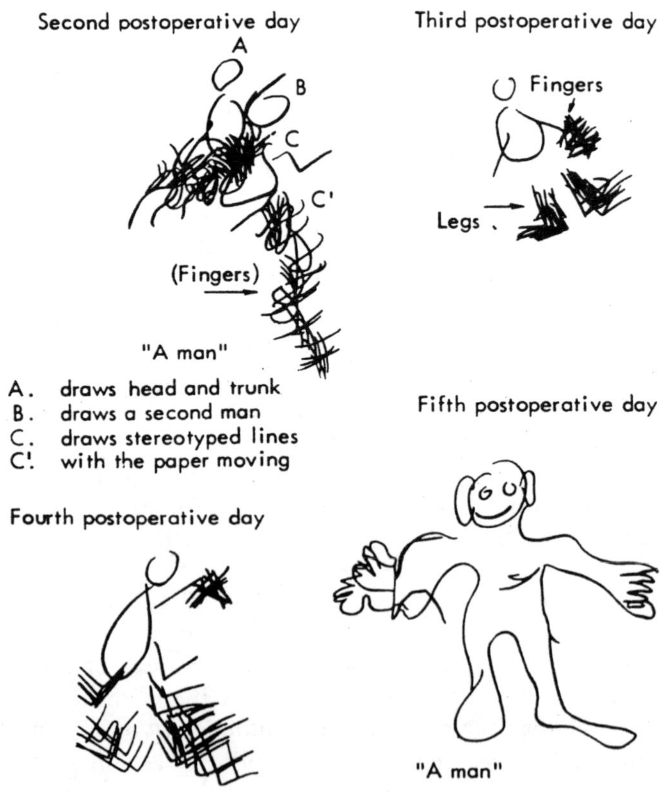
Second postoperative day
A
B
C
C'
(Fingers)
"A man"
A. draws head and trunk
B. draws a second man
C. draws stereotyped lines
C'. with the paper moving
Third postoperative day
Fingers
Legs
Fourth postoperative day
Fifth postoperative day
"A man"

ance of a motor act—its kinesthetic basis, providing the differential composition of complex movements, and its kinetic structure, responsible for the formation of smooth skilled movements in easy consecutive order—a new approach in the analysis of the motor aspect of speech can be adopted and two different components (or two different forms) of motor aphasia can be described.

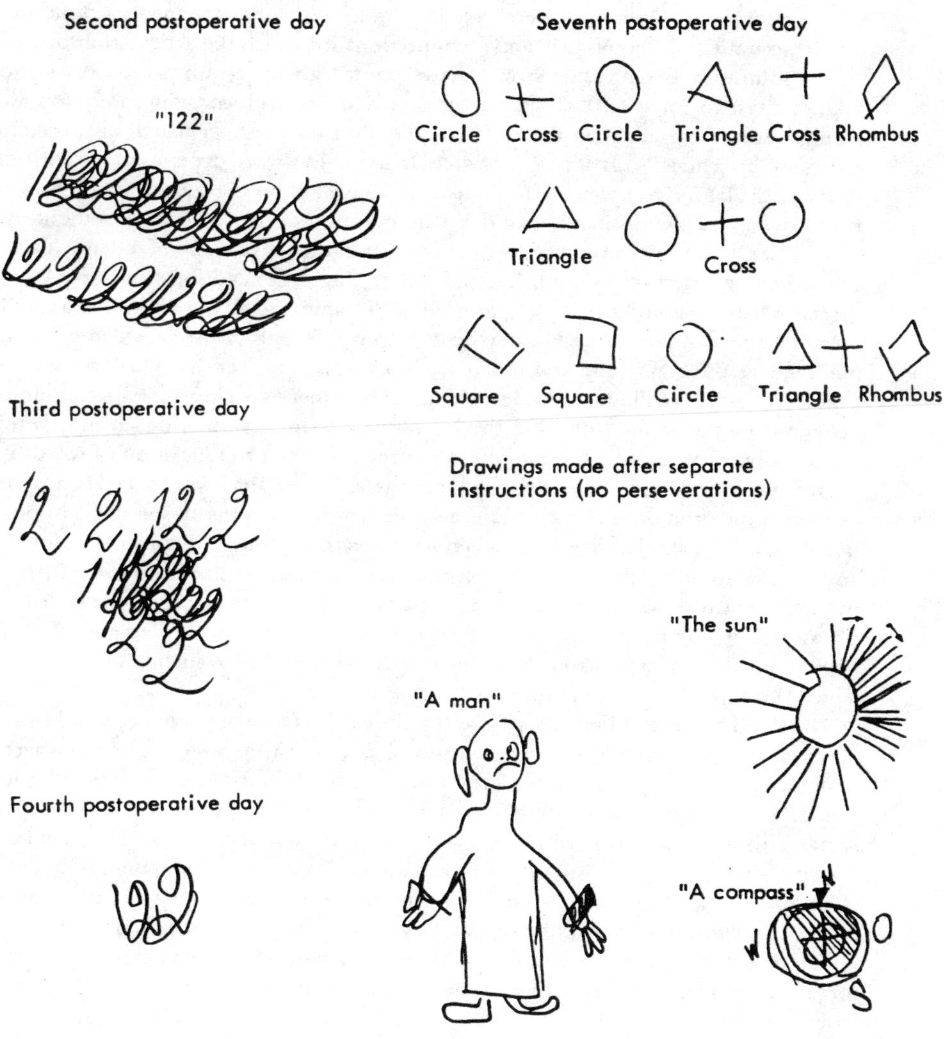

FIGURE 66 Compulsive movements in drawing and writing after removal of an arachnoid endotheiioma of the left premotor region. These tests were performed while the patient had edema. (*a*) Drawing figures. (*b*) Drawing a man. (*c*) Writing numbers. (*d*) Drawing figures 7 days postoperatively.

The role of kinesthetic afferent impulses in articulation has been indicated and the features of kinesthetic (postcentral) motor aphasia have been briefly described. We shall now turn to the analysis of the kinetic components of the act of speech and shall attempt to briefly describe the features of the kinetic (premotor) disturbances of expressive speech that may be found in motor aphasia and to distinguish them as a specific form of motor aphasic disorders.

The motor organization of speech includes much more than the mere identification of the accurately differentiated nerve connections on which the articulation of individual sounds is based. Expressive (motor) speech always requires the presence of a kinetic system (or chain) of articulatory movements, with constant inhibition and modification (depending on the order of the sounds to be articulated) of preceding articulations. The articulation of a particular sound in a word depends on its position in the articulatory complex as a whole and, above all, on the sounds that follow it. For this reason, the distinctions in the pronunciation of the "s" sound in the words "sot," "set," and "sit" are made only if the subsequent articulations are anticipated. These findings are firmly established in modern linguistics and form the basis of the special syllabic method of teaching grammar (El'konin, 1956). On the other hand, the pronunciation of any sound or syllable is possible only if an articuleme can be inhibited at the right time and the articulatory apparatus can be transferred to the next articuleme. It follows that a disturbance of the kinetic system (or the specific motor program) of the whole word and the inability to promptly inhibit each link of this system inevitably leads to a profound impairment of the pronunciation of words.

However, the kinetic schemes of a language are more than words. Jackson (1884) expressed the opinion that the phrase, not the word, is the unit of speech ("propositional speech"). Similar views have been put forward in modern linguistics (Chomsky, 1957) in relation to the whole expression. Every expression possesses some form of dynamic structure with the individual parts requiring specific turns of speech for the phrase to be completed. By means of these dynamic structures, determined at the beginning of each expression, it is possible to foretell fairly reliably the manner in which the expression will continue.

The significance of different words and different parts of speech in the unfolding of the dynamic structure of the whole expression may vary widely. For example, whereas a noun in the nominative case ("a table" or "a book") may determine to a limited extent the subsequent structure of a sentence, verbs such as "lent" or "took" require a more definite system of additives ("lent to someone" or "took from someone"). Finally, auxiliary words (the prepositions "under," "near," etc., and the conjunctions "because," "although," "if," etc.) also possess determinative values and are themselves conceived only within the dynamic system of the whole expression.

There is therefore every reason to believe that language as a whole is an intricately organized dynamic system whose elements (words) are associated with each other in complex series.

It has often been stated in the psychological literature that "internal speech" is of fundamental importance in the formation of the integral system of the sentence. According to Vygotskii (1934, 1956), it is internal speech, with its predicative properties, that performs these dynamic functions and plays a direct part in both the evolu-

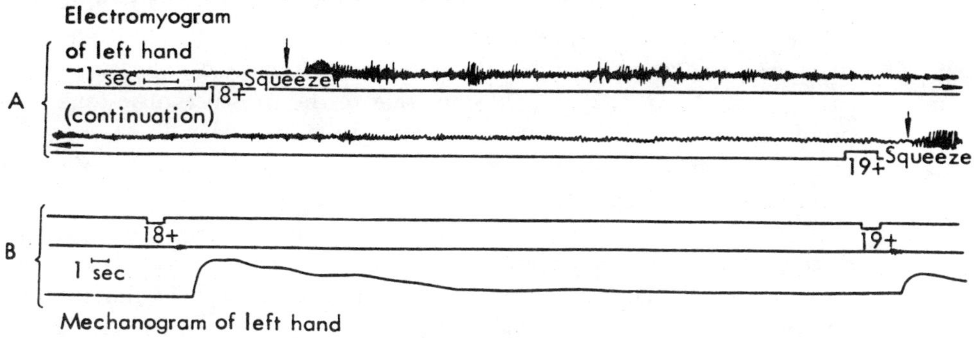

FIGURE 67 Electromyographic signs of static excitation in a patient (Patient P) with a lesion of the premotor region that is part of a pathological process in the right frontal lobe. (*A*) Top line: Electromyogram of the left hand. Bottom line: Stimulus marker. (*B*) Top line: stimulus marker. Bottom line: Mechanogram of the left hand. (*After Grindel and Filippycheva, 1959*.)

tion of the thought into the whole expression and the crystallization of the whole expression into its shortened, conceptual scheme. We can therefore approach speech by using the same criteria we applied to the complex kinetic motor melodies, the only difference being that the structure of the kinetic melodies of speech is based on the structure of language and is thereby incomparably more complex.

Every word can therefore be regarded not only as the bearer of the meaning of a particular object, but also as the unit of expression, with potential connections that unfold as the word is included in the complete sentence.

If we analyze language as a highly complex dynamic system, we can estimate the importance of the premotor zone in the performance of expressive speech and begin to understand the specific disorders found with lesions of that region.

Patients with a lesion of the superior divisions of the premotor zone of the left hemisphere may frequently show characteristic abortive signs of motor disorders of speech. Although they have no difficulty in pronouncing individual words or in naming objects, such patients frequently find coherent speech difficult. Their speech loses its automatism and fluency and begins to be fragmented, so that the pronunciation and sometimes the finding of each word requires a special impulse. Some patients state that their speech has become difficult, that they speak "like a hobbled horse runs." "You say a word," they say, "and then there is nothing to follow it." "Sometimes a word that should come after comes before, you say it, and you don't know what to do next—all the fluency has gone," etc. Because of these difficulties, the speech of patients with lesions of the premotor cortical divisions becomes deautomatized and tense, and the articulation of every word begins to require a special effort. The grammatical structure of speech in such patients may remain intact for a while or may exhibit very slight disturbances.

These disorders of speech are based on disturbances of the dynamic structure of speech processes—those highly automatized skilled movements that, as has been described, disintegrate in the presence of lesions of the premotor region of the cerebral cortex. Additional details on such cases can be found in two publications by the present author (Luria, 1963 [Russian], 1966 [English]).

Whereas a lesion of the superior divisions of the premotor region (not directly related to the speech area of the cortex) gives rise to only very slight impairment of fluent expressive speech, a pathological focus situated in the inferior divisions of the premotor zone of the left hemisphere is associated with disturbances of a very pronounced character.

Despite the fact that there is no strict somatotopic projection in the premotor zone, the individual parts of this zone differ in their significance. The superior and middle divisions of the premotor zone act in unison with other regions of the brain to bring about movements of the limbs. The inferior divisions, comprising part of the speech zones of the cortex, have a different functional significance. There is good reason to include Area 44 with these zones (Broca's area) and to regard this zone as a specialized portion of the premotor region comprising part of the speech zones of the cerebral cortex. This view is confirmed by analysis of the cytoarchitectonic structure of Broca's area, for, although it has much in common with the premotor portion of the cortex, it differs from the latter by the presence of large numbers of cells in the lower part of Layer III that give rise to a powerful system of associative connections with the temporal portion of the cortex. This distinguishing feature of the inferior divisions of the premotor region of the left hemisphere also stands out when the disturbances arising from lesions of this region are analyzed.

At first glance, the syndrome of motor aphasia arising from lesions of the inferior divisions of the premotor zone of the left hemisphere (Broca's area) might seem very similar, if not identical, to the symptomatology of lesions of the inferior divisions of the postcentral region. However, careful examination of this syndrome shows that it is profoundly different.

We have seen that kinesthetic motor aphasia, associated with a lesion of the postcentral divisions of the cortex, is based on disturbances of the kinesthetic (afferent) organization of motor acts, with these disturbances leading to a loss of clarity and responsiveness in articulation. A completely different picture emerges with lesions of Broca's area.

It has been observed (Luria, 1947, Chapt. IV) that patients with motor aphasia due to a lesion of Broca's area do not necessarily exhibit obvious disturbances of oral praxis, frequently being able to pronounce individual sounds. Nor do they show the symptoms of kinesthetic dysgraphia, for they can write individual letters correctly from dictation. There is reason to suppose that the impaired articulation of individual sounds observed in such patients may be partly attributable to pathological inertia in the motor analyzer, interfering with the rapid transfer from one articulation to another, and to secondary influences of the underlying defect on the whole system of articulation. Frequently, these disturbances may also be explained by extensive spread of the pathological process beyond the limits of the premotor zone.

The characteristic speech difficulties of this group of patients are most clearly evident the moment they attempt to pronounce series of sounds or words requiring the formation of a whole kinetic system of smoothly changing articulations. It is then that the fundamental disability of these patients is brought to light, namely, the disturbance in complex consecutive syntheses, encompassing inability to construct complex systems of articulations and difficulty in inhibiting preceding articulations for a smooth transfer from one articulation in a series to the next. These dynamic difficulties constitute the essence of true "Broca's aphasia," or, as it is conventionally called, "efferent (kinetic) motor aphasia."

The disturbance of the system of kinetic syntheses in patients with a lesion of Broca's area is seen most clearly in speech articulation; it is much less clearly defined in those disturbances of complex hand movements that have been described.

Those exhibiting the most severe manifestations of motor aphasia are usually unable to articulate any sound at all and thus cannot pronounce a single word. There are grounds for believing that complete motor aphasia may develop in this form in patients in whom the lesion is not confined to Broca's area but either spreads (as in the classical cases described by Broca himself) over much wider areas of the speech zone or causes marked secondary phenomena by means of diaschisis, deactivating the entire speech system. Such cases will not receive particular attention in this book.

In less diffuse Broca's aphasia the patient is able to articulate isolated sounds but cannot pronounce a syllable or a whole word, for the ability to inhibit individual articulatory impulses and to shift from one articulation to another is extremely limited. The patient has to make a separate, special effort for each sound and therefore cannot articulate a complete word smoothly. As a rule, the pronunciation of an articuleme reveals pathological inertia, and the patient cannot move on to the next sound. For instance, having pronounced "mu," the first syllable of the word "mukha,"* the patient cannot transfer to the next syllable, "kha," and for a considerable time he utters such sounds as "moo . . . moom . . . moo . . . ma" and so on. Only by the use of special methods, in which each syllable is uttered after a long pause or is introduced into a special system (for example, associating "mu" with the mooing of a cow, "kha" with laughter, etc.), can the patient be helped to overcome this pathological inertia.

*Translator's note: "Mukha," pronounced (with a guttural kh) approximately moo-kha, is the Russian for "fly."

In less severe cases this difficulty of switching from one articulation to another may be more latent in form. As investigations by Vinarskaya (1965, 1969) have shown, such patients find it much more difficult than normal subjects to begin to pronounce a flow of consonants, and instead of changing smoothly from one to another (as, for example, when pronouncing the word "solntse"), they jump from one articulation to the next (sol'n'tse). These defects provide important additional evidence for the diagnosis of disturbances of motor speech in subclinical forms of kinetic motor aphasia.

Similar difficulties arise when such patients try to write. Although they can write individual letters correctly, they usually cannot write a syllable or a word for the integral kinetic structure of writing is disturbed. For this reason these patients cannot reproduce the correct order of the letters in a word but repeat several times over the individual elements of a letter or syllable, thereby disrupting the whole process of writing. Examples of this state of affairs are given in Fig. 68.

However, these difficulties in the pronunciation or writing of individual words are not the only speech disturbances associated with marked kinetic motor aphasia. Even after resolution of the pathological process and the gradual disappearance of the gross manifestations of motor aphasia, defects of the same type may be observed when the patient attempts to pronounce complex expressions. These defects are most conspicuous in these patients when they attempt to repeat series of words or a complicated, and even a simple, phrase. Expressions that are complete in themselves give rise to the most severe defects. If, for example, such a patient is requested to repeat pairs of syllables (such as "sha–sa" or "na–da") or series of words (such as "man–dog–cat") and then to change their order, the same pathological inertia of speech movement may be discerned; in the more severe forms of this syndrome the patient is unable to pronounce a single word. Having pronounced one syllable or one word, these patients are unable to make the transition to the next syllables or words and they continue to say, for example, "sha–sha" for "sha–sa" or "man, dog, dan" for "man–dog–cat." If, as a result of training, the repetition of series of words again becomes possible, modification of the acquired stereotype (in the form of a change in the word order) recreates the difficulty. These patients experience still greater difficulty when they attempt to repeat a phrase or to pronounce independent expressions, and it frequently happens that instead of a phrase they say one word or syllable and then try without avail to overcome the ensuing perseveration. Replacement of the phrase "dai pit'" by the helpless repetition of "... tit'... tit'... i ... etc. .. tit'"* is a typical example of this disturbance. The severe disruption and sometimes

*Translator's note: "Dai pit'" (pronounced "dy peet") means "give me a drink." "Tit'" (pronounced "teet") is meaningless.

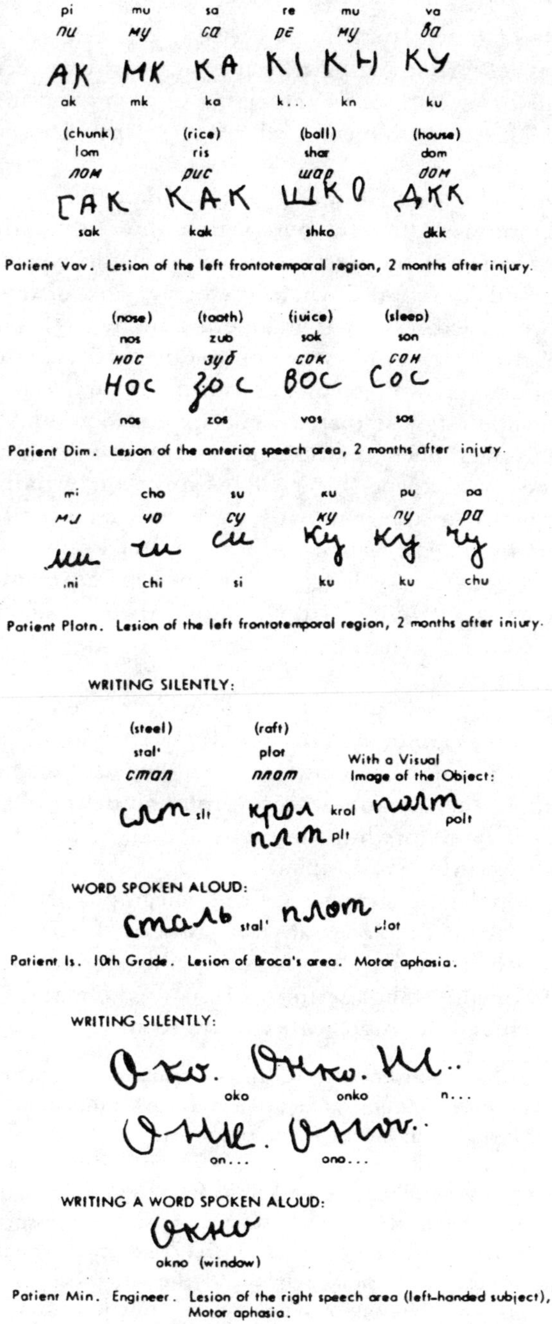

FIGURE 68 Handwriting of patients with "efferent" kinetic motor aphasia.

complete absence of fluent, spontaneous speech, characteristically found in these patients, is not so much the result of a primary disturbance of individual articulatory schemes as the result of a gross disintegration of the kinetics of speech movement and of the dynamic schemes of the expression as a whole.

The disturbances of expressive speech are not limited to difficulties in the pronunciation of phrases. Careful observation shows these difficulties are based on a disturbance of the internal structure of the expression, i.e., on the disintegration of its internal syntactic scheme. This disturbance of the scheme of the whole expression is manifested in the well-known clinical phenomenon of the "telegraphic style" of speech, particularly characteristic of the relatively late stages of recovery from motor aphasia and, in some cases, is the principal sign of that type of aphasia now under discussion. The essence of this phenomenon, whose internal mechanism is not yet clearly understood, is the replacement of the whole expression by individual words, most frequently nouns in the nominative case. For instance, if he wishes to tell how he was wounded, a patient with a gunshot wound of the anterior divisions of the speech area will recite a list of separate names instead of a fluent statement: "Here . . . front . . . and then . . . attack . . . then . . . explosion . . . and then . . . nothing . . . then . . . operation . . . splinter . . . speech, speech . . . speech."

The phenomenon of telegraphic style is difficult to overcome by rehabilitative training, and we cannot yet offer a full explanation for it. It probably is based not only on the disintegration of the "kinetic melodies" discussed earlier in this book, but also on a more profound defect of the scheme of expression, in which all predicative words are especially impaired while isolated nominative words remain intact.

It should be noted that elements of this telegraphic style may also be found in the first form of motor aphasia associated with a lesion of the postcentral region of the cortex, that was described herein. In that context, however, they frequently take the form of "paragrammatical" (incorrectly constructed) speech and are much easier to overcome.

In describing the speech disturbances in motor aphasia, we left aside a problem of the utmost importance although so far it has received little attention. We refer to the *disturbance of internal speech* in various forms of aphasia.

Since the investigations of Vygotskii (1934), internal speech has ceased to be understood simply as "speaking to oneself." Vygotskii described its structural peculiarities and postulated that it has a special function associated with the contraction of the complete sentence into a general conceptual scheme and with the expansion of the general conceptual scheme to the complete sentence. In these investigations, particular attention was directed to discovering whether internal speech is predicative in its structure so that it can subserve the functions outlined above.

The problem of the disturbance of internal speech in the various forms of aphasia has often been referred to (Liepmann, 1913; Pick, 1913; Isserlin, 1936; etc.). The analysis of the extent to which the functions of internal speech are impaired in the different forms of aphasia, however, remains incomplete.

The facts that have been enumerated suggest that disorders in internal speech are particularly prominent in motor aphasia and that in these instances the predicative function is especially severely affected. It is quite possible that the aforementioned disturbances of the scheme of the complete expression and the manifestations of telegraphic style are intimately connected with the disturbance of the predicative function of internal speech that occurs with lesions of the premotor zone.

At the present time, however, no accurate data are available to confirm this suggestion and we can do no more than submit it as a hypothesis requiring special experimental proof.

• • •

One more factor remains to be considered, a very recent discovery that has opened the door to the investigation of the form of kinetic motor aphasia that we have just described. Patients whose active speech has become disordered as a result of acousticognostic defects or defects of the kinesthetic basis of the act of speech show appreciable difficulty in finding the necessary articulations but as a rule retain the general melodic structure of speech. Conversely, in patients with kinetic motor aphasia individual articulations are better preserved but as a rule the melodic structure of speech is lost so that even in the later stages of recovery their speech usually remains melodically inexpressive and retains telegraphic traces.

This deficiency suggests a profound disturbance of the kinetic structure of the expression. It primarily takes the form of a marked disturbance in the accentuation of a phrase, resulting in monotonous speech.

If both groups of patients are asked (as was done by V. :arskaya and Rudaya, unpublished investigation) to pronounce a short phrase with a change of accent (for example, "*I* am going for a walk" or "I *am going for a walk*"), a dynamogram will reveal how easily the melodic organization of the phrase can be changed by those with kinesthetic motor aphasia and how difficult a feat it is for those with the kinetic form. An example of such a recording is given in Fig. 69.

Even though the pathophysiological analysis of the phenomena of motor aphasia is still only in its infancy, some of the factors underlying expressive human speech can be distinguished and the various components of what seemed to be a single form of motor speech disorder can be described.

G. FRONTAL "DYNAMIC" APHASIA

This account of speech disturbances arising from lesions of the anterior divisions of the left hemisphere would be incomplete if one other form of such disorders were not included. What is being alluded to is a disturbance in spontaneous speech that may manifest itself in the last stages of recovery from kinetic motor aphasia. It is sometimes also observed as an independent form of speech disorder arising from a lesion of the regions of the frontal lobe of the left hemisphere situated anteriorly to Broca's area.

This form of speech disorder is related to the disturbances of expressive speech just described in that the scheme of the expression as a whole undergoes important disturbances while disturbances of the kinetics of the act of speech may not be apparent. It differs, however, from the other forms in that disintegration of the grammatical structure of the phrase and elements of the telegraphic style may be absent and the dominant symptom is difficulty in the ecphoria of the whole expression or a disturbance of "speech initiative."

Although it was described some years ago by Kleist (1934) under the name of a "defect of speech initiative" ("Antriebsmangel der Sprache" or "Spontanstummheit"), this form of speech disorder has not yet been sufficiently scrutinized, for the psychological importance of the disturbances observed in these cases is very great.

In contrast to patients with the form of motor aphasia just described, patients with frontal dynamic aphasia have no difficulty in repeating individual words or phrases, in naming objects, or in pronouncing well-established speech stereotypes. Difficulties begin to arise during the performance of sensitive tests and, above all, during the reproduction of series of words or phrases. In patients with frontal dynamic aphasia the familiar derangement of the sequence of the elements of a series and the perseveratory influence of the misplaced elements may sometimes be found. However, these symptoms appear only in special conditions. The greatest difficulties arise when these patients are required to compose their own scheme of an expression and to develop it into spontaneous speech.

Clear evidence of these difficulties may be noticed in the speech of these patients when they are engaged in a dialogue. As a rule, they begin to reply with an echolalic reproduction of the question put to them and render the answer in its shortest, passive form. When the reply is to some extent already embodied in the question, it is given relatively easily, but when the patient has to go beyond the question to form a new system of speech connections, he either makes up for the absence of these connections by echolalia or he refuses to give the required reply at all.

Habitual speech involving automatic series (e.g., recitation of a series of numbers, the days of the week, the months) causes no appreciable difficulty, but as soon as these patients are asked to alter the established order of the series (for example, to recite its elements in reverse) difficulties arise; the patient either continues to reproduce the original order or completely refuses to do what is required. A task that, at first glance, appears easy, such as reciting several words that signify objects with a common property (for example, naming five pointed or red objects) or even naming any five words proves to be beyond the capacity of these patients; they usually give a list of objects in their immediate environment.

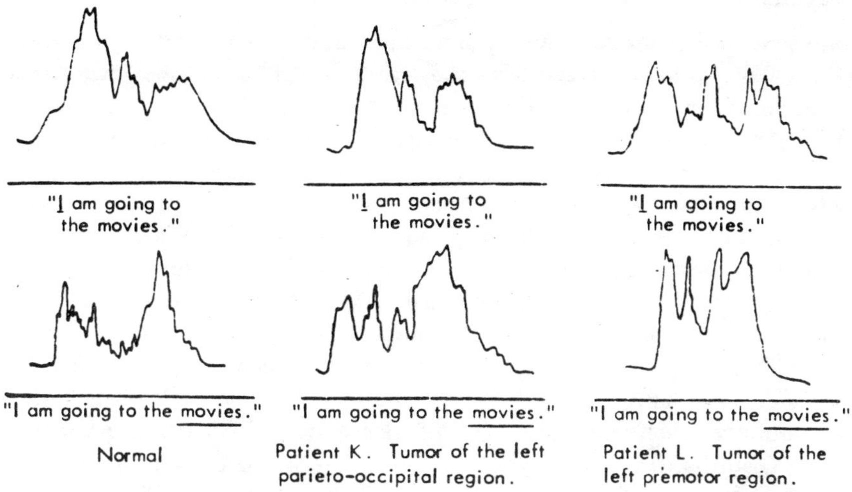

FIGURE 69 Disturbance in accentuation in the speech of a patient recovering from afferent motor aphasia. A characteristic feature is the presence of clear accents in patients with lesions of the posterior divisions of the brain and the absence of such accents in patients with lesions of the anterior divisions. (*After Vinarskaya and Rudaya, unpublished investigation.*)

As has been stated, the disturbances in spontaneous, developed speech are especially prominent in patients of this group. Because of the absence of a scheme of expression, they cannot start to speak or they substitute some habitual, stereotyped expression for what they were going to say. They find little difficulty in making up a story from a series of pictures, but when they try to develop a story from a single picture, they can usually do no more than list the various details or make a very rough guess at its general meaning. They have difficulty in retelling a story that they have read. They can do so only if the story is broken up into parts, so that, instead of reciting the whole story with a consecutive plot, they simply answer a series of questions. They are completely helpless if asked to make a short speech on a particular subject or to expound on a subject initiated by the experimenter. Instead of developing the theme properly, they simply give stereotyped answers. As an example, a patient with a lesion of the posterior frontal region who had traveled considerably in the north was asked to write an essay on the subject of "The North." After prolonged reflection, he wrote: "There are bears up North, which is something I would like to call to your attention."

Another such patient in a similar test said: "The north . . . that means frost" and, after a long pause, he added: "In the north a lone pine grows on the bare hill. . . ." There are grounds for considering that these forms of speech disturbance are based on defects in the ecphoria of predicative speech structures and the associated disturbance of the linear scheme of the sentence.

Special investigations by Luria and Tsvetkova (1968) showed that the patients of this group have appreciable difficulty in recalling verbs, and when asked to name all the verbs they can think of the number they produce is between one-third and one-quarter of the number of nouns recalled. This fact points to a marked, perhaps selective, disturbance of the predicative function of speech, and it explains the disintegration of the linear scheme of the sentence observed in such patients.

In other investigations (Luria, 1963; Luria and Tsvetkova, 1968) patients of this group diligently tried to find the required form of expression but could only manage to pronounce single words (usually substantives), which they were unable to fit into a complete predicative structure.

As Tsvetkova has observed, the long pause, which in these patients precedes the beginning of a spoken expression, is not filled with latent articulatory impulses such as can be recorded electromyographically in normal subjects. Disturbances of this type apparently are based on a profound defect of internal speech. This is a matter for future special investigation.

The essential characteristics of this type of disturbance come to light in the rehabilitation of such patients. As a rule, direct attempts to restore spontaneous speech in these patients are unsuccessful. However, spontaneous narrative speech can be restored if unaided discourse is replaced by a series of questions and answers or if the text to be recited is broken up into separate auxiliary links or pegs on which to hang the unfolding plot. These may take the form of drawings on cards, which the patient may use as external props.*

The essential character of this defect can best be observed during reeducation of these patients when they are given a ready-made linear scheme of expression as an aid. For example, when the patient is unsuccessfully trying to construct a sentence, all that is necessary is to spread out in front of him a series of blank cards (as many as there are words in the sentence), to enable him to pronounce the required sentence by pointing to each card in turn. The contrast that can be observed by comparing the performance of this test with the aid of the cards and the patient's inability to find the required form of expression, a typical feature of such cases, is often striking. An appropriate example is shown below.

a) *spontaneously*

I . . . what can it be? . . . well . . .

b) *with the aid of cards*

I ——→ want ——→ to walk

☐ ——→ ☐ ——→ ☐

c) *spontaneously again*

I . . . can't . . . don't know

Organization of expression with the aid of external support in cases of dynamic aphasia.

*This method of restoration of active speech is examined more fully elsewhere (Luria, 1948).

Such tests can certainly shed considerable light on the precise psychological structure of the speech defect observed in such patients.

This unique syndrome, which most frequently arises from lesions of the posterior frontal region, anterior to Broca's area, cannot yet be adequately explained. There is every reason to suppose that it may be an attenuated variant of kinetic aphasia that is manifested as a disturbance of the formation of new complex dynamic speech connections.

The phenomena of disruption of spontaneous speech, which I have fully described elsewhere (Luria, 1963), will be much better understood after we have analyzed the whole complex of disturbances arising from lesions of the frontal divisions of the cerebral cortex.

• • •

We have described forms of speech disorders that differ essentially from the forms of motor aphasia developing from lesions of the postcentral, temporal, and occipital regions of the cortex. Whereas the basic structure (or code) of the articulatory, phonemic, or conceptual framework of language is disturbed while the kinetic scheme of the expression (or its melody) remains largely preserved in motor aphasia arising from posterior lesions, in the aphasias resulting from a lesion of the anterior divisions of the motor analyzer it is primarily the kinetic organization of speech, its syntactic scheme or melodic structure, that is disordered. We may agree with Jakobson's (1956) distinction between aphasic syndromes centered on a disturbance of the codes of language and those centered on the disintegration of spontaneous "contextual" speech.

At this stage we cannot draw definite conclusions regarding the mechanism of these forms of speech disturbance. The only clear fact is that these disorders cannot be simply regarded as a "disturbance of intention," a "defect of initiative," or a manifestation of "alogical disturbances of the intellect" (Kleist, 1934). They are disturbances of the kinetic organization of speech activity, and defects in "intention" or "initiative" in these cases are specifically related to speech and are not of a general character. Nevertheless, these disturbances in expressive speech are closely associated with the general defects in the kinetic organization of movements arising from lesions of the premotor systems of the brain and are manifested as a failure of integration of serially constructed motor acts. The study of the true mechanisms underlying this disability is a task that remains to be accomplished.

H. DISTURBANCES OF INTELLECTUAL PROCESSES WITH LESIONS OF THE PREMOTOR REGION

Little attempt has yet been made to study intellectual impairment resulting from circumscribed lesions of the cerebral cortex. The study of the intel-

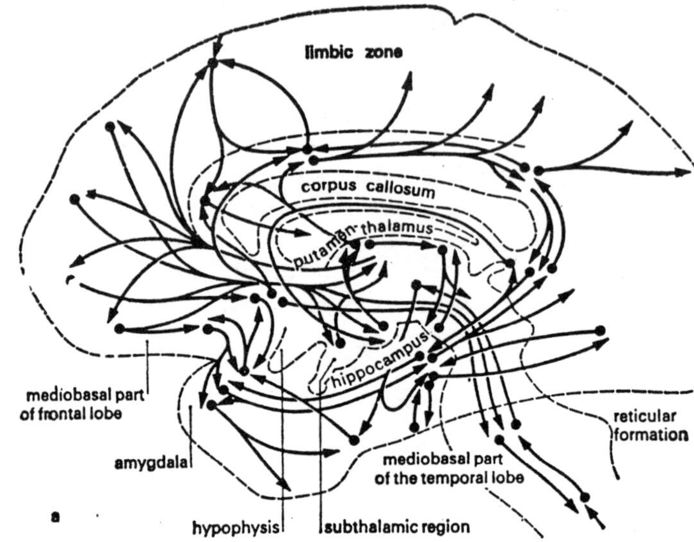

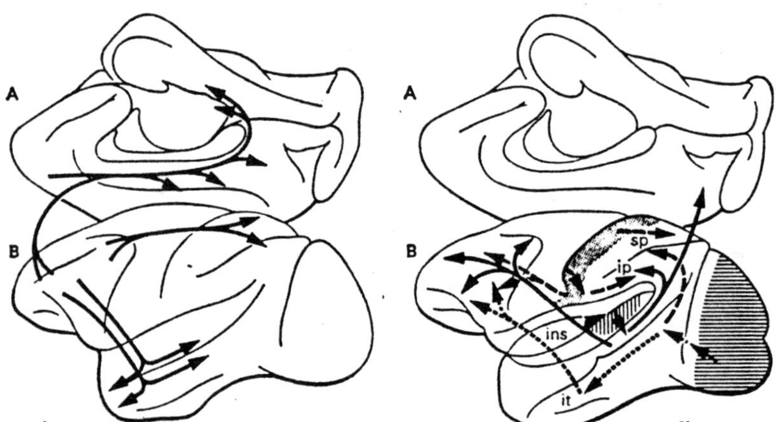

FIGURE 70a Connections of the frontal lobes with other brain structures (after Polyakov).

FIGURE 70b Connections of the frontal lobes with other brain structures (b) after Nauta. (i) efferent connections; (ii) afferent connections, (A) medial surface (B) lateral surface.

From: A. R. Luria; The Working Brain (Penguin, London, 1974).

lectual disturbances associated with the different variants of motor aphasia has likewise been neglected. It follows that we lack the necessary information to describe the intellectual defects arising, in conjunction with kinetic motor aphasia, from lesions of the postcentral divisions of the cortex, and therefore the best that can be done at present is to briefly summarize the data obtained by psychological analysis of the premotor syndrome.

As well as being reflected by disintegration of the smooth kinetic schemes of movement, difficulty in transferring from one element to the next, and inertia of stereotypes once they have been developed, the fundamental defect that we have observed to accompany lesions of the premotor systems is also reflected in the course of intellectual operations. In patients of this group it is not so much the content of the intellectual act that is disturbed (which is more likely to be due to alienation of the meaning of words, to disturbance of the structure of ideas, etc.), as it is the dynamics of the intellectual process.

Detailed psychological studies have recently been made of the dynamic aspect of intellectual processes (Leont'ev, 1959; Gal'perin, 1959; etc.). These investigations have shown that the direct "observation of relationships," which the Würzburg school considered to be an original property of intellectual activity, occurs, in fact, only in the last phase of its development. In developmental terms, intellectual activity begins with a series of fully developed external operations, which are gradually synthesized and automatized, to acquire the character of plastic "mental actions," carried out with the aid of internal speech. It is the synthesizing component of intellectual operations, responsible for the smooth, automatized flow of the series of mental actions, that is apparently seriously disturbed by lesions of the premotor divisions of the cerebral cortex. The existence of these disturbances is clearly brought to light by analysis of the intellectual operations of patients with a lesion of the premotor systems.

Characteristic disturbances are found when *understanding* of complex conceptual systems is called for—written texts, the purpose of problems, etc. In contrast to patients with a lesion of the temporal and inferoparietal (or parieto-occipital) regions of the brain, patients with a lesion of the premotor region have no difficulty in understanding the direct meaning of words; they do not exhibit the phenomenon of extinction of meaning of words or defects in grasping individual logical-grammatical (and, above all, spatial) relationships. The distinctive feature of the intellectual disturbance in these patients is revealed by their difficulty in realizing the significance of complex logical-grammatical structures. They can grasp a problem only after prolonged, detailed, and deliberate operations. This *retardation of understanding* is particularly prominent when the patient is confronted by a relatively long passage with an intricate context. For example, the meaning of a sentence such as: "To rule the country, the monarch relies on the aid of the governing classes, and is subservient to their will" is not immediately appreciated by these patients. They turn it over and over in their minds, repeat it aloud, and introduce the necessary accentuation to make it comprehensible. "I can't understand the first time," such a patient will say, "if I read it through once I grasp only a few words and do not understand what it means .... I have to read it many times, to pick out the ideas and put them together, and then I can understand it . . ." (Luria, 1943, 1963

[Russian], 1966 [English]). There is every reason to suppose that part of the work carried out by means of *internal speech* (in which internal articulation evidently plays a part) is seriously disturbed in the patients of this group. This suggestion is confirmed by the fact that it is difficult or impossible for the patient to understand the general meaning of a passage if he is told to handle it silently without reading it aloud.

Hence, in patients with a lesion of the premotor systems it is not only the process of development of the speech intention that is disturbed (we described this condition when we analyzed the disturbance of the patient's active speech), but also the process of "contracting" the speech structures, which is essential to the understanding of the meaning of a text. In both cases we are dealing with a disturbance of the dynamics of speech processes and not with the disintegration of particular logical-grammatical structures, such as is observed in patients with semantic aphasia.

A disturbance in automatic intellectual operations, or mental actions, may also be observed in other tasks. For example, if a patient with a premotor syndrome is asked to carry out some form of conventional action (fo example, a substitution test, in which he has to insert some arbitrary sign below each of a small number of different signs or patterns), the operation, which is rapidly automatized in the normal subject, remains unautomatized for a long time. Every time he tries to write the sign, the required connection has to be initiated all over again. No general habit is formed. The same situation is seen in simple arithmetical operations. Careful analysis shows that often these operations do not reach the stage of a "contracted" mental action. In addition or subtraction problems, for instance, the patient for a long time shows a tendency to add and subtract by units instead of progressing to automatized, internal tabular computation (calculation with collective groups). In these arithmetical operations it thus takes much longer, sometimes twice as long, if the second number to be added is larger. It thus takes longer, for example, to add 3 + 7 than it does to add 7 + 3 (Luria, 1943).

Disturbances of intellectual processes are also observed when the patient undertakes other logical tasks. Patients of this group can correctly grasp the gist of logical-grammatical relationships that are beyond the comprehension of patients with parieto-occipital lesions. They find it relatively easy to solve problems associated with the spatial arrangement of elements (for example, putting a circle above a cross) by a process of consecutive analysis. However, a characteristic feature of many of these cases is that with repetition of these problems their solution immediately develops into an inert stereotype. The patients cannot perform another operation, even a simpler one. For example, because of the inertia of a stereotype once it has been formed, a patient with a lesion of the premotor divisions of the brain who can correctly carry out such operations as placing a circle below a cross and placing a dot below a minus sign is quite unable to perform a simpler task like placing a cross above a triangle or placing a minus sign above a square.

Similar defects are revealed when the patients are asked to solve problems. For instance, although patients with a premotor syndrome can grasp (with some assistance because the whole problem is broken down into a series of consecutive operations) the scheme of the solution of a problem concerned with proportions, such as "there were 18 books on two shelves, and there were twice as many on one shelf as on the other," they will continue to use the methods that they have adopted even if the conditions of the problem are changed. When, therefore, they go on to solve an easier problem, of the type of "there were 18 books on two shelves, and there were two more books on one shelf than on the other," they continue to use the same method of dividing into parts, which, of course, is incorrect under the new conditions (see Luria and Tsvetkova, 1966).

Whereas disturbances in intellectual operations found with other brain lesions result from a series of special defects in the lexic or semantic aspects of speech, with lesions of the premotor divisions a disorder in intellectual operations is presumably associated with disintegration of the dynamic pattern of speech acts. The changes in the dynamics of intellectual processes that occur with a disturbance of "contracted" mental actions, with the fragmentary solution of problems, and with pathological inertia are particularly well defined in the group of lesions forming the subject of the present discussion. The relatively well-preserved capacity to carry out spatial synthesis and logical-grammatical operations present in these patients distinguishes them from those with lesions of the parieto-occipital systems. Defects in the dynamics of intellectual processes in these cases form a part of the general syndrome of disturbance of the kinetic organization of various motor acts; this accounts for the special character of these disturbances.

The derangement of the dynamics of intellectual processes with lesions of the premotor systems of the brain brings us to a new topic—disturbance of the higher cortical functions accompanying lesions of the frontal divisions of the brain.

5. *Disturbances of Higher Cortical Functions with Lesions of the Frontal Region*

In the previous chapters we examined the structure and function of those parts of the human cerebral cortex that are responsible for the reception and processing of information derived from the outside world and for the formation of differentiated movements by which man responds to external stimuli. We have examined separately those disturbances of the higher cortical functions associated with lesions of the cortical divisions of the auditory, optic, cutaneokinesthetic, and motor analyzers and of the overlapping cortical areas of those zones. Cortical malfunctioning as a result of lesions of the primary and secondary fields of the cortical nuclei of the motor analyzer, the sensorimotor and premotor divisions of the cerebral cortex, was considered. In the present chapter we turn to the analysis of the structure and function of those zones of the cortex which, according to all available information, perform the most complex functions and which have been the subject of detailed investigation for a long period of time. I refer to the functional organization of the frontal lobes and the changes in behavior produced by lesions of this part of the brain.

When we start to consider the functions of the frontal lobes we at once find ourselves in a section of neurology in which the situation differs sharply from that in all other sections of this science. Whereas when we study the functions of the temporal, occipital, and sensomotor zones of the brain we are dealing with regions whose activity is governed by reasonably well-known principles and which, by general agreement, are connected with the reception and processing of the basic types of sensation and the organization of motor acts, when we turn to analyze the functions of the frontal lobes we at once enter a region of unfamiliar and unresolved problems.

Only rarely have the frontal lobes of the brain, which are fully developed only in man, been considered to be connected with the analysis of sensations obtained from various receptors and with the processing of incoming information. Equally rarely the frontal lobes have been regarded as the apparatus directly responsible for motor innervations. Observers have noted that no sensory or motor responses arise to electrical stimulation of the frontal lobes, that epileptic fits caused by irritation of the frontal lobes do not commence with any form of sensory or motor aura, and that even massive lesions of the frontal lobes are unaccompanied by any disturbances of visual, auditory, and tactile sensations and do not lead to any clearly defined disturbances of movement.

On the basis of such observations many workers have concluded that the frontal lobes have no clearly defined function and that, so far as can be deduced from such observations as were possible, they must be regarded as "silent zones" of the cerebral cortex.

However, these observations were contradicted by facts obtained by other investigators. Careful observation of complex forms of animal behavior and, in particular, complex forms of human conscious activity led to completely different conclusions regarding the function of the frontal lobes. When animals were observed after extirpation of the frontal lobes, it was found that complex forms of goal-directed, purposive behavior were disturbed; although the animal could still see and hear, still retained its olfactory and tactile sensation, and had no sign of paralysis, it started to behave inadequately and purposelessly.

Clinicians studying patients with massive lesions of the frontal lobes have described similar facts. These patients were found to preserve all types of sensation, to have no sign of disturbance of movement, and to have no disturbances of gnosis, praxis, and speech; nevertheless, their complex psychological activity was grossly impaired. They were unable to produce stable plans and became inactive and aspontaneous. They could respond to ordinary questions or perform habitual actions, but they were quite unable to carry out complex, purposive, and goal-directed actions. They were unable to evaluate their attempts, they were not critical of their behavior, and could not control their actions; they continued to perform automatic actions which had long ceased to be meaningful, without any attempt at correction. They were no longer concerned about their failure, they were hesitant and indecisive, and, most frequently of all, they became indifferent or they exhibited features of euphoria, as a result of the loss of their critical awareness of their behavior.

All these observations have led many neurologists to conclude that the anterior or "association" zones of the frontal lobes are connected with higher psychological functions and that, as Fulton (1943, p. 418) expresses it, "in approaching the functions of the frontal association areas one is brought face to face with activities which are difficult to describe in physiological terms."

This assessment of the functions of the frontal lobes is linked with the position occupied by the frontal lobes in the general structure of central nervous mechanisms.

There are good grounds for asserting that the function of the frontal lobes, more than the function of any other part of the brain, cannot be expressed by the concepts of the reflex arc as established in classical physiology, and that in order to understand their role in the organization of behavior other ideas, radically different from the classical ones, must be used.

The facts I shall give below indicate that the functions of the frontal lobes (as, indeed, the functions of many other systems) can be expressed only by the concepts of a reflex circuit and the mechanisms of self-regulating systems that have been created in the last decades and have now become firmly established in modern biology.

Preliminary integration of all stimuli reaching the organism and the attachment of informative or regulatory significance to some of this—the formation of the "provisional basis of action," and the creation of complex programs of behavior; the constant monitoring of the performance of these programs and the checking of behavior with comparison of actions performed and the original plans; the provision of a system of "feedback" on the basis of which complex forms of behavior are regulated—all these phenomena in man take place with the intimate participation of the frontal lobes, and they account for the exceptionally important place of the frontal lobes in the general organization of behavior.

On the basis of these ideas the functions of the frontal lobes will naturally continue to be a subject for analysis (ultimately physiological) in the same way as the functions of all other parts of the cortex; psychological and clinical analysis of frontal lobe pathology will still continue to be connected with their physiological study, for this is a basic principle of contemporary science.

I shall be guided by this principle in my description of this section of our investigation.

The history of the investigation of the pathology of the frontal lobes will be traced briefly. With this picture before us we shall go on to consider the disturbances of voluntary movement and actions produced by these lesions, giving special attention to the defects in the complex forms of regulation of movement that are particularly characteristic of this pathological condition. We shall then turn to the findings at our disposal pertaining to the disturbances of gnostic, mnestic, and intellectual processes in association with lesions of the frontal lobes of the brain.

A. HISTORICAL SURVEY

The investigation of the functions of the frontal lobes and of the disturbances occurring with lesions of these lobes began comparatively long ago, in the

1870's, and its course lay in two more or less parallel lines, which rarely came into contact with each other.

On the one hand, it formed a part of a series of experimental physiological and psychological studies whose purpose was to ascertain the changes taking place in an animal's behavior after extirpation of the frontal lobes. These investigations, which began in the period between 1870 and 1890, have become particularly intensive in the past 20 to 30 years and have yielded interesting and valuable results. On the other hand, the behavioral changes of patients with wounds and tumors of the frontal lobes have been studied clinically, principally by psychiatrists and occasionally by neurologists and psychologists. Such studies have yielded clinical data on the changes in human mental activity resulting from frontal lobe lesions. These two lines of investigation have led to an accumulation of considerable, but contradictory, factual evidence.

After Fritsch and Hitzig in the 1870's had identified the motor area of the cerebral cortex, and Panizza (1855), Hitzig (1874), and Munk (1881) had described the optic centers of the cortex, the attention of investigators began to shift to other regions of the cerebral hemispheres, including the frontal lobes. Important mental functions had been attributed to the frontal lobes ever since the time of Gratiolet (1861).

Originally, two main methods were used to study the functions of the frontal lobes, the only ones available at that time (1870–1890): stimulation and extirpation. However, from the start the results obtained by these two methods led to confusion.

It was experimentally shown that electrical stimulation of the frontal divisions of the cortex causes no reaction and that extirpation of the frontal lobes is not followed by paralysis or disturbances in vision, hearing, or cutaneous sensation. The frontal lobe of the brain began to be regarded as the "silent area" of the cerebral cortex. Further, the negative results obtained by investigators led to the view that, in general, the frontal lobes possess no independent functions but are a remarkable example of the "superfluity" created by the evolution of brain tissue.

However, this impression of the total absence of disturbances following extirpation of the frontal lobes quickly gave way to a radically different interpretation. Bianchi (1895, 1920), Bekhterev (1907), Franz (1907), and others discovered that the general behavior of an animal from which both frontal lobes had been extirpated *was* considerably altered, although, indeed, there was no sign of loss of vision, hearing, or general sensation and no gross disturbances of movement. The animal no longer recognized its master, it no longer behaved selectively in relation to food but seized and chewed any object, it no longer actively searched for food but was distracted by any extraneous stimulus, and it no longer moved purposefully but exhibited motor automatisms in the form of walking in circles, automatic "riding arena" movements, etc.

The resulting state of affairs was extremely complicated. The existing physiological concepts were obviously inadequate to explain the complex disturbances that lead to changes in purposeful behavior without affecting the sensory and motor processes. The only course left to workers investigating the frontal lobes in animals was to attempt to express the resulting defect in terms of the contemporary subjective psychology, according to which the frontal lobes are the organ of "abstract intelligence" (Hitzig, 1874), "active attention" (Ferrier, 1876), or "apperception" (Wundt, 1873-

1874). In so doing these investigators reverted to the older idea that the frontal lobes are the site of the "regulating mind" or the "supreme organ of the brain" (Gratiolet, 1861).

Naturally this description could not lead to an adequate scientific explanation of the facts, and the first attempts at psychomorphological interpretation of the functions of the frontal lobes immediately encountered opposition. Some workers, while not casting doubt on the authenticity of the descriptions, were inclined to attribute the behavioral changes observed after extirpation of the frontal lobes to disturbances in the functioning of the brain as a whole and denied that the frontal lobes played any sort of "supreme" role. They regarded the whole brain as the material location of the "intellect." This point of view was adopted by Munk (1881), who accepted the localization of simple sensory and motor functions in the cerebral cortex but could not accept the localization of functions regulating general behavior in any circumscribed areas of the brain. The same view was held by Goltz (1876-1884), a staunch supporter of the antilocalizationists. The assignment of specialized higher mental functions to the frontal lobes was rejected by Loeb (1886, 1902), Monakow (1914), Luciani (1913), and others, who felt that the importance of the frontal lobes in the organization of behavior had been greatly exaggerated.

Another group of workers thought differently. While recognizing the importance of the frontal lobes in mental activity and the profound changes in behavior occurring after their extirpation, they categorically rejected attempts to interpret these facts as the result of a disturbance of the functions of the brain as a whole. They directed their energies toward elucidating the special functions of the frontal regions which, when disturbed, led to such profound disturbances in general behavior.

During the 1880's, Jackson suggested that "the highest motor centres are the most complex and least organized centres and represent widest regions (movements of all parts of the body) triply indirectly." When he speaks of the highest centers as being the "least organized," Jackson (1932, Vol. 2, pp. 53–54, 66) implies that they are the newest divisions and have not yet completed their period of final differentiation. The subsequent development of Jackson's views will become evident as our survey of the history of the study of brain functions continues. They were expressed in a slightly different form and independently by Bianchi (1895, 1920), one of the first authors to systematically study the results of extirpation of the frontal lobes in animals. According to Bianchi (1920), reflex activity is organized at a series of levels, each one higher than the last. The apparatus responsible for the most complex forms of reflex activity is the frontal lobes of the brain. It is these lobes that bring about the widest coordination of sensory and motor elements, utilize the product of the sensory zones to create mental syntheses, and play the same role in relation to the sensorimotor (or kinesthetic) zones that the latter play in relation to the subcortical nuclei. This integrative function of the frontal lobes of the brain is clearly demonstrated by bilateral extirpation of the frontal lobes; as a result of such extirpation the animal's behavior loses its organized character, becoming fragmented and insubordinated to a common synthesis, and ceases to adapt itself to new conditions.

The gaps in Bianchi's arguments, expressed in terms of the typical concepts of that period and anticipating some later research, were filled in by other writers. Some of these stressed that the frontal lobes are the region in which sensory impulses from the body itself are received. Munk (1881), for instance, regarded the frontal lobes as the "Körpergefühlsphäre," while Ferrier (1876) ascribed to them a role in muscle sense and movement perception. Other writers (Goltz, 1884; Loeb, 1886; Luciani, 1913; Libertini, 1895; Polimanti, 1906; etc.) claimed that the frontal lobes play a part in the inhibition of the functions of lower divisions of the brain and saw confirmation of this view in the fact that lower automatisms were revived after extirpation of the frontal lobes.

However, the most interesting development of these propositions must be credited to Bekhterev, who began his series of detailed observations of the functions of the frontal lobes in the 1880's and summarized them in his book, *Fundamentals of Brain Function* (1907), confirming the earlier reports that extirpation of the frontal lobes in dogs causes no defects in vision, hearing, or tactile perception but does cause disintegration of goal-directed behavior. Bekhterev paid particular attention to the fact that animals deprived of their frontal lobes "do not evaluate the results of their actions as they should, cannot correlate new external impressions with past experience, and do not direct their movements and actions to their own advantage." In Bekhterev's opinion, this "loss of successive traces and failure to evaluate these impressions" also leads to a disturbance of that "psychoregulatory activity" which is required for the "correct evaluation of external impressions and the purposive, deliberate choice of movements in accordance with this evaluation"; he regarded this as the principal function of the prefrontal divisions of the brain (Bekhterev, 1907, pp. 1464–1468).

To the previous proposition of the integrative, coordinating, and inhibitory functions of the frontal lobes, Bekhterev added the suggestion that they play an important part in the evaluation of the movements and activities of the body itself. As will be seen, this suggestion subsequently became one of the essential components of the theory of higher nervous processes and functions of the frontal lobes.

The attempt to find objective mechanisms for the higher forms of regulatory activity ascribed to the frontal lobes was a significant contribution by the writers who have been cited. Each of their investigations marked a step forward in the understanding of the disturbance of goal-directed behavior observed in animals deprived of their frontal lobes. Nevertheless, the concept of the psychoregulatory role of the frontal lobes remained without a physiological basis, and in one way or another the psychomorphological interpretation of the frontal lobes as the supreme organ of the brain continued. Further advances had to be made before this viewpoint could be overcome. They took place with the further development of the reflex theory of behavior, associated with the work of Pavlov and his collaborators, and of the physiological ideas of self-adjusting systems.

Pavlov gave an excellent account of the results of extirpation of the frontal lobes in the dog (*Complete Collected Works, Vol. 3*, pp. 175–176). He wrote:

"If you excise the whole posterior part of the cerebral hemispheres of a dog you will obtain an animal to all intents and purposes normal. It wags its tail when you stroke it. It will use its nose and its sense of touch to identify you, or its food, or any other object it may meet. It will show you that it is pleased when it has recognized you with its nose. However, an animal in this state will not react to you if you stand a long way off, for it has not the full use of its eyes. If you pronounce its name, it will not react to this either. You will be forced to the conclusion that such a dog makes only very little use of its eyes and ears, but otherwise is perfectly normal.

"If, however, you excise the whole anterior part of the cerebral hemispheres as far as the boundary of the excised posterior part, you will have a profoundly abnormal animal. It will not behave properly towards you, its fellow dogs, its food (which it will not seek), or to objects in general and to its environment. It is a completely different animal, apparently retaining no trace of purposive behavior. There is thus a vast difference between these two animals: one without the anterior, the other without the posterior part of the hemispheres. You would say that in one case the dog is blind or deaf but otherwise normal, but in the other case that it is a severely disable, helpless idiot."

Pavlov's high regard for the role of the frontal lobes in the "integration of goal-directed movement" is obvious (*Ibid.*, p. 295). In contrast to his predecessors, however, Pavlov started out with a different conception of the functions of the cerebral cortex and its motor divisions, and he was able to make use of a scientific method enabling him to verify his conception experimentally.

As has been stated, (Part II, Section 4A), Pavlov did not regard the motor area of the cerebral cortex as a purely efferent region directing voluntary impulses of an uncertain and nonmaterial nature and responsible for psychoregulatory activity. With the introduction of the concept of the motor analyzer, the cortical motor area came to be regarded as an afferent, analyzing apparatus, connected in the closest way with the other zones of the cortex. In Pavlov's view, the cortical divisions of the motor analyzer possess the same afferent function as other parts of the cortex. Receiving impulses from all other parts of the brain and, in particular, kinesthetic signals giving information on the course of a movement and its effect, these divisions form the afferent basis of voluntary movement. Voluntary movement is thus the result of the "integrated activity" of the whole brain. Pavlov regarded the *frontal lobes as an essential, indeed the most complex, component of the cortical divisions of the motor analyzer*, involved in the selection of necessary goal-directed movements. Extirpation of the frontal lobes, by destruction of important cortical divisions of the motor analyzer, inevitably leads to the disintegration of complex motor syntheses and to impairment of the animal's goal-directed movements. At the same time, as investigations by Pavlov's school have shown, relatively simple forms of conditioned-reflex activity, as exemplified by secretion tests, remain unaffected (Tikhomirov, 1906; Demidov, 1909; Saturnov, 1911; Kuraev, 1912; Shumilina, 1949) or are only partially disorganized (Shustin, 1956, 1959; Brutkowski, Konorskii, *et al.*, 1956).

After Pavlov's death, experimental investigations of the behavior of dogs and monkeys after extirpation of the frontal lobes were continued by Anokhin (1949), Shumilina (1949), and Shustin (1955, 1959) in the Soviet Union, by Konorskii (1956, 1957) and his collaborators in Poland, and by American workers (Jacobsen, 1935; Malmo, 1942; Kennard and co-workers, 1941; Orbach, 1956, 1959; Pribram 1958*a* and *b*, 1960, and co-workers 1954, 1956; Mishkin and co-workers 1955, 1956, 1958; etc.).

Various experimental techniques of behavioral study were used. These investigations made an important contribution to the accurate definition of the defects caused by destruction of the frontal lobes of the brain. They showed, and this is particularly true of the investigations of Anokhin (1949) and Shumilina (1949), that extirpation of the frontal lobes leads to a *gross disturbance in the preliminary syntheses of individual signals* that precede movement and that constitute the "prerelease" or "orienting" afferent organization (Anokhin, 1949). That is why, according to Anokhin, a dog without its frontal lobes may react directly to one conditioned signal but cannot differentiate between two signals, requiring *two different motor reactions* (known in psychology as a "choice reaction"). If dogs deprived of their frontal lobes are confronted by two feeding bowls, they do not simply run to the one containing food but begin to run aimlessly from one bowl to the other, carrying out stereotyped "pendulum movements." The application of reinforcement at one point does not lead to a selective reaction, for dogs deprived of their frontal lobes can no longer correctly assess the meaning of reinforcement. Their behavior ceases to be regulated by signals on the success or failure of the corresponding reaction and their movements lose their adaptive character.

Similar conclusions regarding the disintegration of forms of behavior demanding a preliminary synthesis of signals have been reached by American workers studying the behavior of monkeys whose frontal lobes were resected. In the situation created in Köhler's experiment, a monkey deprived of its frontal lobes could use a stick to reach a bait only if the stick and bait were in the same field of vision; it could not do so if they were placed on different platforms, although before the operation this had been easily done (Jacobsen, Wolf, and Jackson, 1935). Similar results were obtained in puzzle-box experiments. The animals were able to solve simple problems consisting of one motor operation, but this contrasted sharply with the gross disintegration of serial operations requiring preliminary synthesis of the situation (Jacobsen, 1935; Finan, 1939; Malmo, 1942; etc.). The results obtained by Pribram (1959*a* and *b*, 1960) are of fundamental interest. In a series of special experiments, he showed that reinforcement of one of the motor reactions in a situation involving a complicated choice does not bring about the required changes in an animal's behavior. He accordingly concluded that disregard of the effect of its own movement ("success signal" or "mistake signal") is an essential sign of disturbed behavior due to resection of the frontal lobes of the brain.

As the investigations of Pribram and others have shown, the behavior of animals whose convex portions of the frontal lobes were resected differs significantly from that of those with resection of the posterior divisions and from animals deprived of the mediobasal regions of the frontal lobes. The latter operation causes considerable change in general activity but does not give rise to the type of behavioral disturbance that has been described.

The findings obtained by different workers suggest that one of the essential results of destruction of the frontal lobes in animals is a *disturbance of the preliminary (what Anokhin calls "prerelease") syntheses underlying the regulation of complex forms of motor operations and the evaluation of the effect of their own actions, without which goal-directed, selective behavior is impossible.*

These workers believe that in animals deprived of their frontal lobes the traces of previously established systems of connections do not persist for long and that the animal is easily distracted by extraneous stimuli, so that the active state of readiness for a particular action (called "intention" in psychology) does not develop. Defects in these processes were studied in experiments involving delayed reactions (Jacobsen, 1935, 1936; Pribram and co-workers, 1952–1959; Mishkin and co-workers 1955–1958; Rosvold, 1959; Rosvold and Delgado, 1956; Orbach, 1959; etc.). These investigations revealed two very important facts. Whereas in a normal animal a delayed reaction may be formed relatively quickly and maintained for a long time, in a monkey deprived of its frontal lobes there is much less likelihood of the formation of a stable delayed reaction. The production of delayed reactions either becomes totally impossible or is disturbed by the action of any extraneous stimulus. And, as the latest observations of Pribram (1959*a* and *b*, 1960) have shown, the "expectancy" of reinforcement produced in a normal animal by presentation of a signal completely disappears after extirpation of the frontal lobes. Jacobsen (1935) and others convincingly showed that it is impossible to produce conflicts or experimental neuroses in monkeys by extirpation of their frontal lobes.

A possible explanation for many of these findings may be found in the fact that resection of the frontal lobes leads to a marked increase in the animal's motor activity. This is clear from several investigations (Jacobsen, 1931; Jacobsen *et al.*, 1935; Richter and Hines, 1938; Kennard *et al.*, 1934; and, in particular, Konorskii and co-workers, 1956). In these studies it was observed that delayed reactions are disinhibited and elementary (subcortical) automatisms that are revived in animals after resection of the frontal lobes.

• • •

The experimental work on the role of the frontal lobes in the behavior of animals has been briefly surveyed. Notwithstanding the extreme complexity of the problem, these investigations have led to certain hypotheses and have indicated possible ways of study of the disturbance of behavior in animals with lesions of the frontal lobes.

The experimental investigation of the function of the frontal lobes in animals has been beset by a number of difficulties, but the study of the pathology of the frontal lobes in man has produced even more complex and contradictory data. The pathological changes in human mental activity associated with lesions of the frontal lobes have usually been studied by psychiatrists, who have confined their activity to describing the clinical manifestations that they have observed. Very few experimental studies have been undertaken on the disturbances of the higher cortical functions associated with these lesions.

Because of the complexity of the observed phenomena, the investigation of mental disturbances accompanying lesions of the frontal lobes in man, while it has yielded many (and quite contradictory) empirical facts, has not yet led to the discovery of general principles. Systematizing the observations and devising suitable experimental techniques to explain the accumulated data remain to be done.

The history of the clinical study of the pathology of the frontal lobes in man will now be briefly reviewed. Following this review, the results obtained from experimental psychological research will be described.

One of the first accounts of the changes in human behavior arising from a lesion of the frontal lobes was given by Harlow (1868), who described a case of a severe wound of the frontal lobes that was followed by marked personality changes, the release of primitive animal instincts, and the disturbance of the "balance between intellectual and animal traits." Starr (1884) and Leonora Welt (1888) published similar accounts of gross disturbance of emotional life after injury to the basal portions of the frontal lobes. Jastrowitz (1888) and Oppenheim (1890) reported that tumors of the pole of the right frontal lobe, spreading to the orbital surface, are accompanied by a syndrome of dementia with a characteristic euphoria at the climax of the disease.

Following these reports, many psychiatric articles were published in which profound disturbances of volitional, intellectual, and affective life resulting from trauma or tumors of the frontal lobes were described. The authors of these articles specified a disturbance of initiative as typical of the mental changes associated with lesions of the frontal lobes. They described this type of disturbance as a disintegration of the plan of successive actions, which in severe cases leads to an apathetic akinetic-abulic syndrome, long regarded as specific for lesions of the frontal lobes. They also concluded that lesions of the frontal lobes are characterized by gross intellectual deterioration, disturbance of abstract thought, and reversion of behavior to primitive "concrete" forms.

Finally, these authors reported that the behavior of patients with a marked "frontal syndrome" is distinguished by profound disturbances of the complex emotions and, in particular, by emotional conflicts. In patients with the severest forms of this syndrome the critical attitude toward their own actions and the conscious evaluation of their behavior are impaired.

All of these investigations yielded a rich store of data, and the subject of mental disturbance from lesions of the frontal lobes now forms one of the best documental branches of psychiatry. These data have been summarized at various times by Feuchtwanger (1923), Baruk (1926), Kleist (1934), Brickner (1936), Rylander (1939), Freeman and Watts (1942), Halstead (1947), Haeffner (1957), Ajuriaguerra and Hécaen (1960) and others, so that we need not consider them further.

As with the experimental studies of frontal lobe functions in animals, analysis of the accumulated data pertaining to man presents considerable difficulties. Many clinicians and psychopathologists suggested that the weakening of the intellect and the change in the emotional life and general behavior described by the aforementioned authors are not so much the result of a lesion of the frontal lobes as a symptom referable to the brain as a whole. That there is no detectable loss of discrete functions (sensation, movement, speech), as various writers have reported, and the fact that the intellectual impairment and gross changes in behavior are especially prominent in those cases in which a tumor of the frontal lobes is accompanied by severe symptoms of general cerebral disturbances tend to support this hypothesis. The doubts about the local nature of the observed defects expressed by Schuster (1902), Pfeiffer (1910), Monakow (1910, 1914), and others were apparently reinforced by the negative findings of Penfield and Evans (1935), Hebb (1942, 1945,) and others who described cases in which resection of large areas of the frontal lobes caused no appreciable defects in behavior. Finally, to these remarks must be added the details of the large number of observations of patients after prefrontal leukotomy or topectomy. Tests on these patients gave no results that would clearly indicate the presence of specific changes attributable to a disturbance of the functions of the frontal lobes (Mettler, 1949; Scoville *et al.*, 1953; Le Beau and Petrie, 1953; Tizard, 1958). A curious situation developed, in which some authors looked upon the frontal lobe as one of the more important sections of the human brain, as the "organ of civilization" (Halstead, 1947) or as the seat of "abstract intelligence" (Goldstein, 1936, etc.), whereas others were inclined to deny it any special function in human mental activity. Notwithstanding these contradictions in the clinical analysis of the functions of the frontal lobes, clinicians succeeded in giving a more or less general description of the frontal syndrome appearing especially in extensive lesions of the frontal lobes.

Neurological analysis of frontal lobe lesions reveals a relatively poorly defined pattern of disturbances. These patients have no gross loss of sensation and no apparent paresis. Investigation of the motor functions often reveals signs of ataxia (due to a disturbance in the frontocerebellar connections), disturbances in posture and gait, signs of asynergia and of ataxia of the trunk, and, finally, increased tone leading to spasticity. Perseveration of movement is also observed and is particularly pronounced when the lesion spreads to the subcortical formations. In the latter cases a revival of elementary automatisms (in the form of defensive, grasping, or sucking reflexes) may often be observed; sometimes a disturbance of the function of the pelvic organs together with a generalized adynamia is seen, which in extensive lesions of the frontal lobes may lead to a total loss of spontaneous activity.

To this account must be added the distinctive forms of epileptic attack observed with lesions of the frontal lobes, as a rule without any sensory or motor aura and accompanied by a general loss of consciousness. As Penfield (1954) suggests, this indicates a connection between the frontal region and the underlying structures of the reticular formation. With this, the basic neurological symtomatology of frontal lobe lesions is practically exhausted.

The picture of disturbance of *mental processes* accompanying frontal lobe lesions is a much richer one. These disturbances take different forms depending on the severity of the lesion, the extent to which the subcortical formations are involved by the pathological process, and the severity of the general cerebral manifestations.

In relatively mild cases of lesions of the prefrontal divisions of the brain, clinicians (Khoroshko, 1912, 1921, etc.; Feuchtwanger, 1923; Kleist, 1934; Rylander, 1939; Denny-Brown, 1951; etc.) have invariably observed that, although the "formal intellect" is intact, these patients show marked changes in behavior. Sometimes the whole picture of the disease is superimposed on depression, in which case the patients lack in initiative, curtail their circle of interests, and develop the defect of activity that Kleist called "Mangel an Antrieb" (lack of drive). If the disease is accompanied by signs of irritation, the picture is complicated by uncontrollable impulsive actions, which the patient performs without proper realization of their probable results or concern with their consequences. Often both of these states may coexist in the same patient, in which case the loss of spontaneous activity is superimposed on a background of either diminished or increased excitation.

Besides disturbances of organized, goal-directed behavior, these patients also exhibit emotional changes. These changes have been described by practically all workers who have investigated cases of frontal lobe lesions. Clinicians have pointed out that patients with frontal lesions are emotionally unstable; failure does not cause any prolonged emotional reaction, and they begin to show indifference toward their surroundings. A particularly important observation is the lack of marked emotional conflicts in patients of this group, whereas other types of brain lesion are accompanied by such conflicts.

Clinical observation shows that when the lesion has spread to the basal divisions of the frontal region emotional disturbances with a tendency toward impulsive actions, trivial jokes, and euphoria may exist without any significant change in formal intelligence (Jastrowitz, 1888; Welt, 1888; etc.). When the pathological process involves more extensive areas of the convex portion of the prefrontal cortical area, this picture is supplemented by intellectual disorders in the form of impaired "intellectual syntheses" (Brickner, 1936), impaired awareness and relationship toward a complex situation (Lhermitte, 1929; Rylander, 1939; etc.), and impaired abstract, categorical behavior. According to Goldstein (1936, 1944) and others, *the latter* occupies a central position in the pathology of mental activity in the frontal syndrome.

It must be stated that, besides the disturbance of initiative and the other aforementioned behavioral disturbances, almost all patients with a lesion of the frontal lobes have a marked loss of their "critical faculty," i.e., a disturbance of their ability to correctly evaluate their own behavior and the adequacy of their actions. All these features of the frontal syndrome are firmly established in clinical psychiatry.

The frontal syndrome is especially prominent with extensive lesions of the frontal lobes associated with general cerebral manifestations. In these cases the disturbances in initiative turn into gross adynamia and the emotional changes, into complete loss of critical appraisal and emotional indifference. Lucid consciousness gives way to confusion, and the unity of the personality is destroyed.

The phenomena that, in the opinion of psychiatrists and neurologists, contribute to the frontal syndrome distinguish it both from syndromes produced by lesions of the posterior divisions of the brain and from those produced by lesions of the premotor zone.

Although there is a wealth of clinical material in the literature on mental disturbances caused by frontal lesions, these descriptions can by no means be regarded as constituting a scientific analysis of these complex phenomena. Moreover, attempts to show that a lesion of the frontal lobes causes a disturbance of intelligent behavior as a whole, and yet leaves the more elementary processes unchanged, has the inevitable result that the functions of the frontal lobes begin to be regarded as different in principle from the functions of the other parts of the brain. The frontal lobes themselves begin to be interpreted psychomorphologically as the supreme organ of mental life or as the organ of active thought, critical awareness, etc. This point of view is a reflection of the actual complexity of the problem. However, to a large extent, it is bound up with the fact that until now the changes in mental activity arising from lesions of the frontal lobes have usually been the object of psychopathological observation conducted without recourse to specialized psychophysiological analysis; the results obtained have continued to be analyzed in the light of obsolete concepts. There is no doubt that the introduction of various modern experimental neuropsychological techniques into the study of frontal lobe function and the interpretation of the results from the standpoint of modern ideas on self-regulating systems will shed fresh light on the functions of the frontal lobes and will enable the facts obtained to be fitted into a system of adequate scientific concepts.

I shall discuss briefly the basic information on the structure and functional organization of the frontal lobes before going on to examine their role in the regulation of states and complex forms of human activity.

B. STRUCTURE AND FUNCTIONS

The frontal division of the cerebral cortex, which in man accounts for up to one quarter of the total cortical mass, together with the inferoparietal region constitutes the most complex and, phylogenetically, the newest structure of the brain. It possesses a very fine structure, it matures later than the rest of the brain, and it has the richest and most varied system of connections.

There is no need to give a full account of all the aspects of its structure in this book. Only those special features that will contribute to the accurate placement of the frontal lobes in the general functional organization of the cerebral hemispheres will be considered.

The prefrontal divisions of the cerebral cortex are situated anteriorly to the motor (Area 4) and premotor (Areas 6 and 8) areas and comprise a series of formations (Areas 9, 10, 11, and 46) situated on the convex portion or mediobasal surface of the frontal lobe. As has been explained (Part I, Section 2C), anatomists now regard this region as one of the most phylogenetically recent tertiary regions; it possesses the finest structure and displays the most varied connections with all the remaining structures of the cerebral hemispheres.

The prefrontal divisions of the cerebral cortex are formed only in the latest stages of phylogenesis. They start to differentiate into separate fields only in the lower monkeys and attain a considerable level of development in primates; only in man, however, do the convex portions of the prefrontal region become adequately differentiated in structure, with the appearance of a series of distinct new fields not present in the immediately preceding stages of animal evolution. Comparison of the cytoarchitectonics of the cerebral cortex of rodents, the lower and higher monkeys, and man shows at once the extent of the evolutionary development of the frontal lobes, some sections of which may with justification be regarded as specifically human divisions of the cerebral cortex.

The distinctive features of the frontal divisions of the cerebral cortex also stand out clearly when their fine anatomical structure is examined. It was stated (Part I, Section 2C) that in the early stages of embryogenesis the frontal lobe is distinguished by its radial striation, which definitely differentiates it from the cortex of the posterior divisions of the brain and relates it genetically to the motor cortex of Areas 4 and 6. This confirms the important conclusion that the cortex of the frontal region together with the motor and premotor areas is the cortical end of the motor analyzer.

The prefrontal divisions of the cortex differ in a number of respects, however, from the fields of the motor and premotor areas constituting part of the cortical nucleus of the motor analyzer. Knowledge of these differences is important for the understanding of the specialized functions of the frontal lobes.

In contrast to Areas 4 and 6, the prefrontal divisions of the cortex have a distinctive structure, for they do not contain giant pyramidal Betz cells. Compared to Area 6, they show a much more powerful development of the second and third (association) layers, where the neurons are finer in structure. To this must be added the fact that the system of vertical connections of the prefrontal division of the cortex with the subjacent divisions of the thalamus differs significantly from the connections of the cortical nucleus of the motor analyzer.

Meyer (1950) and Meyer and Beck (1954), Pribram (1960), and workers at the Moscow Brain Institute (1949) showed that the central field of the cortical nucleus of the motor analyzer (Area 4) is connected with those thalamic nuclei that are directly related to the motor periphery and that are, consequently, relay nuclei. In contrast, Areas 9, 10, 11, 45, and 46 of the prefrontal region are connected with other nuclei of the thalamus (in particular, with the structures of the medial nucleus), having no direct relationship with the motor periphery and belonging to the more complex, "internal" part of the apparatuses of the central nervous system (Fig. 22).

Hence, the prefrontal divisions of the cerebral cortex can be considered the cortical portion of the motor analyzer. Accordingly, they have a much more complex structure and system of afferent-efferent connections than do Area 4 and even Areas 6 and 8.

The complexity of the neuronal structure of the fields of the prefrontal region is confirmed by the fact that they develop much later in ontogenesis. Flechsig (1920), the first to use the myelogenetic method, showed that the fibers of these cortical divisions are the last to myelinize and that this region of the cortex begins to function later than the other regions. Investigations at the Moscow Brain Institute, notably by Kononova (1940, 1948), showed that, whereas in the first (intrauterine) stages of ontogenesis the fields of the cortical nucleus of the motor analyzer (Areas 4, 6, and 8) develop at a much faster rate than the fields of the prefrontal region, in later (extrauterine) stages this is no longer so. The fields of the prefrontal region begin to develop much faster than those of the postfrontal divisions, so that the size of the territory occupied by them increases rapidly.

Very important data have been obtained in studies of the early phylogeny of the brain involving a detailed study of the endocranium in man at successive stages of prehistory. As Kochetkov has shown in his remarkable book *Paleoneurology* (1973), the frontal lobes, the volume of which is very small in archianthropoids, start to develop substantially only at comparatively late stages in paleoanthropoids, and reach a considerable size only in modern man.

It must be realized that the prefrontal divisions of the cerebral cortex, which begin to function in the last stages of development, are at the same time the most vulnerable and the most prone to undergo involution. Their higher (association) layers atrophy particularly rapidly in diffuse diseases such as Pick's disease or general paralysis.

The complexity of the functional organization of the frontal cortex and the wealth of its connections are confirmed by neuronographic investigations, notably those undertaken by McCulloch (1943) and his co-workers. The results summarized in Table 2 demonstrate that the cortical fields of the prefrontal region possess very rich connections with almost all of the more important parts of the posterior divisions of the cortex. It is especially important to note that some fields (for example, the oculomotor Area 8) possess specific afferent-efferent connections with the optic areas whereas others (Areas 10, 45, and 46) are connected by a system of analogous afferent-efferent connections with Areas 22, 37, and 39 of the parietotemporal region and with those sections of the superior temporal region (Areas 42 and 22) constituting part of the system of speech zones.

These data indicate the structural complexity of the prefrontal divisions of the cerebral cortex and the diversity of their connections with other divisions of the cerebral hemispheres. It may be concluded that not only do the prefrontal divisions belong to the cortical system of the motor analyzer, but also, provisionally, that they play an important role in the afferent organization of movement. Since they receive afferent impulses from nearly all of the more important parts of the cerebral cortex, they must be instrumental in the sorting of these impulses and in the transmission of them to the system of the motor analyzer.

All the facts mentioned above indicate the high morphological complexity of the frontal lobes, of their connections, and their late phylogenetic development.

However, there is one other factor that must be taken into account. As the most recent investigations of Ravich-Shcherbo, consisting of a comparative analysis of differences between pairs of uniovular and binovular twins, have shown, electrophysiological studies by the evoked potentials method reveal evidence of a high level of genotypic determinants in the sensomotor regions of the cortex but only a very low level of genotypic determinants in the functions of the frontal lobes. This important fact shows convincingly that variability in the work of the frontal lobes, with their complex

Table 2

Results of Neuronographic Investigation of the Prefrontal Divisions of the Cortex*

Afferent connections	*Efferent connections*
8←19, 22, 37, 41, 42	8→18
9←23	10→22
10←22, 37, 38	46→6, 37, 39
44←41, 42, 22	47→38
45←21, 22, 23, 37, 41, 42	24→31, 32
47←36, 38	

*This table was compiled from figures obtained by pooling the results of investigations by Dusser de Barennes and co-workers (1941), McCulloch (1943), Sugar, French, and Ghusid (1948, 1950), and others.

functional organization, is much more closely connected with external (paratypical) than with genetically determined (genotypic) factors (Ravich-Shcherbo, unpublished investigation).

The foregoing remarks particularly apply to the convex cortical divisions of the frontal lobes. When the mediobasal divisions are considered, different characteristics come to light and a special description is therefore called for. As has been mentioned (Part I, Section 2D), the modern view of the central nervous apparatus is that it consists of two mutually interacting systems, one concerned with the analysis and synthesis of exteroceptive and proprioceptive impulses and the other more closely related to the analysis of interoceptive impulses and directly responsible for the regulation of the internal conditions of the organism, with the maintenance of homeostasis, and with the equilibration of the internal environment.

The first of these systems is based on a chain of isolated neurons, reacting rapidly, differentially, and in accordance with the "all or nothing" law. The second system consists of a complex of neurons, morphologically united into a single network; the reactions of this system take place more slowly, gradually, and in a less differentiated manner (Pribram, 1960). At the lower levels of the central nervous system these systems constitute the apparatuses known as the reticular formation of the brain stem and thalamus. At higher levels they are components of the mediobasal divisions of the cerebral cortex, namely, of the limbic lobe and of the mediobasal divisions of the frontal and of part of the temporal regions of the brain.

Various reports (Klüver and Bucy, 1939; Klüver, 1952; Masserman, 1943; Hess, 1954; Olds, 1955; Olds and Olds, 1958; Rosvold *et al.*, 1956; Rosvold, 1959; Pribram and co-workers, 1954–1956; Pribram, 1958, 1959) have shown that these mediobasal divisions of the cortex, particularly the formations hitherto known as the "olfactory brain," possessing rich connections both with the hypothalamic region and with the frontal divisions of the brain, have specific and far more complex functions than had been realized.

Experiments have demonstrated that stimulation of the limbic lobe and of the structures connected with it leads to marked changes in autonomically regulated processes (metabolism, body temperature, and the rhythm of sleeping and waking). They have also shown that any disturbance of the normal working of the limbic lobe of the hippocampus (i.e., of the primitive and intermediate mediobasal formations) may lead to marked changes in the affective state of an animal, characterized by the development of uncontrollable aggressive outbursts (which may probably be regarded as both fright and attack reactions [Klüver and Bucy, 1939; Masserman, 1943; etc.]). Finally—and we consider this particularly important—observations made in recent years have shown that disturbances of the normal activity of the limbic lobe are also reflected in the animal's general behavior and have thereby bridged the gap to the pathology of behavior associated with lesions of the frontal lobes.

For instance, in the experiments of Weiskrantz (1956), destruction of the amygdaloid body in a monkey led to a change in its behavior in regard to food. Starvation no longer made the animal search actively for food. The starving monkey did not even start to eat food placed before it. However, once it had begun to eat, it continued to do so, whether or not it was sated. It appears that the urge to eat, as well as the feeling of satiety, was not transmitted to the brain in the presence of this lesion. Similar results were obtained by Olds (1955) and Fuller, Rosvold, and Pribram (1957). They resected the mediobasal divisions of the forebrain of an animal and observed the same phenomenon of constant eating continued beyond satiety. Stamm (1955) surgically destroyed the medial areas of the cortex in rats and found that when the female rat had finished collecting its young, scattered all over the cage at the outset, into its nest, it could not stop the activity but continued to shift them about from place to place.

These findings indicating profound disturbances of complex behavioral acts in the presence of lesions of the mediobasal divisions of the cortex have been confirmed by electrophysiological investigations. For instance, Lissak *et al.* (1957) and Lissak and Grastyan (1959), Adey (1959), McLean (1959), and others have shown that a change in the state of the organism associated with the development of an arousal reaction is accompanied by electrical activity in the limbic lobe. This activity disappears in the course of habituation. However, when an animal is confronted with a puzzle box, and gives a wrong response which does not produce the required effect, the activity reappears.

From these and other findings it may be concluded that the mediobasal cortical divisions, which are closely connected with the underlying structures of the reticular formation and hypothalamic region, participate in the regulation of the body state and reflect changes taking place in that state. From all evidence, the structures of the limbic region, the hippocampus, and the closely connected frontal divisions of the brain appear to work as a single system. This concept provides a new and significant line of approach to the functions of all these sections of the cerebral hemispheres.

• • •

From the foregoing it is possible to make certain assumptions regarding the role of the frontal lobes in the organization of mental activity that should be taken into account when the changes resulting from a lesion of these parts of the brain are analyzed. The fact that the frontal portion of the cortex is very similar in structure to the motor and premotor areas and the fact that all the evidence suggests that it is a component of the system of the central divisions of the motor analyzer indicate that it is very closely involved in the analysis and synthesis of the impulses of excitation lying at the basis of *motor processes*.

On the other hand, the frontal lobes have the closest connections with the reticular formation, from which they receive impulses continuously and to which they send corticofugal discharges, so that they are an important organ for the regulation of active states of the individual. This function of the frontal lobes is particularly important because the frontal lobes themselves have intimate relations with all other parts of the brain, and they are the means whereby impulses are dispatched to lower subcortical formations after preliminary processing with the aid of the most complex cortical mechanisms. The fact that the frontal region is closely connected with the underlying structures of the limbic lobe, and through them with other nervous apparatuses concerned with interoception, gives reason to suppose that it receives signals of the various changes taking place in the organism and that it is intimately involved in *the regulation of body states.* Evidently, changes in body state occur not merely because of the appearance of new stimuli, evoking arousal reactions, but also because of the body's response activity. It may be postulated that these changing states may lead to corresponding further changes in the activity of the body. There are, therefore, important grounds for believing that *the frontal lobes synthesize the information about the outside world received through the exteroceptors and the information about the internal states of the body* and that *they are the means whereby the behavior of the organism is regulated in conformity with the effect produced by its actions* (as demonstrated experimentally by Anokhin, 1949, 1955, and Pribram, 1959*a* and *b*, 1960).

The investigation of the functions of the frontal lobes is the most difficult aspect of the study of the physiology of higher nervous activity; the amount of scientific evidence is still very limited. However, there can be no doubt that in all future attempts to study their functions, we will have to apply the same principles that have served us in our study of other parts of the cerebral cortex. This means we must try to discover the relatively elementary factors directly connected with the activity of these divisions of the brain, disturbance of which leads to the disintegration of the more complex functions; we must also conduct a careful analysis of the forms of afferent synthesis that are affected by lesions of the frontal lobes and of those defects of the complex and specifically human afferent organization of motor acts by speech produced by these lesions.

Since we do not possess all the necessary information for such an analysis, our choice of subject matter is limited to those changes in the regulation of active states in whose production the frontal lobes play a most intimate part, and to types of disturbance of voluntary movement and activity and of perceptual activity that are characteristic of lesions of the frontal lobes. Of these we have made a special study.

C. THE FRONTAL LOBES AND REGULATION OF STATES OF ACTIVITY

The fact has long been familiar in clinical medicine that patients with massive lesions of the frontal lobes are as a rule in a state of reduced activity, that their attention is easily distracted by irrelevant stimuli, and that it is usually impossible to organize their attention and to keep it focused on a definite plan.

This basic fact has often been described by neurologists and psychiatrists who have observed patients with massive frontal lesions (Kleist, 1908, 1930, 1934; Feuchtwanger, 1923; Rylander, 1939; Leonhard, 1964, 1965; Hécaen and Ajuriaguerra, 1956), but it did not receive a thorough systematic investigation.

It is only recently, since advances in neurophysiology have indicated the closest relations between the frontal lobes of the brain and the reticular formation of the brain stem and thalamus (Part II, Section 5B), and as a result of the introduction of precise neuropsychological and psychophysiological tests into clinical practice, that the role of the frontal lobes in the regulation of states of activity became amenable to scientific analysis.

The frontal lobes are heterogeneous in structure, reflecting their functional plurality. One of the most important anatomical features of the frontal lobes is the richness of their afferent and efferent connections with the various nonspecific structures of the brain: the thalamus, the hypothalamic region, and the reticular formation of the brain stem.

According to Pribram (1968), part of the prefrontal cortex on the medial and orbital surfaces of the frontal lobes should be included in a single "frontal-limbic" system. Nauta (1971) also contends that the prefrontal cortex is the "cortical modulator of the limbic system." The prefrontal cortex has rich connections with the formations of the limbic system, the nonspecific thalamic nuclei (especially the dorso-medial nucleus), with the mesencephalic reticular formation, and with other special formations, as a rule bilaterally (Fig. 70); this is evidence, on one hand, of the wide inflow of nonspecific and highly heterogeneous information into the cortex of the frontal lobes, and, on the other hand, of the possibility that the frontal cortex can influence nonspecific formations at different levels.

The second important anatomical feature of the prefrontal cortex is that it contains numerous cortico-cortical and commissural pathways connecting it with other parts of the cortex in the posterior regions of the brain and with the synonymous anterior zones of the opposite hemisphere. Through these pathways the prefrontal cortex receives highly integrated information belonging, evidently, to all sensory modalities.

Finally, in the prefrontal cortex in man specialized cortical areas exist for controlling the activity of the speech system. All these anatomical data point to the special role of the frontal lobes in the regulation of activation processes or in the activity of nonspecific brain structures and the special relationship of the speech system with these processes.

According to the results of neurophysiological investigations on animals and man (French, Segundo, Penfield, Pribram, Sager, Narikashvili, and others) electrical stimulation of the anterior zones of the cortex (sensomotor and anterior oculomotor areas, medial frontal and temporal cortex) evokes a typical picture of the orienting reflex as reflected in behavior and the electroencephalogram, indicating the existence of corticofugal influences arising from the anterior zones of the cortex. The cortex of the posterior zones has far fewer such connections. Within the anterior zones of the cortex the prefrontal region plays the dominant role as regards corticofugal influences on the various nonspecific formations (French, Segundo, Nauta, Pribram, Sager, Szentagothai, et al.).

Physiological investigations by the classical conditioned-reflex or instrumental method have shown that after extirpation of the frontal lobes in animals (lower and higher mammals and primates), regulation of the levels of wakefulness is disturbed; this is manifested as hyper- or hypoactivity, phenomena of de-inhibition or omission of the classical conditioned and instrumental reflexes, a disturbance of delayed reactions, and so on (Konorski, Brutkowski, Stempin, Pribram, et al.). In animals without their frontal lobes various disturbances of orienting and investigative behavior arise in the form, in particular, of hyperreactivity, i.e., increased reactivity to the novelty factor (Malmo, Mishkin, Gross, Pribram, Weiskrantz, et al.). Removal of the frontal lobes leads to changes in the system of aggressive and defensive unconditioned and conditioned reflexes (Fulton, Kennard, Brutkowski, Anokhin, Shumilina, et al.).

On the whole, two different pathophysiological syndromes have been shown to exist in patients with frontal lobe lesions—one connected mainly with lesions of the medial and orbital surfaces of the frontal lobes, the other with lesions of the dorsolateral zones of the prefrontal cortex. Disturbances of the activity of the nonspecific system (changes in the level of wakefulness, disturbances in the system of orienting, defensive, food-getting and sexual unconditioned and conditioned reflexes) as a rule follow a parallel course and are observed mainly in lesions of the mediobasal zones of the frontal lobes. The fact that the medial and orbital cortex of the frontal lobes is predominantly concerned with the regulation of nonspecific forms of activation is also confirmed by the similarity between the effect (behavioral and conditioned-reflex) arising in lesions of these parts of the cortex and of certain formations belonging to the limbic system in the anterior part of the gyrus cingulus, hypothalamus, amygdala, and hippocampus.

Clinical neuropsychological investigations of patients with frontal lobe lesions have led to the differentiation of two basic groups of neuropsychological syndromes associated with lesions of the frontal lobes: (a) the syndrome of a lesion of the lateral, and (b) the syndrome of a lesion of the mediobasal zones of the frontal lobes. Lateral frontal syndromes (premotor, prefrontal) are characterized mainly by various forms of deautomation of motor, speech, and intellectual acts while states of consciousness and memory functions remain relatively intact. Mediobasal frontal syndromes (basal, medial) are characterized by disturbances mainly of the emotions and personality, disturbances of consciousness, of memory processes, and the selectivity of psychological functions, whereas motor functions and formal logical and speech operations remain relatively intact.

On the basis of clinical neuropsychological data, it can thus also be deduced that the mediobasal zones of the frontal lobes are predominantly concerned with the regulation of nonspecific activation processes.

This problem has been studied in special investigations by Khomskaya and her colleagues (1966, 1970, 1972, 1973, 1977). Their work has shown that the mediobasal zones of the frontal lobes play a direct part in the regulation of two types of nonspecific activation processes: short-term orienting reactions and longer changes in the level of activation or of the functional state of the brain.

Four groups of subjects were studied: healthy people (control); patients with lesions of the mediobasal zones of the frontal lobes (Group I); patients with lesions of the lateral zones (Group II); and patients with local lesions either of the cerebral hemispheres outside the frontal lobes or outside the hemispheres altogether (Group III). The parameters chosen for analysis were: autonomic indices of the orienting reflex (vascular and psychogalvanic reflexes), frequency-amplitude indices of the EEG, and changes in shape of the EEG waves in two experimental situations: (a) in response to uninformative and informative stimuli (acoustic and photic), and (b) during intellectual tests (mental arithmetic, etc.). The first experimental situation studied short-term processes of nonspecific activation (orienting reflex); the second situation explored longer processes (functional state of the brain or level of activation).

The experiments showed that when uninformative stimuli are given informative value by means of a spoken instruction (for example, when the subject is instructed to count the number of sounds in a series), the autonomic and electroencephalographic components of the orienting reflex, when previously extinguished by repeated presentation of the stimuli, are firmly restored in healthy subjects and cannot be extinguished for a long time.

Examples are given in Figs. 71, 72, and 73, where psychogalvanic, vascular, and electroencephalographic responses to interrupted acoustic stimuli obtained in tests on healthy subjects are shown. It will be clear from these figures that by means of a verbal instruction presenting healthy subjects with a problem to solve, stable orienting reflexes to informative stimuli can be evoked. Short-term activation processes during active problem solving are characterized not only by their greater intensity, but also by differences in their qualitative composition. Figure 73 shows that during problem solving high α-frequencies and β-frequencies play a more active role in the orienting response, whereas the reactivity of the slow waves of the EEG spectrum is reduced.

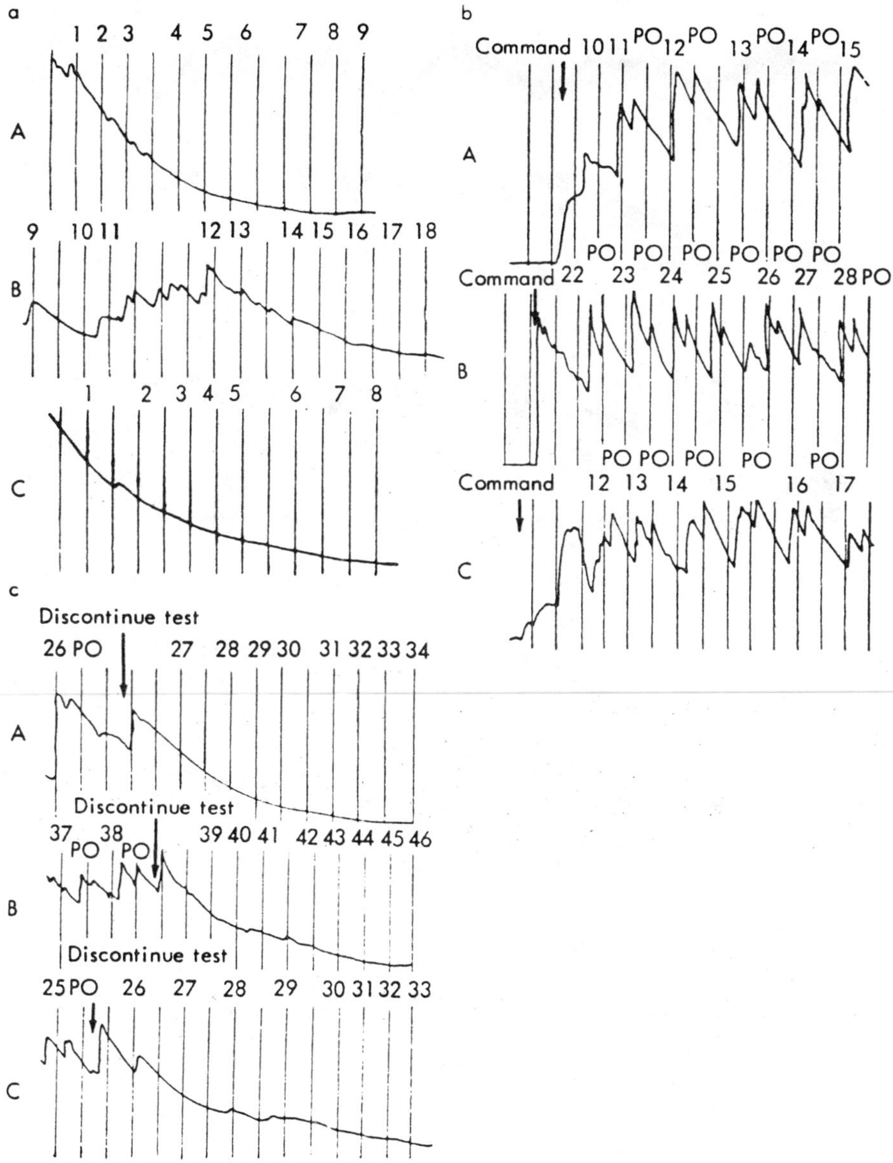

FIGURE 71 Restoration of psychogalvanic components of orienting reflex to sounds by means of a verbal instruction in normal subjects (after Khomskaya): (a) extinction of psychogalvanic reflex to interrupted sounds (60 dB) in three subjects. Three types of extinction are shown: (A) rapid extinction, (B) prolonged extinction, (C) absence of PGR to sounds. Numbers indicate order of stimuli; (b) restoration of orienting psychogalvanic reflexes after addition of instruction to count the number of sounds in each interrupted stimulus. Arrow indicates addition of instruction. "VR"—subject's verbal response; (c) disappearance of orienting psychogalvanic reflexes after stopping instruction.
KEY: 1) Stopping instruction
2) Instruction

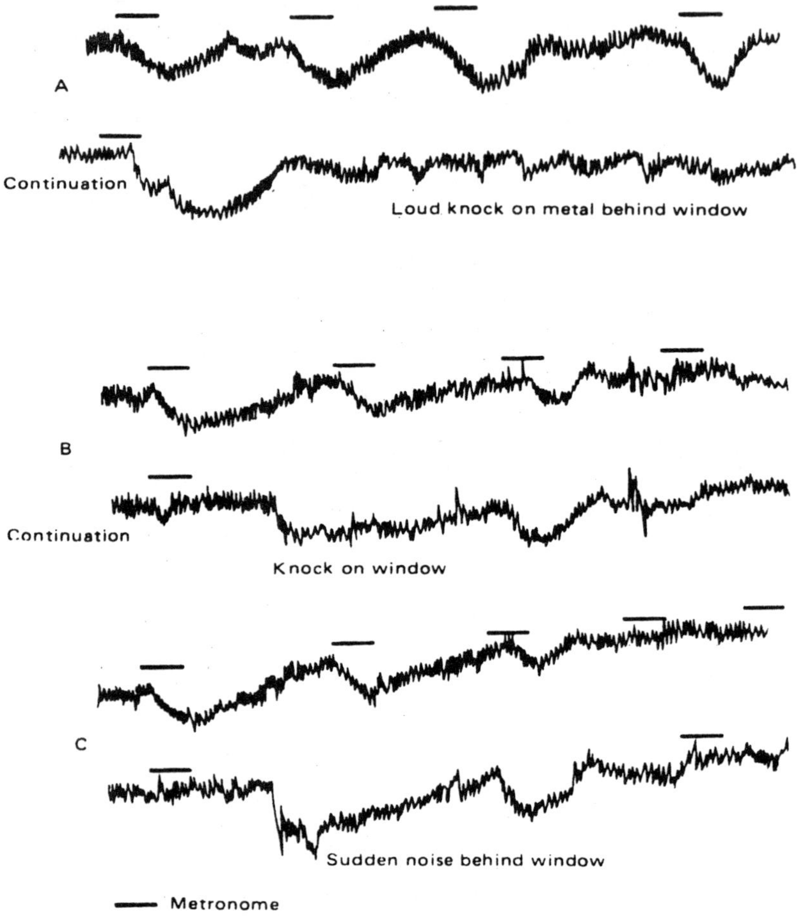

FIGURE 72 Inhibition of vascular responses to irrelevent stimuli after formation of a dominant focus by verbal instruction (after Vinogradova). (A) Experiment with normal subject. Weak informative sounds evoke a stable orienting reaction (top line); loud knock on window evokes no response (bottom line). (B) and (C) Experiments with oligophrenic children. Weak informative sounds quickly cease to evoke a response (both top lines). Loud knock on window evokes a well-marked reaction (both bottom lines).

During sustained intellectual efforts (for example, when performing serial calculations) healthy subjects develop prolonged changes in the level of activity or of the functional state of the brain (Fig. 74, I); these changes are expressed as a disturbance of the rhythm of changes in the second values of asymmetry of the EEG waves and the appearance or strengthening of spatial synchronization of fluctuations in asymmetry of the EEG waves (Fig. 74, II). Periodic changes in the second values of asymmetry of the EEG waves (G-waves), and also spatial correlation of asymmetry values in

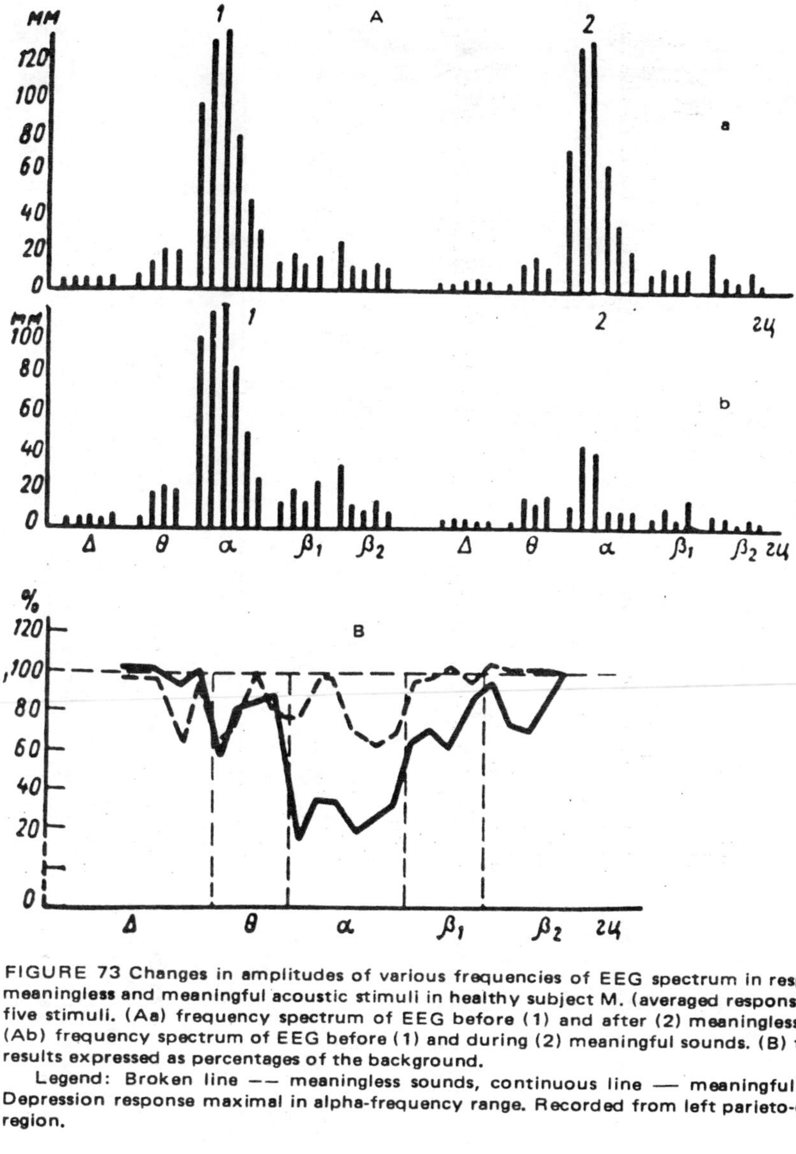

FIGURE 73 Changes in amplitudes of various frequencies of EEG spectrum in response to meaningless and meaningful acoustic stimuli in healthy subject M. (averaged response to first five stimuli. (Aa) frequency spectrum of EEG before (1) and after (2) meaningless sounds; (Ab) frequency spectrum of EEG before (1) and during (2) meaningful sounds. (B) the same results expressed as percentages of the background.

Legend: Broken line –– meaningless sounds, continuous line — meaningful sounds. Depression response maximal in alpha-frequency range. Recorded from left parieto-occipital region.

different regions of the left and right hemispheres, are known to be indicators of the functional state of the brain (Artem'eva and Khomskaya, 1966; Khomskaya, 1972). Elevation of the functional state is accompanied by a regular "break" in the G-waves, or shortening of their period, and an increase in the spatial synchronization of the asymmetry indices. In healthy subjects intellectual exertion is thus regularly accompanied by elevation of the level of activity of the functional state of the brain.

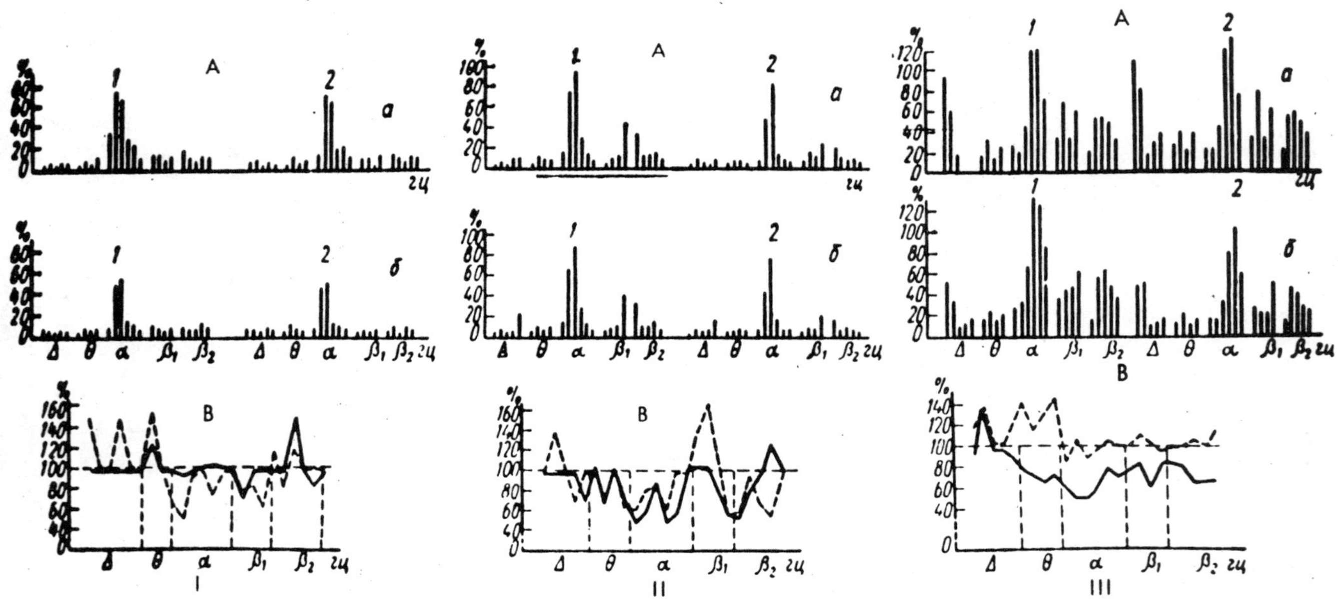

FIGURE 74 Changes in EEG frequency spectrum during application of first 5 meaningless and meaningful acoustic stimuli in patients of first (I), second (II), and third (III) groups: (I) Patient K-v (intracerebral tumor of both frontal lobes spreading to corpus callosum, septum pellucidum, and basal ganglia); (II) Patient D-i (intracerebral tumor of left frontal lobe); (III) Patient S-n (intracerebral tumor of left occipito-parietal region). Legend as in Fig. 73. Parieto-occipital recording from "sound" hemisphere.

Patients with lesions of the mediobasal zones exhibit serious disturbances of the regulation of nonspecific activation processes by the speech system. A verbal instruction no longer restores or strengthens short-term nonspecific activation processes. The verbal instruction has no effect on the autonomic and electroencephalographic components of the orienting reflex (Fig. 75). In the patients of the first group (Fig. 75, I) with a lesion of the mediobasal zones of the frontal lobes, the effect of strengthening of the activation reaction, predominantly in the alpha-range, characteristic of healthy subjects was absent after introduction of the verbal instruction; or a response of opposite sign occurred within the alpha-range (exaltation instead of depression). In the patients of the second group, with lesions of the lateral zones of the frontal lobes, the activation response to informative stimuli was better preserved, just as it also was in patients with lesions outside the frontal lobes (Group III; Fig. 75, II and III).

Patients with lesions of the mediobasal zones of the frontal lobes also showed gross disturbances in the system for the regulation of long-term changes in the level of brain activity. The performance of serial calculations was not reflected in the dynamics of changes in the second values of asymmetry of the EEG waves in this group of patients (Fig. 76, I) or in the spatial correlation of the indices of asymmetry of the EEG waves in different regions of the brain (Fig. 76, II), by contrast with the patients of the other groups.

The facts I have just described are evidence that the mediobasal zones of the frontal lobes are mainly concerned with higher forms of regulation of short- and long-term processes of nonspecific activation, taking place with the aid of the speech system.

Another series of investigations by Khomskaya and her colleagues (1977) showed that the mediobasal zones of the frontal lobes constitute the apparatus whereby the brain controls *local,* selective forms of nonspecific activation. A lesion of this apparatus leads to the omission (or to severe disturbance) of local forms of change in the level of brain activity.

Generalized changes and local, selective changes in brain electrical activity, or general and local activation processes during the performance of different types of psychological perceptual tests (voluntary memorizing of words, differentiation between volleys on the basis of duration and intensity, proofreading tests, serial arithmetical operations, and so on) were examined. Changes in the EEG spectrum and in the parameters of the evoked potentials and spatial correlations of the shape of the EEG waves in different parts of the brain, namely the index of generalized spatial synchronization (SS) and the index of local SS, were recorded. In healthy subjects, any type of voluntary perceptual activity was found to be accompanied by two types of activation processes from the standpoint of their spatial distribution: those with generalized changes, correlating with the

A

B

C

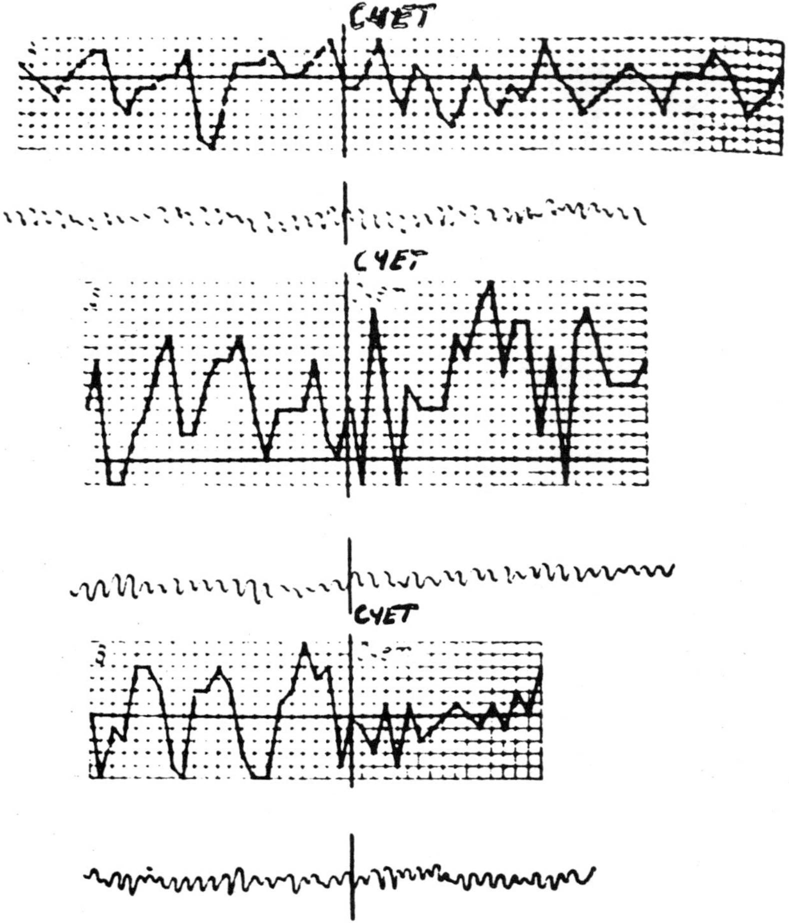

FIGURE 75 (I) Disturbance of rhythm of changes in second values of asymmetry of EEG waveforms (G-waves) in healthy subjects during mental calculations. (A,B,C) different subjects. Beneath each graph 3-sec cuts of the EEG are shown. Vertical line marks beginning of calculating (multiplying two-digit numbers). EEG recorded before and after beginning of

A

B

C

D

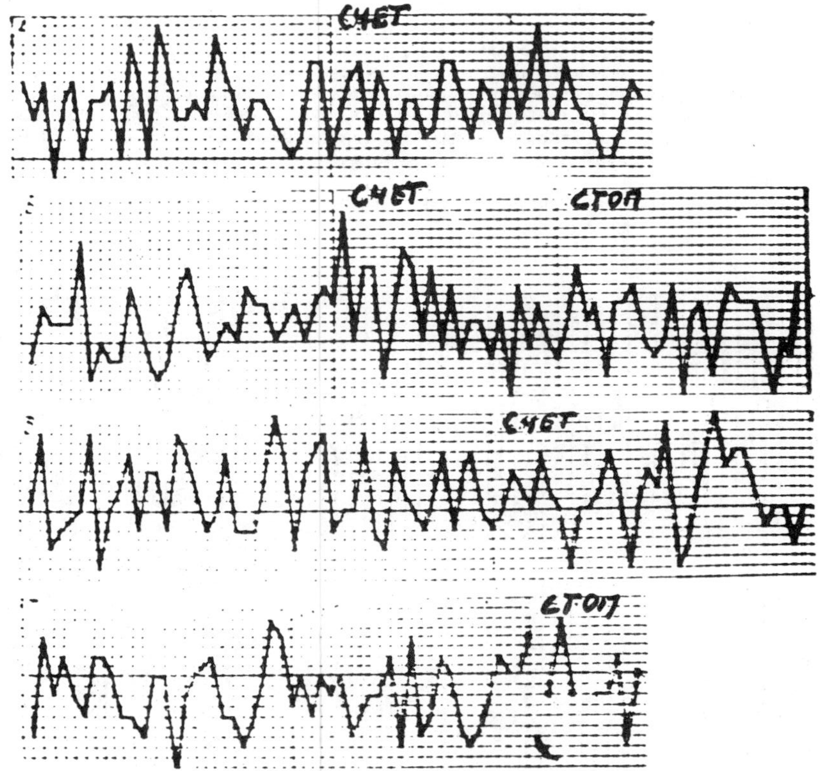

activity visually indistinguishable. (II) Dynamics of changes in G-waves in patients with various brain lesions during mental arithmetic: (A) patient A-li belonging to Group I (intracerebral tumor of basal zones of left frontal and temporal lobes, replacing gyrus rectus and orbital gyrus of left hemisphere); parieto-central recording from right hemisphere, subtraction from 100 in 7's; (B and C) Patient K-v of Group II (astrocytoma of posterior frontal zones of right hemisphere, parieto-central recording from left hemisphere, repetition of 7 times multiplication table; (D) Patient S-v of Group III (arachnoencephalitis with features of occlusive hydrocephalus), left parieto-central recording, subtraction from 100 in 7's. (III) Spatial synchronization of G-waves in different brain regions of healthy subjects performing different tasks. (A) subject L., subtracting from 100 in 7's; (B) Same subject, subtracting from 219 in

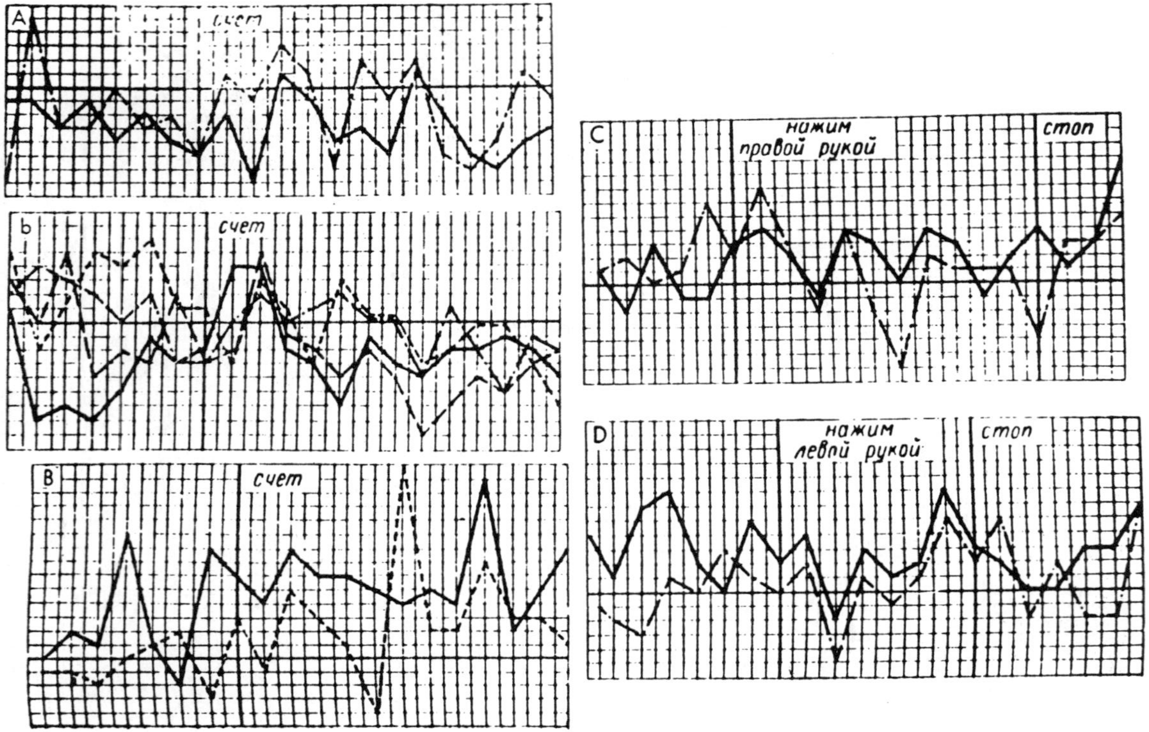

7's; (C) Subject K., subtracting from 100 in 7's; (D and E) Subject T., imaginary pressing with right and left hand.

Legend: (A and B) continuous line — right parieto-occipital region; line of dots and dashes and broken lines .——. same recordings on left side; (D and E) continuous line — right occipito-parietal recording; line of dots and dashes .——. same recording on left side. (IV) Spatial correlation of G-waves in different brain regions of patients with various brain lesions during arithmetical operations. (A) Patient Ch-a of Group I (state after rupture of aneurysm of left anterior cerebral artery); (B) Patient P-v of Group II (state after removal of intracere-

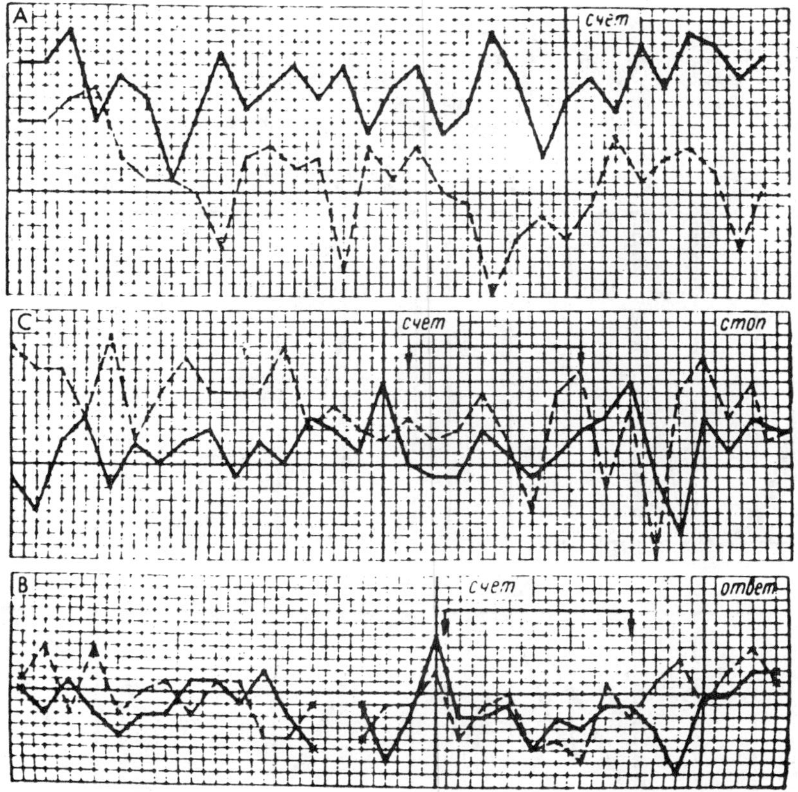

bral tumor of left frontal lobe). Continuous lines indicate parieto-central recording from left; broken line –– the same from right hemisphere; subtraction from 100 in 7's; (C) Patient S-v of Group III (arachnoencephalitis with features of occlusive hydrocephalus); continuous line — recording from left occipito-postfrontal region; broken line –– same recording from right hemisphere. Problem: multiply 78 by 3.

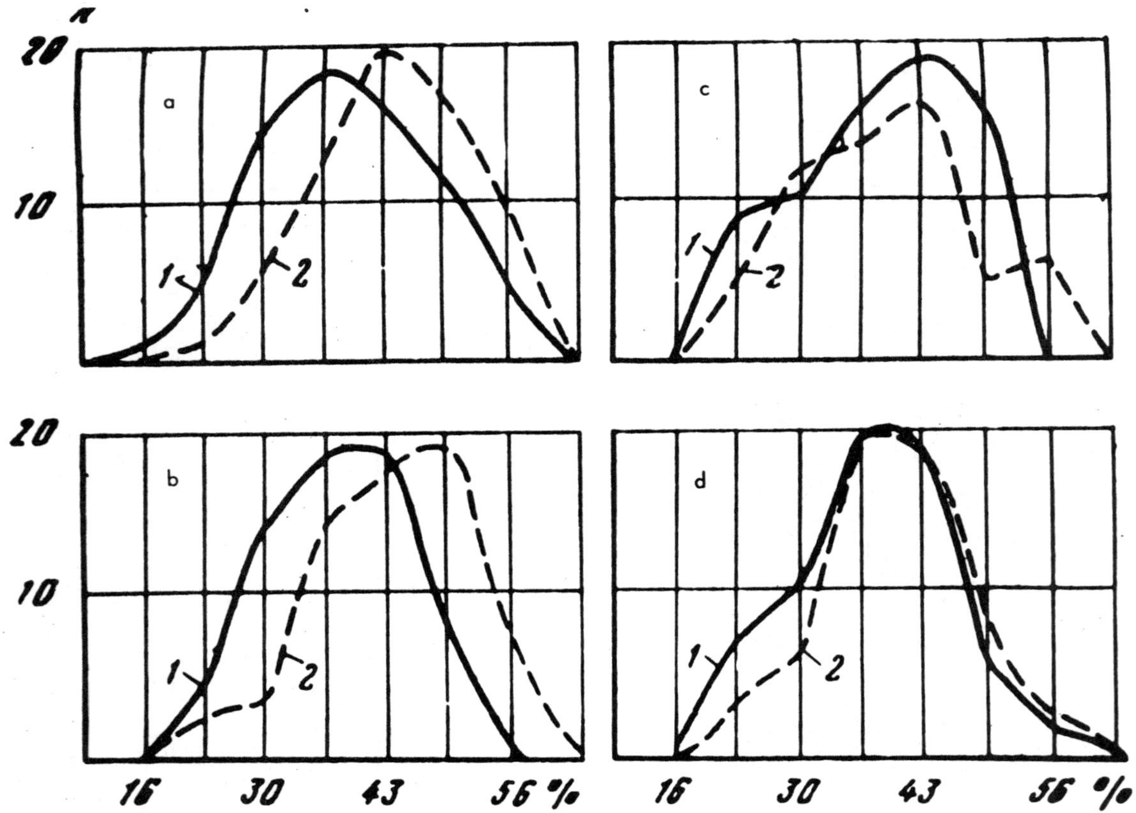

FIGURE 76 Distribution of values of index of local spatial synchronization of G-waves (local SS) in background recordings of EEG of healthy subjects and during performance of verbal tests requiring concentration of voluntary attention: (a) frontal, (b) parieto-occipital zones, (c) middle zones of left hemisphere, (d) middle zones of right hemisphere; (1) background EEG, (2) during problem solving. Shift of distribution to the left signifies increase in local SS values and vice versa.

degree of difficulty of the problem for the subject; and local or selective changes, correlating with the character of the activity to be performed, with its meaning. For instance, normally voluntary word memorizing is accompanied by small general changes in the level of activation (in the form of an increase in the index of generalized SS) and by local changes (in the form of an increase in the index of local SS in the frontal zones) (Fig. 77). During the performance of verbal tests (thinking of words in accordance with an assigned program) in healthy subjects, not only general activation but also local activation arises in the middle zones of the left hemisphere and in the frontal zones. A different distribution of foci of local activation is observed during the performance of gnostic tests, tests of sustained intensity of acoustic attention, and so on.

Under normal conditions voluntary perceptual psychological activity is thus characterized by the distribution of local activation processes among systems in different parts of the brain, by strengthening of interhemispheric asymmetry of brain electrical activity, and by the regular involvement of the frontal zones and in the left hemisphere, just as in healthy subjects.

The study of patients with local brain lesions has shown that generalized and local activation are controlled by different brain structures. The first type of activation is associated chiefly with the activity of the lower levels of the nonspecific system, the second with the mediobasal zones of the frontal lobes and with the activity of the fronto-limbic level of the nonspecific system.

In patients with lesions of brain-stem structures local changes in activation processes during the performance of verbal tests are recorded chiefly in the frontal zones and in the left hemisphere, just as in healthy subjects.

Regular changes of local activation are not found in patients with lesions of the mediobasal zones of the brain (Fig. 78). Disturbances of the regulation of local activation processes during various forms of psychological activity by patients with lesions of the mediobasal zones of the frontal lobes are clearly manifested in experiments in which evoked potentials (EP) are used as electroencephalographic indicators of brain electrical activity.

Evoked potentials are known to reflect local changes in activity and, at the same time, they are also indicators of the general functional state of the brain. A connection between the parameters of EP (amplitude and time) and processes of attention has now been proved in physiology. During the mobilization of attention as a rule there is an increase in amplitude and a decrease in the temporal parameters of the late components of EP, reflecting local strengthening of activation processes.

Experiments in which EP were recorded simultaneously in the premotor and parieto-occipital zones of the left and right hemispheres in healthy subjects (Simernitskaya, 1970; Simernitskaya and Khomskaya, 1966; Demina and Khomskaya, 1976) showed that the attraction of attention to stimuli

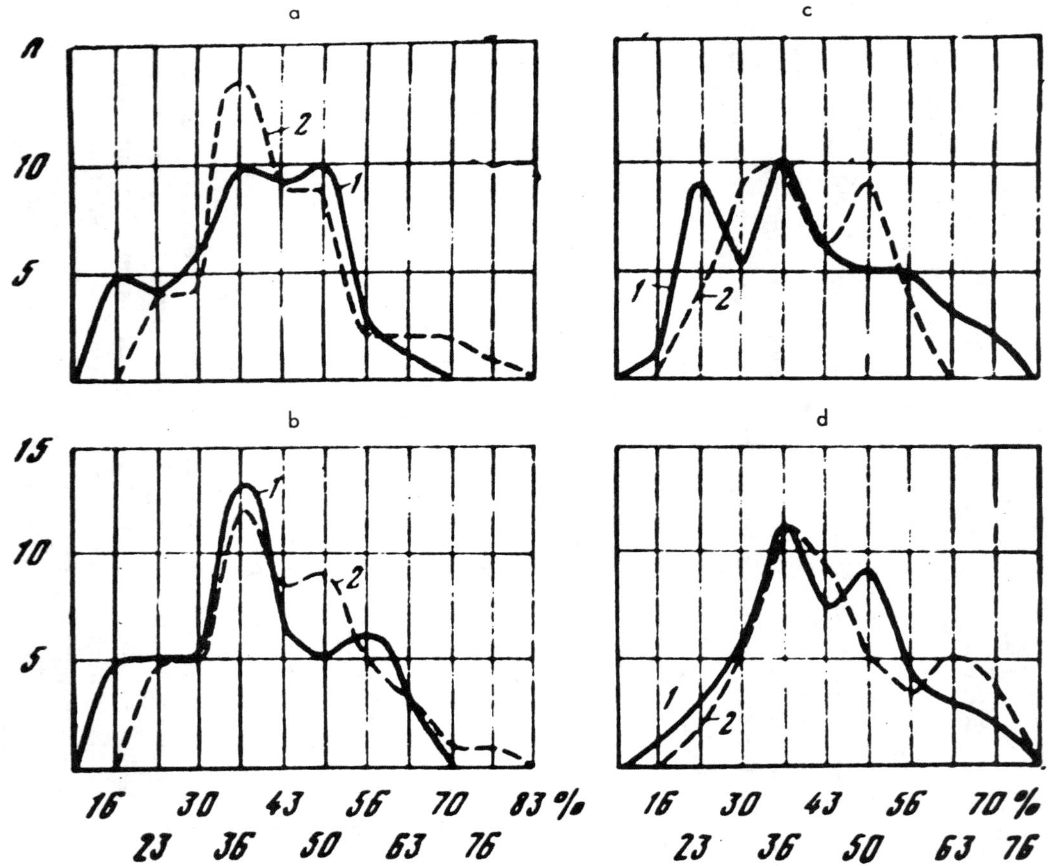

FIGURE 77 (I) Distribution of values of local SS index in different brain regions of patients with lesions of mediobasal zones of frontal lobes in background EEG and while solving verbal problems: (a) frontal zones, (b) parieto-occipital zones, (c) middle zones of left hemisphere,

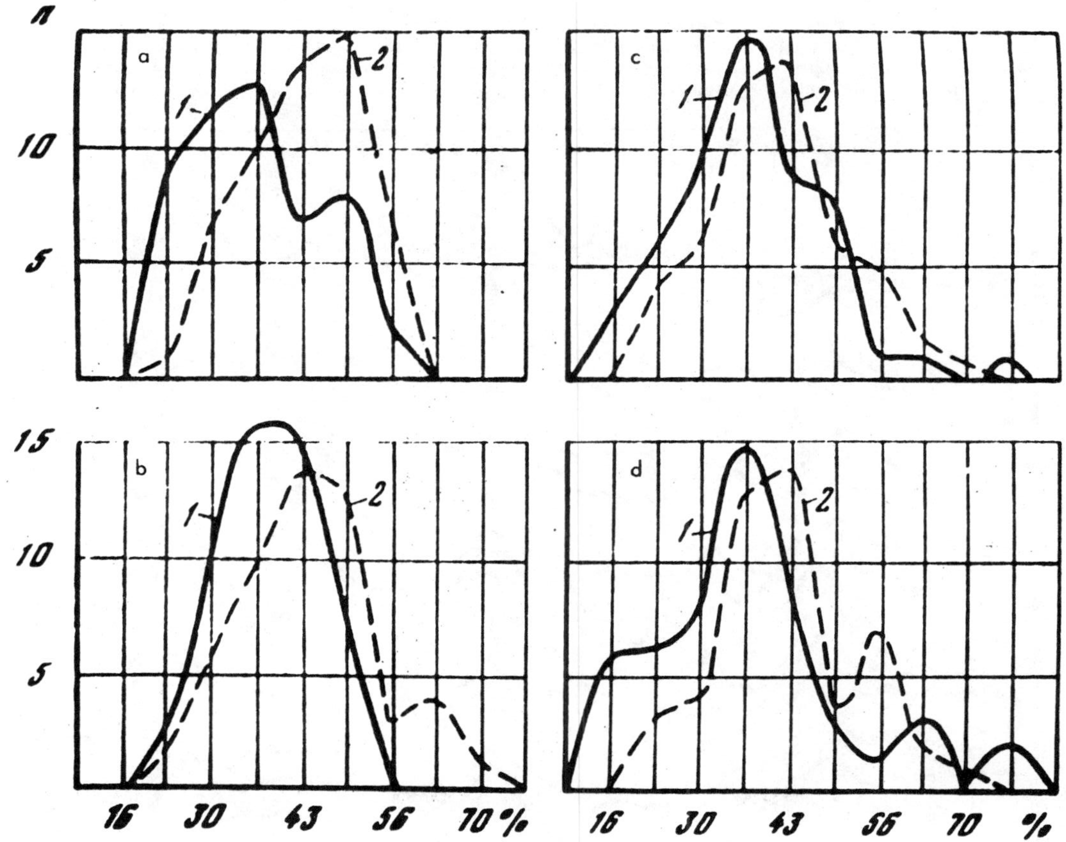

(d) middle zones of right hemisphere; (1) background ECG, (2) during problem solving. Shift of distribution to the left implies increase in values of local SS and vice versa. (II) Distribution of values of local SS index in various brain regions of patients with lesions of brain-stem structures, in background EEG and while solving verbal problems. Legend as in Fig. 77 (I).

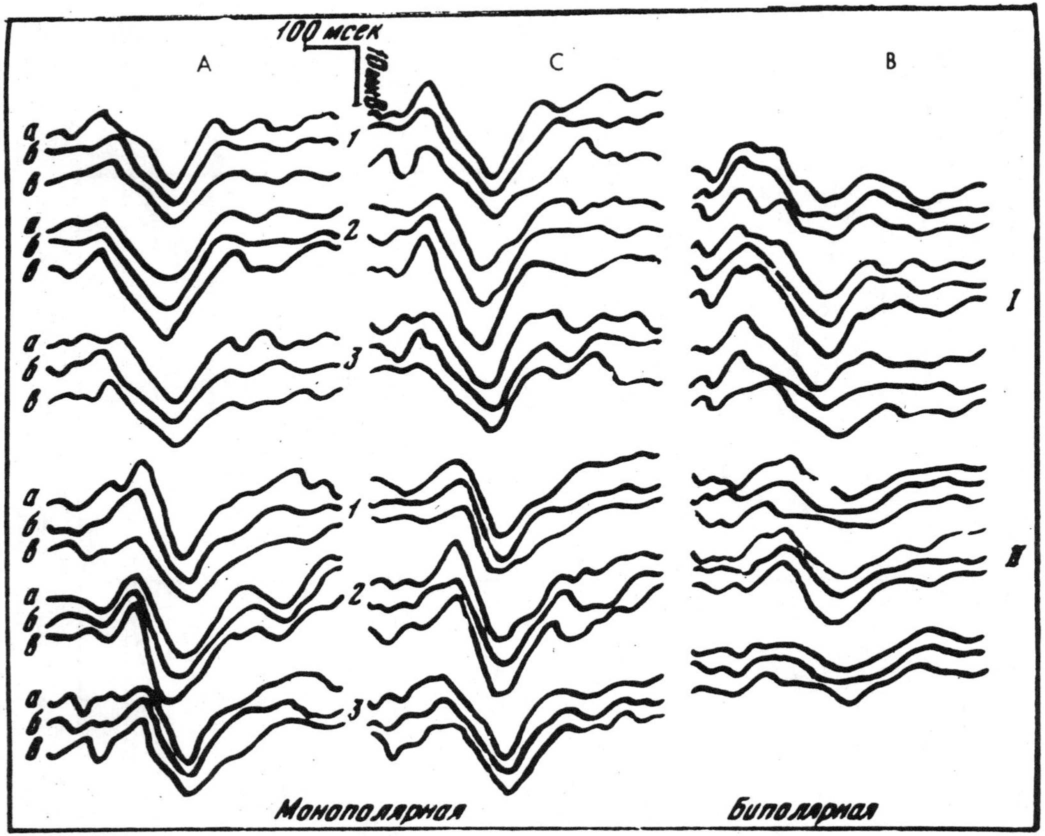

FIGURE 78 (I) Dynamics of late EP waves in healthy subjects during involuntary (1,3) and voluntary (2) attention, in parieto-occipital and premotor zones of left and right hemispheres recorded by monopolar and bipolar methods. (I) Parieto-occipital zones, (II) premotor zones, (A and C) left hemisphere, (B) right hemisphere, (a,b,c) consecutively averaged EP (for responses 1-10, 11-20, and 21-30). (II) Dynamics of late EP waves in patients with lesions of mediobasal zones of frontal lobes during involuntary (1,3) and voluntary (2) attention, in

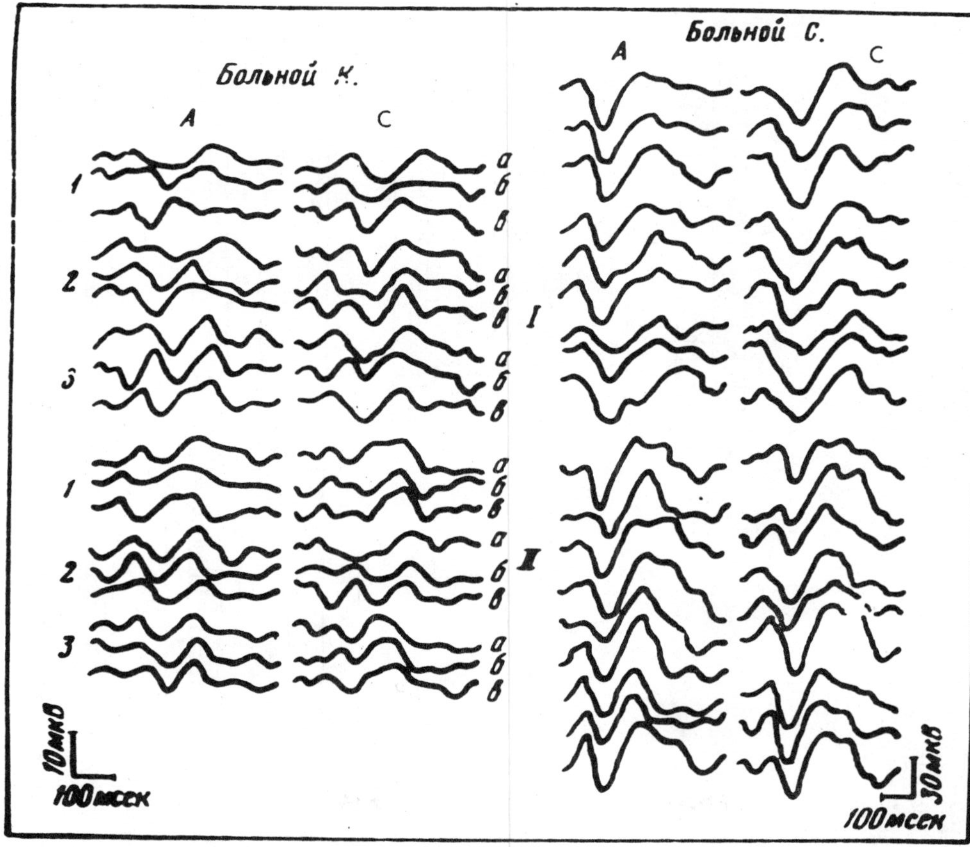

parieto-occipital and premotor zones of left and right hemispheres. Monopolar recording. (A) left hemisphere, (B) right hemisphere; (a,b,c) consecutively averaged EP (for responses 1-10, 11-20, and 21-30). Patient K., diagnosis: astrocytoma of right frontal lobe spreading to basal ganglia and to left frontal lobe; Patient S., diagnosis: traumatic injury to right frontal lobe with evidence of involvement of left frontal lobe, sequelae of head injury.

(flashes) by means of an instruction (for example, "Tell me which of two flashes is the shorter," "Press the key with your right hand as quickly as possible after each flash") leads to a change in the amplitude and temporal parameters of the EP in regions of the brain corresponding to the character of the test. During tests of assessment of the duration of flashes (i.e., during the concentration of "sensory" attention) changes in the EP parameters were mainly in the posterior zones, especially in the right hemisphere. During tests involving responding as quickly as possible to flashes with the right (or left) hands (i.e., during the concentration of "motor" attention) changes in the EP parameters were observed mainly in the anterior zones of the brain, especially in the left hemisphere (Fig. 79).

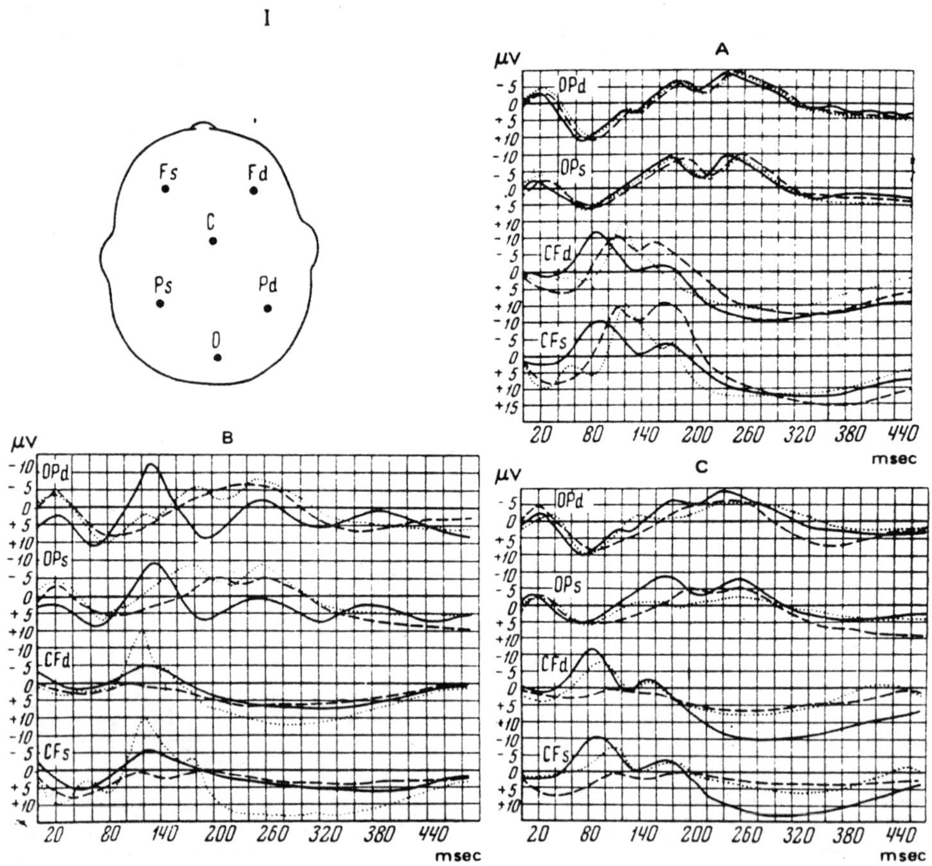

FIGURE 79 Changes in parameters of evoked potentials (EP) in response to various instructions in a normal subject and in patients with frontal lobe lesions (after Simernitskaya and Khomskaya, 1966). (I) Changes in parameters of EP in healthy subject E in response to various instructions. (A) "After the 8th to the 10th flash you will get an electric shock in your left arm"; (B) "Note which flashes are longer than the others"; (C) "As soon as you see a flash press as quickly as you can on the button with your left hand." Occipital-parietal derivation in top two curves; central-frontal derivation in bottom two curves. Continuous line shows EP

Mobilization of voluntary attention in healthy subjects thus leads to an increase in the local activity of different brain structures depending on the character of the activity performed.

Simultaneously, with the mobilization of attention, interhemispheric differences in electrical activity, reflected in the EP parameters, are increased. Interhemispheric asymmetry of EP during the concentration of "sensory" and "motor" attention under conditions of lateral (unilateral) stimulation of the left or right cerebral hemisphere is particularly well defined (Demina, 1957). During passive perception of the stimuli the highest amplitudes and lowest values of the temporal parameters of EP are recorded in the hemisphere contralateral to the side of stimulation. During the active perception of stimuli the original interhemispheric asymmetry of the EP parameters is

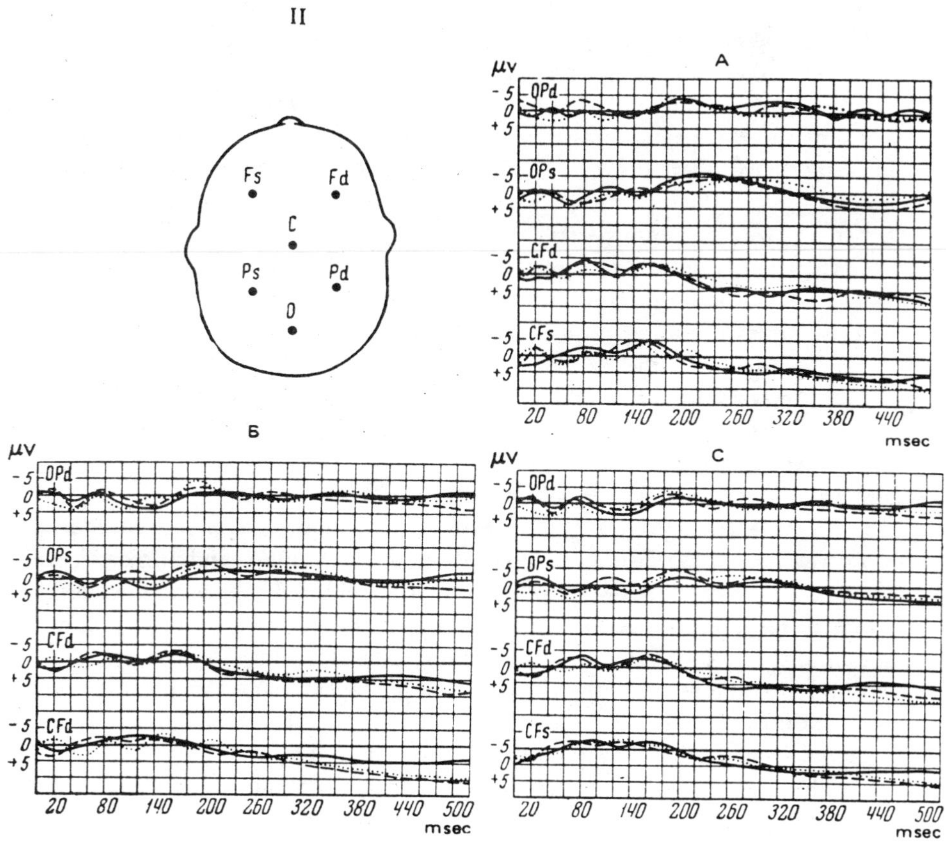

during performance of test. Line of dots and line of dashes indicate EP before and after performance of test. After a visually perceived instruction local changes take place in EP in parietal-occipital derivation (B). In response to other instructions local changes in EP are found in central-frontal derivation (A) and (C). (II) EP in patient U (tumor of anterior region of right falciform process) after various instructions. By contrast with the normal subject the specific character of a verbal instruction does not affect the character of electrical activity.

accentuated even more as the result of the preferential strengthening of local activation in the right parieto-occipital zones during the performance of sensory tests and the premotor zones of the left hemisphere during the performance of motor tests. These facts indicate differences in the relations of the left and right hemispheres to voluntary gnostic and motor activity.

In patients with lesions of the mediobasal zones of the frontal lobes the regulation of local activation processes is severely disturbed, as reflected by the EP parameters (Fig. 80). As a rule, the mobilization of "sensory" and "motor" attention is not reflected in the EP parameters. Areactivity of the EP indices is observed during the performance of both types of tests in both the anterior and posterior zones of the brain. When patients of this category mobilize their voluntary attention, the normal interaction between the hemispheres characteristic of healthy subjects is disturbed. Either a complete absence of interhemispheric differences or, on the contrary, a sharp but pathological increase in interhemispheric asymmetry, manifested as an increase in the amplitude and shortening of the temporal parameters of EP both on the side of the lesion and in the relatively sound hemisphere, is observed in them. Interhemispheric asymmetry of EP is particularly characteristic in the premotor zones of the brain. Disturbance of interhemispheric interaction is combined in these patients with areactivity of the EP indices during the performance of various tests.

In patients with lesions of the pituitary gland and structures lying at the level of the posterior cranial fossa, just as in patients with lesions of the posterior zones of the hemispheres, the regulation of local activation processes (i.e., a change in the EP parameters during the concentration of "sensory" and "motor" attention) remains relatively intact. Areactivity of the EP indices can be observed only in the region of the pathological focus or in the affected hemisphere.

Other workers have also observed similar facts.

Observations by Grey Walter (1966) have shown that expectation of an instruction evokes distinctive slow waves in the human cerebral cortex which he called "expectancy waves." Grey Walter observed these slow waves, arising in response to the instruction to await the appearance of a conditioned stimulus, as the signal for performing a movement, in the frontal lobes only; the intensity of these "expectancy waves" varied depending on the probability of appearance of the signal; when the instruction to await the signal was withdrawn, these waves disappeared (Fig. 81).

These observations (together with the facts obtained by Pribram when studying the "expectancy response" in monkeys and its changes after extirpation of the frontal lobes, already mentioned earlier) are a further indication of the role played by the frontal lobes in the maintenance of stable active states of the organism.

Similar facts were obtained by M. N. Livanov and his collaborators (Livanov, Gavrilova, and Aslanov, 1966). These workers found that when they recorded electrical activity simultaneously from a large number of points on the cortex, any human activity (for example, solving difficult arithmetical problems) causes a considerable increase in the number of synchronously working cortical points; moreover, a marked increase in correlation of electrical activity of the working points first appears in the frontal lobes.

Similar results can be observed in patients with the paranoid form of schizophrenia, in whom a continuous state of stress, associated with static points of excitation, is also manifested as an increased number of synchronously working points in the frontal cortex. Administration of chlorpromazine, reducing this state of stress, was also shown to sharply reduce the large number of synchronously working points just described above in the frontal cortex. These observations are illustrated in Fig. 82.

The study of nonspecific activation processes and their regulation by means of various verbal instructions, presenting different problems for solution, thus shows that the frontal lobes and, in particular, their mediobasal zones occupy an important place in the system of mechanisms responsible for the normal course of psychological processes. Their function is to regulate, with the aid of the speech system, short-term and long-term and, in particular, local and selective activation processes that are the neurophysiological basis for the activity of brain systems.

D. THE FRONTAL LOBES AND REGULATION OF MOVEMENTS AND ACTIONS

What I have just said above about the role of the frontal lobes in the regulation of states of activity prepares us for an examination of an even more difficult problem: the role of the frontal lobes in the regulation of voluntary movement and action and in the programming of the most highly organized forms of human activity.

As I stated then, it is not only the fact that they have the most intimate connections with structures of the reticular formation that distinguishes the frontal lobes. As many workers (see 4A) have shown, the frontal lobes are particularly closely connected in their origin and structure with the cortical apparatus controlling *movement;* for that reason, they were regarded by some workers, including Pavlov, as an essential part of the cortical zones of the *motor analyzer*.

There is thus every reason to suppose that they are very closely concerned

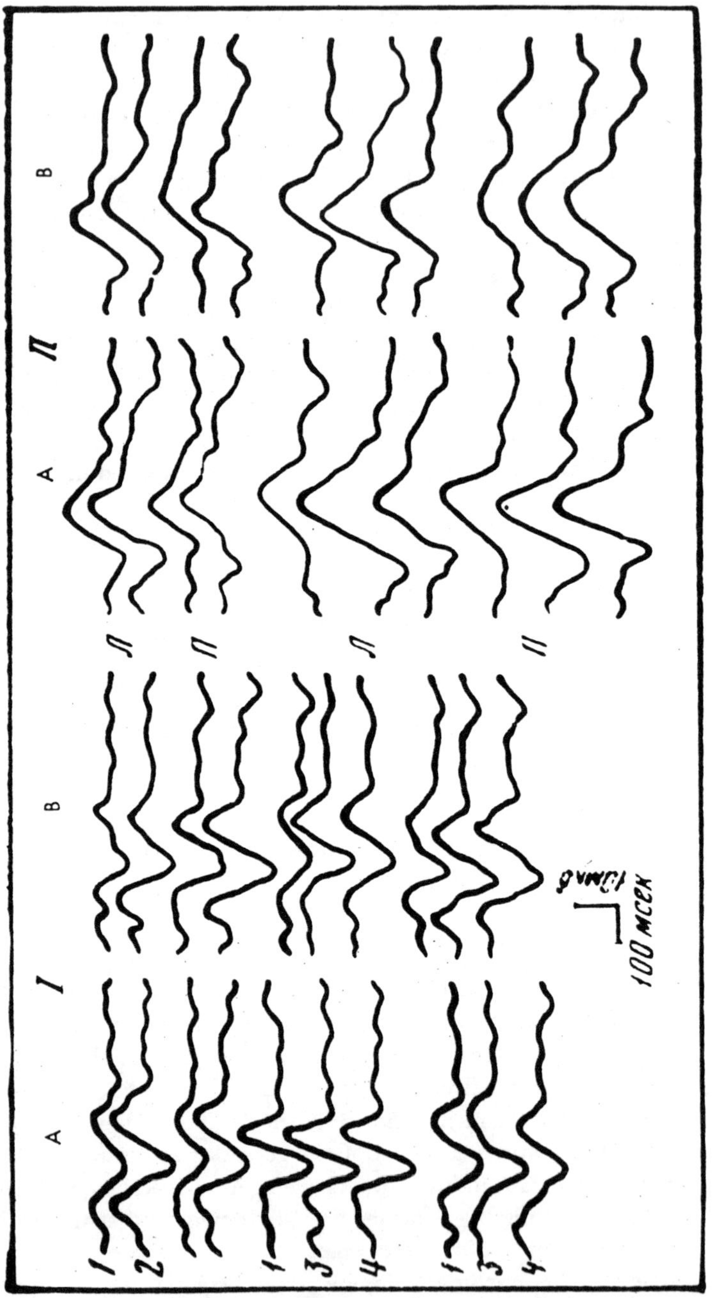

FIGURE 80 (I) Examples of averaged EP of healthy subjects in parieto-occipital and premotor zones in response to photic stimuli applied consecutively in left (A) and right (B) fields of vision during involuntary attention and during solving of problems requiring "sensory" attention (distinguishing flashes by duration) and "motor" attention (responding to flashes as quickly as possible with the right or left hand). (A) left-sided stimulation, (B) right-sided stimulation; (I) parieto-occipital zones, (II) premotor zones; (1) involuntary attention to flashes, (2) "sensory" attention, (3) "motor" attention to right hand, (4) "motor" attention to left hand. (L) left hemisphere, (R) right hemisphere. (II) Principal

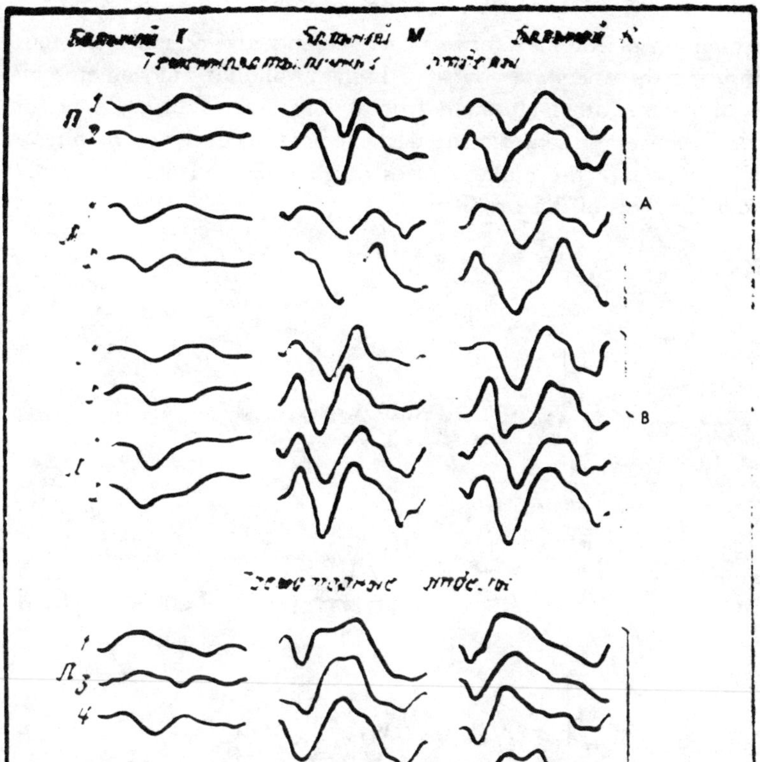

forms of disturbance of interhemispheric asymmetry of late EP waves during involuntary and voluntary attention in patients with frontal lobe lesions. (A) left, (B) right hemisphere; (L) flashes presented in left visual field, (R) in right visual field; (1) EP during involuntary attention, (2) during "sensory" attention, (3) during "motor" attention to right hand, (4) during "motor" attention to left hand. Total duration of recording 500 msec. Patient Kh., diagnosis: intracerebral tumor of mediobasal zones of frontal lobes, more especially on right; Patient M., diagnosis: meningioma of the wing of the left sphenoid bone; Patient K., diagnosis: intracerebral tumor of left frontal lobe.

with the regulation of complex forms of movements and action and, above all, with ensuring the adequate course of human voluntary movements and actions. At the same time, although frontal lobe lesions produce no appreciable disturbances of sensation and movement, effects are manifested there as disturbances of the highest forms of goal-directed activity. I shall now turn to an analysis of this problem.

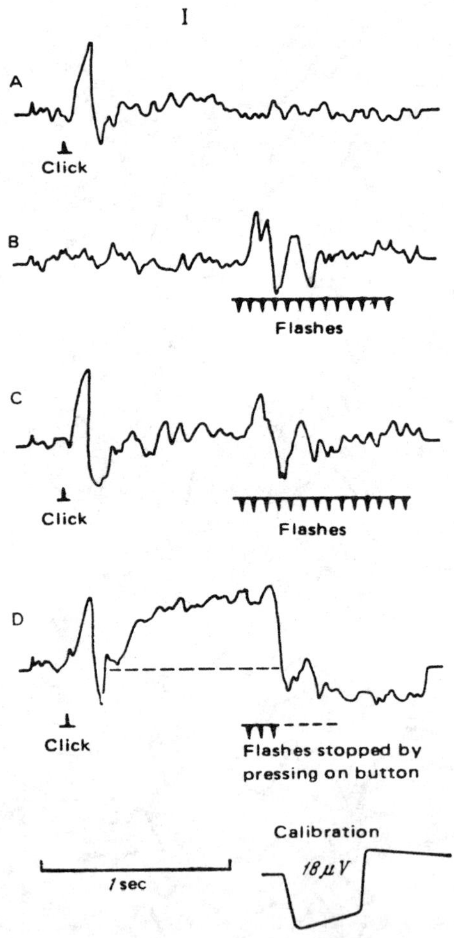

FIGURE 81 Dynamics of expectancy waves under different experimental conditions (after Grey Walter, 1966). (I) Comparison of responses: (A) isolated acoustic stimuli; (B) isolated visual stimuli; (C) association of stimuli; (D) combination of stimuli with patient's response. "Expectancy waves" observed only in the last case. (II) Effect of withdrawal of the trigger stimulus: (A) control connection with "expectancy waves"; (B) averaged record of first six presentations without trigger signal; "expectancy waves" reduced; conditioned response can be seen at the moment when the trigger signal is expected to appear; (C, D, E) consecutive averaged record showing gradual disappearance of "expectancy waves"; (F) rapid recovery of "expectancy waves" on repeated presentation of trigger signal. This particular subject can be

II

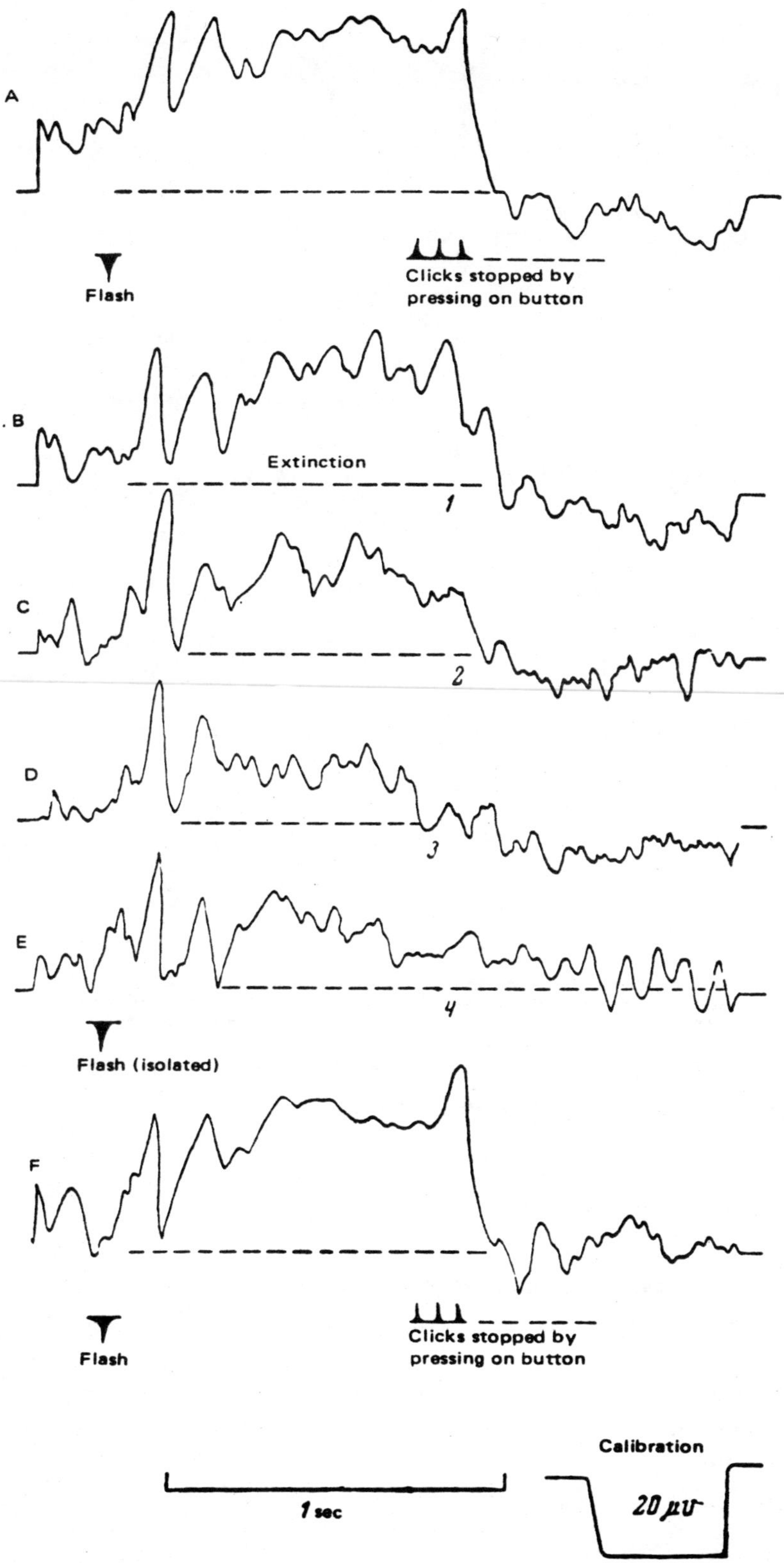
A
Flash
Clicks stopped by
pressing on button
B
Extinction
1
C
2
D
3
E
4
Flash (isolated)
F
Flash
Clicks stopped by
pressing on button
1 sec
Calibration
20 μV

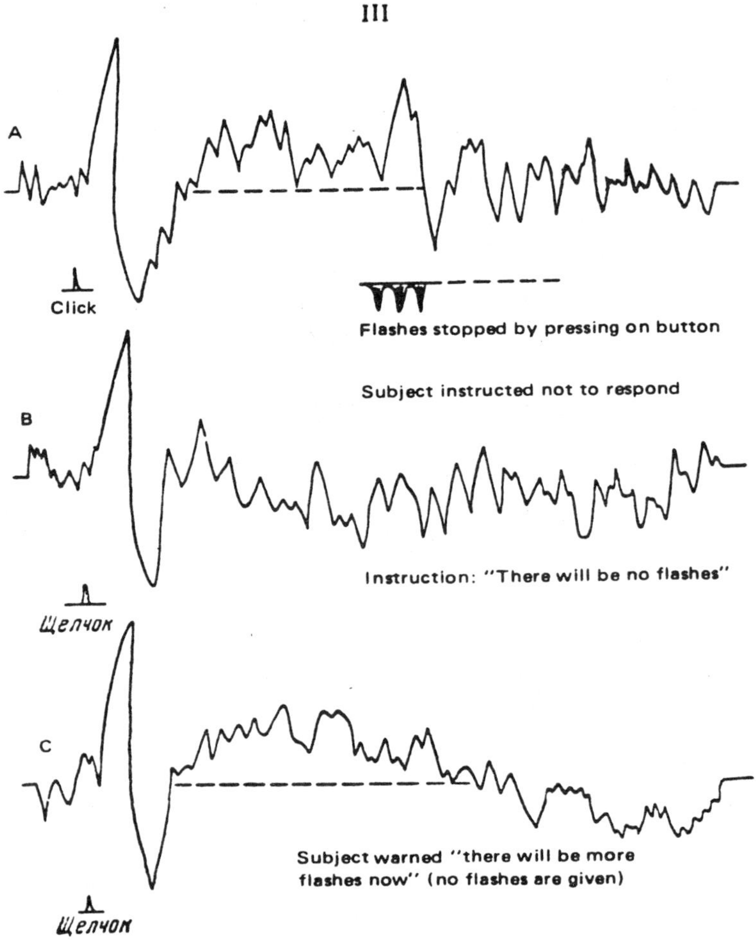

classed as a "sanguinic" because he adapts himself easily to the changing situation. (III) Effect of the situation (preparation for the signal) on appearance of "expectancy waves": (A) subject decided not to press the button; "expectancy waves" disappear; (B) subject is warned that there will be no trigger signals; "expectancy waves" immediately disappear; without the instruction they become extinguished after 30-50 presentations (see II); (C) subject is wrongly warned that flashes will appear again; "expectancy waves" indicate a compromise between trust in the instruction and immediate experience.

i) The structure of voluntary movements and actions

Voluntary movements and actions are a specifically human feature. Although they develop on the basis of the so-called voluntary movements of the animal, they differ from them in many essential features, and without a careful analysis of those features it is impossible to understand their structure.

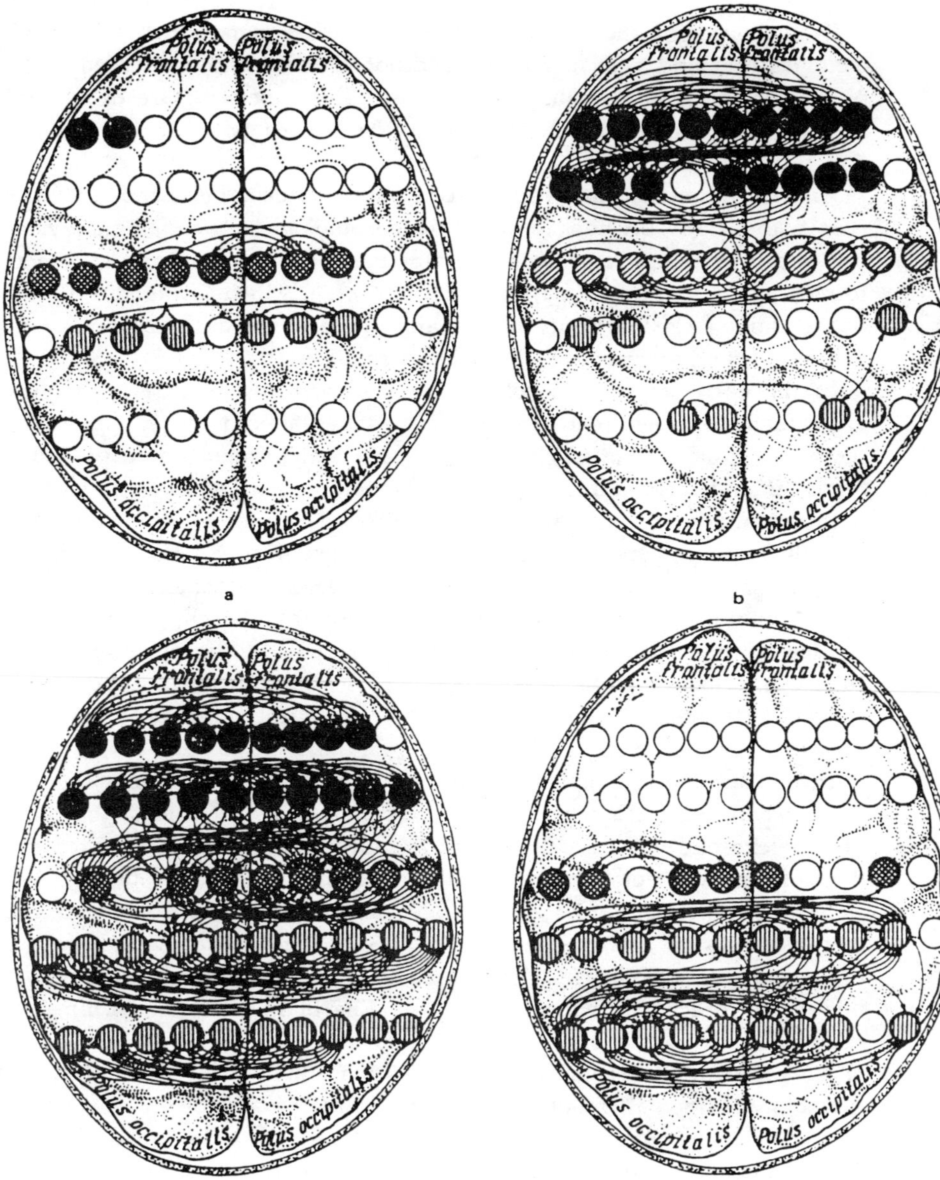

FIGURE 82 Correlation between synchronously working points of the frontal cortex in states of stress (after Livanov, Gavrilova, and Aslanov, 1966). Above: temporal correlation between biopotentials from cortical points of healthy subject S. E.: (a) in state of rest; (b) at 5th second of solving arithmetical problem; circles on chart of cortex denote electrodes applied to surface of scalp. Electrodes located in anterior frontal zones shaded black; those in motor area cross-hatched; those in posterior zones of cortex shaded vertically. Legend to subsequent figures the same. Arrows connect cortical areas correlating for a high percentage of the time. Below: temporal correlation between electrical activity of cortical points of patient with paranoid form of schizophrenia under treatment with chlorpromazine; (a) during solving of arithmetical problem before taking chlorpromazine; (b) while solving similar problem 1 h 15 min after taking chlorpromazine.

Each movement and action of an animal arises in response to a certain biological demand, which is its unconditioned basis, and is satisfied in the process of the animal's subsequent actions. The superstructure of the animal's conditioned-reflex behavior cannot be formed without this unconditioned-reflex basis.

Human voluntary movement and actions, on the other hand, can arise even without any previous "unconditioned" biological basis. A great number of our voluntary movements and actions arise on the basis of a *plan,* formed with the intimate participation of *speech,* which formulates the aim of the action, relates it to its motive, and indicates the basic scheme for the solution of the problem with which the person is faced.

In the early stages of development, as Soviet psychologists (Vygotskii, 1956, 1958; Leont'ev, 1959; Zaporozhets, 1960; Gal'perin, 1957, 1959, 1964) showed, a child's voluntary action is determined by demands expressed in the command of an adult. Later, this "action shared between two people" becomes an action which starts to be controlled by the child's own actions: initially by his perceptual activity, later by his extended external speech and, finally, very much later, by the contracted ideas and schemes formulated with the aid of his internal speech. It is this internal speech, contracted and condensed in the adult, which plays an active part in the processing of incoming information and in the formulation of what Bernshtein (1947, 1957) called the "motor task," singling out the aim of the action and providing a general scheme for it.

In the case of the simplest or the most usual voluntary action, when the necessary movement is determined unambiguously by the aim of the action and the external situation, the role of the speech components is limited simply to formulation of the idea and the triggering of the appropriate motor stereotypes. In more complex cases, when formulation of the motor task no longer ensures the unambiguous appearance of the required action, the role of the speech components of the voluntary motor action is more complex. In such cases speech participates in the recoding of information reaching the subject, the distinguishing of its most important features, and the inhibiting of irrelevant possible courses of action arising either under the influence of direct environmental stimuli or as a result of inert traces of previous experience. By picking out the essential system of connections and creating the internal scheme of action so that it becomes dominant and inhibits all irrelevant, inadequate actions, the speech component becomes the basis of the most complex forms of regulation of the voluntary motor act.

However, the controlling influence of external or internal speech is not restricted to the creation of a general scheme or program of action, which, as Bernshtein (1947, 1957) showed, can subsequently be carried out by any motor operation, the available assortment of which varies flexibly depending on the situation. Throughout the performance of a voluntary action internal speech helps to monitor the course of the action; it compares the action as performed with the original plan, gives out signals indicating their agreement or disagreement, corrects any errors made, and either ceases to act as soon as the aim has been achieved or resumes its activity if the aim has not been achieved. This monitoring function of speech, a component of the "action acceptor" (Anokhin, 1949, 1955) mechanism or the T-O-T-E (Miller, Pribram, and Galanter, 1960) mechanism, during the performance of complex voluntary actions, makes it an important component of the "system with the highest level of self-regulation," as human voluntary activity may be described.

The systems of connections evoked by the plan retain their dominance, and all irrelevant connections not corresponding to the motor task are inhibited. Even a slight decline in the state of cortical activity is sufficient to make the dominant role of these fundamental connections unstable; the irrelevant connections arising under the influence of direct external stimulation or inert traces of previous experience become equal in strength to the selective connections evoked by the plan, and the subject's behavior loses its goal-directed and selective character.

All this suggests that although the frontal lobes do not participate in the performance of the simplest and most usual actions, they can and must play a decisive role in the preservation and realization of the programs of all complex forms of activity; they maintain the dominant role of the program and inhibit irrelevant and inappropriate actions.

Presumably, therefore, when a lesion of the frontal lobes has led to a decline in the state of activity, the precise performance of motor programs will be substantially impaired, selective actions and movements corresponding to the task will no longer occupy a dominant place, and inadequate and irrelevant actions will arise just as easily and will no longer be inhibited. The patient's motor activity as a whole will start to lose its selective character.

After these introductory remarks we can begin our analysis by first considering the distinguishing features of the disturbance of behavior observed in patients with frontal lobe lesions in the course of ordinary clinical observations, and we can then go on to consider the facts obtained by special neuropsychological tests.

ii) Disturbance of behavior and of the structure of action in lesions of the frontal lobes

The disturbance of complex forms of goal-directed behavior has always been regarded as one of the principal manifestations of a frontal lobe lesion. As I stated above, psychiatrists have usually described these defects as disturbances of spontaneity and of critical judgment. As a result of closer observation it is possible to give more precise characteristics of these defects.

A frontal lobe lesion is not accompanied as a rule either by symptoms of paresis or ataxia or by a disturbance of well-consolidated manipulations with objects. Such patients can perform customary actions perfectly well and show no evidence of apraxia during their performance.

A disturbance of voluntary movement and actions arises only when the action has to begin in accordance with a preformed plan and, in particular, when there is ambiguity in its character, and its performance requires inhibition of other actions which are irrelevant and inappropriate to the task.

In patients with the mildest forms of frontal lobe lesions these defects may be manifested as signs of a decline in the patient's activity, described by the patient's companions as "losing interest." Frequently the patient ceases to take an active part in social life, becomes inactive and "inattentive," and does only the simplest and most mechanical actions. When asked to perform relatively more complex actions, in the course of which the subject is exposed to many types of stimuli and has to inhibit irrelevant actions, his behavior often loses its selectivity; his goal-directed actions are easily replaced by irrelevant stereotyped reactions or by uncontrollable perseverations. I recall one of my patients, with a slowly growing tumor of the frontal lobes, whose first manifestation of his illness occurred when, on going to the station one day to catch a train in one direction, he got into the train which happened to arrive first, although it was going in the opposite direction. Not until later did he realize that he had behaved purely on impulse and had given way to the influence of the immediate situation. Another patient, chancing to see the button which operated the bell, involuntarily performed the stereotyped action and pressed it, but when the nurse came to him he did not know what to say.

In yet another of my patients, a housewife with a slowly growing tumor of the frontal lobes, goal-directed behavior was replaced by grossly incorrect actions; for example, she would sweep the burning hot stove with a broom, or put pieces of string into the soup pan instead of vermicelli.

A similar form of behavior disturbance occurred in a patient with a wound of the frontal lobes who, when working in the carpenters' shop of the hospital for the purpose of rehabilitation, inertly went on planing a piece of wood until nothing remained of it. Even then he did not stop planing, but continued to plane the bench itself. In another similar case, the neighbors noted that a patient, in whom a tumor of the frontal lobes was later found, shut herself up in the bathroom for a long time and inertly went on scrubbing the same place over and over again while leaving the rest untouched. Another example of this category of disturbance of behavior concerned a patient in whom a tumor affecting the functions of both frontal lobes was subsequently found, who had to make a speech but simply repeated part of it over and over again and, on returning home, asked his son the same question repeatedly, immediately forgetting every time that he had done so. Many such examples of impulsive actions by patients with massive frontal lobe lesions (including some patients with wounds of the frontal lobes even after their discharge from the hospital) complete the details of this picture. In all these cases goal-directed selective behavior was replaced by habitual stereotypes based on the direct action of a particular stimulus which the patient did not compare with the original plan and did not inhibit.

The disturbance of complex forms of activity connected with the performance of a particular program and the ease with which the necessary actions are replaced by irrelevant stereotyped acts, unconnected with the underlying task and depriving the activity of its selective character, constitute the characteristic features of patients in the early stages of the development of the "frontal syndrome." Disturbance of a critical attitude toward these defects of behavior and failure to correct incorrect actions distinguish these symptoms from all the other forms of disturbance of movements and actions that may arise in patients with lesions of other parts of the brain. These facts are well described in the literature (Kleist, 1934; Brickner, 1936; Rylander, 1937), and there is no need to dwell further on them here.

• • •

The disturbance of the selective character of voluntary actions and its replacement by more elementary forms of motor acts, observable in the course of general observation of the patient, is seen particularly clearly during *clinical tests* of the type which patients usually undergo in the course of neuropsychological investigation.

The patient with a frontal lobe lesion can easily perform the test of repeating simple positions of the hand (Part III, Section 3B); however, if requested to reproduce the position of the hand of the physician facing him, he often has difficulty and easily substitutes for the required position its mirror image (for example, when the physician points with his index finger he responds by pointing with his little finger, the one whose position corresponds to the direct impression). This "echopraxic" response is performed by the patient without any preliminary "recoding" of the position as he perceives it, and he is unaware of his mistake. Only when the examiner draws the patient's attention to the mistake and explains it is the correct movement performed, but the mistake is repeated in the next test. Frequently the performance of the required movement is disturbed by a pathologically inert stereotype; having once performed the required action, the patient cannot inhibit it and introduces components of it into the next test.

Similar observations can be made on patients with a "frontal syndrome" during Head's test (reproducing the position of the hands of the physician sitting in front of him); this requires the recoding of the position of the hands as directly perceived and the performance of "cross" movements (Part III, Section 3B). In these tests the patient with a frontal syndrome easily omits the essential recoding of the pattern as perceived and produces an echopraxic mirror image of the physician's posture, with no misgivings about either the correctness of his performance or the awareness of his mistakes. Only sometimes, by extended verbal decoding of the required movements ("I lifted my right hand; your right hand is on the other side compared to mine; you should have lifted this hand"), can a mistake be corrected; but when the test is repeated the echopraxic "mirror-image" responses occur again.

Disturbances of the performance of motor acts by patients with a frontal syndrome can be seen if we ask them to repeat a *series of movements,* such as clenching the fist, then stretching out the thumb, and finally, extending the palm, or placing the hand in three successive positions as instructed (Part III, Section 4B). In such cases a patient with a severe disturbance of frontal lobe function will easily abandon the program or simplify it and perseverate one component of it, or he will make no attempt whatever to analyze the task presented to him and will start to perform haphazard movements. The same results can be seen when the patient is instructed to tap out rhythms (Part III, Section 4B); I shall return later to the analysis of the disturbances arising in such patients.

In all the cases described above, the disturbances observed in patients with frontal lobe lesions are similar in character: the program of movement issued to the patient is not analyzed as carefully as it should be, and it is not preserved as the dominant scheme of the action. It is easily replaced by the performance of other, more elementary programs, not requiring preliminary recoding of the task, and by the appearance of *echopraxic actions or perseverations,* which the patient does not inhibit. Unawareness of the mistakes and failure to correct them, as I said above, are additional features of this syndrome.

• • •

Although the disturbance of goal-directed behavior assumes such distinct forms in relatively mild cases of the "frontal syndrome," it is particularly noticeable in patients with massive lesions of the frontal lobes, for example, tumors of this region associated with increased intracranial pressure. Careful observation of the general behavior of these patients reveals the picture of disturbance of active, goal-directed activity already described above, but this time in a particularly severe form.

Such patients usually exhibit gross forms of inactivity: they make no request and perform no purposive movements. They are dirty; sometimes they do not request the bottle to urinate, or do not take it if it is by the bedside. Even if hungry or thirsty, they make no active attempt to take food or drinks placed on their table.

Despite the severe disintegration of their active behavior, they are visibly aware of any change taking place in the ward; someone coming in, the squeaking of a door, or coughing by the patient in the next bed arouses a strong orienting reflex, most frequently manifested as movements of the eyes, or sometimes turning the head toward the stimulus. They answer questions monosyllabically and inactively, but they will readily join in a conversation which the physician is holding with the patient in the next bed, adding their own retorts and then again relapsing into silence. Usually they find it almost impossible to perform a definite action in response to an instruction; they cannot raise their arm, shake the physician's hand a definite number of times, or point to a specified object (especially if their hands are under the bedclothes and they have first to take them out), but usually they tug at the sheet, pick up with their fingers the towel lying on the bed, or scrape the wall near the bed; often they are involuntarily attracted by a small spot on the wall and they make attempts to clean it, not stopping even if they are told not to do so. They will not take the physician's hand if it is a few inches away from their own, but if the physician puts his own hand into theirs they will grasp it and are often unable to terminate this grasping reflex. In response to the instruction to shake the physician's hand three times, they either give one continuous, tonic shake of the hand or they repeat the hand shaking over and over again, unable to stop the automatic movement once they have begun. Often they repeat echolalically after the physician: "Yes, I must shake it three times . . ." but even so they continue with their automatic action quite regardless of the instruction they have just received. In short, they can neither start nor stop an action in response to a spoken command, and the revival of their elementary orienting reflexes or automatism is in sharp contrast to the gross disintegration of their voluntary activity or actions evoked by a spoken instruction.

Equally clear disturbances arise in such patients during manipulation of objects. A simple task involving an object (for example, striking a match, rolling a cigarette) may be completed relatively well; if, however, the patient is instructed to perform a less familiar action or an action in conflict with a well-consolidated, familiar motor act, he very quickly abandons the assigned program for the familiar action, if some common link can be found between it and the action he was instructed to perform. Examples of such disturbances can be seen in patients with severe lesions of the frontal lobes investigated by Filippycheva (1952). If one of these patients were given the program for an action consisting of several consecutive stages (for example, lighting a candle with a match), he often performed only one fragment of the action (for example, striking the match and then immediately putting it out), or he replaced this relatively complex and unfamiliar program with another simpler version; putting the candle in his mouth, he tried to light it with the match just as he would light a cigarette. In one typical case a patient with a massive tumor of the frontal lobe (previously a well-mannered person), whose sister was eating with a spoon, took her hand, which was close to the patient's lip, and politely kissed it, without expressing the slightest emotion. The replacement of the complex action programs by a well-consolidated stereotype, quite unrelated to the basic program, is the most typical feature of the disturbances of voluntary activity in this group of patients.

The structure of the disturbance of voluntary actions in patients with massive lesions of the frontal lobes is seen particularly clearly if such a patient is asked to draw a simple pattern, for example, a circle, a triangle, or a cross, or if he is given an instruction requiring him to perform a more complex action program (for example, to draw two crosses, a circle, and a minus sign).

If a lesion of the frontal lobes spreads into the deep zones of the frontal region to affect the subcortical ganglia and to disturb the inhibition of primitive automatisms, the task of drawing a simple figure is easily interrupted by the revival of elementary motor automatism; having started to perform a particular task, the patient is unable to give up, and the performance of the action is interrupted by bursts of uncontrollable automatism. The difference between these disturbances and the motor perseverations observed in patients with deep lesions of the premotor zones is that whereas in the latter the program of the action remains intact and the disturbance affects only the motor performance of the action, in frontal lesions the evoked motor automatisms very easily cause the action program to disintegrate and the patient's movements to lose their connection with the task. Examples of such cases are given in Fig. 83.

If the lesion extends into the anterior zones of the frontal lobes, the disturbance of drawing patterns may assume a different character. Such a patient may show no sign of revival of elementary automatism; he can easily carry out simple tasks and draw a figure shown to him. However, if the visual afferentation (copying) is replaced by a spoken instruction, and if the patient is asked to draw a number of different figures, having drawn the first figure correctly, he will very often be unable to switch to the second and third and will draw the same figure over and over again, quite unaware of his mistake and making no attempt to correct it (Fig. 84).

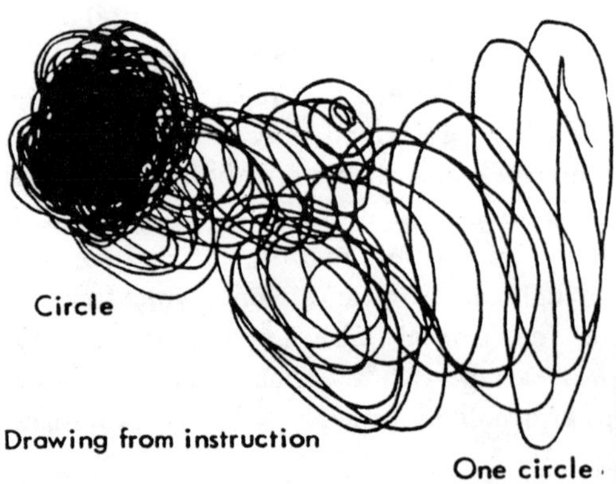

FIGURE 83 Gross disintegration in the performance of an action with replacement by motor perseveration in a patient (Patient Kur.) with an extensive lesion of the frontal lobes (bilateral intracerebral tumor).

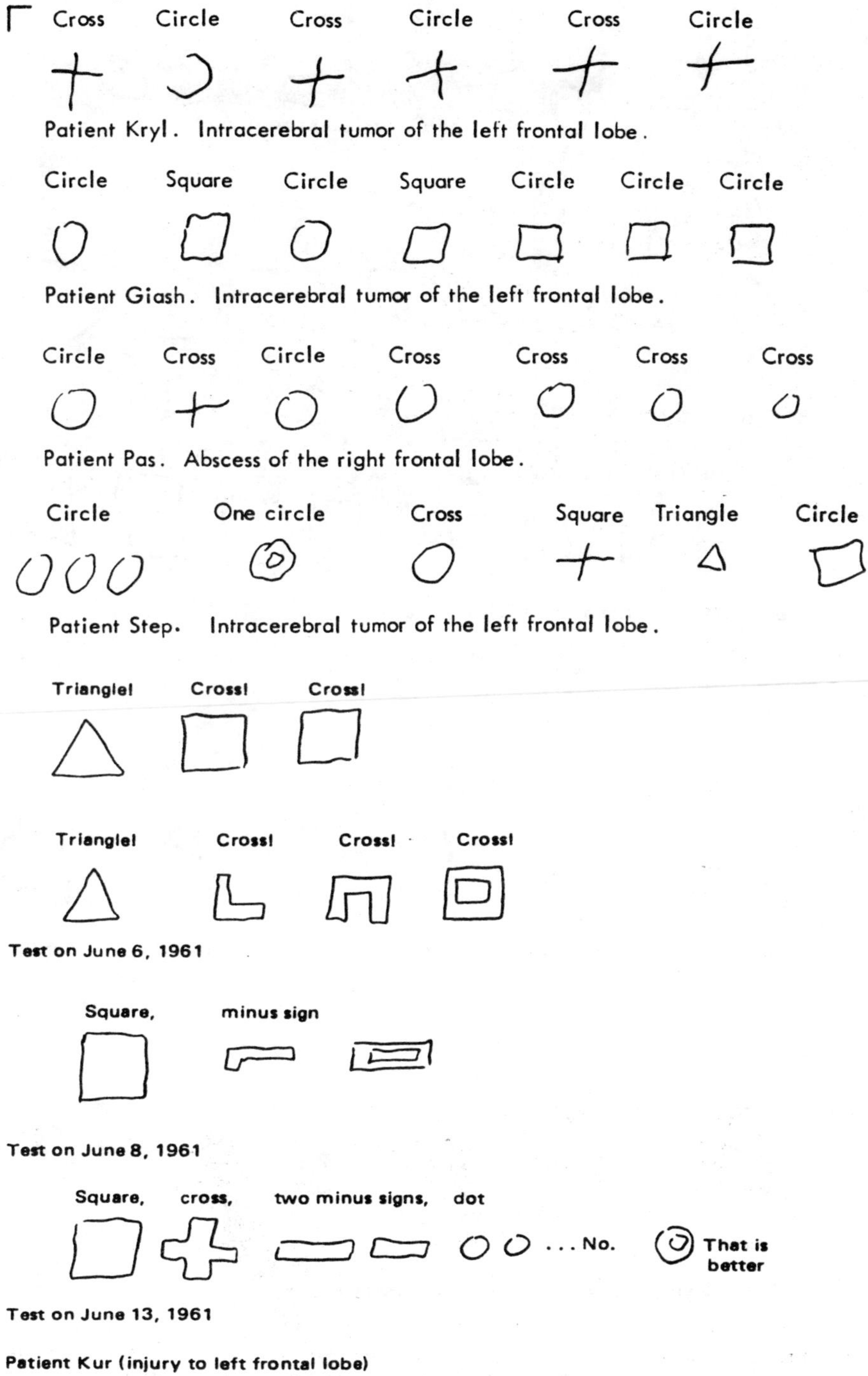

FIGURE 84 Disturbance of the performance of single tasks as a result of pathological inertia of action in patients with extensive lesions of the frontal lobes.

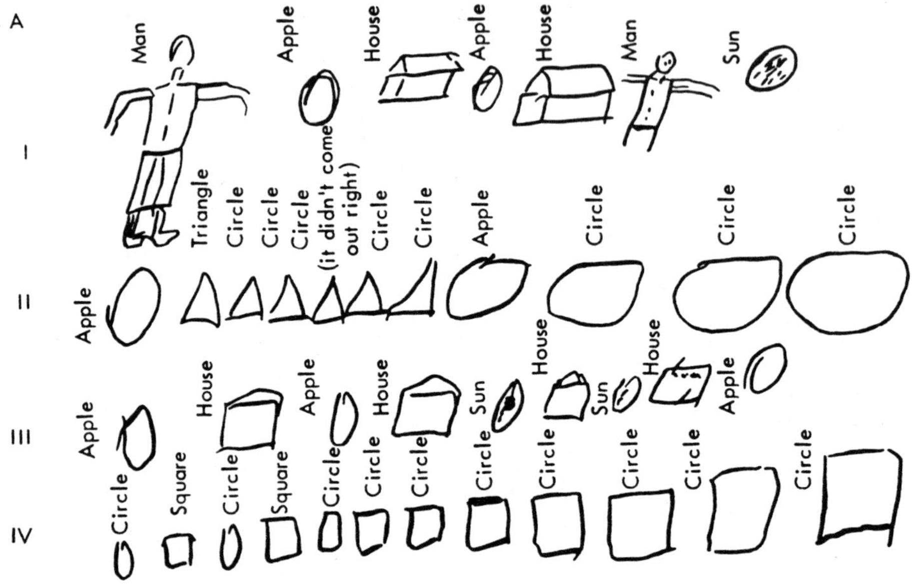

Patient Giash. Tumor on left frontal lobe.

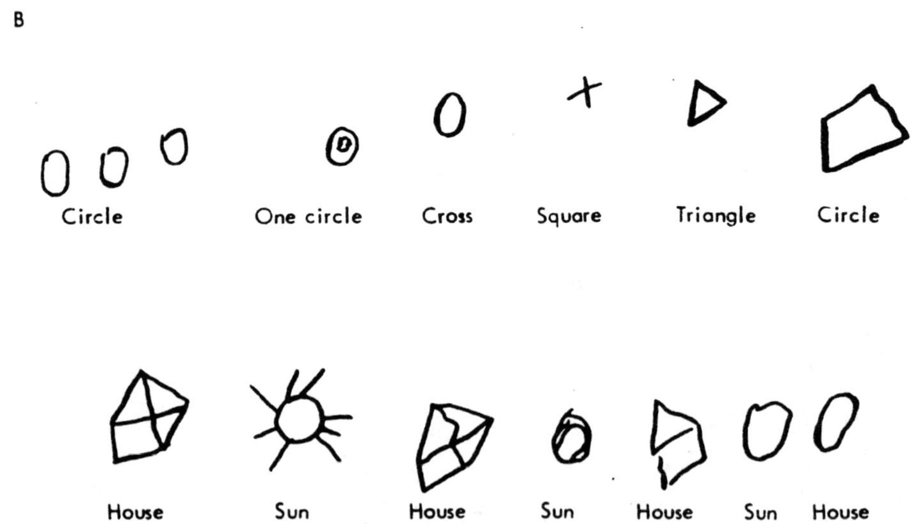

Patient Step. Tumor of left fronto-temporal region.

FIGURE 85 Disturbance of performance of single tasks during changes in the afferent organization of movement in patients with extensive lesions of the frontal lobes. Giving the instruction in concrete form overcomes the inert stereotype.

Only if the patient is instructed to draw patterns which differ very greatly, and with the aid of their visual content, can this pathological inertia be overcome (Fig. 85). However, this compensatory effect of transferring the motor act to a higher (manipulative) semantic level, to which I have just drawn attention, is by no means always possible, and in some cases of the largest frontal lesions (for example, massive bilateral frontal tumors), not even transferring the action to a higher semantic level can produce the required effect. The inertia of the stereotype manifested in the drawing of simple geometrical shapes remains unaltered.

This disintegration of the performance of the essential action program and its replacement by an inert stereotype is seen still more clearly during the performance of sequential tasks—if, for example, the patient is instructed to draw two circles, a triangle, and a cross all at once.

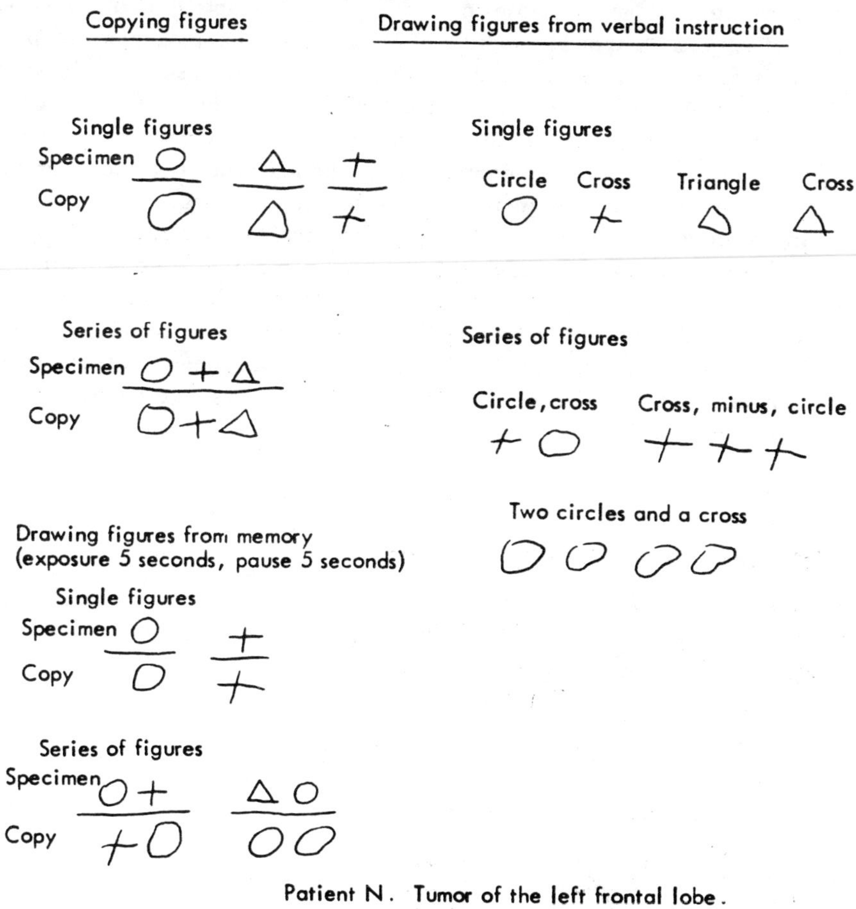

FIGURE 86 Disturbance of the performance of serial tasks by command in patients with extenisve lesions of the frontal lobes.

In such cases the program as instructed has to be carried out in response to traces of a spoken instruction, and the patient finds it particularly difficult to subordinate his actions to such traces. Inert stereotypes arising during the performance of the first stage of the program are so much stronger than the traces of the spoken instruction that the performance of the program as a whole is easily abandoned. Instead of a complex series of actions one stage is repeated inertly. As Fig. 86 shows, although such patients can copy a series of figures, the performance of an action program on the basis of traces of a spoken instruction is immediately replaced by the repetition of one stereotyped action.

A characteristic feature of the disturbance of complex actions in patients with lesions of the frontal lobes is that once the stereotypes have arisen, their pathological inertia can sometimes become very complex in character and be manifested as perseveration, not of single motor acts, but of whole systems of actions. A typical example of these highly complex types of perseveration found in patients with massive frontal lobe lesions is shown by the patient who, having once signed his name or having written a word, is unable to switch from the act of writing to that of drawing; when asked to draw a certain shape, or sometimes even when instructed to copy or even to trace a certain shape, he inertly repeats the act of writing.

An example of this perseveration of systems can be seen in Fig. 87. Characteristically, whereas the typical feature of patients whose pathological focus is situated in the postfrontal zones of the brain and spreads to the subcortical ganglia is inertia of their movements, the typical feature of patients with massive lesions of the anterior frontal zones is perseveration of complete systems. The results of tests of two corresponding patients are compared in Fig. 88.

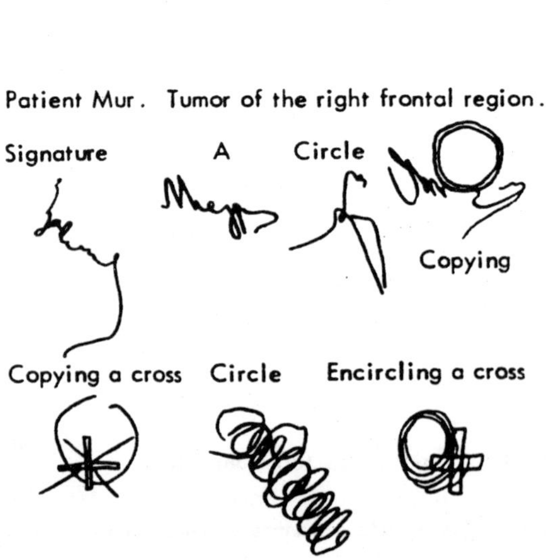

FIGURE 87 Inertia of action in a patient with an extensive lesion of the frontal lobes.

A

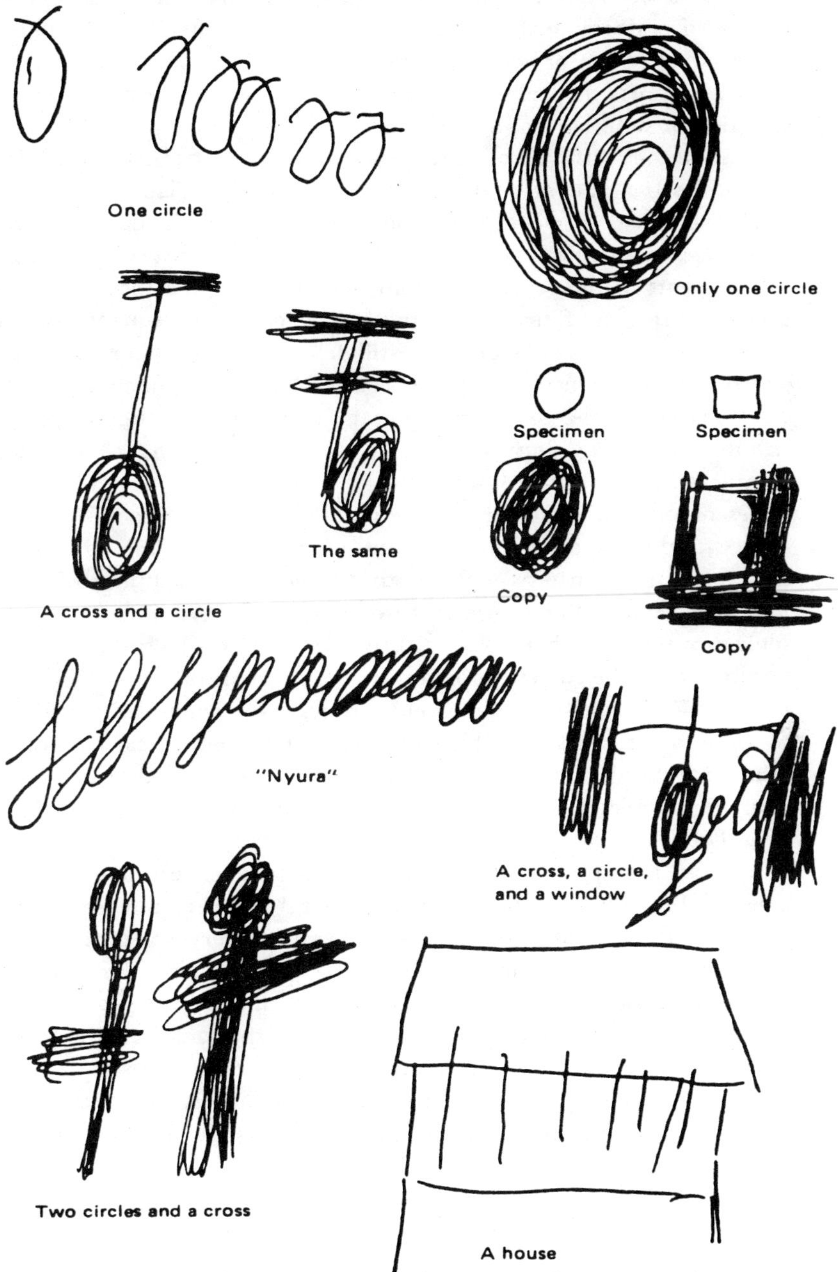

FIGURE 88 Two types of perseveration in patients with frontal lobe lesions (Luria, 1965): (a) motor perseverations in a patient with a tumor of the basal zones of the frontal lobes,

The disturbance of complex action programs under the influence of pathological inertia sometimes assumes particularly interesting forms. In these cases the inertia of a stereotype, once it has arisen, is so great that instead of performing the complex program, the patient simply perseverates a preceding action or one component of it; as a result either in part or in whole, he starts to perform not the current instruction but a previous instruction or subprogram included in it.

Examples of this type of disturbance of action performance are illustrated in Fig. 89. If a patient with a massive tumor of the right frontal lobe (Fig. 89a) was asked to write down the figure 3, he could do so. If, however, he was asked to write down "122" he wrote "333" instead, thus combining the elements of the recent program with those of the inertly perseverating previous program. The same thing happened in subsequent tests; even if he was asked to copy figures, he still fell under the influence of the inert stereotype and copied (relatively correctly) "122," which he repeated as 121, mixing up the necessary program with the inert stereotype and substituting the inertly perseverating "2" for the specimen "4" shown to him. Characteristically, the same patient was unable to write his name ("Fesenko"), but when asked to write the word "okno" (window), he started to do the earlier problem and wrote his own name. Similar observations were made in tests with another patient with a tumor of the frontal lobe (Fig. 89b). Having drawn three circles and five lines in response to a spoken command, when instructed to insert ten dots he drew ten lines (contamination of the current program by the previous one). And in response to the next instruction—"Insert twelve crosses"—he continued to draw a series of lines, in the course of which he even lost the numerical part of the program; naturally, therefore, in the next test, when he had to draw three circles, he completely failed to do so and inertly drew rectangular figures (Fig. 89b).

A clear example of the pathological inertia of previous stereotypes is given in Fig. 89c. A patient with a bilateral lesion of the frontal lobes following ligation of the anterior communicating artery was instructed to draw a "cross" (as on a church). He did so without difficulty, but was then unable to switch to drawing a star and continued inertly to draw a cross. After he had successfully drawn "a pair of spectacles" he was unable to switch to drawing "a watch," but continued to draw the spectacles; only when his mistake had been pointed out did he draw a pair of spectacles with a watch drawn in the center of one lens. He could draw "a comb" easily,

---

affecting subcortical motor ganglia, when patient attempts to draw. (b) pathological inertia of stereotypes, once they have arisen, in a patient with a massive injury of the postfrontal zones and a severe "frontal syndrome."

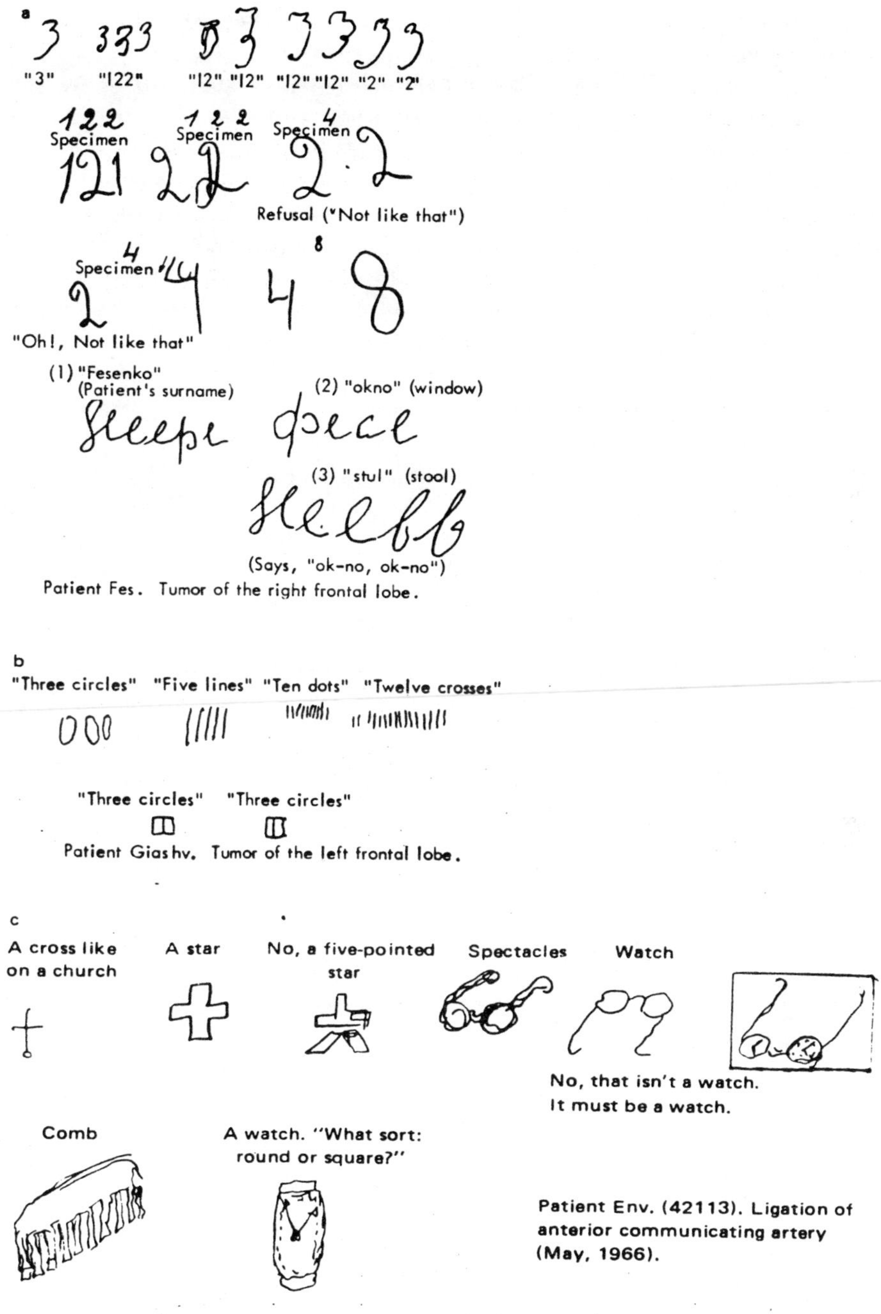

FIGURE 89 Inertia of stereotypes during drawing by patients with lesions of both frontal lobes (note the inert repetition of the previous drawing or pattern).

but when he then was asked to draw "a watch," the watch he drew was not round but rectangular, repeating the shape of the comb.

In the cases I have just described the patient was unable to perform his action program because of the influence of traces of previous actions. However, it is typical of patients with massive frontal lesions that the performance of assigned programs may be disturbed by the influence of the immediate situation, on the one hand, and by inert stereotypes of past experience on the other. This can be illustrated by two very clear examples.

A patient with a severe traumatic lesion of both frontal lobes, followed by the development of a cyst which replaced the brain tissue in the frontal region, when asked to draw a square, drew three squares, thereby filling the top line of the paper (Fig. 91). When asked to draw one square, he drew lines all around the edges of the paper. At this time the doctors were talking to each other a little way off. The patient picked up the word "pact" from their conversation and thereupon wrote the words "Act No." When one doctor murmured to the other, "It is rather like the experiments with animals, after extirpation of the frontal lobes," the patient picked up the word "animal" ("zhivotnoe" in Russian) and wrote down the words "o zhivotnovodstve" (meaning "about stock breeding"). When the doctor asked the nurse, in a whisper, the patient's name, the patient immediately wrote it down—"Ermolov." Thus, the patient's whole behavior was determined not by specialized, selective systems of connections, but by irrelevant stimuli, which he perceived without any kind of discrimination and which quickly evoked a motor reaction.

Another patient with a tumor of the frontal lobe, a chauffeur by occupation, was asked to draw two triangles and a minus sign. As Fig. 92 shows, he did this without difficulty. However, he drew the minus sign in the form of a

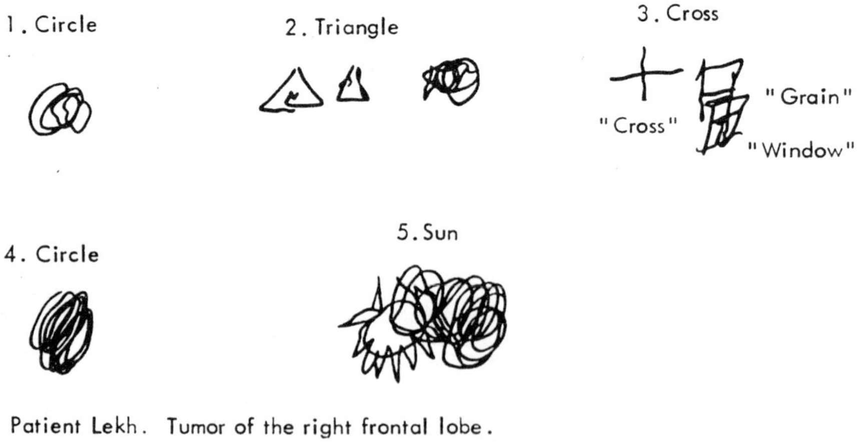

FIGURE 90 Disturbance of selectivity of action systems in a patient with an extensive lesion of the right frontal lobe.

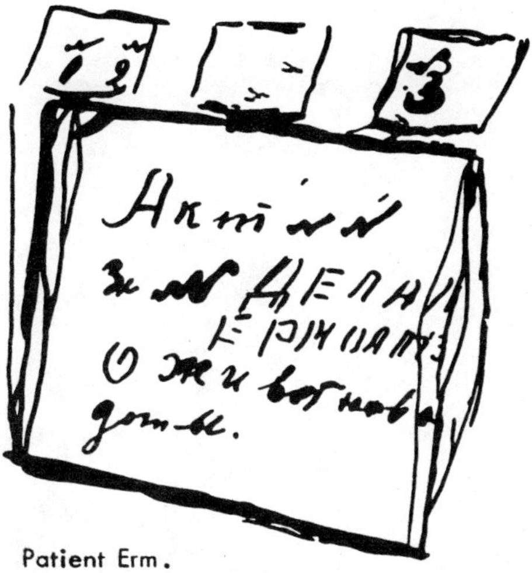

Patient Erm.
Injury to the frontal lobe
with cyst formation.

FIGURE 91 Disturbance of the selective performance of a task by fragmentary reactions to external stimuli in a patient with severe trauma to both frontal lobes followed by a cyst that replaced the brain tissue in this region.

closed rectangle (perseveration of the previous action). When he was then asked to draw a circle, he drew the same figure in the middle of the circle, and then, clearly under the influence of the familiar image of a street sign stating "No Entry," he wrote beneath the figure the words "No Entry."

Some preliminary conclusions can be drawn from the observations described above relating to the disturbances of voluntary movements and actions in patients with massive lesions of the frontal lobes.

The waking state of the cortex, maintained by the normally functioning frontal lobes, enables complex systems of voluntary actions to be carried out under the control of plans formulated in speech. The system of connections evoked by the plan is so dominant that the influence of all irrelevant stimuli (including traces of actions evoked previously) is inhibited as the activity acquires its selective and oriented character. However, lesions of the frontal lobes depress the state of activity and disturb the essential conditions for the performance of complex action programs. The influence of irrelevant stimuli and of traces of actions performed previously becomes practically as strong as that of the connections arising under the influence of the assigned program; traces of that program cease to be dominant and the future activity loses its selective character. These investigations provide a new approach to the detailed analysis of the role of the frontal lobes in the regulation of voluntary movements and actions, whose disturbance is one of the main symptoms of frontal lesions.

As we have already seen, a lesion of the frontal lobes gives rise to noticeable disturbances of the regulation of a state of activity, and especially to disturbances of the stable activation of the cortex by spoken instructions. Is this basic fact reflected in the power of exerting firm control over move-

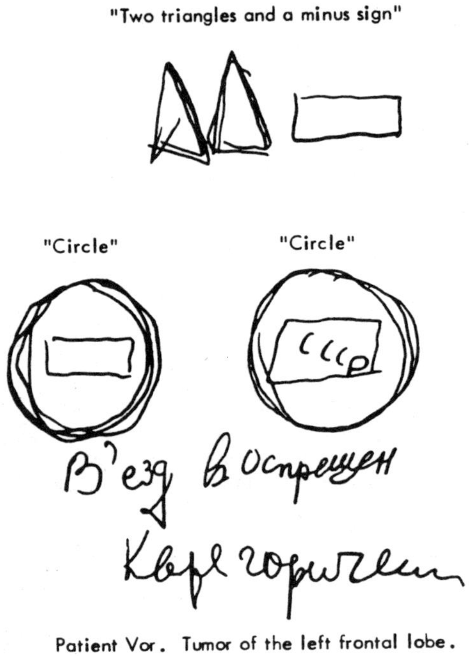

FIGURE 92 Disturbance of the selective performance of tasks by introduction of habitual connections (on the basis of occupation) in a patient (a chauffeur) with an extensive lesion of the left frontal lobe.

ments and actions and subordinating them to a complex program formulated with the aid of speech? The above observations suggest that frontal lobe lesions do in fact disturb complex forms of regulation of movements and actions; however, the mechanisms of this disturbance require special investigation. Let us now examine the relevant facts.

Investigations (Luria, 1956, 1958, 1961; Zaporozhets, 1960) have shown that at the age of 1.5–2 years a child is not yet able to subordinate his actions to an instruction spoken by an adult. The adult's spoken instruction may indeed trigger off certain movements, but it cannot make the actions performed in obedience to the spoken instruction sufficiently stable; nor, in particular, can it stop an activity which has already started. A child at the age of 1.5–2 years can easily start to carry out an adult's instructions (e.g., an instruction to take a named object), but if in the course of the action another brighter or novel object is encountered, the program evoked by the adult's instructions collapses and the child's hand is drawn to the irrelevant but brighter or more novel object. It is almost impossible to inhibit this direct orienting reaction by means of a spoken instruction. It is just as difficult to stop the child's action, once it has started, by means of a spoken instruction or to change it into a different action. For instance, if the child has started to put a ring on the peg of a toy pyramid, the instruction to take a ring off the peg will in some cases make the child continue to act as before even more vigorously, rather than switch to a new action.

Attempts to subordinate the child's actions to a more complex *conditioned program,* formulated in speech, meet with even greater difficulty. Investigations by Yakovleva (1958) and Tikhomirov (1958) have shown that if a child aged 2–2.5 years is given a hollow rubber bulb and is told: "When the light shines you must squeeze it," this merely evokes a direct orienting reaction (a search for the "light"), or a direct motor response (squeezing the bulb), which often cannot be inhibited. The system of connections (the program) arising under the influence of the spoken instruction is easily replaced either by actions in response to the direct impression (the orienting reflex) or by inert continuation of the previous movement (perseveration). Not until the age of 3.5–4 years does the action program evoked in the child by a spoken instruction become strong enough to ensure the necessary action without distraction and to inhibit irrelevant activities.

This brings us to an important conclusion: *The ability to subordinate one's action to a program formulated in a spoken instruction and to inhibit more elementary forms of actions arising in response to direct impressions or as a result of perseveration of previous actions is formed only gradually and is the product of prolonged development.*

These complex forms of programming of movements and actions require a constant waking state of the cortex, so that traces of selective connections evoked by the instruction can be preserved and irrelevant responses inhibited. Naturally these complex forms of voluntary movements and actions are disturbed by lesions of the frontal lobes which depress the state of cortical activity.

The fact that the frontal lobes, with their intimate connections with the reticular formation, are also closely connected with the motor cortex (Part I, Section 2C), and also with the anterior zones of the speech area, with an important role in the formation of internal speech (Part II, Sections 4F, G), makes the frontal lobes a particularly essential part of the apparatus for complex programs of movements and actions. There are therefore good grounds for expecting that the stable performance of programs on the basis of the *signal function of speech* will be particularly severely disturbed by lesions of these parts of the brain.

It was on the basis of these considerations that I began a series of experiments in my laboratory which lasted many years (1950–1965) and was devoted to the analysis of disturbances in the programming of movements and actions of varied complexity in frontal lobe lesions. The aim of these experiments was to study the disturbance of regulation of voluntary movements and actions arising in frontal lobe lesions under the simplest "model" conditions and to examine the essential mechanisms of this disturbance.*

* The results of these investigations were published in: A. R. Luria and E. D. Khomskaya, eds., *The Frontal Lobes and Regulation of Psychological Processes* (Moscow: Moscow University Press, 1966).

If a patient with a massive lesion of the frontal lobes is given a simple instruction (for example, to raise his hand or press a hollow bulb), he can carry it out easily enough (sometimes after a longer latent period and by a slower movement than normally); only patients with the severest symptoms of aspontaneity are unable to do so. If, however, the patient's hands are beneath the bedclothes or they are holding the edge of the blanket, he finds it difficult to carry out even this simple instruction. Because this patient has first to carry out a preliminary subprogram (to take his hands from under the bedclothes or to inhibit his grasping reflex) before going on with the second subprogram (the performance of the action as instructed), he finds it impossible; the spoken instruction leads simply to the appearance of general excitation which is not channeled into the necessary movements. Even when the patient's hand is in the necessary position initially, it is not easy to obtain a stable motor response to the instruction.

Observations by Meshcheryakov (1953, 1966) and Filippycheva (1952, 1966) showed that in response to a direct instruction "squeeze the bulb" such a patient often performs the correct movement, but at the second or third repetition of the same instruction the movement becomes slow, its intensity is diminished, and the patient quickly ceases to produce the required motor response: he will begin by repeating in echolalic fashion the words of the instruction "Yes, yes, press . . . ," but make no movement, and finally he will cease to respond at all. Clearly the verbal instruction quickly loses its conditioned regulatory role, and the motor response is very quickly extinguished, behaving like an orienting reflex which is not supported by additional stimulation. Frequently in these tests defects of a different type appear. After starting to press the bulb in response to the instruction, the patient perseverates the movement he has started and cannot stop, even when told to press *only* in response to the spoken instruction. In that case perseveration of the initiated motor responses and the inert excitation cause the adequate performance of the instruction to disintegrate. Examples of both types of disturbances are given in Fig. 93.

The disturbance of performance of actions in response to a spoken instruction in patients with frontal lobe lesions is also demonstrated in a more complex series of tests aimed at studying the performance of *conditioned motor responses* to a spoken instruction. The patient is told to press the button whenever he hears a tap or whenever the light shines. As a rule, the patient with a massive frontal lobe lesion grasps this spoken instruction clearly and retains it well; however, as the experiments of Meshcheryakov (1953, 1966) and Filippycheva (1953, 1966) showed, he very soon ceases to make the necessary movements, and in response to the corresponding conditioned stimulus he says: "Yes . . . I must press . . . ," but fails to carry out the movement required.

The same result is obtained if attempts are made to produce a conditioned motor reflex in such a patient with the aid of continuous verbal rein-

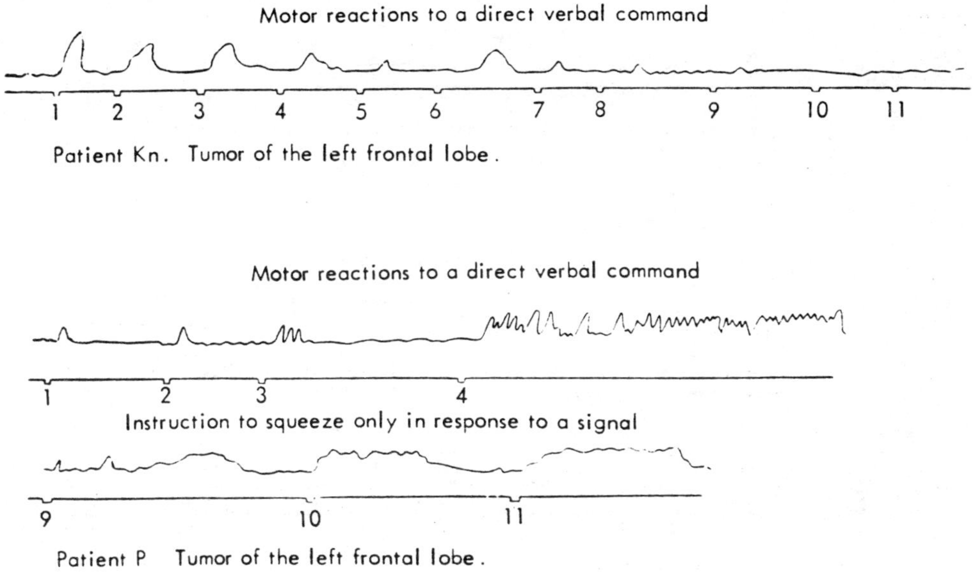

FIGURE 93 Motor reaction of a patient with an extensive lesion of the frontal lobes to a command. Upper line denotes mechanogram of movement of the hand; lower line denotes signals. (*After Meshcheryakov, 1953.*)

forcement. As a rule, if a normal subject (or a patient with a local lesion of the posterior part of the brain) is shown a conditioning stimulus (for example, the flashing of a lamp) several times to accompany the instruction "Press!" he will very quickly respond regularly to each stimulus by the required movement; the stimulus acquires conditioning significance (in this case, formulated by the subject himself), and any subsequent presentation of these conditioning stimuli will start to evoke a stable motor response for which further reinforcement is unnecessary.

This effect does not arise in patients with massive lesions of the frontal lobes. As the experiments of Meshchervakov (1953, 1966) and Filippycheva (1952, 1959, 1966) demonstrated, the stimulus does not acquire its conditioning role, the patient does not establish the necessary connection between the stimulus and the accompanying verbal instruction, and he does not form a stable conditioned motor reflex. This conclusion is illustrated in Fig. 94.

The phenomena I have described above rest on a precise physiological basis. Observations by Grindel and Filippycheva (1959) and Filippycheva (1966) have shown that the dynamics of nervous processes in the pathologically changed cortex is profoundly modified in patients with massive frontal lobe lesions and that normal relations between the cerebral cortex and the subcortical motor ganglia are severely disturbed.

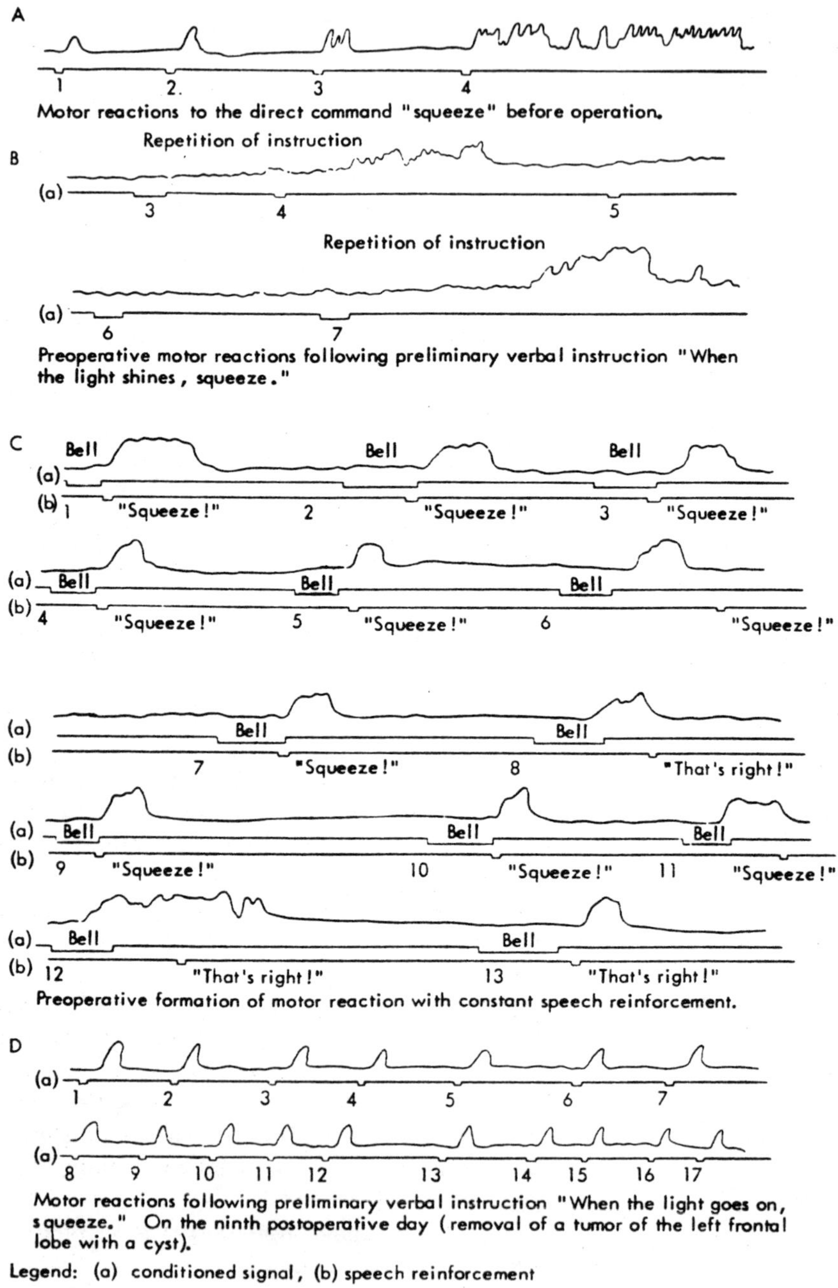

FIGURE 94 Conditioned motor reactions of a patient with an extenive lesion of the frontal lobes. Upper line denotes mechanogram of movements of the hand; lower lines denote (*A*) signals and (*B*) reinforcement. (*After Meshcheryakov, 1953.*)

In one group of these patients the signal or spoken instruction evokes a persistent and inert focus of excitation; for that reason every irrelevant exteroceptive stimulus (something touching the patient's hand, the click of an instrument, the creaking of a door, or sometimes even a simple command: "Pay attention!" or "Get ready!") evokes an immediate motor response or potentiates a movement already started. Naturally in such patients uninhibitable responses between stimuli may also be frequently observed.

In another group of patients, in whom a focus of static excitation is evidently in a state of parabiosis, a different picture may be observed. Often even a direct command fails to evoke the necessary motor response, but the introduction of irrelevant stimuli causes a decrease in the amplitude or even the complete disappearance of motor responses.

The mechanisms I have just described are seen particularly clearly in tests of a more complex type, when attempts are made to form a *complex system (or program)* of motor responses either with the aid of continuous speech reinforcement or after a preliminary spoken instruction.

The simplest type of such test is that involving the formation of a *system of differentiated motor responses to two different stimuli.* In this test the subject is shown two signals, one (for example, a red light) accompanied by the instruction "Squeeze!" and the other (for example, a green light) accompanied by the instruction "Don't squeeze!" One or two reinforcements are sufficient for the normal subject to form a system of connections expressed by the rule: "I must squeeze when the red light shines but not when the green light shines," and all his subsequent behavior will be guided by this rule.

A complex program of behavior such as this is not formed by a patient with a massive lesion of the frontal lobes. As the experiments of Meshcheryakov (1953, 1966), Ivanova (1953, 1966), and Filippycheva (1966) showed, this generalized informative meaning of stimuli, formulated in a general rule, is extremely difficult, and sometimes impossible, to produce in patients with massive lesions of the frontal lobes. Even if the necessary conditioned reflex can in fact be formed (which is by no means always the case), these patients cannot formulate the appropriate rule. When questioned, they cannot say why they gave a motor response to one signal but refrained from doing so at the appearance of the other signal. Frequently they are not even aware that they gave a motor response to the signal when it appeared, and when asked why they pressed, they answer: "Because you told me to." Because of these circumstances the formation of a conditioned motor response takes a very long time in these patients (sometimes scores of combinations are necessary); the system of responses ultimately formed is very unstable and easily breaks up under the influence of distracting conditions. For instance, alternately applying the two stimuli (positive and inhibitory) is sufficient to produce in the patient an inert stereotype of a response

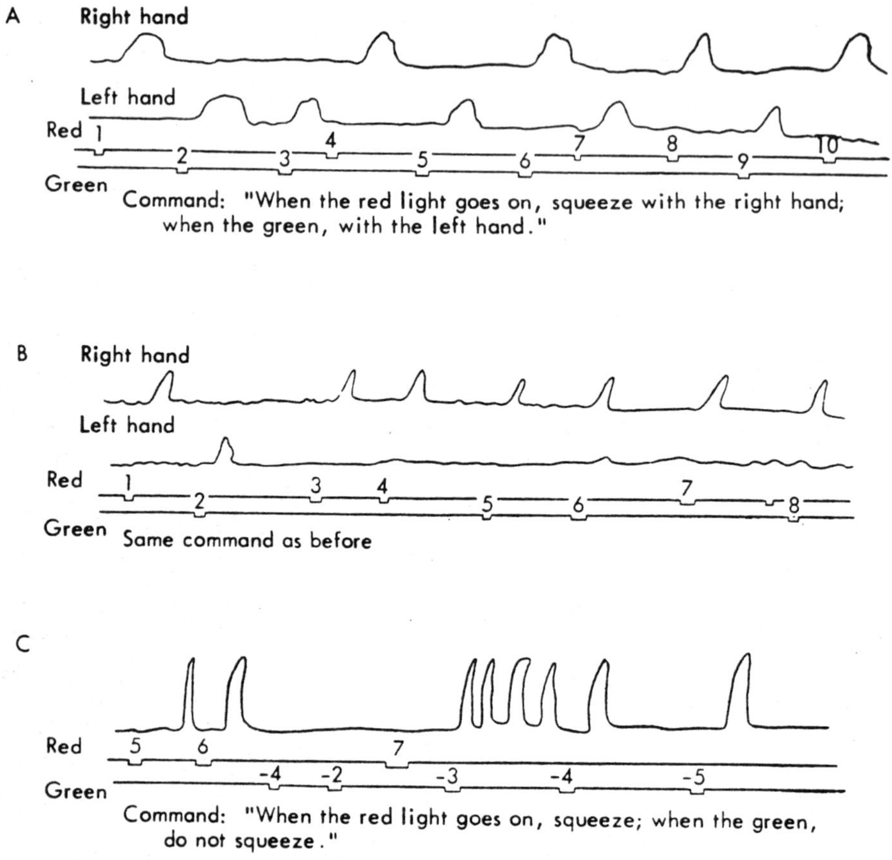

FIGURE 95 Disturbance of the "choice reaction" in patients with tumors of the left frontal lobes. (*A*) Patient T. After the fifth signal correct reactions are replaced by alternate reactions of both hands. (*B*) Patient S. After the fourth signal correct reactions are replaced by stereotyped reactions of the right hand only. (*C*) Patient Yan. After a series of signals there is haphazard pressing in response to inhibitory stimuli (see signals 3 and 4). (*After Ivanova. 1953.*)

to time, and when further stimuli are applied the patient will squeeze to alternate signals inertly, without matching his response to the type of signal.

Disturbances of the formation of complex systems of responses as described above are seen equally clearly in cases when we do not expect that a program of appropriate responses has been formulated by the patient himself, but he is given a ready-made program of action in the form of a spoken instruction. An example of this is the test in which the patient is instructed: "When the red light shines you must squeeze the bulb, when the green light shines you must not squeeze it," or, in another more typical program: "When the red light shines you must squeeze with your right hand, when the green light shines you must squeeze with your left hand."

In normal subjects such an instruction is easily retained, the appropriate system of connections is formed, and it at once starts to control the subsequent course of the responses. We also know that the action program formulated is so strong that no changes in the conditions of the test (introduction of irrelevant stimuli acting as external inhibition, a change in the order of presentation of the stimuli, or the formation and subsequent disruption of stereotyped alternation of the responses) can destroy the action program formulated on the basis of the spoken instruction. A similar stability of action programs once formulated can be observed in patients with lesions of the postcentral or occipito-parietal zones of the brain.

Observations by Ivanova (1953, 1955) and Filippycheva (1960) showed that patients with frontal lobe lesions as a rule have considerable difficulty in retaining such action programs and putting them into effect. Patients with massive lesions of the frontal lobes and the most severe type of frontal syndrome are unable to retain a differentiated spoken instruction firmly; pathological inertia in their speech system is so strong that they will either repeat the verbal construction given to them ("When the red light shines you must squeeze the bulb") or they deform the instruction and deprive it of its logical, differential character. Naturally such patients cannot give a selective system of actions, or they start to squeeze the bulb in stereotyped fashion without the stimulus, or they fail to respond at all.

Patients with a less severe frontal syndrome may succeed in understanding and retaining the spoken instruction satisfactorily, but the instruction does not evoke stable performance of the necessary program. Most frequently such patients carry out the necessary actions once or twice; however, very soon the action program required by the instruction disintegrates, the actions performed fall under the influence of other irrelevant factors, so that a patient who has once been given two signals alternately will continue to respond in stereotyped manner to whatever stimuli are presented by alternate movements of the right and left hand, or he will begin to respond to all stimuli inertly by repeated movements of the same hand (Fig. 95). Characteristically, in all these cases, the spoken instruction did not disappear and the patient could easily repeat it; it simply lost its regulatory significance. The influence of the inert motor stereotype was frequently so strong that even reinforcement of the spoken instruction did not have the desired effect.

This conclusion was demonstrated by a series of experiments carried out by Ivanova (1953, 1966) and Khomskaya and co-workers (1961), in which a patient was instructed to respond to every stimulus by naming the action called for by the instruction (for example, on the appearance of the red light the patient had to say "Right!" and he had to respond to the green light by saying "Left!") while, at the same time, performing the corresponding action. Their observations showed that it was very difficult for patients with lesions of the frontal lobes to perform this test; even if they succeeded in pronouncing the necessary spoken answers, their answers did not perform their essential regulatory function; the patients continued to exhibit stereotyped motor responses which did not match the spoken instructions which they themselves uttered.

One fact is characteristic of all the cases described: an action program formulated in speech, even if given in ready-made form, easily loses its regulatory role; the stimulus presented rapidly loses its informative significance; and the patient's actions fall under the influence of an inert stereotype, so that the selective character of the patient's behavior is disturbed. This inability of the patient to control his actions by means of a program given as a verbal instruction is seen particularly clearly in the next series of tests which I shall now describe.

In these tests the conditioned meaning of stimuli assigned by a spoken instruction conflicts with the direct meaning of the stimulus. In order to carry out the assigned program the subject has to inhibit any tendency to obey this direct meaning of the stimulus, and he must organize his actions in accordance with the spoken program. A typical example of this series is the test in which a patient must give a *weak* response to a *strong* stimulus and a *strong* movement in response to a *weak* stimulus, or he must give a *short* squeeze in response to a *long* acoustic stimulus and a *long* squeeze in response to a *short* acoustic stimulus. Other similar tests of a clinical nature are those in which the patient has to raise his hand *twice* in response to *one* tap and *once* in response to *two* taps or, finally, when he must show his *finger* in response to a clenched *fist* and show his *fist* when the examiner raises his *finger* (Part III, Section 3D).

These tests, providing particularly difficult conditions for the patient and requiring the preliminary decoding of the stimulus as directly perceived and the inhibition of echopraxic responses, can reveal disturbances of complex forms of regulation of actions and disclose defects of this regulation even in patients with a relatively latent or asymptomatic frontal syndrome.

As Khomskaya (1959, 1960, 1966) observed, a patient with a frontal lobe lesion who has been instructed to squeeze the bulb weakly in response to one signal and to squeeze it strongly in response to another signal will remember the instruction well but in practice he is governed by the direct meaning of the stimulus and not by the assigned program, pressing strongly in response to a strong signal and weakly in response to a weak signal. This replacement of the "conflicting" response demanded by echopraxis frequently arises after only the first two or three responses. If the test goes on for a long time it completely replaces the action program, thereby clearly demonstrating that the regulation of actions of a patient with a frontal syndrome is at a lower level, it is no longer recoded in accordance with the assigned program, and it is dominated by the immediate situation. Characteristically, this echopraxic character of movements is still found even in tests in which the patient is instructed each time to repeat the assigned condition (whenever a strong stimulus appears, to say "weak!" and whenever a weak stimulus appears, to say "strong!") and so give himself the necessary instructions. In such cases patients with a frontal syndrome will give themselves the correct spoken instruction but will continue to be governed by the direct meaning of the stimulus. This distinguishes patients with a frontal syndrome from those with lesions of the parietal cortex, in whom the defects of the kinesthetic control of movements can be corrected by additional spoken instructions given by the patient himself. This conclusion is illustrated in Fig. 96.

Similar results were described by Maruszewski (1959, 1966), who observed how patients with frontal lobe lesions had difficulty in carrying out a program involving responding to a long stimulus by short movements. The tendency to fall under the direct influence of the stimulus and to make the duration of the movement correspond to the duration of action of the stimulus proved so difficult to overcome in such patients that even the introduction of additional verbal reinforcement failed to give the required effect. Fig. 97 shows the distinction between a patient with a parieto-occipital lesion, who has no difficulty with this task, and a patient with the frontal syndrome, for whom this task was impossible.

Similar clinical observations were described by Luria, Pribram, and Khomskaya (1965), who observed the difficulty of patients with frontal lobe lesions in carrying out "conflicting" instructions requiring them to respond to one movement by another different movement, and how easily such patients (even though they remembered the instruction given to them) began to make their movement a copy of the experimenter's own movement. Characteristically, as these experiments showed, a patient with a marked frontal syndrome could retain the instruction given to him perfectly well: "When I show you my fist you must show me your finger, when I show you my finger you must show me your fist," but soon stopped performing the necessary recoding and started to make their own movements a copy of the experimenter's. A patient with a relatively mild frontal syndrome can correct these mistakes only when he repeats the instruction and recodes the stimulus aloud. Even this method does not have the desired effect in a patient with a massive frontal syndrome, for although instructing himself aloud: "finger!" he still continues to show his fist and copies the experimenter's movement echopraxically.

Another typical feature of patients with frontal lesions is that their ability to control the process of preparing for a movement, on the one hand, and of stopping a movement, on the other, also is appreciably disturbed. Ob-

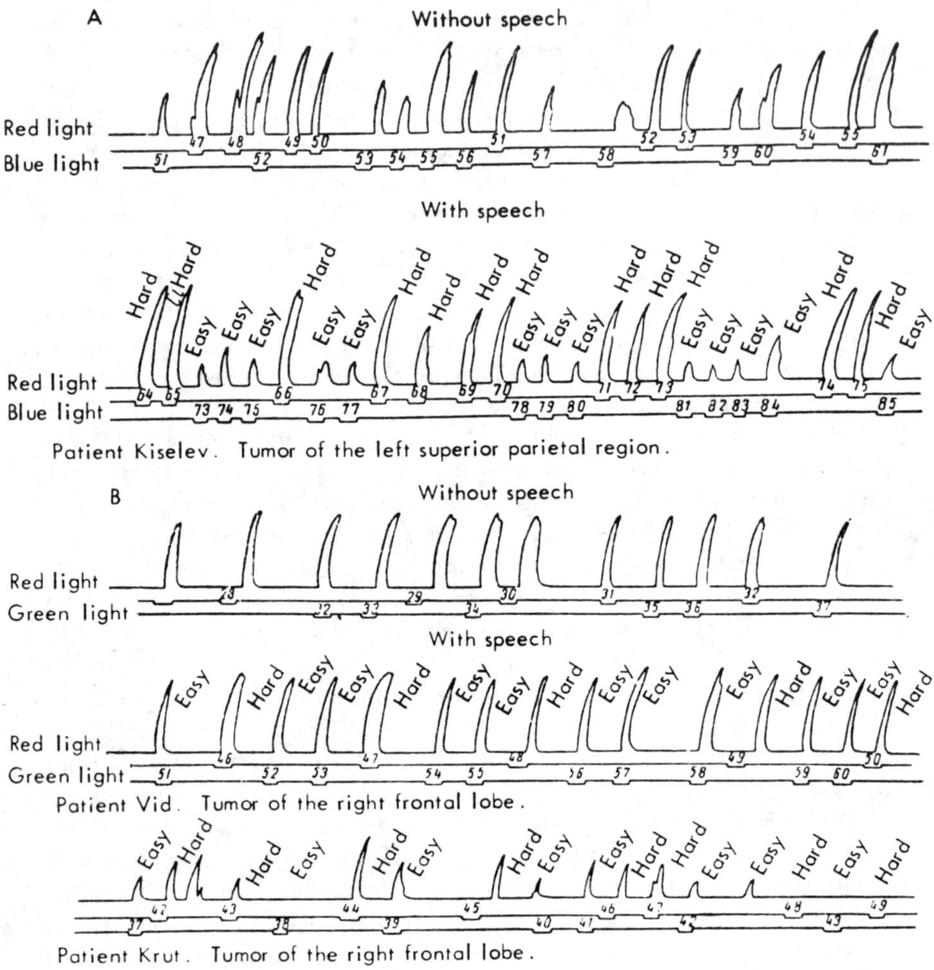

FIGURE 96 Various types of speech regulation of motor reactions in patients with lesions of the parietal and frontal divisions of the brain, as revealed by the reaction to the command, "Squeeze hard when the red light goes on and easy when the blue light goes on." Captions above the mechanogram indicate the patients' speech responses. (*A*) Positive influence of speech on motor reactions in a patient (Patient Kis.) with a tumor of the left superior parietal region. (*B*) Negative influence of speech on motor reactions in patients (Patient Vid. and Patient Krut.) with intracerebral tumors of the right frontal lobes. (*After Khomskaya, 1959.*)

servations have shown that if a normal subject is given the signal "Get ready!" changes appear in his electromyogram, indicating that preparations for movement have taken place (Bassin, 1956), and the latent period of the

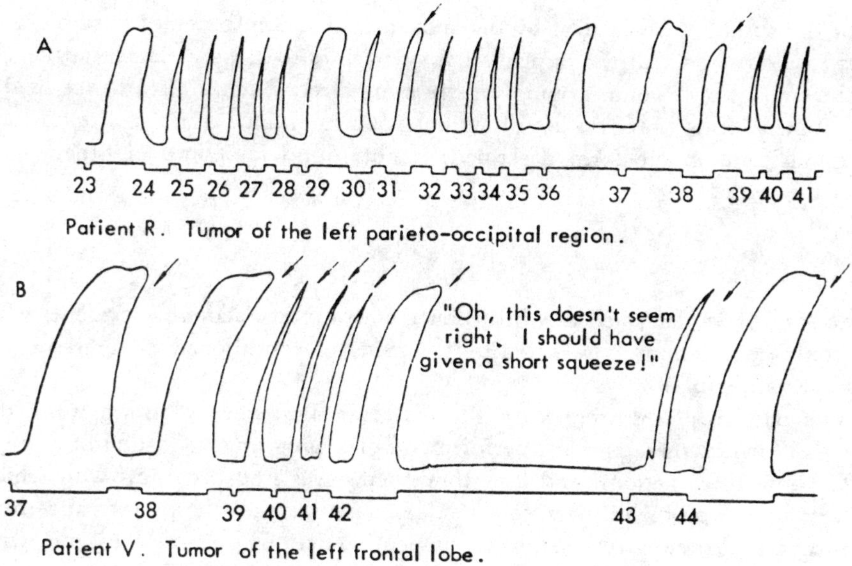

FIGURE 97 Disturbance of the speech regulation of motor differentiation in conditions of conflict in a patient with a lesion of the frontal lobes, as revealed by the reaction to the command, "Squeeze slowly in response to a short signal and quickly to a long signal." The arrows denote incorrect reactions. (*After Marushevskii, 1959.*)

motor response is appreciably shortened (Ioshpe and Khomskaya, 1966). This effect cannot be found in patients with a massive frontal lesion. The speed of their motor response is not appreciably changed.

Similar observations have shown that such patients also have difficulty in controlling the aftereffect of a motor response. A motor response during which, for example, the patient has to perform a movement which lasts as long as the stimulus applied, evokes a definite motor aftereffect. If, however, the subject is given an exteroceptive stimulus (acoustic, for example), informing him of the degrees of contraction of his muscles, this "feedback" about the movement will sharply reduce the duration of the aftereffect of the motor response. As Ioshpe and Khomskaya (1966) showed, this effect does not take place in patients with frontal lesions, and the control of their movements by preliminary warning or "feedback" is ineffective.

We can draw some important conclusions from these facts. A pathological state of the frontal lobes, depressing the active state of the cortex, causes the patient's actions to cease to be firmly programmed by a spoken instruction, and they easily fall under the influence of the direct message of the stimulus or of an established inert stereotype. The conditioned meaning of the stimulus, given to it by the spoken instruction, becomes unstable and is easily lost, so that the patient's behavior sinks to a more elementary level; the control over voluntary movement is impaired. Such a disturbance of the complex forms of regulation of actions is an essential feature of frontal lobe lesions and, in the form described, is not found in lesions of other parts of the brain.

• • •

So far I have described the disturbance of voluntary actions in patients with frontal lobe lesions as revealed by the study of conditioned motor responses to certain stimuli.

The pattern of disturbances is no less clear, however, when we study the way in which these patients perform complex programs consisting of a series of consecutive actions, and how they themselves find programs with which to solve the problems given to them. We soon see that the performance of a program consisting of a series of consecutive actions presents the brain with particularly complex demands. The subject performing such a program has first to retain the visual or verbal instruction given to him; he must grasp the necessary scheme of the action and analyze its subsequent action into a series of successive subprograms; he must constantly check each component of the action as he performs it against the original program and correct mistakes which may arise in the course of its performance. Finally, if the program consists of a group of successive subprograms, it must inhibit the inert aftereffect of each particular act as it arises and must switch at the proper time to the next component of the action; if the cortex is in the pathological state characteristic of massive lesions of the frontal lobes, this will be particularly difficult.

The performance of a sequential action program can be studied by various methods. The patient can be instructed to perform a series of rhythmic movements, such as tapping out a certain rhythm either in response to an audible example or in accordance with a spoken instruction (Part III, Section 4D); he may be given the task of performing a series of definite actions, also in response to a visual pattern or to a spoken instruction (Part III, Section 3B, D). In both cases the patient has to retain the program given, to keep the necessary sequence of subprograms he has to perform, to be able to switch from one to the other, and to inhibit the tendency to fall under influences not connected with the program. Experience shows that the performance of such an action program is particularly difficult for a patient with a frontal lobe lesion.

These difficulties are clearly seen even during relatively simple tests of the repetition of assigned rhythms. Unlike patients with disturbances of acoustic gnosis, accompanying lesions of the temporal lobe, and unlike patients with a disturbance of kinetic melodies, connected with lesions of the premotor cortex, patients with frontal lesions have no difficulty whatever in grasping melodies presented to them by ear or in switching smoothly from one component of the motor program to another. The essential disturbances which arise in these patients are connected with the retention and performance of motor programs given to them.

Patients with the most massive lesions of the frontal lobes are in general unable even to begin to perform programs assigned to them. They listen to the rhythm and then start to tap on the table at random, or they fidget with their fingers, sometimes slipping into continuous nonrhythmic tapping. Patients with less serious frontal lesions will start to tap out a rhythm, but the assigned program is quickly disturbed by perseveration of its individual elements (or subprograms). Or, the patient will substitute a simplified program. For instance, if such a patient is asked to tap out a rhythm consisting of one strong and two weak beats (/″) or of two slow and three fast beats (//‴), the necessary "asymmetrical" program will soon give way to a symmetrical program (// // //), or it will distintegrate as the patient gradually increases the number of taps (Fig. 98).

Characteristically the patient may have equal or even greater difficulty in carrying out a program if the direct pattern (repetitive tapping perceived by ear) is replaced by a spoken instruction. In that case if the patient is instructed to "give one strong and two weak taps," he will retain the spoken instruction and at first will repeat it successfully throughout the test; very soon, however, he will cease to perform the test correctly and will either replace it by a simplified program or he will fall under the influence of an inert stereotype.

Disturbances of performance of an assigned program are particularly well-marked in patients with frontal lobe lesions if the conditions of the test require them to switch from one program to another. In such cases the

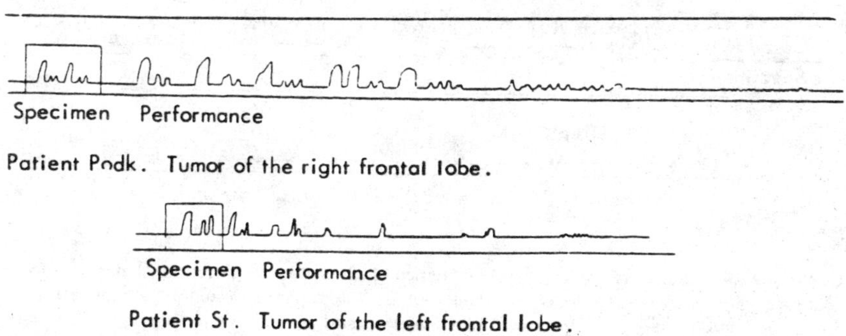

FIGURE 98 Disturbance of the performance of motor rhythms in a patient with an extensive lesion of the frontal lobes. (*After Knyazhev.*)

stereotype arising during performance of the first program is so inert that even after the patient has received a direct or verbal instruction to tap out a different rhythm, he inertly continues to repeat the first one; he will retain the new instruction (given to him verbally), but will not notice that he does not perform the corresponding program.

The characteristic fact that patients with frontal lobe lesions do not check the performance of their actions against the assigned program, but easily simplify it or fall under the influence of an inert stereotype, is seen particularly clearly if, in order to consolidate the assigned program, it is suggested to the patient that he repeat the rhythm aloud—for example, by saying to himself aloud: "one, two; one, two" or "strong, weak, weak," and so on. Getting the patient with a relatively mild frontal syndrome to repeat the spoken instruction aloud in this way may improve the performance of the program; if it is omitted, the same defects arise as before (Fig. 99).

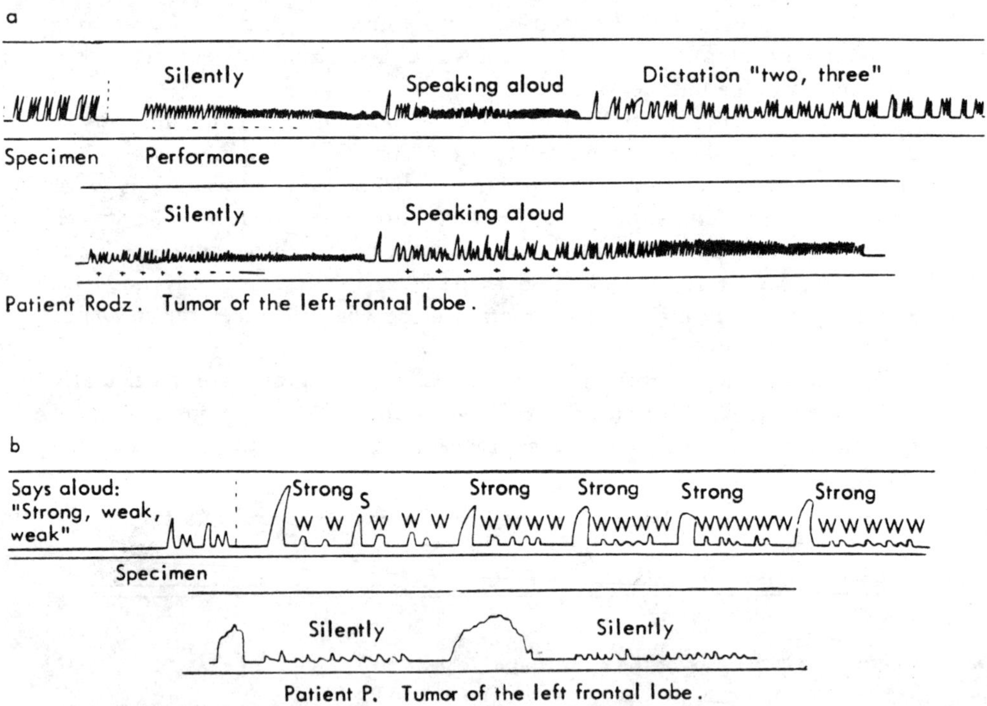

FIGURE 99 Disturbance of the regulatory influence of speech on the performance of motor rhythms in patients with extensive lesions of the frontal lobes. The patient is asked to reproduce the motor rhythm, one strong tap and two weak ones, silently and to the accompaniment of the speech reactions "one, two, three" and "strong, weak, weak." (*a*) Saying the rhythm aloud ("one, two; one, two, three") does not lead to the desired effect. Dictation by the experimenter restores the motor rhythm. (*b*) Pathological inertia of the speech reactions during performance of motor rhythms (the number of "weak" speech responses is increased). When speech reactions are eliminated the motor rhythm disintegrates completely. (*After Knyazhev.*)

Even when patients with a severe frontal syndrome recite the program aloud, they continue to fall either under the influence of factors disturbing the performance of the task or under the same pathological inertia. But this time the inertia extends also to the speech system; in this way the program itself is altered and the patient begins to perseverate the individual elements of the instruction (Fig. 100).

Similar observations can be made in a series of tests suggested by Luria, Pribram, and Khomskaya (1965) and analyzed in detail by Lebedinskii (1966). If patients with a frontal lobe lesion are instructed to continue setting out a series of tokens, in the form of alternation of "asymmetrical" components (e.g., white, black, black), a patient with a massive frontal lobe lesion will at first continue the series correctly as it was begun, but later will either replace it by a series of "symmetrical" components (black, black; white, white), or will begin to set out tokens of the same color. The patient characteristically does this, although he retains the assigned instruction and even corrects any mistakes made by the investigator should the latter do the test himself and ask the patient to point out any mistakes he might make. However, when the patient performs the program himself,

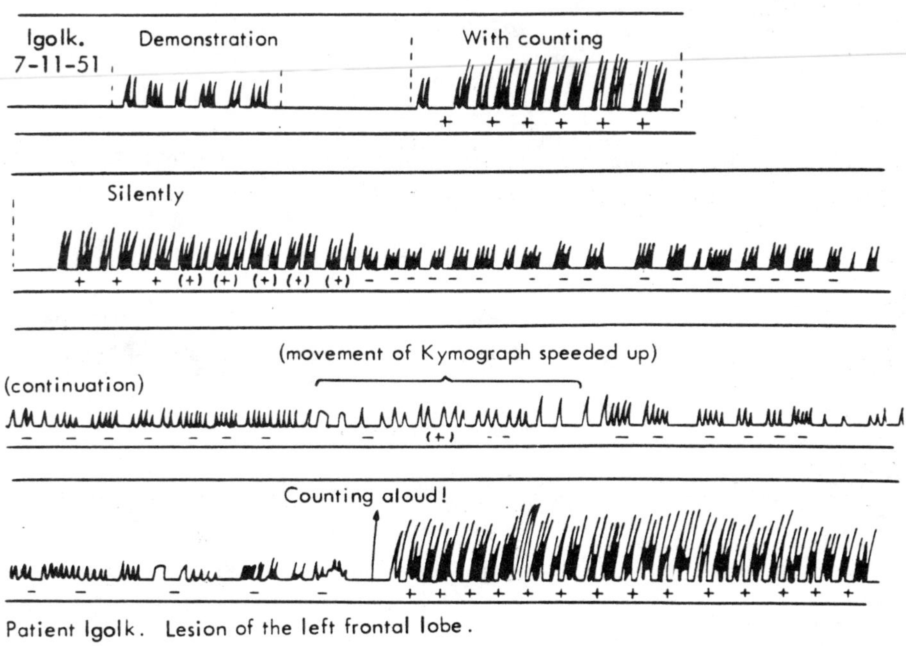

FIGURE 100 Regulatory influence of loud speech on the performance of motor rhythms in a patient with a mild frontal syndrome. Performance of the motor rhythm silently may lead to disturbances of the motor reactions and the rhythm rapidly disintegrates. The motor rhythm is restored by telling the patient to say aloud "one, two; one, two, three." (*After Knyazhev.*)

all the defects described above are found, and he is unaware of his own mistakes. Correspondingly, even if the patient speaks the program aloud this often will not help him; a patient with a massive frontal lobe lesion, who has correctly dictated to himself the words "black, white, white," will continue to oversimplify the program, setting out a series of tokens of the same task or a series consisting of alternate pairs of white and black tokens (Fig. 101).

Even more obvious disturbances are found when a patient with a massive frontal lesion is instructed to draw a series of figures consisting of alternating asymmetrical components (for example, two crosses and one circle). In these cases the performance of the complex program, composed of two subprograms (retention of the numerical index and alternation of the two different figures) is easily oversimplified. Although the patient retains the spoken instruction, in practice he deforms the program, readily replaces it by a simple (symmetrical) program, or falls under the influence of an inert stereotype (Fig. 101b). In this case also, the patient does not compare his performance with the program assigned, and he is not sufficiently aware of his mistakes.

In contrast to massive frontal lesions, a lesion in other parts of the brain never, as a rule, presents such a syndrome of disturbance of the regulation of complex action programs.

• • •

The above observations illustrate the difficulty experienced by patients with massive brain lesions when retaining and performing programs given to them

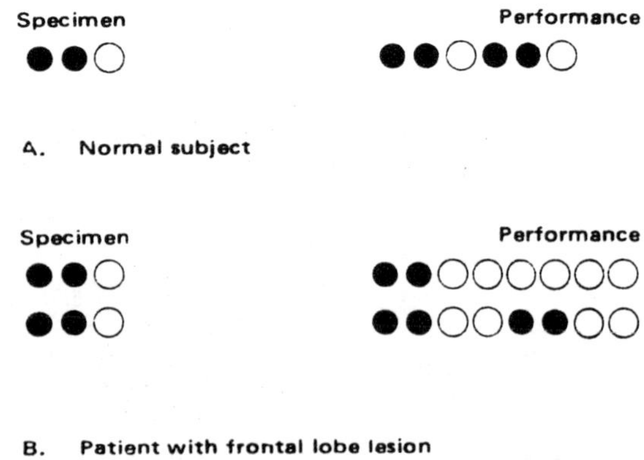

FIGURE 101 Simplification of assigned program of arranging tokens by a patient with a massive frontal lobe lesion

and the ease with which they replace them by simplified programs or by inert stereotypes. Equally marked disturbances are seen in situations in which patients with a frontal syndrome have to find their own essential program and subordinate their future actions to that program.

Recent investigations (Newell, Shaw, and Simon, 1956; Reitman, 1966; De Groot, 1965) have shown that the finding of the necessary programs in cases when the subject has no ready-made solutions obeys the laws of stochastic analysis. After analyzing the situation as it has arisen, the subject distinguishes those components of it which are most likely to lead to a solution; later, it is these methods of solution (generalized by the subject and put into the form of an hypothesis) that determine his subsequent actions. The actions corresponding to these hypotheses, or these heuristic courses, begin to arise with the greatest probability; actions not corresponding to these hypotheses are inhibited, and the probability of their occurrence is reduced.

These investigations showed that the formation of such goal-directed actions passes through several stages and incorporates many inappropriate actions, starting with those stages when the search is extended in character and ending with those in which the search begins to take place in a contracted manner, requiring only a few "heuristic" features, each carrying maximal information and determining the future organized course of the action.

Perhaps the most convenient model with which to investigate the formation of such heuristic action programs is that suggested by Sokolov (1960). The subject is instructed to touch a group of elements (e.g., tokens), forming letters, with his eyes closed. In some cases, letters (e.g., P and R) differ in only a few minor features. These features (e.g., the place where the "tail" begins) possess the greatest heuristic importance and ultimately are sufficient to decide into which category the suggested structure belongs. Tests have shown that normal subjects, after touching such structures, at first make many searching movements, but later they conduct their search in a manner adequate to the program, reduce their movements, and begin to pick out the heuristic points selectively, and so quickly reach the necessary solution (Sokolov, 1960; Arana, 1961).

The process of finding the necessary search programs is totally different in character in patients with a marked frontal syndrome. Observations by Tikhomirov (1961, 1966) have shown that patients with frontal lobe lesions start to solve this problem by touching the letters presented to them, but their search is chaotic in character and their searching movements are not guided by definite hypotheses. These patients do not begin to pick out elements carrying the greatest information and providing evidence of the most likely solution to the problem of which of the two letters they must identify. Having touched the whole of the letter and obtained the necessary solution, they do not form a suitable program for the subsequent search, and they do not contract their movements. Their search remains chaotic and easily falls under the influence of irrelevant and nonheuristic factors: they begin to trace mechanically the outline of the structure (falling under the influence of the immediate situation), or they repeat over and over again movements they have begun, replacing active searching by an inert stereotype.

In all these respects they differ sharply from patients with lesions of the parieto-occipital zones, whose difficulties are of a different character and can easily be overcome with external assistance. These observations are illustrated in Fig. 102.

Similar results can be obtained in another series of tests in which the subject has to discover under which of twelve squares an object is hidden. Tests carried out originally by Bruner (1956) and later in a modified method by Tikhomirov (1964) show that normal subjects gradually contract their search by forming appropriate action programs which are guided by "stochastic prediction" of the position of the original object. However, observations on patients with massive lesions of the frontal lobes, undertaken by Tikhomirov and Poznyanskaya, show that the necessary action programs are not formed; instead patients continue to search for the object by random movements, or (much more often) they subordinate their movements to irrelevant, nonheuristic factors, and turn over all the squares or inertly reproduce actions they have performed before (Tikhomirov, 1966). These tests yield results very similar to those of Pribram, who investigated the character of searching movements in monkeys after removal of the frontal lobes (Pribram, 1954, 1961, 1966).

Examination of the structure of purposive voluntary movements and actions thus shows that patients with frontal lobe lesions lack firm control of programs formed on the basis of speech, that such programs are formed

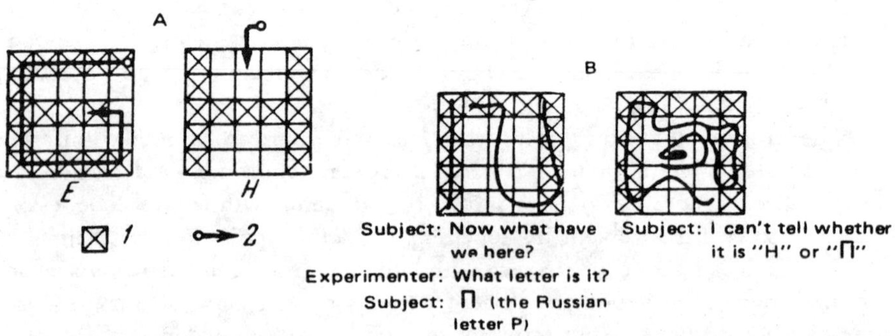

FIGURE 102 Searching movements while fingering letters (A) by normal subjects and (B) by patients with frontal lobe lesions (after Tikhomirov): (1) occupied square of the board; (2) trajectory of movement of subject's finger.

only with difficulty by these patients, and they do not regulate the subsequent course of their activity. The facts I have just described show how easy it is for these programs (which in normal subjects firmly control their actions) to be disturbed under the influence of external factors or inert stereotypes; and how quickly the actions of patients with massive frontal lesions lose their goal-directed, selective character. We do not yet know the physiological mechanisms that cause this disturbance of behavior. However, there is reason to suppose that it is based on a change in the structure of voluntary acts, including a disturbance of the state of cortical activity, as a result of which programs created with the aid of external or internal speech readily lose their dominant character and are no longer stronger than the action of irrelevant stimuli and inert stereotypes of previous actions. The disturbance of the regulatory function of speech, which can be identified by special study of patients with frontal lesions is, in all probability, the most important consequence of these changes.

Frequently, the influence of irrelevant associations is so considerable in such patients that the sharp line of division between one activity and another is disturbed and a characteristic "contamination of activity" develops. A patient with a massive tumor of the right frontal lobe (Fig. 90) was asked to draw a series of patterns named by the experimenter (a circle, a triangle, a cross, etc.). At first he could do this easily. However, when he came to draw the cross, he drew it and then without any instruction he began to draw a whole series of figures, saying as he did so "cross, window, grain" and so on. This action became understandable when it was discovered that two days before an experiment had been carried out, to test his word memory, in which the word "cross" followed by the words "window," "grain," and so on had appeared. This one common link between the two completely different activities was sufficient for one of them to be replaced by the other.

E. GNOSTIC DISTURBANCES

The literature on disturbances of mental processes that are produced by lesions of the frontal lobes contains only isolated references to concomitant sensory changes. A few authors have mentioned that with lesions of the frontal lobes interoceptive and proprioceptive sensations are impaired. On the basis of such observations, Munk (1881) and others postulated that the frontal lobes are concerned with the analysis of internal stimuli and that they may be interpreted as the "Körpergefühlsphäre." However, no further observations have been made in this direction and these findings must be subjected to a detailed analysis in future research.

Equally little attention has been paid to the changes in exteroceptive (for example, optic) perception in patients with frontal lobe lesions. An exception is the work of Teuber (1959, 1964) who found definite defects of this nature in patients with frontal lobe lesions. These defects were discovered in connection with the assessment of the position of lines in space if their axes did not coincide with the position of the patient's body. Such a patient could evaluate the coordinates of external space correctly if his body was in the normal vertical position but made gross errors when the position of his own body was changed.

The scarcity of investigations on the sensory changes associated with frontal lobe lesions is due to the fact that in classical psychology it had become more or less traditional to approach perception as a complex but relatively passive process, carried out primarily by the sensory divisions of the cerebral cortex and not by the brain as a whole. Another factor contributing to this state of affairs is the fact that the frontal lobes were regarded more from the point of view of their motor than of their sensory functions. However, there is every reason to suppose that a lesion of the frontal lobes, like a lesion of other parts of the cerebral hemispheres, is accompanied by changes in the various forms of perceptual activity, although such changes are very different from the disturbances in patients with lesions of the temporal, occipital, and postcentral regions of the cortex.

We know that optic perception is not a passive reflection of signals reaching the eyes; it is an active search process manifested as the selection of the most informative points and their comparison with each other. Besides sensory it also possesses motor components, in the form of active movements of the eyes that "palpate" the object being perceived and that thus enable the essential elements to be distinguished; it is this motor component of perception, responsible for the complex work involved in the analysis and integration of the optic stimuli, that is primarily affected by lesions of the frontal lobes.

The findings obtained in the study of patients with frontal lobe lesions (Luria, 1939, 1963; Andreeva, 1950; Filippycheva, 1952) have led to the specification of a group of symptoms indicative of a profound disturbance in perceptual processes and attributable to these lesions. The changes in optic perception observed in patients with a frontal lobe lesion will now be briefly considered.

In certain lesions of the cortex, especially of its occipital zones (Part II, Section 3C), in visual-field defects, and so on, visual perception may be substantially disturbed: however, in these cases, the defect of visual analysis and synthesis may, to some extent, undergo compensation, particularly as a result of activation of orienting movements of the gaze. For instance, as has been shown (Part II, Section 3C), a patient with tunnel vision can orient himself satisfactorily in visual space so that his defect is almost unnoticed by others.

The results are completely different in patients with lesions of the frontal lobes. The disturbances of optic perception found in such patients are most frequently associated with substantial disturbance of the active searching activity which, under normal conditions, creates the "orienting basis of actions" (Gal'perin, 1959, 1965). In patients with frontal lesions this defect is often manifested as a disturbance of the active process of examination of the object, with disturbance of active fixation. These defects of the motor aspect of optic perception form the basis of the syndrome of disturbed gnostic processes observed in patients with lesions of the frontal lobes. That is why a patient in whom an extensive frontal lobe lesion has led to optic atrophy, as frequently occurs with such tumors, cannot compensate for the diminishing visual acuity and the narrowing of the visual field by means of active scanning movements; his optic perception thus acquires that inactive character so often described by investigators. That is why a patient with a frontal lobe lesion perceives far fewer details of a picture shown to him than a patient with a lesion of the posterior divisions of the brain. These observations (Luria, 1963), which are in agreement with common clinical findings, have recently been verified by a special method that enables the movements of the eyes to be fixed during the prolonged examination of an object. Disturbances of the searching scanning movements arising from frontal lobe lesions have also been described by Teuber in a personal communication.

Closely connected with the disturbance of scanning movements is the second symptom of the pathology of optic perception produced by lesions of the frontal lobes — difficulty in perceiving fast-moving objects. If a patient's gaze is fixed on a certain object and the object is suddenly shifted elsewhere, he sometimes will continue to fixate the same point in space inertly and be unable to find the object (Luria, 1963). This inertia of gaze is also related to the phenomenon, described in the literature, of impairment in "fluctuation of attention," or of the variation in perception during the examination of figures marked by unstable equilibrium of their component elements (such as Rubin's figures). The investigations of Teuber (1960*b*), Cohen (1959), and others have shown that patients with severe, especially bilateral, lesions of the frontal lobes do not exhibit the normal fluctuations of visual attention, that for periods of several minutes they see only one of two competing optic structures. Similar findings were obtained earlier by the present author (Luria, 1939). Closely connected with these observations is our discovery that the perception of Weigl's (several conceptual elements introduced into a single entity) or Poppelreuter's figures (a group of shapes superimposed on each other) by patients with frontal lobe lesions is characterized by persistent inert attention on only one detail of the pattern, reflecting the patients' inability to move from one component to another as easily as they should.

The disturbance of optic perception in patients with frontal lobe lesions may also be revealed when they examine Gottschaldt's figures, in which individual details are masked by a general geometrical structure. These methods will be described subsequently (Part III, Section 6B). The patient with a lesion of the frontal lobes is unable to actively pick out the required part of the pattern from the whole, even if first shown to him. Similar results were described by Teuber and Weinstein (1956) and Strauss and Lehtinen (1946) in tests involving the distinguishing of figures from a homogeneous and structurally organized ground or field. Patients with frontal lobe lesions showed considerable difficulty in all such tests, readily slipping back to the "strong" structure. It is especially interesting to analyze the method by which such patients solve the problem of distinguishing a particular structure from the homogeneous background. In the technique originally described by Revault d'Allones (1923), a patient with a frontal syndrome is asked to pick out a certain structure (for example, a white cross) from a chessboard. This patient invariably will continually wander to other squares, unable to fix his attention on the problem and distracted by irrelevant stimuli. The graphic record of the attempt by a patient with a frontal lobe lesion to solve a problem of this type demonstrates the instability of the system of optic connections formed by the preliminary instruction and the ease with which such patients yield to the influence of directly acting visual factors (Fig. 103). The disturbance of optic perception in frontal lobe lesions is thus associated not only with a disturbance of scanning movements. It may be assumed that this symptom is based on the pathological inertia of the nervous processes, which is clearly apparent in both the sensory and motor spheres in patients with a frontal syndrome.

These suggestions have been confirmed by special experiments (Luria, 1963). If a patient with a severe frontal sydrome is presented with a number of different geometrical figures, among which there are letters (or numbers), in a tachistoscope, he will begin to perceive the figures incorrectly but will perseverate and will inertly transfer the properties of one figure to another. An example of this lack of mobility of perception is shown in Fig. 104. It can be seen that the elements of one of the figures (the sun with its rays) have been transferred inertly by the patient to the other figures, so that he begins to picture them with similar rays and even to transfer this feature to the letters. A similar manifestation of the pathologically inert aftereffect of a stereotype is the replacement of a geometrical figure, after three or four presentations in a tachistoscope, by another. The inert aftereffect of the first figure persists for a long time in the patient with a frontal syndrome and the drawing of the new figure retains elements of the one formed previously (Fig. 105).

This phenomenon cannot yet be described in sufficient detail. It is possible that, besides inertia in the sensory sphere, there are manifestations of pathological inertia in motor processes influencing the drawing of the

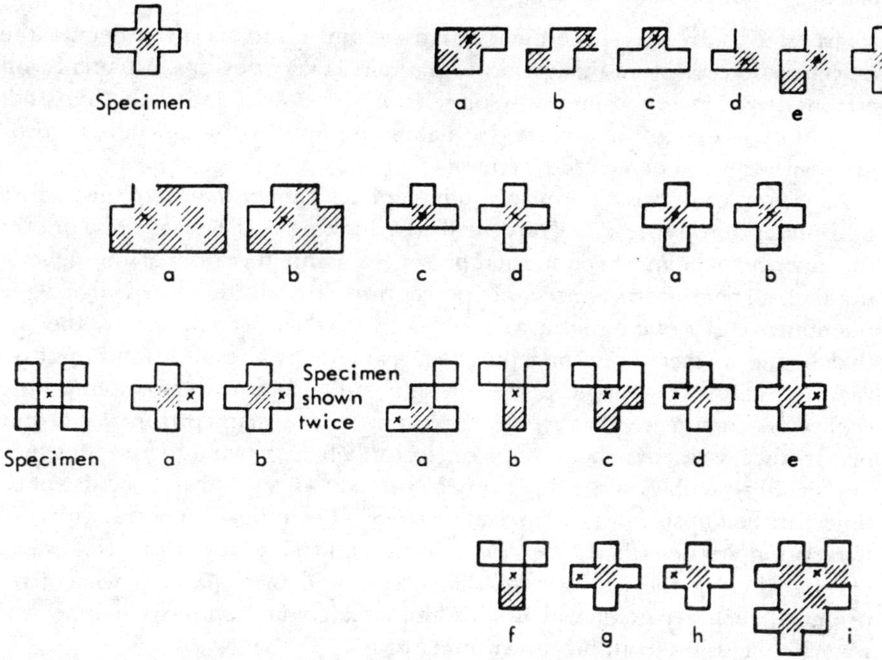

FIGURE 103 Distinguishing of a given structure from a homogeneous background by a patient (Patient Sar.) with an extensive tumor of the left frontal lobe with cyst formation. The diagrams indicate the trajectory of the movements of the patient's finger during the attempt to distinguish the required figure from a chessboard. The cross (X) denotes the square in question which was indicated each time by the experimenter.

structure as perceived by the eye. Several factors, however, suggest that pathological inertia of the sensory processes is fundamentally involved. This conclusion is confirmed by the observations of Zislina (1955), who described a considerable increase in the duration of successive visual images in patients with a frontal syndrome.

• • •

We have described the series of disturbances arising in a patient with a frontal syndrome in relatively simple processes of visual perception. However, there is every reason to suppose that the more complex the activity of perception, the more it necessitates a preliminary, planned approach to the material perceived, the more severely will the process of perception be disturbed in patients with frontal lobe lesions. Analysis of clinical findings shows this view to be correct.

When a patient with a frontal sydrome is instructed to examine the picture of an object lying in an unusual position or a complicated picture that can be interpreted only after preliminary analysis and synthesis of its details, the defect of perception in this group of patients is very obvious. A patient with a frontal sydrome examines only one detail of the picture shown to him and, instead of analyzing the picture, he makes an impulsive judgment in accordance with the one perceived fragment.

As examples of these impulsive judgments, a patient may take the picture of a butterfly to represent a bird or fly (by looking at the wings only) or take the picture of a mushroom to represent a lamp (because of the general outline). These disturbances of perception are distinguished from the phenomena of optic agnosia (described in Part II, Section 3C) by the fact that in the former the wrong judgment is made as a result of an impulsive verbal reaction to a single perceived sign and that usually no attempts are evoked to correct it. That is why a patient with a marked frontal sydrome nearly always reaches the wrong conclusion when shown a picture in which one detail resembles some other object, for example, if shown a picture of an object turned upside down. (Special methods of investigation of this aspect of perception are described in Part III, Section 6.) In the latter instance, instead of first altering the position of the picture and then deciding what it represents, such a patient will usually immediately and impulsively reach the wrong conclusion from his direct impression.

If this disturbance in analytic-synthetic activity is accompanied by pathological inertia of a previously given verbal evaluation, the manifestations of the dynamic "frontal agnosia" will be intensified, so that a patient with a severe frontal syndrome who has, for example, decided that a picture represents an apple will begin to describe all pictures subsequently shown to him

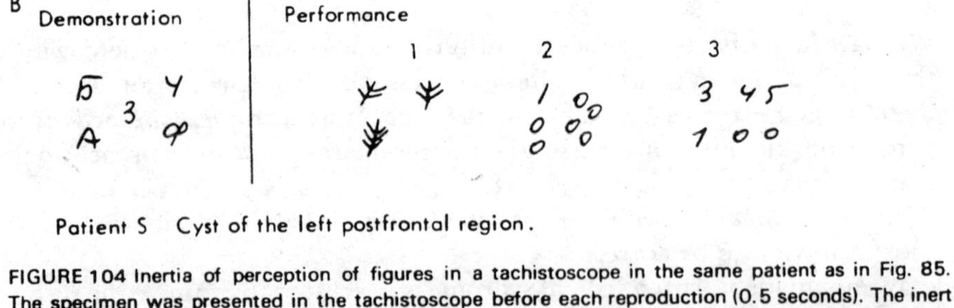

FIGURE 104 Inertia of perception of figures in a tachistoscope in the same patient as in Fig. 85. The specimen was presented in the tachistoscope before each reproduction (0.5 seconds). The inert stereotype of the Christmas tree should be noted (perseveration from the drawing of the sun's rays), as well as the inert stereotype of the circles.

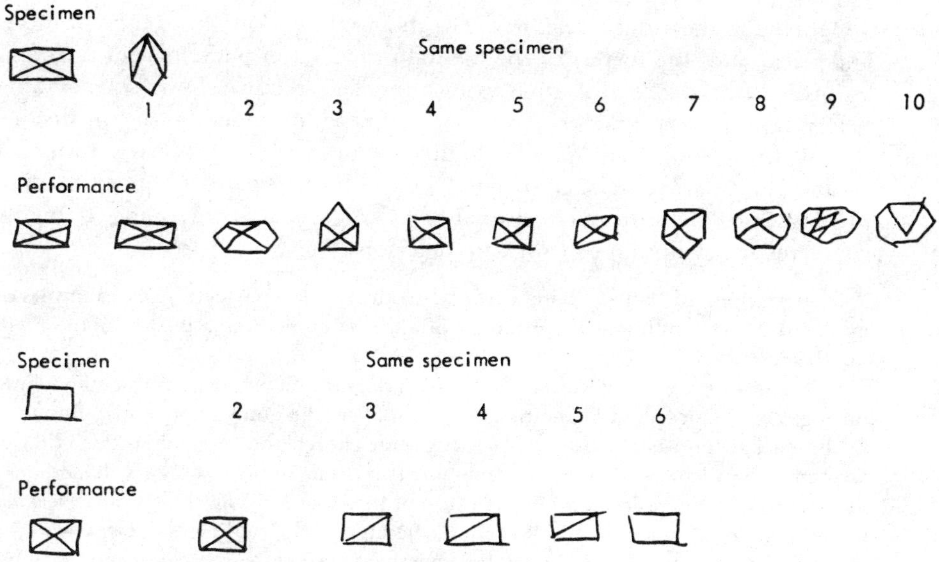

Patient S. Cyst of the left postfrontal region.

FIGURE 105 Inert aftereffect of a perceived structure in a patient with a lesion of the frontal divisions of the brain (the same patient as in Figs. 85 and 86). Specimen was presented in a tachistoscope before each reproduction (0.5 seconds).

as fruit, regardless of what they actually represent. It seems that the changes in perception exhibited by patients with a "frontal syndrome" reflect disturbances inherent in these patients in any form of purposive activity. If, therefore, the conditions of perception are made more complex, these defects will stand out with special clarity.

The characteristic disturbance in perceptual activity found in a frontal syndrome is seen most clearly during *analysis of the meaning of thematic pictures*. Understanding of the meaning of a story told in pictures (for example, the sort of event forming the subject of most works of art of this type) is the result of a complex psychological process. It begins with the perception of the individual details of the picture, a search for its "centers of meaning," and the formation of a hypothesis concerning the general meaning of the picture, and it continues with the synthesis of the individual conceptual elements and the correction of unsatisfatory hypotheses until the overall meaning of the picture becomes clear (Bruner, 1957). If the picture is simple and represents a familiar situation, the process of perception is soon complete and the meaning is grasped at once. If it is complicated and requires the formation of new systems of connections before it can be understood, the process involves a prolonged examination and stage-by-stage analysis of the subject matter.

Because of these difficulties in the formation of preliminary generalizations and because of the inertia of the mental processes in patients with a frontal syndrome, the process of analysis of a thematic picture shows considerable deterioration. The patient gives way to random judgments, conclusions drawn from individual parts of the picture, irrelevant associations of meaning, or inert verbal stereotypes. These tests of the patient's understanding of thematic pictures may justifiably be regarded as revealing a highly characteristic symptom of frontal lobe lesions.

Investigations of patients with a frontal syndrome have yielded many examples of impaired understanding of the meaning of a thematic picture, and some of these will now be described.

A patient with a marked frontal syndrome is shown a picture depicting a man falling through the ice; people are running to help him, near the pond a sign reads "Danger", in the background is the outline of a city with church towers, and so on. Without analyzing the picture as a whole he may interpret it as showing "high-voltage lines" or "wet paint" or "wild animals" (because of the "Danger" sign) or "war" (because of the people running) or "the Kremlin" (because of the outline of the city with the spires in the background), and so on. It is characteristic that these irrelevant connections formed by the patient are not inhibited or analyzed critically and that the one detail perceived by him is sufficient for him to reach a conclusion about the whole picture.

Sometimes a disturbance in the perception of the meaning of a picture may occur in patients with a relatively mild frontal syndrome. For instance, we have seen many such patients interpret Klodt's painting *The Last Spring* (depicting a dying girl sitting in an armchair, while her aged parents look at her anxiously and her sister stands by the window in an attitude of profound grief) as "a wedding" (because of the white dress) or "given in marriage" (because of the pose of the old people watching the girl from behind the door, reminiscent of the details of Fedotov's picture *The Major's Courtship*), and so on. Instead of a true analysis, there are only irrelevant associations, evoked by individual fragments of the picture. We have also observed defects in the understanding of the expressive elements of a picture. For example, such patients thought that a widow, standing by a coffin in an attitude of profound despair, was "a woman with a handkerchief in her hand... yes, of course, she has a cold" (Evlakhova, unpublished investigation).

Particularly clear evidence of a disturbance of the active examination of complex objects in patients with frontal lobe lesions can be obtained by a careful study of the patient's eye movements throughout the period of examination. Several methods can be used for investigations of this kind (Part III, Section 6A). In particular, eye movements can be traced by recording movements of a beam of light reflected from a mirror attached to the patient's eye (Yarbus, 1965) or by a photoelectric method (Vladimirov and Khomskaya, 1962).

Investigations of this kind (Yarbus, 1965) have shown how the examination of a complex picture by a normal subject includes complex searching movements of the eyes, picking out the most informative features and comparing them with one another. A change in the instruction controlling the process of examination significantly modifies the direction of these movements so that the subject's eyes begin to pick out more and more new features reflecting the tasks set by the instruction (Fig. 106). Examination of Repin's picture "The Unexpected Return" reflects this highly complex system of searching movements of the eyes which themselves aid in analyzing the meaning of the picture; it also shows how the character of the search varies when the instruction presents the subject with fresh problems (Fig. 106, A, B).

The picture is completely different if the eye movements of a patient with a marked frontal syndrome are recorded as he examines a complex picture. Examples of the record of eye movements during examination of the same picture by patients with frontal lesions are given in Fig. 106, C, D. These records show that when the patients examine the picture they do not make the necessary searching movements with their eyes; they pick out just one detail (which they fix for a very long time) and, on this basis, they guess the meaning of the picture as a whole; later their eye movements either continue to fix this same detail or they follow a chaotic course. It is interesting to note that even if different instructions are given to the patient ("Tell me what the people in the picture are wearing?" "How old is the man?" "How well off do you think the family is?" "How long has the man who has returned been away from home?" and so on), there is no change in his eye movements; either they remain chaotic in character or, most frequently of all, the patient inertly continues to fix one particular point (Luria, Karpov, and Yarbus, 1965).

The disturbance of visual analysis of complex pictures may assume different forms in patients with frontal lobe lesions, but in every case there is a profound disturbance of the programs of active analysis of the material presented.

A patient with a frontal lobe lesion meets with even greater difficulty when he attempts to understand the meaning of a series of pictures depicting the stages of a story. The establishment of a single logical chain of thought relating to several pictures requires careful analysis of details and subsequent integration, which may be particularly difficult for patients with a frontal lobe lesion. Zeigarnik (1961) found that this task brings to light gross perceptual disturbances in patients with a frontal syndrome, and instead of finding a single chain of meaning between the pictures, they merely describe the individual pictures or their details.

Hence, the processes of visual perception in patients with a frontal lobe lesion are not always as fully preserved as it might seem. However, the disturbances in visual perception in these patients differ significantly from those in patients with optic agnosia caused by lesions of the occipital and occipitoparietal regions of the brain for in the latter the disorder is based on a defect in visual-spatial synthesis.

Very little is known about the factors associated with impaired gnostic activity in patients with frontal lobe lesions. There is no doubt, however, that in these disturbances, as in others, an important role is played by pathological inertia of the nervous processes, as revealed in the motor and, possibly,

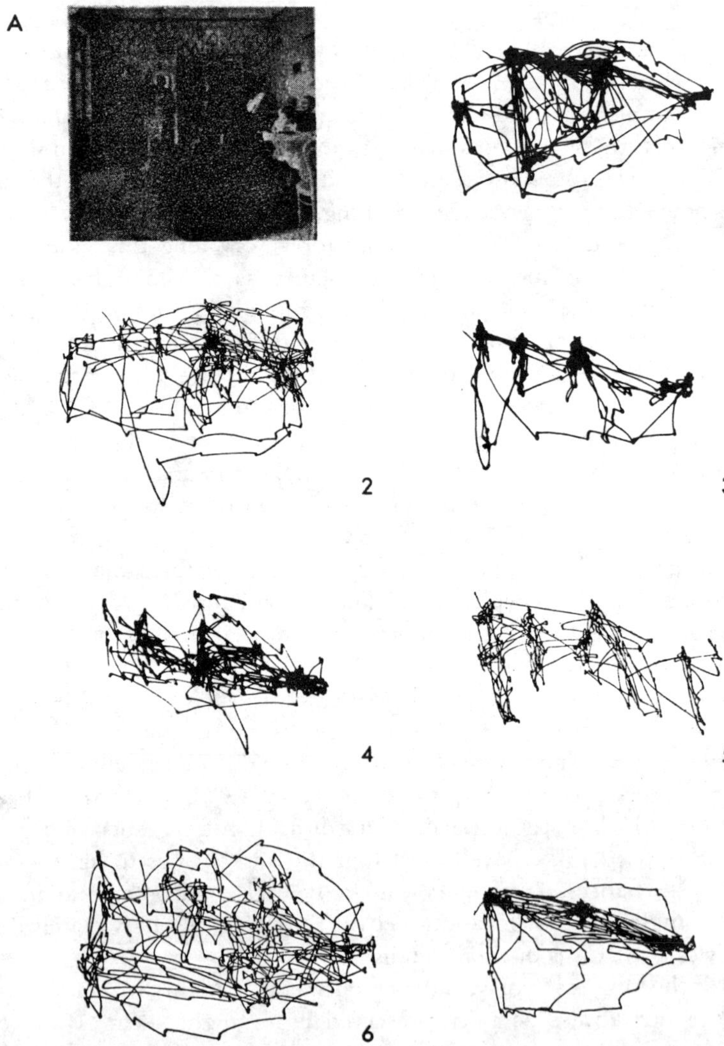

FIGURE 106 Patient T. Left parieto-occipital lesion with syndrome of simultaneous agnosia: searching movements of eyes intact. (C) Patient U. Intracerebral tumor of right

sensory spheres; this influence is chiefly manifested in defective preliminary, orienting scanning movements, which have been discussed. It is possible that these disturbances in gnostic activity are also based on disturbances in successive proprioceptive syntheses, about which little is known and which must be the subject of special investigation. Finally, it appears that a derangement in the process of comparing the actual object with the subjective evaluation

B

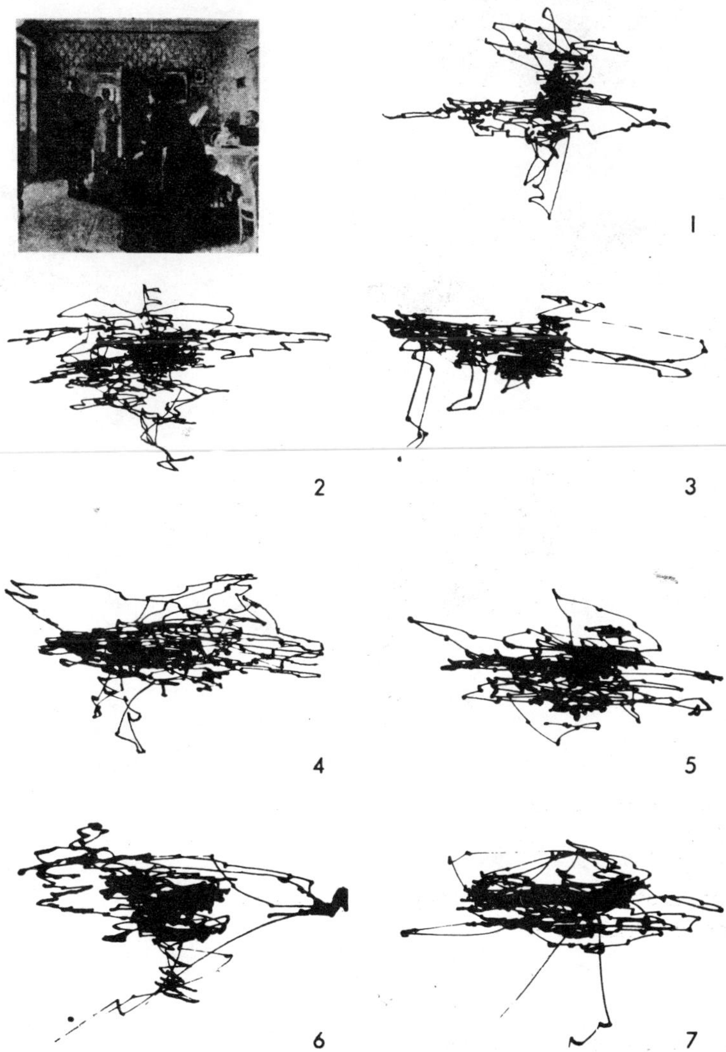

frontal lobe with severe frontal syndrome: searching movements of eyes absent. (D) Patient G. Injury to frontal region with atrophy of the substance of one frontal lobe and a severe frontal syndrome: searching movements of eyes completely absent.

C

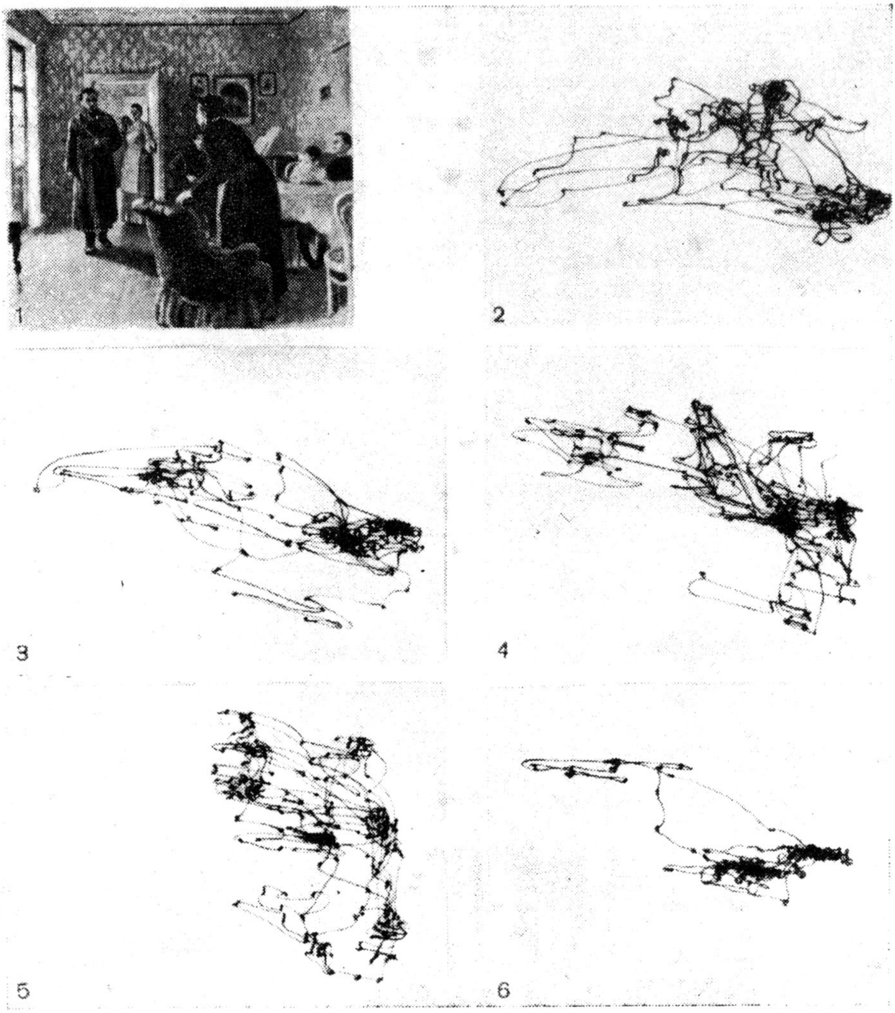

FIGURE **106** (Continued)

of it, leading to failure to correct mistaken conclusions, is fundamental to these gnostic disorders.

F. MNESTIC DISTURBANCES

A disturbance of mnestic processes is observed in patients with lesions situated in various parts of the cerebral cortex. However, the character of these disturbances varies considerably with their situation.

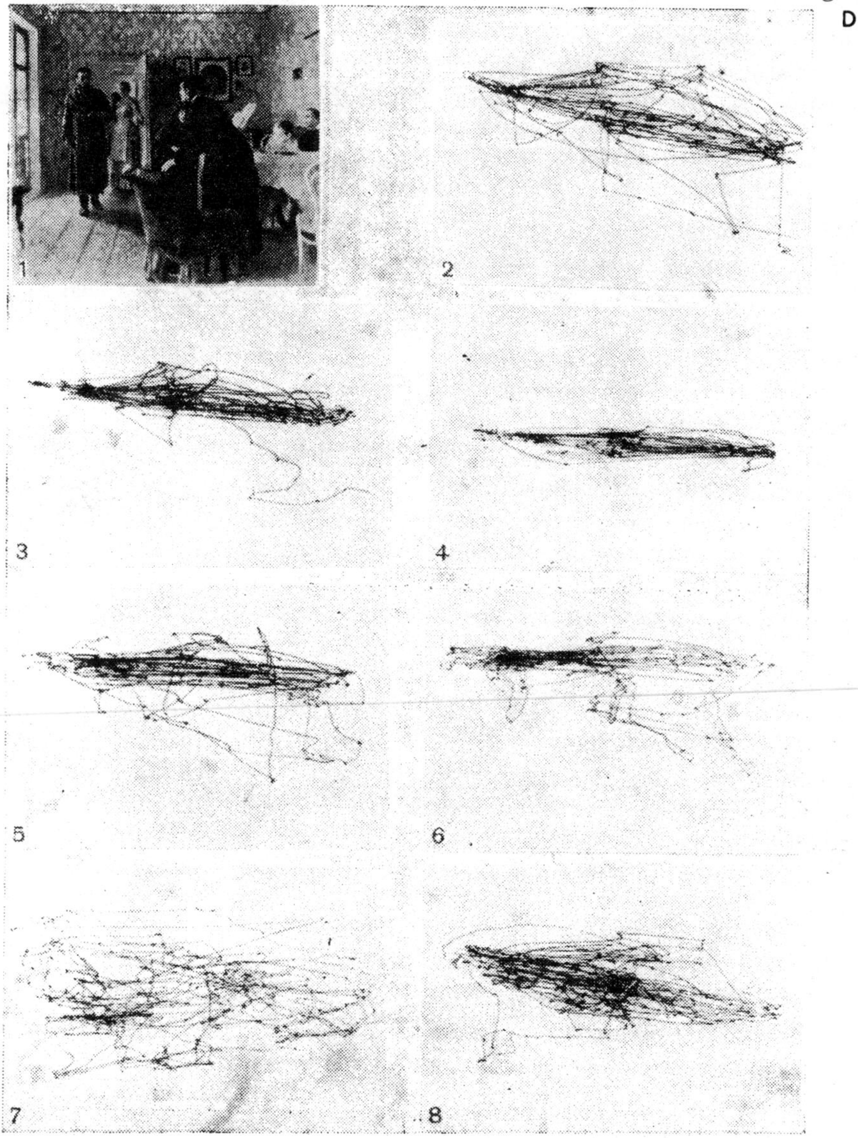

FIGURE **106** (Continued)

As has been explained, disturbances of mnestic processes arising from lesions of the cortical divisions of the auditory, optic, and cutaneokinesthetic analyzers are, as a rule, of a very special character and constitute an inseparable part of sensory and gnostic disturbances. For instance, mnestic disorders in patients with a lesion of the left temporal region are most conspicuous in connection with acoustic (or combined acoustic and verbal) images and are successfully compensated for by the intact optic or tactile images. In patients with a lesion of the occipital and occipitoparietal divisions of the brain, however, they show more of the properties of optic or optic-spatial defects and may be compensated for by the system of acoustic or motor images. And, as stated previously, even the special character of disturbances of sequential processes at higher levels of activity is maintained in such patients, and the compensation for defects by means of intact analyzers remains the basic principle of rehabilitative training.

We do not yet know how far this principle of greater involvement of mnestic processes of a particular modality extends to cases of frontal lobe lesions. It is possible that a disruption in the stability of interoceptive and motor images is more prominent in these cases, but this is a problem for future investigation.

At this stage we may dwell in rather greater detail on the disturbance of the mnestic processes associated with frontal lobe lesions because the impairment of the selective structure of activity typically found in these patients leads to obvious impairment not only of the gnostic, but also of the mnestic, processes. The profound derangement of the processes of voluntary memorizing is a no less important symptom of a lesion of the frontal lobes than the disturbance of voluntary action of that of selective, intelligent perception.

Mnestic disorders manifested by a disturbance in delayed reactions were observed in animals after extirpation of their frontal lobes. Disturbances of delayed reactions were particularly prominent when irrelevant stimuli acted on the animal in the interval between the conditioned signal and the reaction. When no irrelevant stimuli were applied during the experimental procedure, the selective delayed reactions were much better preserved (Mishkin, 1957; Pribram 1959*a*; etc.).

Disturbances of mnestic processes in patients with lesions of the frontal lobes have been studied in considerable detail and have been investigated clinically. Patients with a severe frontal syndrome accompanied by a generalized loss of cortical tone may exhibit gross memory defects in the form of a disturbance of the selectivity of images, which has already been discussed. Such patients can "recognize" the doctor when he approaches, but very often this recognition is not sufficiently precise. Often one simple sign (spectacles, hair color, etc.) is enough to make the patient take the doctor for somebody else. The reproduction of pre-existing verbal connections is a similar manifestation of this defect. For example, instead of his present address, the patient may give the name of the town where he lived previously or the name of a town that sounds like that of the one in question. In fact, the effect of irrelevant (but more firmly established or possessing a similar component link) connections is frequently so strong that patients of this group are unable to give even a most elementary personal history. The system of images associated with the patient's personal experiences is particularly severely affected.

The character of the disturbance of mnestic processes accompanying frontal lobe lesions becomes particularly clear in the course of special psychological testing of the processes of *voluntary memorizing*. Defects in the mnestic functions are obvious under these conditions even in those patients who have no marked general cerebral symptoms. However, they are not as apparent when different aspects of the function are investigated. The *ability to recognize* a previously indicated object is usually more intact in these patients than is active reproduction.

Even patients with a relatively extensive frontal syndrome can name the object in a picture shown to them or can find the picture among several others.* However, no sooner is the range of the material widened or no sooner is the material presented under conditions requiring a change from one system of connections to another, than it is apparent how easily the mnestic processes are influenced by the pathological inertia of the images or by irrelevant, previously formed connections. For example, once a patient with a severe lesion of the frontal lobes has given a name to a picture shown to him, he will call all other pictures by the same name, without correcting his mistakes.

The disturbance of the selectivity of the systems of connections stands out particularly clearly in experiments involving the active reproduction of material. As has been described (Part II, Section 5C), patients with a severe frontal syndrome may be able to perform a single task easily (for example, draw a circle or cross) but when successive tasks are called for often perseverate in the preceding action instead of carrying out the new task. These patients show signs of confusing the afterimages of the new and the previous instruction if the scope of the activity is widened.

Similar findings may be obtained in classical experiments involving the reproduction of a series of four or five presented words or numbers (after a single presentation). Patients with a lesion of the frontal lobes will easily reproduce a series of three or four words or numbers presented to them. If, however, after a single reproduction of the series, a series of different words or numbers is presented or the same elements are presented in a different order, they have considerable difficulty in reproducing the new series. The afterimages of the preceding series are inert and begin to interfere with the reproduction of the new variants. Adequate reproduction of the new series is replaced by repetition of the old patterns.

This observation can be seen particularly clearly if a patient with a frontal lobe lesion is asked to memorize and recall a series of 3 or 4 words, and he is then asked to memorize a second series of the same number of words. Frequently the inert traces of the previous series becomes intermingled with the recall of the second series; the patient will start to recall a series con-

* An exception is found in cases with extensive lesions where disturbances of the frontal systems are associated with disturbances of the limbic and diencephalic regions.

sisting of some words of the first and some of the second series. This defect may be seen even more clearly if, after learning the second series of words, the patient is then instructed to recall the first series again. The inertia of the previous traces in such cases is so strong that he will recall a mixed series with contamination by elements of both. This defect is particularly pronounced in patients with lesions of the fronto-temporal zones or in patients in whom the syndrome of a lesion of the medial zones of the brain is superposed on the background of general depression of memory processes (Part II, Section 2G).

These manifestations are distinguished from the symptoms of inertia that have been described in connection with motor aphasia by the fact that patients with a marked frontal syndrome are usually completely unable to take account of the mistakes in their reproduction of words and cannot correct a wrongly reproduced series.

The pathology of mnestic activity is made particularly apparent in patients with frontal lobe lesions by experiments involving the learning by heart of large series of elements (for example, ten or twelve words or numbers). In order to facilitate the learning by heart of such a series presented several times in succession, a normal subject compares the actual series with the one he has reproduced, pays particular attention to words he has missed, and gradually increases the number of words memorized. A patient with a frontal syndrome performs this task in a completely different manner. As a rule, he at once memorizes a few words (no more than three or four) and on subsequent presentations of the series continues to repeat the same elements as before, without comparing the result with the original series. Once he makes a mistake, he inertly continues to repeat it without correcting it. The entire subsequent process of memorizing becomes nothing more than the simple reproduction of the group immediately learned, with no active attempts to increase the number of memorized elements. The "memorizing curve" thus becomes plateau-like and remains at a low level (three to five words or numbers memorized), showing no tendency to rise. A few such curves, plotted by the author from the results of Zeigarnik's experiments, are shown in Fig. 107.

The impairment of the active character of the mnestic processes in patients with a lesion of the frontal lobes is revealed by the profound change in their "strategy" of learning by heart that is revealed in the memorizing experiments. The experiments of Hoppe (1930) showed that when a normal subject is about to undertake a particular task he sets for himself a "level of aspiration," taking account of the success or failure of his previous actions. For instance, having memorized six words, the subject will not aim at memorizing ten or twelve words at the next presentation of the series. Unless he sets a suitable target for himself, allowing him to successfully accomplish the task, he will not increase the level of future demands on himself.

Although the strategy involving the level of aspirations is usually maintained by patients with lesions of the posterior divisions of the brain, it is severely disrupted in patients with a frontal syndrome. The requirement pattern is abnormal in such patients; when asked how many words they expect to memorize, they continue to repeat the same number even though it does not match the results already achieved. This abnormality is an essential aspect of the disturbance of mnestic activity in these patients. An example of this pathological change in the dynamics of the level-of-aspiration formulation is given in Fig. 108.

The profound disturbance in the structure of the mnestic activity of patients with a frontal lobe lesion is particularly marked in experiments

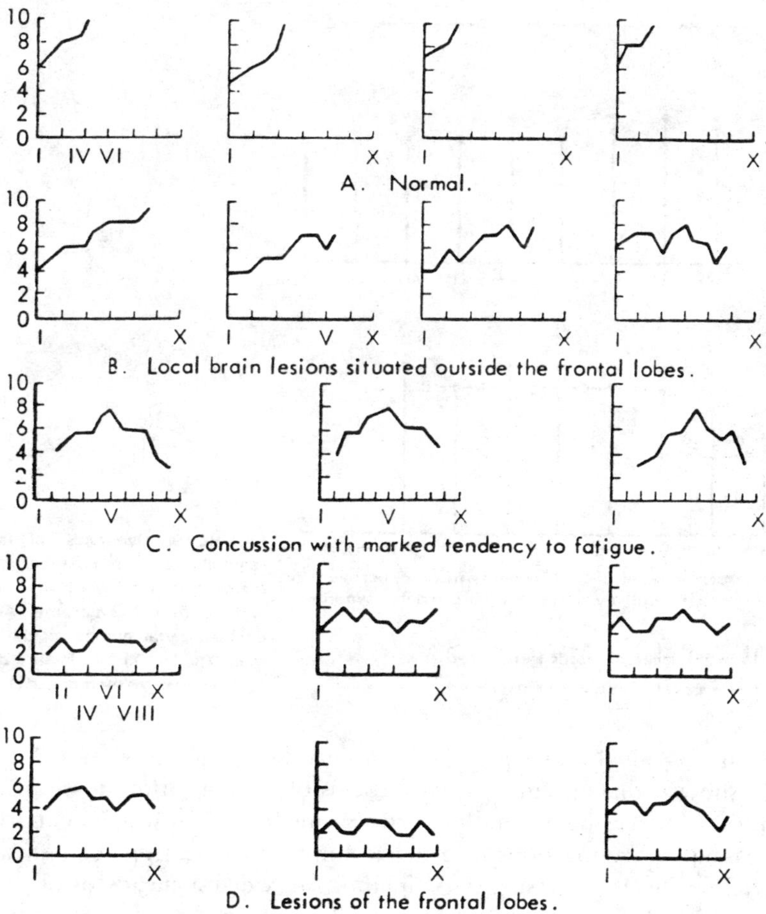

FIGURE 107 Memorizing curves of normal subjects and of patients with lesions of the frontal lobes. The curves indicate the results of attempts to memorize a series of ten words during ten successive presentations. Abscissa denotes serial number of the experiment (I to X); ordinate denotes number of words memorized (1 to 10). (*Devised from data presented by Zeigarnik.*)

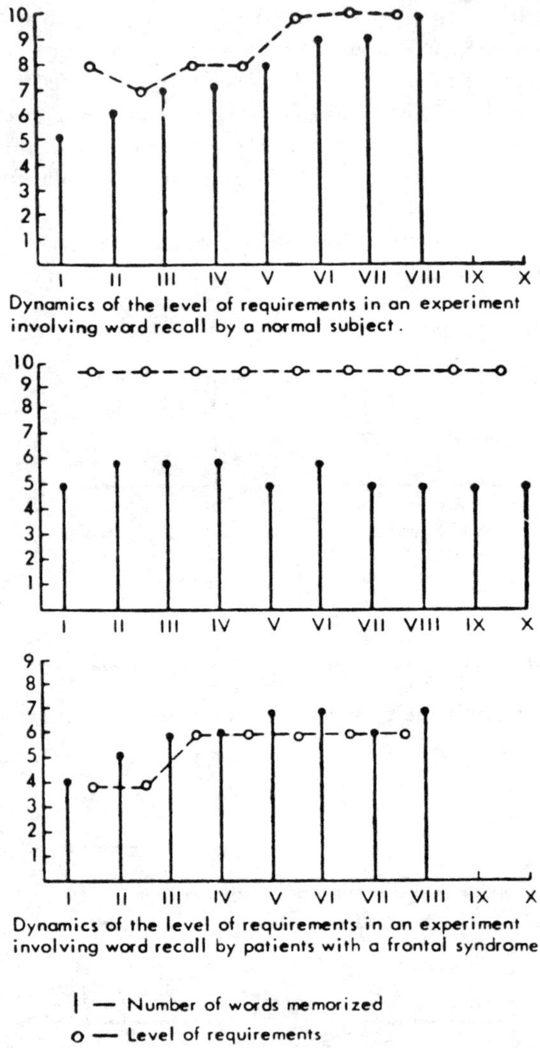

FIGURE 108 Dynamics of level-of-requirement formulation during memorization of words in a patient with a frontal syndrome. Abscissa denotes serial number of the experiment (I to X); ordinate denotes number of words memorized (1 to 10).

involving so-called "indirect memorizing." Some 30 years ago, Leont'ev (1931) showed that in children the process of memorization develops along the lines of increasingly complex forms of mediation, by which he meant the use of auxiliary connections in order to improve the learning of a particular material by heart. His suggested method provided a means of objectively investigating the use of this process and its effectiveness. The experiment consists essentially of the following: A subject is asked to memorize a series of words, each time choosing a picture or making a conventional mark on a piece of paper. Subsequent examination of the picture he has chosen or the mark he has made should bring back to his memory the auxiliary connection he has formed, and by means of this connection he should be able to reproduce the desired word (Part III, Section 7D).

Experiments carried out by means of this technique on patients with lesions of the posterior (temporal and parieto-occipital) divisions of the brain showed that, in principle, the use of auxiliary connections for memorizing is still possible. Moreover, a form of rehabilitative training incorporating these auxiliary connections can be devised for these patients (Luria, 1948). In contrast, patients with a lesion of the frontal lobes give completely different results in these experiments. The process involved in the formation of auxiliary connections, required as future aids in the reproduction of a given word, is grossly deranged, and as a rule such patients do not even associate a particular word with the appropriate picture. The subsequent presentation of the picture, therefore, does not restore the required word, and it may even act as a source of irrelevant associations.

Experiments involving indirect memorizing thus demonstrate that the basic mnestic defect in patients with lesions of the frontal lobes does not *reside* so much in the appearance of verbal connections and associations as in the *selective utilization of these connections in accordance with the patient's requirements*. Hence, a breakdown in the mnestic process when a series of auxiliary devices is offered is an important sign of a disturbance of higher mental activity in patients with lesions of the frontal lobes (see below, Part III, Section 7).

I shall again examine below some of the features distinguishing disturbances of semantic memory characteristic of patients with a severe frontal syndrome.

G. INTELLECTUAL DISTURBANCES

We shall conclude our account of the disturbances of the higher mental processes arising from frontal lobe lesions by analyzing the characteristic changes in intellectual processes developing in these patients.

The neurological and psychopathological literature contains comparatively few references to intellectual disturbances in patients with lesions of the frontal lobes, and such details as may be found are contradictory. According to these reports, these contradictions are reflected clinically. While indicating the marked changes in the behavior of these patients, and noting that one of the more important signs of the "frontal syndrome" is a characteristic dementia with associated disturbances of mental activity, clinicians have at the same time reported the preservation of the "formal intellect" of such patients. Some writers, for example Hebb (1942, 1945), state that resection of a large portion of the frontal lobe may not be followed by any appreciable lowering of intellectual functioning.

The experimental psychological literature repeats these contradictions in clinical observation. Many authors who have used quantitative psychometric intelligence tests when studying patients with lesions of the frontal lobes obtained inconsistent results. For instance, the investigations of Mettler and co-workers (1949), Hebb (1950), Crown (1951), Klebanoff *et al.* (1954), Le Beau (1954), and others show that frontal topectomy and leukotomy are not necessarily followed by any obvious decline in the level of performance in these tests and that, therefore, there are no grounds for assuming that any significant change in the intellectual processes takes place because of lesions of the frontal lobes.

In sharp contrast to these findings are the results obtained by psychological qualitative analysis. Of the comparatively few studies of this type, one of the first to be published was that of Kleist (1934), who described a frontal lobe syndrome whose central feature was a change in intellect. In Kleist's opinion, a lesion of the frontal lobes leads to the development of a passive, alogical intellect, in that the intellectual activity of these patients ceases to comprise a chain of logical operations by means of which the patient carries out certain tasks. As a rule, abstract, logical intellectual activity is replaced by the alogical reproduction of randomly formed associations.

A closely similar position, although based on different philosophical concepts and experimental findings, was taken by Goldstein (1936, 1944), who claimed that a lesion of the frontal lobes of the brain is accompanied by a lowering of "abstract orientation" and of "categorical behavior." Klages also (1954), adopted this viewpoint; he noted that patients with a lesion of the frontal lobes are unable to understand definite logical relationships.

Halstead (1947) obtained instructive results from his experimental investigation of the intellectual processes in patients with a lesion of the frontal lobes. He found that the classification of objects, which is based on abstraction, is beyond them. The patients he studied had considerably lowered performance ratings in respect to special tests, devised by himself, involving abstract intellectual operations. These tests are described in Part III, Section 12C. One of the most detailed investigations of the nature of the intellectual disturbance in a patient who has undergone bilateral resection of the frontal lobes was undertaken by Brickner (1936); the patients he investigated demonstrated considerable intellectual deterioration. Finally, Zeigarnik (1961), in her careful investigation of the intellectual processes in patients with frontal lobe lesions, not only discovered considerable changes in the intellectual processes of such patients, but also analyzed them qualitatively.

What are these disturbances of the intellectual processes observed in the so-called frontal syndrome? Part of the answer to this question may be given by a recitation of the results of investigations carried out in recent years.

• • •

During gross preliminary investigation of patients with a frontal syndrome no constant failure to understand the meaning of words or phrases or logical-grammatical relationships, such as observed in the different forms of aphasia, is apparent. However, both processes quickly begin to undergo profound changes in these patients when perceptual activity is required. Special attention must therefore be paid to the investigation of the disturbances of intellectual processes in patients with a frontal lobe lesion.

Psychological investigations have shown that intellectual activity begins when the goal cannot be attained by available methods and where a definite *task* arises.

The first stage of intellectual activity is analysis of the conditions of the task and the identification of its most important elements. This stage, creating the "orienting basis of actions," may be extended in character to begin with, and supported by external aids; later it acquires the character of an internal "intellectual action," which has recently been a subject for psychological study (Gal'perin, 1959, 1966).

The whole subsequent process of intellectual activity, built up on the basis of this preliminary orientation, assumes the planned character that has also been studied in the course of recent investigations of heuristic processes (Vygotskii, 1956; Bruner et al., 1956; Newell, Shaw, and Simon, 1958). These investigations have shown that the hypotheses based on this orienting activity give the subsequent course of intellectual processes their goal-directed, selective character. Systems of connections corresponding to these hypotheses are more likely to appear, whereas those not corresponding to the hypotheses are less likely to appear; irrelevant connections not embodied in the hypotheses or in conflict with them are inhibited. If to this we add the fact that the whole process of searching for hypotheses and putting them into effect is accompanied by comparison between the attempts made and the original plans, the complex and selective character of intellectual activity will be relatively clear (Part III, Section 12A).

In patients with frontal lobe lesions, with the behavioral features I described above, this complex process of intellectual activity is severely disturbed.

Such patients as a rule do not begin to analyze the situation created by the task presented to them. The orienting basis of the intellectual action is either completely omitted or greatly contracted; the individual elements of the task are not compared with one another; and no hypotheses are put forward on their basis, whereby the more appropriate connections would be more likely to arise and the less appropriate, not corresponding to the hypothesis, would be inhibited. For this reason heuristic connections are no longer stronger than irrelevant, random, or perseverating connections, and the whole process of intellectual activity loses its selective character. The process of comparing the action performed with the conditions of the task as a rule is omitted. No effort is made to ascertain if the action corresponds to the original purposes.

Let us attempt to trace the characteristic features of the disturbance of intellectual processes in patients with frontal lesions by first analyzing how the processes of practical or constructive intellectual activity are modified in these patients. We shall then go on to describe the disturbances of the "verbal intellect" observable in such cases.

• • •

A typical example of practical (or nonverbal) intellectual activity is the solution of constructive problems. In these cases the subject is requested to perform a certain constructive task (for example, to build something out of bricks). The task has no direct solution but requires preliminary familiarization with the available material and the performance of certain preliminary calculations; only then, when a scheme or program for solving the problem has been created, can the subject begin to carry out the task with the aid of the auxiliary operations he has found.

One such example is given by tests widely used in clinical practice to study constructive praxis (for example, to construct particular designs out of matches, requiring the formation of a preliminary scheme of solution). Special methods developed in psychology have also been employed in which a large tube of one color is made up from a group of small tubes, painted different colors on different sides (Link's test). Or, patterns can be made by arranging tubes, as in Kohs' test (Part III, Section 6D).

Usually these tests are used to investigate patients with lesions of the parieto-occipital zones of the brain and a syndrome of constructive apraxia. However, they can also serve as useful methods for the investigation of disturbances of intellectual activity in patients with frontal brain lesions.

To solve a constructive problem the subject has first to familiarize himself with the conditions of the problem and with the material available. In the test involving construction of a Link's cube, the subject must calculate the number of small cubes with different colored sides required and verify that a sufficient number of these cubes are available. Analysis of the material and its preliminary classification are thus essential components of the adequate solution of the problem. Only after this preliminary stage can the subject proceed with the stage of creating a scheme of a possible solution, to which all his subsequent actions will be subordinated.

As was pointed out above (Part II, Section 3E), patients with parietal-occipital lesions and with a syndrome of constructive apraxia can retain the instruction given, and they can make the necessary attempts to familiarize themselves with the conditions of its performance. The only difficulties they experience are those connected with the disturbance of their orientation in the spatial relations which they have to use.

The picture in patients with frontal lesions is totally different. As Gadzhiev (1951, 1965) observed, patients with a frontal lobe lesion and a marked frontal syndrome do not begin to solve the constructive problem by preliminary familiarization with its conditions; only 3 of the 28 patients whom he studied from this group preserved the normal scheme of the intellectual act by first familiarizing themselves with the conditions of the task, classifying the available material, and composing a preliminary program for the solution. The overwhelming majority of patients at once started to attempt to solve the problem by placing one cube against another, without noting the number of cubes with sides painted the correct color, and they prematurely used up cubes which they should have kept for future stages of the construction. Naturally these immediate attempts, not under the control of a program drawn up beforehand, could not lead to the desired result and, after several attempts, the patient abandoned the task.

Investigation of the formation of an assigned pattern from Kohs' blocks by patients with lesions of the frontal lobes (Luria and Tsvetkova, 1965; Tsvetkova, 1966) yielded similar results.

It will easily be seen that Kohs' test requires the subject to examine the pattern he has to make from the individual blocks and to pick out the necessary constructive elements which, as close analysis of this test shows (Part III, Section 6D), do not coincide with the elements of direct impression. The task can be correctly undertaken only after a preliminary recoding of "elements of expression" into "elements of construction."

As I stated above (Part II, Section 3E), patients with lesions of the parieto-occipital zones make persistent attempts to carry out this preliminary phase of constructive activity, and they experience difficulty only in the spatial analysis of the material. They are clearly aware of their difficulties and they attempt to correct their mistakes.

In contrast, as Tsvetkova (1966) showed, patients with frontal brain lesions and a marked frontal syndrome make no attempt to familiarize themselves first with the conditions of the task and to distinguish the essential constructive elements. Having perceived directly one fragment of the pattern shown, they immediately begin to attempt to assemble it from the available blocks; they never compare their attempt with the original pattern and never correct their mistakes. As a result of this work, which lacks its "orienting basis," the patient makes constructions which do not correspond at all to the patterns shown. Yet they are often quite satisfied with the results they achieve.

The character of the disturbance lying at the basis of defects of constructive activity of this type can be seen if Tsvetkova's method of programming the behavior of these patients is used. In some cases, all that is necessary is to pick out the successive stages of the patient's disturbed activity and to suggest to him a program which will control each subsequent set of his behavior: (1) Look at the first row of the pattern (2) Tell me how many blocks it consists of (3) Pick out the first block (4) Find the block which matches it (5) Put it in the right place . . . and so on. Thus, the whole program of the patient's behavior is exteriorized in order to replace his absent "internal program" of action, thereby giving the patient's constructive activity an organized character so that the problem becomes soluble (Fig. 109).

• • •

Substantial disturbances are found in patients with frontal brain lesions during various types of verbal thinking. I shall begin my account of the relevant data by showing how the analysis of a written text and of logical-

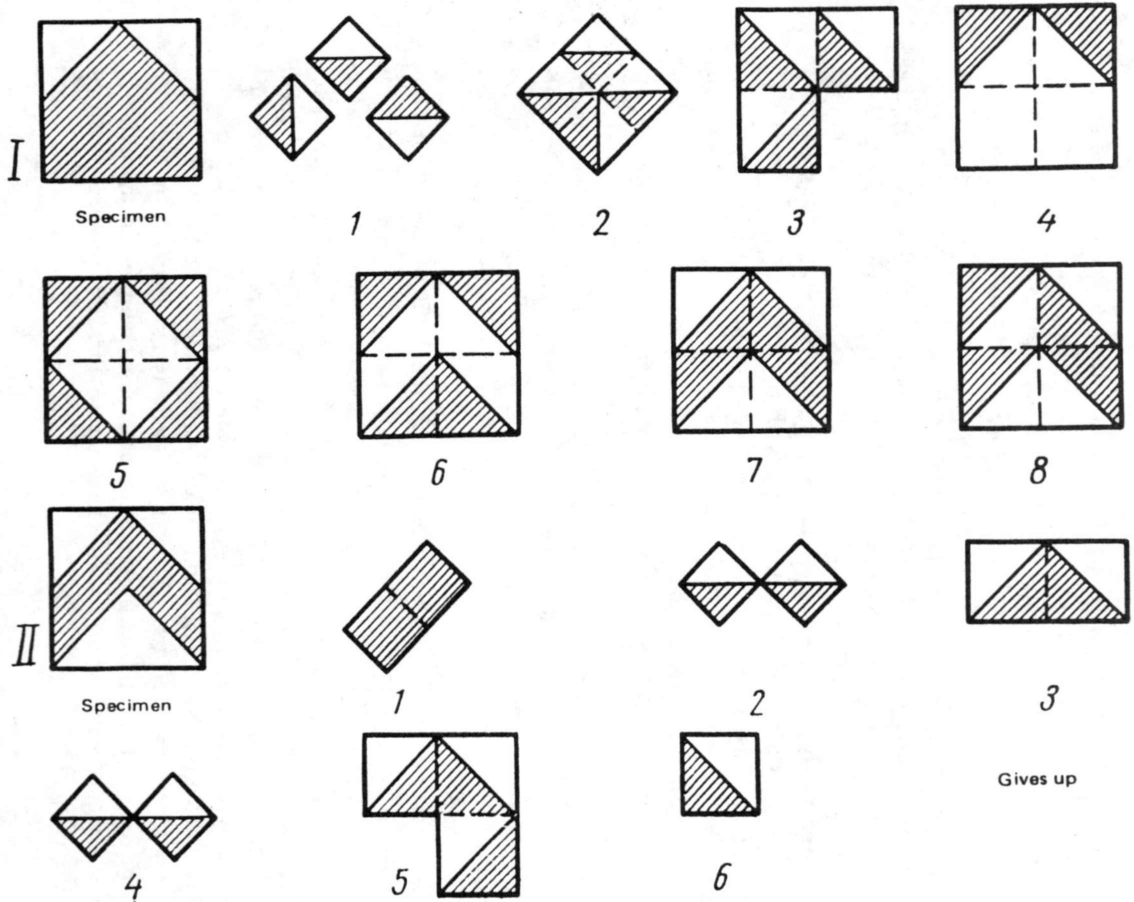

FIGURE 109 Performance of Kohs' test (forming structures from single blocks) by patients with massive frontal lobe lesions. Successive attempts to solve the problem are illustrated. The impulsive character of these attempts will be seen. The first patient develops an inert stereotype. (I) Patient A (tumor of right frontal lobe). (II) Patient B (intracerebral tumor of left frontal lobe).

grammatical relations is disturbed in these patients, and I shall end it by examining the disturbances observed in these patients when they try to solve arithmetical problems.

Lesions of the frontal lobes, as we know, do not disturb the understanding of the meaning of complex logical-grammatical structures which bear the slightest resemblance to those found in patients with lesions of the parieto-occipital zones. However, the understanding of relatively simple meaningful structures may give rise to considerable difficulty. These difficulties are not manifested when the expressions are unambiguous in character; however, they may be quite conspicuous when a semantic structure can have different interpretations and when the correct understanding of its meaning involves making a choice from several possible alternatives.

As many investigators have shown (Goldstein, 1936; Scheerer, 1949; Zeigarnik, 1961), the first substantial difficulties arise in patients with frontal brain lesions in the understanding of transferred meaning (metaphors, proverbs, and so on). Any expression with a figurative meaning, as we know, can have many (or at least two) meanings: its direct meaning is determined by the direct meaning of its component elements; its metaphorical meaning is determined by the conventional meaning attached to the given expression. For the metaphorical meaning to be correctly understood a choice must be made between the two alternatives; the direct meaning of the elements composing the expression is inhibited, and the probability of appearance of connections reflecting the metaphorical meaning is thereby increased.

This process of choosing a necessary meaning can be disturbed in several mental diseases; in patients with lesions of the frontal lobes it is particularly severely disturbed. However, as observations have shown, the correct understanding of the metaphorical meaning is disturbed, in this case, not because of defects of abstract thinking, as Goldstein (1936) thought (for a patient with a frontal lesion can understand complex abstract expressions perfectly well), but because such patients are unable to make the necessary choice from several possible alternatives. Having inhibited the irrelevant alternatives, they are left with the meaning concealed behind the metaphorical expression.

This can be observed particularly clearly if such a patient is instructed to analyze the meaning of a proverb by choosing from a number of sentences offered by the examiner the one whose meaning corresponds to the proverb. If, as Zeigarnik (1961) did, when testing the patient's ability to understand the proverb "A fine cage does not feed a hungry bird," the examiner suggests that the patient choose one of three possible sentences which corresponds most closely to the meaning of the proverb—"You must look after the cage to keep it fine," "A good housewife must know how to make tasty dishes," and "You must judge a person not by his outward appearance but by his inner qualities"—the patient with a frontal syndrome will find it difficult to choose, or will consider that all the sentences offered are equally suitable for expressing the meaning of the proverb. The situation arising as a result of analysis of the meaning, namely that one alternative becomes more probable and the rest become less probable, does not apply, and it is impossible for the patient to make the necessary choice.

The disturbance of analysis of semantic structures in patients with frontal brain lesions is seen more clearly still when they are required to analyze a complex written text and pick out its essential meaning. The understanding of any written text, narrative, descriptive and, in particular, a text containing a hidden meaning, requires considerable work on the analysis of its component parts, their synthesis, and the identification of the most important semantic elements and inhibitions of irrelevant associations which arise during reading of the text. Only if this active process is preserved intact can a complex text be understood properly (Part III, Section 12B). However, as will be clear from all I have said above, it is this process which is particularly severely disturbed in patients with frontal lesions.

Such patients neither work on analyzing the text into elements and their comparison nor do they create hypotheses for subsequent verification. Instead they draw conclusions regarding the meaning of the text as a whole from the meaning of fragments perceived directly; they may replace the essential semantic units of the text by irrelevant meanings and considerably simplify the semantic program embodied in the text. Naturally a complex moral or general meaning of the text, the recognition of which, as psychological investigations have shown (Morozova, 1953), requires considerable effort, most frequently remains unnoticed, and the understanding of the text loses its essential depth.

However, a particularly important fact is that the depressed state of cortical activity, of which I have spoken above (Part III, Section 5C), causes equalization of the relative strength of the essential and irrelevant traces, so that the identification of the essential elements of meaning is often disturbed by a surge of irrelevant associations. The fact that the patient cannot control this surge of associations disturbs the selective character of transmission of the meaning of the text severely and leads the patient widely astray from its true semantic structure.

This observation can be illustrated by a typical example chosen from my extensive series of such cases.

A patient with an extensive lesion of the frontal lobe (an arachnoid endothelioma) was asked to explain the meaning of Tolstoi's tale "The Hen and the Golden Eggs."* After it had been read to him three times, he gave the following account: "A man had a hen. . . . It walked about and grew fat. . . ." The story

* Taken from Tolstoi's *School Stories*: "A man had a hen which laid golden eggs. He wished to obtain more of the gold at once, and killed the hen. But he found nothing inside. It was just like any other hen."

was again read to him, whereupon he told it as follows: "A man had a hen. . . . It lives like any other hen, pecked grain, kept busy, and so was able to live." The patient was asked to relate the moral of the story. "The moral is that things are not what they seem . . . the proof of the pudding is in the eating . . . and that was certainly true in this case. There are thousands of examples of this sort of thing. The man was greedy. . . . He went after big game and tried to take advantage of other people. . . ."

It is clear that this patient continually wandered off into irrelevant associations and habitual stereotyped expressions of speech. However, he answered individual questions of a concrete nature correctly: "What did the hen lay?" "Eggs." "What sort of eggs?" "Golden." The patient then slipped into irrelevant associations. "What did the man do?" "He registered them and informed all the hens as they arrived about the rapid. . . ."

The same type of disturbance was revealed (Khomskaya, 1960) by a patient with a severe frontal syndrome in regard to the short story "The Crow and the Doves."* The story was read three times to the patient, but he could not retell it unaided. The experimenter then took recourse in individual questions; nevertheless, the replies did not disclose the meaning of the text.

"What did you read about?" "About a crow." "What happened?" "What happened [echolalia] was that it did not get what it wanted and did not throw out [fragment of the text] what it wanted." "Did the crow make itself white?" "Into a squirrel [contamination between Russian words "galka" (crow) and "belka" (squirrel)]. The story was read to the patient again, and he was asked to relate it. "A crow could not understand about its money. . .so that it. . .the rabbits [instead of doves] took it in, but didn't know what to do with it." "What is the moral of the story?" "The moral is different. The doves could not take it in and it could not fly away from them, and it did not get what it wanted. . . .So it ran. . .[his eye fell on the book] Books!" "Where?" "To its own home. . .and picked a white color. . .then it painted itself with whitewash. . .it didn't like it. . .you don't do anything here—the face doesn't quite match [associations from his occupation: he was a barber], it should be painted differently, and the crow made it the way it was before. . . ." "What does the story teach?" "The point is that it was impossible to fool this cat [instead of crow], but it did not want to be like the others. . .It came home, stuck to its own business, and it did not like them. . ." "Like what?" "The kittens. . .that about tells the story. . . .It wanted to take the part of another animal, but it could not." "What did?" "The cat." "Not the crow?" "Yes, the crow. It wanted to be taken for something white." This extract shows that the patient could answer individual questions but not without constantly bringing in irrelevant associations.

This loss of selectivity of systems of connections is seen more clearly still when, in the course of tests, I read a patient first one fragment, and then another fragment of a text, and then ask the patient to recall the first and to say what it was about. The current and previous traces in this case are equal in strength. But the patient with a frontal brain lesion (especially

*The story is as follows: "A crow heard that the doves had good stocks of food, and so he painted himself white and flew to the dove cote. The doves thought he was one of them and took him in. However, he could not help cawing like a crow. The doves then realized that he was a crow and threw him out. He went back to live among the crows, but they did not recognize him and would have nothing to do with him."

a lesion of the medial zones of the frontal region) loses the selective character of recallable associations and confuses the elements of the two fragments. The examples given above will serve as illustrations.

These examples show that *a fundamental defect in patients with a frontal syndrome is* not so much a distortion of the meaning of the abstract ideas contained in a text as *an inability to remain within the limits of the selective system of connections given by the text, a ready emergence of irrelevant connections, and an inability to inhibit these irrelevant connections*. All these aspects of defective textual understanding in patients with a frontal lobe lesion were studied in detail by Andreeva (1950) and by Tsvetkova (1966), who described many of the disturbances that have been described herein.

The fact that patients with frontal brain lesions are unable to carry out the necessary analysis of a text and to pick out its most informative components is seen particularly clearly in the observations of Tsvetkova (1966), who showed that whereas such patients are able to relate the meaning of a story read to them, they are quite unable to form a plan of a dictated fragment. Instead they will continue in echolalic and stereotyped fashion to relate something they have just heard.

I mentioned above the disturbance of active recall of a text found in many patients with lesions of the frontal lobes (Part II, Section 5G).

From experiments on the understanding of a text it is but a short step to the analysis of the distinctive features of one of the most important aspects of the intellectual activity of patients with frontal lobe lesions, namely, the disturbance of operations with concepts and logical relationships.

As previously stated, the opinion has been expressed in the literature that, more than any other lesion of the brain, a lesion of the frontal lobes leads to disturbances of "abstract orientation" and "categorical behavior" (Goldstein, 1944) and that the processes of classification lose their categorical character and, instead, become processes of introduction of a given object into a visually perceived situation. Similar views were expressed by Kleist (1934) when he spoke of the "alogical" character of the intellectual activity of patients with frontal lobe lesions. The findings at our disposal give no grounds for subscribing to this opinion but, rather, suggest that the nature of the impairment of operations with concepts in patients with frontal lobe lesions is considerably more complex.

Clinical observations have revealed that even patients with a severe lesion of the frontal lobes do not manifest total disintegration of the system of abstract ideas. In such patients relationships like "part, whole" or "whole, part" and "family, species" or "species, family" and relationships involving opposites were found to be adequately comprehended. When instructed to find a word bearing a definite logical relationship to a given word, most patients were able to do so correctly. In fact our results show that in certain conditions even the logical operation of analogy is within the capacity of a patient with a severe frontal syndrome.

The principal difficulty observed in these patients is in inhibiting irrelevant associations. For instance, although they can perform simple analogies (such as, "bird - flies," "fish - swims"; "father - son," "mother - daughter") they experience great difficulty in coping with irrelevant associations. The appearance of such irrelevancies prevents them from finding the required relationships. For example, when a patient with a tumor of the left frontal lobe, an engineer by training, was given the problem of completing the analogy "sheep - wolf, mouse - ?", he replied: "Of course, it must be fur, they all have a fur.... No... sheep - wolf, mouse... cat... this is the analogy; although there is a mouse fur.... I don't know."

This wandering into irrelevant associations and the instability of the selective aspect of logical operations are revealed by tests requiring the selection of one of a group of three words that bears the same relationship to a given word as exists between a given pair of words (Luria and Lebedinskii). In this variant of the experiment each of the suggested words elicits certain associations with the given word. As a rule, the patient is unable to choose the necessary association from all that spring up. For instance, in the analogy question "lamp–light: stove–(heat, night, fire)?", a patient replied: "They all fit: stove and heat . . . lamp–light . . . stove–night . . . no, that doesn't fit . . . light is the product of the lamp, and fire is the product of the stove, and you can read by it when the door is open. . . ."

The aforementioned intellectual peculiarities of patients with a frontal syndrome may be classified as a disturbance of selective logical operations. This defect is especially obvious when certain logical operations have to be carried out unaided and the governing principle, if identified, has to be employed in further systematization of the material.

Experiments on the classification of objects or the formation of ideas are especially suitable to detect this type of disorder, and several variants of these have been developed by Vygotskii (1934), Weigl (1927), and others. They have been widely used by Goldstein and Scheerer (1941) and Halstead (1947). In these experiments the subject is instructed to classify a series of objects (geometrical figures, drawings, or actual objects) in accordance with the principle identified. In the opinion of Goldstein, Halstead, and others, patients with lesions of the frontal lobes find the solution of these problems particularly difficult. They are unable to discern the necessary principle or to retain it in a sufficiently stable form to enable them to classify the material in accordance with it. Observations made by Soviet psychologists (notably Zeigarnik, 1961) have led to an analysis of the difficulties experienced by patients with frontal lobe lesions when performing these tasks.

Patients with relatively mild frontal lesions frequently begin to classify the objects correctly and to identify some kind of principle (usually firmly established by past experience) for their systematization. However, this system of classification usually cannot be retained by these patients, and they slip off into irrelevant associations. As a result, they categorize into one group all the objects present in a common, concrete situation of the objects related to one another by certain external associations. Therefore, in order for such patients to successfully solve classification problems, they must be constantly stimulated by the experimenter and there must be constant repetition of the initial principle of systematization.

From her study of a large number of patients with massive lesions of the frontal lobes, Zeigarnik (1961) concluded that the instruction to classify objects does not generally evoke any goal-directed, selective activity. Even if the patients repeat the command correctly, they begin to manipulate the objects (or pictures of objects) haphazardly. And even if they are initially successful in classifying objects in accordance with the principle presented to them, this ability is soon extinguished and they begin to select objects in accordance with various signs, usually those most conspicuous to the eye. Similar conclusions were reached by Halstead (1947), who also believes that the ability to distinguish abstract signs and to classify objects in accordance with these signs is particularly impaired in patients with lesions of the frontal lobes.

Although these findings are completely reliable, certain doubts remain: Are these disturbances in the complex forms of intellectual activity observed only with lesions of the frontal lobes or do they also appear in association with general cerebral (of whatever cause) changes in mental activity? Their local significance therefore requires further attention.

The disturbance of the processes of verbal thinking in patients with lesions of the frontal lobes is seen extremely clearly in tests involving solutions of arithmetical problems, which can be regarded with full justification as typical models of intellectual activity.

The absence of a necessary plan for solving the problem, the omission of the phase of preliminary investigation of its requirements, and the replacement of true intellectual operations by fragmentary impulsive actions are all typical of the behavior of patients with a frontal syndrome.

As has been repeatedly mentioned, patients with a frontal lobe lesion show no signs of a primary disturbance in arithmetical skill. As a rule, they retain the categorical construct of number and can carry out individual, well-established operations of addition and subtraction without special difficulty. Important disturbances begin to appear when the task extends beyond the limits of simple and habitual arithmetical operations, i.e., when the problems consist of a series of successive, mutually dependent components and therefore constitute a complex intellectual activity. Typically, these patients experience difficulty during mental arithmetical operations involving the carrying over to the tens column, especially in operations composed of several stages (for example, 31–17 or 12+9–6). In these instances a series of actions, in which the result of the first action is the starting point for the second, must be carried out. For example, having subtracted 17 from 30, the patient must then add 1 to the remainder or, having added

12 and 9, he must then proceed to the next action, 21–6. It is easy to see that such serially constructed arithmetical operations require the memorization of the results so far obtained and their utilization in subsequent actions.

It is this sequential ordering of intellectual activity that is apparently disrupted in patients with a lesion of the frontal lobes, being replaced by fragmentary operations. The patient usually simplifies the proffered task, merely performing fragments of the problem or only one of the necessary operations.

Defects in arithmetical calculation become especially obvious when such patients "mentally" solve problems comprising a consecutive system of operations. One such test widely used in clinical practice is that of counting backwards from 100 in 7's (or, in the more complicated version, in 13's). In this problem, the patient must make the first result the starting point for the next operation of subtraction and continue in this manner until the remainder is less than 7. He must continuously carry over to the tens column, memorize the result obtained, and keep the instructions in mind for a long time.

Because of the disturbance of the selective system of association that has been described, patients with lesions of the frontal lobes begin to make a series of mistakes during the performance of this task. One typical mistake is the simplification of the operation by performing one fragment of it instead of the whole series of actions. For instance, when subtracting 7 from 93, the patient will sometimes answer "84," the explanation for this being that, having split 7 into its components (4 and 3), he carries out the operation 93 – 3 and then simply adds the remaining number of units (4) to the next lower number of tens and obtains the result 84. Another typical mistake is the abandonment of the required arithmetical operation, replacing it by a series of stereotyped responses based on one of the operations (for example, 100—93—83—73—63—etc.). Some patients with lesions of the frontal lobes may obtain the correct solution to the problem if the mental calculations are converted into a series of consecutive operations in which all the actions are constantly denoted aloud (100 – 7 = 93, 93 – 7 = 86, 86 – 7 = 79, etc.). However, in those with a severe form of frontal syndrome this method may not have the desired result.

Hence, the difficulty patients with a frontal lobe lesion experience in carrying out arithmetical operations is of evidently the same nature as the disturbance of the mnestic processes, i.e., disintegration of complex intellectual activity. It is thus different from the disturbance in primary acalculia (Part II, Section 3G).

The disturbance of intellectual activity in patients with a frontal syndrome is particularly marked, however, in the solution of relatively difficult arithmetical problems. As stated previously, the solution of an arithmetical problem is a model of an intellectual act. The goal, set out in the problem to be solved, is achieved under definite conditions; preliminary investigation is required, and the correct method of solution must be found before the necessary operations can be carried out. The performance of these mutually dependent stages of the process is especially difficult for patients with lesions of the frontal lobes.

Patients with lesions of the occipitoparietal divisions of the brain also experience appreciable difficulty in the performance of arithmetical operations but they may retain some idea of the general method of solving the problem. The investigations of Filippycheva (1952), Andreeva (1950), Rudenko (1953), Maizel' (1949) and, in particular, of Tsvetkova (Luria and Tsvetkova, 1966; Tsvetkova, 1966) showed that, in contrast, patients with severe lesions of the frontal lobes characteristically wholly or largely *omit the phase of preliminary investigation of the requirements of the problem and fail to form a general plan for its solution.* Without a strategy, the process of solution of the problem is converted into the combination of individual numbers, with each result usually bearing no relation to the final solution.

Many patients with frontal lobe lesions cannot even remember the terms of the problem, and when repeating them they display that fragmentation which has often been mentioned before. As repeated by these patients, the conditions of the problem do not reflect the logical system of associations from which conclusions must be drawn; often during the repetition of the conditions their most important part—the question which enunciates the problem—is omitted and is replaced by the echolalic repetition of one element of the conditions. For example, the problem "There were 18 books on two shelves, and there were twice as many books on one as on the other. How many books were on each shelf?" is repeated as follows by the patient: "There were 18 books on two shelves . . . and twice as many again. . . . How many books were on the two shelves?" Even if such patients repeat the problem correctly, a correct solution does not ensue.

The following are two examples of how problems are characteristically "solved" by patients with a frontal syndrome.

A patient with a lesion of the left frontal lobe was given the problem just stated ("There were 18 books on two shelves, and there were twice as many books on one as on the other. How many books were on each shelf?") Having heard (and repeated) it, the patient immediately carried out the operation $18 \div 2 = 9$ (corresponding to the portion of the problem "There were 18 books on two shelves"). This was followed by the operation $18 \times 2 = 36$ (corresponding to the portion "there were twice as many on one shelf"). After repetition of the problem and further questioning, the patient carried out the following operations: $36 \times 2 = 72$; $36 + 18 = 54$, etc. Characteristically, the patient himself is quite satisfied with the result obtained.

More complex problems, such as "A son is 5 years old; in 15 years his father will be twice as old as he. How old is his father now?" are completely beyond the grasp of such patients. Without listening to the conditions, they at once begin to make such calculations as 15 × 5 = 75 or 3 × 15 = 45, without forming even an approximate plan for solving the problem. It is interesting to note that if the investigator breaks the problem up into individual questions and puts t' em consecutively to the patient, the problem can be solved. However, if the patient is subsequently given a similar problem to solve by himself, the same difficulties arise.

It is obvious that problems involving "conflicts" (Part III, Section 12D) cannot be solved by such patients. For example, in response to a problem of the type "A pedestrian takes 30 minutes to reach the station, while a cyclist goes 3 times as fast. How long does the cyclist take?" the patient at once answers "30 × 3 = 90 minutes" or a reasonable facsimile thereof.

The fact that the ability to perform individual arithmetical operations that have been firmly established by past experience is preserved has no bearing on the solution of even simple arithmetical problems. Such problems cannot be solved because preliminary investigation of the elements of the problem does not take place because the system of consecutive actions corresponding to a general plan is replaced by random operations with numbers. As stated, these defects are typical of the type of intellectual disturbance developing in patients with lesions of frontal lobes.

Characteristically, therefore, the exteriorization of all forms of behavior that are essential for the successful solution of the task and the use of methods of "programming" of the patient's behavior, which were described in connection with the study of their constructive activity (Part II, Section 5G), can be used with success to compensate for defects arising in the solution of arithmetical problems. Investigations by Tsvetkova (1966) showed that the disability in a patient of the group I have described can be overcome by providing a rigid program of the actions required (e.g., (1) Read the conditions of the problem. (2) Repeat the words of the problem. (3) Look and see whether the necessary data are already available. (4) Look and see what must be done to obtain these data, and so on). In some cases this is sufficient to restore up to a point the patient's disturbed process of problem solving.

It should be noted that such fragmentary "solutions" to problems are not confined to patients with frontal lobe lesions. Patients with a severe general cerebral hypertensive-hydrocephalic syndrome also may evince signs of a similar disintegration of complex intellectual activity. In these cases, however, the defect in the intellectual operations is different in structure and, what is particularly important, is part of a different syndrome.

I have discussed the disturbance of problem solving in patients with frontal lobe lesions in a special monograph (Luria and Tsvetkova, 1966). I therefore shall not deal with it further here.

• • •

A number of features distinguishing the intellectual impairment disturbances of those with frontal lobe lesions have been discussed. As might be expected, these disturbances are closely related to the defects that may be observed in the composition of even relatively simple voluntary movements and actions as well as in that of the gnostic and mnestic processes of patients with lesions of the frontal lobes.

In all patients with lesions of the frontal lobes, the definite changes in mental processes are superimposed on a background of considerable modification of the dynamics of the nervous processes, lowering of cortical activity, and of manifestations of pathological inertia in the cortical divisions of the motor analyzer. Characteristically, the preliminary investigative stage required for a complex activity is omitted or becomes too unstable, the system of associations that should regulate the subsequent course of the mental process is not formed, and the patient's actions fall under the influence of inert afterimages of past experience or of extraneous stimuli and, consequently, irrelevant associations. In the absence of continuous comparison between the plan of action as prescribed by the instruction and the results actually obtained, the mistakes that arise are not rectified by the patient himself.

To recapitulate: The frontal syndrome is characterized by an inherent contradiction—the potentially preserved "formal intellect" and the profoundly disturbed intellectual activity.

H. PRINCIPAL VARIANTS OF THE FRONTAL SYNDROME

The choice of the foregoing facts was dictated by the purpose of the account—to distinguish the basic type of disturbance arising from lesions of the frontal lobes. Naturally, considerable simplification was thereby introduced, and no attention was paid to those variations in the frontal syndrome that are produced by lesions differing in localization, nature, and severity.

However justifiable such a simplification may be in the initial presentation, continuation of this policy would be dangerous. Our clinical analysis must therefore embrace not only the unity, but also the diversity, of the symptoms arising from lesions of the frontal lobes. However, sufficient data have not yet accumulated to provide a full enough account of all the variants of the frontal syndrome that are encountered in clinical practice. Also, it must be recognized that these variants are very numerous and that among patients with frontal lobe lesions there are some who are grossly disoriented and who show gross abnormalities of behavior as well as others in whom no appreciable disturbance can be found even after the most careful investigation. Within the compass of this book, only the principal variants of the frontal syndrome can be discussed, and only in the briefest possible manner. The differences in the manifestation of the frontal syndrome owe both to the fact that different parts of the frontal lobes subserve different functions and to the fact that the nature and extent of the lesion affect the nature and severity of the disorder. As has been pointed out, the frontal region of the cerebral cortex is clearly divided into three large sections, differing in structure, connections, and function. There are the premotor divisions (Areas 6 and 8), constituting the secondary fields of the cortical end of the motor analyzer; the prefrontal convex divisions (Areas 9, 10, 11, and 45); and the mediobasal, or orbital, divisions (Areas 11, 12, 32, and 47), which are very closely related to the transitional (from the paleocortex to the neocortex) structures of the limbic lobe. Lesions of each of these divisions of the frontal region of the brain lead to different functional changes.

The syndrome arising from lesions of the *premotor divisions* of the frontal portion of the cortex has been described (Part II, Section 4E). It was pointed out that its central features are a disturbance of skilled movement and a disintegration of complex kinetic melodies. If the lesion is situated in the left hemisphere and extends to the middle and inferior segments of the premotor region, the same defects will be present in the motor organization of speech processes.

The syndrome due to a lesion of the *convex divisions of the prefrontal region* is essentially different from the premotor syndrome. All that has so far been described in the present section pertains to this particular syndrome. The principal features of this syndrome are a disturbance of voluntary movement and action, resulting from pathological changes in the neurodynamics of the cortical portions of the motor analyzer; difficulty in the formation of preliminary syntheses, a process necessary for the direction of the subsequent course of the mental activity; and ready formation of irrelevant associations, disturbing the selectivity of any form of activity. The essential feature of this syndrome is the lack of continuous comparison between the plan of action and the results actually attained, and this is evidently responsible for the "disturbance of critical values" familiar to clinicians in patients with the frontal syndrome. If the lesion is situated in the left prefrontal region, next to the speech areas, the syndrome may possess features of the "aspontaneity" of speech that has been classified in this book as "frontal dynamic aphasia" (Part II, Section 4G).

Unfortunately, very little can be said about the syndrome associated with a lesion of the right frontal lobe. As a rule, with lesions of this region the speech disorders and the phenomena associated with speech "aspontaneity" are relegated to the background. The aforementioned disturbance of action patterns is complicated by the symptom of anosognosia, which, in the course of observation, has been found to be especially prominent with lesions of the right hemisphere. Examination of this important problem is outside the scope of this book.

Considerable differences from the picture just described are found with lesions of the *mediobasal divisions* of the frontal region and, in particular, of the *orbital part of the frontal cortex*. As has been pointed out, these divisions are especially closely connected with the limbic lobe and, through it, with the hypothalamus. In all probability because of this, with lesions of this region the center of the syndrome shifts toward affective disorders (a phenomenon established both by experiments on animals and by clinical observation). The gross changes in the affective sphere leading to disturbances of character and personality, first described by Welt (1888), are well-known clinical features of this type of lesion.

The syndrome caused by a tumor of the olfactory fossa, which has been adequately studied by neurologists and neurosurgeons, is a special case of a lesion of the orbital divisions of the frontal region. It consists of disturbances in vision and olfaction and marked changes of character, with disinhibition of primitive drives and appreciable disturbances in the affective sphere.

All the defects described above are clearly brought to light by neuropsychological investigation. Although gnosis, praxis, and speech remain largely intact, these patients often show increased impulsiveness during tests of their praxis, usually without any sign of pathological inertia of established motor stereotypes, but often their motor responses arise impulsively (sometimes even in the form of premature movements). The same impulsiveness is revealed in their memorizing and intellectual activity; they often give fragmentary, impulsive responses when recalling series of words, when assessing the meaning of a thematic picture, and during arithmetical operations, although the operations themselves remain potentially intact.

Only in very severe lesions (e.g., very large meningiomas of the olfactory fossa), as a result of the pressure of the tumor on the frontal lobes and of dislocation, these defects may be made more severe and may assume the form of a massive "frontal syndrome" such as I have described above.

In the light of the information concerning the parts played by the structure, connections, and functions of the mediobasal divisions of the frontal lobe in the regulation of states of excitability, the difference between this syndrome and the syndrome caused by lesions of the convex divisions of the frontal lobes becomes more easily understood. It should be noted, however, that particularly marked symptoms arise from *bilateral lesions* of the frontal regions, possibly because in the case of unilateral lesions the intact portion carries on the functions of the affected portion.

Disturbances of higher cortical functions arising in lesions of the medial (parasagittal) zones of the frontal region are particularly interesting. These lesions may arise as the result of meningiomas of the falx, or through spasm of the anterior communicating arteries supplying blood to the medial zones of the frontal lobes.

In these two cases the picture observed may be very different. In patients with parasagittal meningiomas the changes in higher cortical functions may be varied in character. If the tumor arising from the falx is small in size and does not exert any significant pressure on the frontal lobes, the lesion may give rise to no noteworthy symptoms. If, however, it begins to exert pressure on the anterior zones of the corpus callosum, symptoms of a disturbance of the coordinated function of the two hands typical of these cases arise, reciprocal coordination of movements is disturbed, and coordinated hand movements begin to show signs of motor deautomatization. Finally, if the tumor attains a large size and displaces the frontal lobes of both hemispheres, the same picture of a massive frontal syndrome as that already described above again arises.

A syndrome of exceptional severity appears following spasm of both anterior cerebral arteries, which frequently accompanies aneurysms of the anterior communicating artery and hemorrhages resulting from them. In such cases, which I have described in detail elsewhere (Luria, Konovalov, and Podgornaya, 1970; Luria, 1976a), a disturbance of the blood supply to the anterior zones of the limbic region leads to marked disorders of memory, combined with general confusion of the patient, loss of a critical attitude to his disabilities, confabulations, and so on. These disturbances are manifested particularly clearly both in the patient's general orientation in his surroundings and his own state, and in the recalling of the text of stories, which is marked by contamination and confabulation. All these defects are frequently superposed upon a state of general euphoria with preservation of praxis, gnosis, and speech.

Where these defects arising from spasm of the two anterior cerebral arteries are compensated by the collateral circulation or by abolition of the spasm, this picture gradually disappears. If, however, the vascular disorders persist, or if branches of the anterior cerebral arteries running to the deeper structures of the limbic region are damaged during surgical operations, these disturbances of direct memory may become permanent in character, and they may sometimes lead to the formation of a chronic Korsakov's syndrome.

The description of the principal variants of the frontal syndrome would be incomplete without some mention of the *regional syndromes* associated with lesions involving neighboring regions of the frontal lobe in addition to the frontal lobe itself. Foremost in this group is the syndrome produced by *frontoparietal lesions*, in which the marked symptoms of the deautomatization of movement and impairment of skilled movement are combined with sensory disorders, indicating that the parietal divisions of the cortex are involved. Also to be mentioned in this connection is the syndrome of the frontotemporal lesion, arising when tumors of the frontal region have spread into the pole of the temporal lobe or with tumors of the anterior divisions of the fissure of Sylvius, which compress both the frontal and temporal regions. The leading symptom of this syndrome (if the tumor is situated in the left hemisphere) is a composite of the components of the frontal syndrome with distortion of the meaning of words and aphasic disturbances. This combination may gravely complicate the manifestations of adynamia of speech observed with lesions of the frontal lobes and may cause especially severe and intractable forms of speech disturbance. Finally, this group includes the manifestations of the very complex, and as yet inadequately studied, frontodiencephalic syndrome. This syndrome is distinguished by the fact that the aforementioned disturbances in the complex forms of mental activity are superimposed on profound cognitive disorders, mnestic defects, and disorientation in time and place. These adjuvant disturbances apparently accrue from a sharp lowering of cortical tone, which results from a disturbance in the tonic and activating role of the reticular formation.

All these syndromes are of great clinical interest and their careful study is an essential task in clinical psychoneurology. As has been stated several times, variants of the frontal syndrome are contingent not only on the location of the lesion, but also on its nature, on the extent of frontal dysfunction, and on the severity of the accompanying general cerebral symptoms.

Uncomplicated gunshot wounds of the frontal lobes (especially perforating bullet wounds and circumscribed, depressed fractures of the skull with slight changes in the underlying gray matter) usually do not cause gross disturbances of the higher cortical functions. The vast majority of the "symptom-free" lesions of the frontal lobes described in the literature belong to this group. In contrast, expanding lesions, especially if large and accompanied by changes due to increased intracranial pressure, are usually accompanied by well-defined symptoms. This particularly applies to rapidly expanding intracerebral tumors, which not only cause those changes that are based on size and toxic effects, but also, as a result of the rapid rate of growth, prevent the brain from adapting itself to the new conditions. For this reason, slowly growing extracerebral tumors (meningiomas, for instance) may be associated with much less marked symptomatology; in some cases (when the period of growth of the tumor is measured in years) no changes in the higher cortical functions can be detected until a certain critical point in development.

Very little is still known about the variants of the frontal syndrome associated with cortical and intracerebral lesions. The differential diagnosis of extracerebral and intracerebral tumors of the frontal region (as, indeed, in other regions) is often very difficult. It may be noted, however, that the gross changes of tone and the well-marked perseverations that have been alluded to are found more frequently in intracerebral lesions of this region. Among the symptoms of great importance in the differential diagnosis are the changes in cognitive functions, which are most in evidence with lesions of the frontodiencephalic connections.

The problem of variants of the frontal syndrome and their neuropsychological and surgical assessment is still very incompletely studied, and special combined investigations are necessary.

It remains for us to mention one further feature of the functional organization of the frontal lobes, which must not be forgotten in the study of their pathology. As Jackson (1884) pointed out long ago, the frontal region of the brain is the youngest and, at the same time, least differentiated formation of the cerebral hemispheres. The ability of its parts to assume the functions of other parts is therefore much greater than is that of such highly differentiated formations as the sensorimotor, optic, or auditory cortex. It is possible that this factor may help to explain the clinical picture associated with lesions of the frontal region, which still remains the most baffling section of psychoneurology.

6. *Disturbances of Higher Cortical Functions in Deep Brain Lesions*

This section of neuropsychology was not discussed in the previous edition of this book because the practical application of neuropsychological methods to the study of patients with deep brain lesions has hitherto encountered a number of difficulties. Not even the extensive developments in stereotaxic operations on deep brain structures in the last decades, which have yielded so much new information about their functions, have removed the chief difficulties in the way of analysis of the changes arising in cortical activities when the normal work of these deep brain zones is disturbed.

Although the "vertical" principle of organization of brain activity has been firmly established now for a long time in neurology, since the classical studies of Moruzzi and Magoun (1947), Magoun (1958), and Lindsley (1960), there is no longer any doubt that the work of the cerebral cortex depends essentially on impulses which reach it from the brain stem via the reticular formation, modifying the tone of its activity.

But analysis of the changes in higher cortical processes (gnosis and praxis, speech and thinking) in patients with *deep* brain lesions immediately meets with a distinct difficulty: all these processes remain basically intact in these patients and there may be no disturbances whatever of gnosis and praxis or of speech and intellectual processes.

Patients with tumors of the pituitary gland (and with parahypophyseal tumors), and patients with relatively early tumors of the third ventricle spreading also to the limbic region of the cortex usually show no symptoms of a disturbance of gnosis and praxis; they retain their speech, and are able to perform relatively elementary intellectual operations. The only symptom clearly manifested by these patients may be a certain lowering of the tone of psychological processes, a certain slowness and proneness to fatigue, which is equally manifested in all the spheres of their activity.

Only in patients with massive tumors of the third ventricle is the situation substantially altered: such patients may exhibit gross disturbances of consciousness, states intermediate between sleep and waking, and sometimes a long-lasting state of pathological sleep, which changes easily into phenomena of gross disorientation about place and time, about their immediate environment, and about their own state. Such patients often cannot say where they are when asked; they say that they are evidently "at the factory," "at the command post," or "at the station" (i.e., indicating some sort of temporary, transit place); they confabulate, stating for example that in the morning they visited several institutions, or were at the sawmill. One patient stated that his wife visited him (she was at that moment in the next room), and so on. The whole of this picture has been adequately described in psychiatric literature.

Perhaps the most important fact is that, against the background of this clearly abnormal state of consciousness, the special higher cortical functions of these patients may remain intact. They may have no difficulty in performing tests of praxis, repeating given movements, recognizing pictures, repeating sounds or words, or reading and writing, and they can perform relatively simple arithmetical operations.

This dissociation between the depression of cortical tone and transition to an oneiroid state and the integrity of formal operations constitutes perhaps the most significant feature of these patients.

The first symptoms of a disturbance of higher cortical functions in the patients of this group were brought to light very clearly as soon as their memory was investigated. The results of the tests showed that many patients with pituitary tumors (spreading beyond the sella turcica and becoming parasellar in character) showed no signs of lowering of cortical tone. They were apparently mentally completely healthy, yet they showed clear modality-nonspecific disturbances of memory. This defect was not fully revealed by tests of simple learning of word series but only by the use of a method, which will be described in detail below (Part III, Section 7C), to study the stability of traces of the word series given to these patients and the extent to which the recall of these traces was inhibited by interfering factors.

A patient was given a series of three or four words which he had to repeat; he was then immediately given another similar series of words which he also easily repeated. When, however, he was then asked to recall the first series of words, he was unable to do so, stating that he had forgotten them or that he could recall only one or two of the words of the first series. This problem, indicating instability of traces and their increased susceptibility to inhibition by interfering factors, was nonspecific in character and was manifested equally during the recalling of series of words, geometrical shapes, movements, and so on (Kiyashchenko, 1973).

Characteristically, in relatively mild cases of this syndrome of a deep brain lesion, the difficulty described above was the only symptom that could be found by testing the higher cortical functions of these patients. Another characteristic was that, on the change from the recall of isolated elements (words, numbers, etc.) to the recalling of organized structures (sentences or stories), these phenomena of increased trace inhibition by interfering factors disappeared. This pointed to the complete integrity of higher forms of cortical activity and to the possibility of using complex organization of material as a factor for the compensation of the original defect.

A substantially different picture arises in patients with massive lesions of deep brain structures, such as tumors of the third ventricle spreading to the hypothalamic region or to the hippocampus, causing severe dysfunction of psychological processes. The syndrome of memory disturbances in these cases is superposed upon a sharp lowering of cortical tone and serious disturbances of consciousness, often accompanied by oneiroid states, disorientation in the surroundings, and confabulation.

The way this syndrome is manifested in experimental investigations of memory is that the increased inhibition of traces by interfering factors occurs not only in tests of memorizing and recalling series of isolated elements (words, figures, shapes) but also in experiments on memorizing organized semantic entities (sentences, stories). In this case the compensating effect of the complex level of semantic organization of the material is absent. The patient who is asked to repeat one sentence, then another, and then go back and repeat the first sentence cannot do so and generally abandons the task or mixes up the two sentences (e.g., after repeating successfully the two sentences: "Apple trees grew in the garden behind the high fence" and "The hunter killed a wolf at the edge of the forest," when asked to recall the first sentence, said: "In the garden . . . at the edge of the forest . . . grew . . . no, killed a wolf!").

Even more serious defects arise in these patients when their ability to memorize and recall complete stories is tested.

In the severest cases of deep brain lesions it may be almost impossible for the patient to repeat one simple story (such as "The hen and the golden egg" or "The jackdaw and the pigeon") but even more difficult to repeat a more complicated story consisting of two semantic themes (e.g., "The ant and the pigeon"); such patients will either recall separate fragments of the story or will wander off into irrelevant associations and lose the thread of the story. For instance, when relating the first story he might say: "Well, let me see . . . this was . . . about a hen . . . the hen was killed. . . ." *Who by?* "One of the farmer's enemies . . . no, the farmer turned the hen out . . ." and so on. Naturally the patient's recall of the first story after hearing the second was deeply flawed; the result was a mixture of elements from both stories and a flood of uncontrollable irrelevant associations. (For instance, if the patient was asked to recall the story "The jackdaw and the pigeon," after the other story "The ant and the pigeon" had also been read, he would say: "Let me see, . . . what was this? . . . a pigeon fancier . . . decided to catch a pigeon and laid a net . . . but a dove was caught in the net . . . he then decided to set a trap . . . he put some wheat in it . . . and the pigeons . . . the pigeons were taken in by the deception . . ." and so on.)

Correspondingly, if lesions of deep brain structures spread to the frontal zones of the brain (as can happen, for example, with craniopharyngiomas), such a patient will be even less able to restrain the floods of uncontrollable irrelevant associations or inert stereotypes, the organized system organized to block interfering influences will become "open" to all irrelevant influences (direct impressions, uncontrollable associations), and any meaningful recall becomes quite impossible.

The characteristics of the memory disturbances described above in patients with deep brain lesions have been discussed in detail elsewhere (Popova, 1972; Kiyashchenko, 1973; Kiyashchenko et al., 1975; Luria, 1976), and it is therefore unnecessary to dwell on the matter.

Two characteristic features distinguishing the syndromes of memory disturbance in deep brain lesions must be mentioned. First, patients of this group when trying to recall material presented previously as a rule will continue to be aware of the inadequacy of their attempts; they will state that they have "forgotten," that "they cannot quite recall what was told to them," that they "cannot recall it exactly," and so on. As a rule it is this feature which distinguishes these patients from those with a massive frontal syndrome, in whom this critical attitude toward their defects is absent.

The second feature distinguishing the syndrome arising in deep brain lesions is instability or fluctuation of the defects described. All these defects may fluctuate considerably: some days (or even hours) they may be present in more serious forms, on other days (or hours) in milder forms—further evidence that all these defects are connected primarily with a disturbance of general cortical tone.

The reason why these defects are manifested most clearly in memory may perhaps be that, as recent investigations have shown (Vinogradova, 1974), neurons of the limbic region are closely concerned with the act of comparing traces, so that they are intimately related to mnestic activity. Impairment of this activity is an inevitable consequence of a lesion of the "circle of Papez," of which the structures mentioned above are a part.

• • •

What are the disturbances of the affective sphere and the *primary disturbance of activity* that can often be observed in the patients with deep brain lesions? Clinicians are well aware that lesions of certain parts of the thalamus and adjacent structures can give rise to serious affective changes which, in the presence of pathological excitation of these structures, lead to sharp accentuation of protopathic sensation, in which the changes of sensation are indissolubly connected with emotionally charged experiences. The functional blocking or degeneration of these structures may lead to marked disturbances of the affective sphere and to the appearance of primary indifference and disturbances of activity. This may be of very great importance for the course of the higher cortical processes.

All types of conscious psychological activity are known to begin with certain motives, which subsequently acquire a concrete form as definite plans, which are, in turn, carried out as a successive chain of operations (Leont'ev, 1959). Obviously if there is primary depression of cortical tone, and the constant inflow of energy-yielding impulses from the deep subcortical formations is interrupted, the whole course of psychological processes will be substantially altered.

These changes are manifested as a sharp primary lowering of activity, and they can be observed in all psychological functions starting from the simplest motor act and ending with complex forms of cognitive, speech, and intellectual activity.

Patients with such disturbances usually lie passively and respond weakly to irrelevant stimuli; they are frequently in a drowsy, oneiroid state. When instructed to raise their hand or clench their fist, they remain passive and either make no action at all or a very weak movement which quickly dies away. When asked to name an object or tell the story represented by a picture, they either remain inert or whisper a fragmentary answer which immediately dies away. The same result is found when their intellectual operations are tested (e.g., an elementary calculation, or a simple arithmetical test such as counting backward from 100 in 7's), invariably, they give either a whispered echolalic response or, at best, they perform only one stage of the required operation. The slightest effort on their part causes them to fall asleep.

Electrophysiological investigations by many different workers (in the USSR, by Faller and Filippycheva, 1975, 1977) have shown that these states are reflected in a very distinctive pattern. Whereas any problem requiring activity leads to desynchronization or depression of the alpha-rhythm of the EEG in normal subjects, in the patients of this group such problems either give rise to no electrophysiological response whatever or, what is particularly important, they may lead to the paradoxical appearance of pathological slow waves, showing that in such cases every effort evokes pathological inhibitory responses.

The phenomena of *primary inactivity* described above, found in lesions of the superior part of the brain stem, differ essentially from the *secondary inactivity* exhibited by patients with lesions of the frontal lobes, already described above. "Frontal inactivity" arises as a rule when the patient is given relatively difficult tasks requiring the formation of a plan and an action program; in contrast, the primary inactivity of patients with lesions of the brain stem is unaffected by the difficulty of the task. In patients with frontal lesions this inactivity is manifested either as echopraxia and perseveration or as the appearance of fragmentary impulsive actions; however, nothing of the kind is found when patients with massive deep brain lesions are so tested. The primary inactivity in patients of this last group reflects only a general lowering of tone and is manifested in the waking-sleep parameter, with a clear tendency to switch from the former to the latter.

The differential diagnosis between primary (brain-stem) and secondary (frontal) disturbances of activity is by no means always easy, but it is one of the most important tasks in clinical neuropsychology.

Syndromes of gross nonspecific disturbances of memory and consciousness, primary inactivity, and disturbances of the emotional sphere (such as the symptoms of the oneiroid state and disorientation, superposed on general integrity of the higher cortical functions of gnosis, praxis, and speech which I described above), arise as a rule in patients with lesions of the upper part of the brain stem, hypothalamus, mammillary bodies, and hippocampus, forming part of the "circle of Papez." These syndromes also arise in patients with extensive tumors of the third ventricle, the influence of which spreads to the structures listed above.

A completely different picture is found in lesions confined to higher levels and, in particular, to the structures of the immediate subcortex (the thalamostriate system). As has recently been discovered (and which I shall mention again below), the structure of the thalamus is extremely complex; it includes groups of specific "relay" nuclei and groups of nonspecific nuclei, whose function has been studied much less thoroughly than that of the individual parts of the cortex. There are good grounds for supposing that all the functional structures represented in the cerebral cortex are also present at the deep level in the thalamus, but in a more compressed and condensed form. If the idea of "vertical structure" of the functional systems of the brain is accepted, it can be assumed that isolated lesions of individual areas (or nuclei) of the thalamus will affect the course of the higher cortical functions in a completely different manner from lesions of lower structures, and that their effects will be much more selective in character.

However, the neuropsychological data on the role of these structures in the course of higher cortical functions are far less abundant than the data on functional organization of the cortex, possibly because isolated lesions of these structures are much more difficult to observe. I shall therefore dwell very briefly on the ways in which the investigation of this problem has developed.

Hitherto we have regarded the deep subcortical formation (including the thalamus, hypothalamic region, and individual parts of the "old brain") as a nonspecific system responsible simply for controlling the states and modulating the tone of the cortex.

In the last decades, however, evidence has been obtained that impulses traveling to the cortex from these formations are not necessarily nonspecific. This view was expressed in the USSR by Anokhin (1968), who pointed out that if impulses traveling from the brain stem to the cortex are not modality-specific in character, this by no means implies that they are nonspecific, or that they may be connected with different and highly specific cravings (sexual desire, hunger, thirst, and so on). This finding can be supported by biochemical analysis of the corresponding structures and investigation of the forms of activation evoked by them.

Even more interesting results were obtained very recently by Bekhtereva and her colleagues (1970, 1971, 1974). By the use of a sensitive method of recording action potentials from individual groups of neurons located in the various thalamic nuclei, these workers showed that such groups of neurons respond differently to different semantic codes of language, and that, consequently, the highest degree of selectivity of cortical function is reflected actually at this deep level. Selectivity can evidently descend in a vertical direction and obtain reinforcement from the selective activity of neurons in deep brain structures.

The presence of these highly selective "vertical" connections running from the formations of the brain stem to the cortex sparked off another series of investigations associated with the names of Ojeman (1968, 1971, 1976), Van Buren et al. (1975), and Ricklan et al. (1971, 1975), who first raised the question of the role of deep subcortical structures in speech activity and inquired into the disturbances of speech activity arising in lesions of these structures.

Most of the results obtained by stereotaxic operations relate to either the stimulation or the coagulation of individual thalamic nuclei. Characteristically, neuropsychological investigations of these patients have been of a relatively special nature, and most frequently they have been restricted to changes in short-term forms of visual and verbal memory arising in the course of these operations. However, despite this fact, the investigations mentioned above have yielded very important results.

Coagulation of individual nuclei of the left thalamus has been shown to cause the unexpected appearance of speech disorders (e.g., stoppage of speech, or, sometimes, paraphasia).

There is no doubt that the complexity and high degree of differentiation of these formations, with which we are already familiar, must very specifically affect the modulation of higher cortical processes, but further research is necessary before a reliable answer can be given to this question. The data pointing to the role of individual thalamic nuclei in the course of higher cortical processes and the psychological changes arising in response to their stimulation and coagulation are still very limited.

Significantly more severe disturbances can be observed in the relatively rare cases of operations performed for the removal of an aneurysm on the thalamus. This operation has become possible only recently as the result of advances in neurosurgery. In these cases, destruction of part of the posterior regions of the left thalamus can give rise to distinctive speech disturbances which, at first glance, resemble aphasia but which are in fact "quasi-aphasic" disorders. The patients of this group partly lose their ability to understand speech addressed to them. Characteristically, they hear and understand some questions correctly and give the correct answers; others they do not hear properly, and their answer consists of irrelevant expressions, quite incomprehensible and unconnected with the question. Similar defects may arise in the naming of objects and the repetition of words. Whereas in some cases both these tasks are performed quite adequately, in others unexpected and completely irrelevant answers are given, which surprise even the patients themselves. For instance, one such patient, when asked to repeat the word "pencil" exclaimed: "Uncle Tom's cabin," and immediately added: "What on earth put that into my head?!"

These disturbances of speech continue for two or three weeks after the operation and then gradually regress. The possibility cannot be ruled out that these unique disturbances are based on gating defects affecting the inhibition of irrelevant associations and impairing the selectivity necessary for the appropriate course of speech processes.

Phenomena of this sort (which have also been observed by other workers, notably Ojeman) must naturally receive careful investigation. Only then will the role of structures of the thalamus and the deep structures of the left hemisphere in speech activity become clear.

7. *On Functional Interaction Between the Hemispheres*

I mentioned above that the two hemispheres of the brain differ in importance and that one of them (the left hemisphere in right-handed persons), which is directly connected with the right hand and speech, is dominant (Part II, Section 1B). However, in the first edition of this book I refrained from a more detailed examination of the problem of the functional organization of the two hemispheres for the perfectly valid reason that at that time little was known about the character of this functional organization and the real forms of interaction between the two hemispheres in the mechanism of higher cortical functions.

In the last 10 to 15 years, however, this has been the subject of much research. New facts have been obtained which justify a closer look at the question of functional interaction between the hemispheres. I shall try to present this new information in its most general features without attempting in any way to survey the world literature on the problem (which now numbers many hundreds of titles). My aim will be simply to discuss some of the basic principles and facts obtained in the last few years in my own laboratory (chiefly by E. G. Simernitskaya and her colleagues).

As I stated above, since the time of Broca (1861) and Wernicke (1874) it had been firmly established that the dominant (left) hemisphere is directly related to speech and the attendant operations, whereas the nondominant (right) hemisphere is unrelated to speech and remains "dumb." This interpretation naturally aroused misgivings, and consequently many neurologists actively supported Hughlings Jackson's (1876) idea that the nondominant (right) hemisphere is directly related to visual perception, in the organization of which speech plays no part.

Although a similar view is held by most contemporary researchers who attempt to explain how functions can be "localized" in the dominant (left) and nondominant (right) hemispheres, it must now be regarded as unacceptable.

On Functional Interaction Between the Hemispheres

As was stated earlier (Part I, Section 1, 3–4; Part II, Section 1), I hold views which are diametrically opposite to those just described above. Unlike the classical authors, who attempted to relate each particular higher psychological "function" to a particular area of the brain and to "localize" it in particular brain structures (areas of the cortex, groups of neurons, or even single neurons), I have argued from a totally different standpoint.

I have always regarded a higher psychological "function" as a complex *functional system,* the organization of which in the brain involves the participation of a dynamic "constellation" of collectively working parts of the brain and areas of the cortex; every part of the brain or every area of the cortex makes its own *specific contribution* to the operation of this functional system. A lesion of any part of the brain or of any cortical area can thus lead to disintegration of the functional system as a whole. However, the disturbance of the whole functional system will differ in character each time, and that is why we can ask the fundamental questions: What factors are included in the organization of this functional system? What is the role which each part of the brain plays in its organization?

We have no grounds for rejecting this view when we examine the problem of the functional role of the two hemispheres. I therefore consider that the principle just enunciated must be accepted in this case also and that the question to be asked is not what functions are "localized" in the dominant (left) and the nondominant (right) hemispheres, but instead, considering that each complex psychological process takes place with the participation of *both* hemispheres, *What specific contribution is made by each hemisphere to the performance of higher psychological processes?*

Modern scientific psychology and the modern theory of development of higher psychological processes, the foundations of which were laid by Vygotskii (1956, 1960, 1962) not only provide a direct approach to this problem, but they also enable the formulation of a concrete hypothesis that can serve as the starting point for the explanation of the contribution made by each of the two hemispheres to the mechanism of psychological functions.

All perceptual processes, as we know, incorporate in their composition the "sensitive tissue" of the reflected world (visual impressions and their traces); this "sensitive tissue" of psychological processes, as we know, is not only their basis, but it predominates clearly in the early stages of the psychological development of the child. During the child's psychological development, he acquires speech. Since speech is completely different in its origin (social) from the "sensitive tissue" of experience, the child reconstructs in speech this "sensitive tissue" of experience on a new basis, creating complex forms of perception embodied in certain verbal-logical codes, complex forms of logical voluntary memory, active attention, and abstract thinking.

None of these processes can be understood as a product of the natural development of the "sensitive tissue" of experience, or as a form of verbal-logical activity separated from its basis.

This complex character of "higher psychological functions," which are themselves a synthesis of the direct "sensitive tissue" of experience and its verbal organization, is the basis for the understanding of the structure of all complex forms of psychological activity. This initial statement can provide the key to the understanding of interaction between the two hemispheres which lies at the basis of the construction of higher psychological functions, and the answer to the questions: What specific contribution is made by each hemisphere to the course of these functions? and What form does their disturbance take when one hemisphere no longer plays its part in their organization?

The contention established by classical neurology that the dominant (left) hemisphere, for reasons not yet sufficiently understood (possibly connected with interaction between the right hand and cue signals in speech formation), is responsible for the learning of the codes of language and for their use, whereas the nondominant (right) hemisphere does not have this role, still remains valid. However, it by no means follows that all the components of speech are "localized" in the dominant (left) hemisphere and all the components of visual sensory experience are "localized" in the nondominant (right) hemisphere.

What I said above regarding the structure of all higher psychological processes as systems, and the role of speech in the formation of higher forms of perceptual activity, suggests that they all (including speech itself) depend on functional interaction between the two hemispheres, but that in a lesion of each hemisphere these processes (including speech) are affected differently. Careful analysis of the previous statements can not only clarify the role of each hemisphere in the functional organization of higher psychological processes but, at the same time, it can provide new ways of looking at the intimate structure of these processes. Let us turn to the information presently available.

Lesions of the cortex of the dominant (left) hemisphere and, in particular, of its "speech areas" lead to different forms of disturbance of speech and also of gnosis and praxis, which take place through the close participation of speech. These facts have been described in detail by clinicians, and their investigation is a fundamental part of neuropsychology.

The manifestations of a lesion of the nondominant (right) hemisphere and, in particular, of its posterior (temporo-parieto-occipital) zones are much less clear. Although in the last decade very many investigations have been made of this symptomatology—and the symptoms arising in these cases have been recently summarized by Levy (1974), and Babenkova (1976)—it is still very difficult to express in definite, generalized, logical categories.

We can say in general that lesions of the right hemisphere, as many workers have stated, lead to a disturbance of psychological processes which have relatively little connection with speech codes but which are of the nature of direct experiences, assessments of the perceptual situation and direct monitoring of actions while they are in progress.

It was noted quite a long time ago that massive lesions of the posterior zones of the nondominant (right) hemisphere lead to a condition of anosognosia, known for a long time as "Anton's syndrome" (after the person who described it first in 1893; later it was described by Redlich and Bonvicini in 1908 and 1911). Patients with these lesions are unable to appreciate their defects: patients with left-sided paresis frequently are unaware of it; and patients with left-sided hemianopsia often do not suspect that they do not perceive the left half of the visual field, and they are unaware of the left side of a picture or text. When they draw objects they ignore the left side (this phenomenon of "ignorance of the left side" was described some years ago by Critchley, Zangwill, and others; and the condition of unawareness of the left half of the visual field or "left-sided fixed hemianopsia" was described by me in 1950 and in Part II, Section 3C).

Another and very important fact has been observed by many investigators: patients with a lesion of the nondominant (right) hemisphere often show definite signs of disturbance of direct orientation in their own body and in the immediate surrounding space. Many of them identify parts of their own body incorrectly, their limbs appear abnormal in size to them, the body schema is disturbed, and their direct perception of space is impaired (metamorphopsia); they have difficulty in assessing time and their immediate surroundings; in patients with more massive lesions this phenomenon assumes the form of gross disorientation, so that they are uncertain of their whereabouts at any given moment. In some cases I have found such a severe disturbance of direct orientation in these patients that in the course of the same conversation they said they were in two different cities and were quite unaware of the contradiction (one such patient was a scientific worker whose formal speech operations were well preserved, and when the physician remarked that a person could hardly be in two different parts of the country simultaneously, he replied: "Why, what does it matter? It all depends on your point of view: what about the theory of relativity! . . ."). If we add to this the fact that all the phenomena described above can be superposed upon marked affective changes (if the pathological process affects the deep zones of the right hemisphere), the picture of the disturbance arising in lesions of the nondominant (right) hemisphere will be even more conspicuous.

It would be wrong to imagine that the changes I have just described in these patients are limited to the direct awareness of their own state. Definite defects may also characterize their perception of the outside world.

It has been known for some time that in lesions of the posterior (occipito-parietal) zones of the nondominant (right) hemisphere there is a unique type of disturbance of direct perception, especially of its integral forms which do not require special operations of analysis and correlation with a certain system of codes. For instance, clinicians have described the condition of agnosia for faces (prosopagnosia), accompanying lesions of the right hemisphere (a phenomenon originally described by Charcot), as well as severe disturbances of drawing (manifested not only as unawareness of the left side, but also as a disturbance of perspective and of the general scheme of the picture as a whole (Kok, 1967; Korchazhinskaya and Popova, 1977). And many workers have emphasized the role of the nondominant (right) hemisphere in the condition of object agnosia—inability to identify objects even when pictured realistically.

Defects connected with lesions of the nondominant (right) hemisphere in the auditory sphere are supported by frequent reports in the literature on this subject. Although these patients retain normal speech, the musical components of hearing are impaired, and they are unable to identify or reproduce melodies.

Finally, there are data which indicate that lesions of the right hemisphere may be accompanied by changes in speech activity in which, although all the phonemic, lexical, syntactic, and semantic components (in other words, all the codes of language) are preserved, the speech of such patients becomes overexpanded, they drift too easily into minute details, the regulation of speech is impaired, and it becomes "over-reasoned" in character. Our observations relative to this fact have not yet been published.

It is difficult at present to classify all these diverse symptoms of lesions of the right hemisphere into definite categories, and they may perhaps be described as disturbances of processes not requiring verbal encoding, but of a more direct character (i.e., connected with the direct sensory basis of psychological activity).

A noteworthy addition was made to these clinical observations when Sperry and co-workers (1961, 1964, 1967, 1969), Gazzaniga (1970), and Gazzaniga, Bogen, and Sperry (1967) conducted experiments with division of the corpus callosum, so that the functions of the two hemispheres could be observed in isolation.

The patients of this group, receiving information in one hemisphere only, exhibited quite different symptoms. Whereas stimuli directed toward the left hemisphere could readily be named and read, visual stimuli directed to the right hemisphere could be recognized but not named, and words directed to the occipital zones of the right hemisphere could not be read, although in these cases the corresponding objects could be correctly chosen. (I shall return to this last observation again later.)

• • •

So far the description has been concerned only with the intrinsic functions of each hemisphere and has indicated the contribution which each hemisphere can make to the combined activity of the whole brain. We must now turn to observations directly connected with the problem of changes arising in the same psychological process in lesions of the dominant (left) and nondominant (right) hemisphere.

It would perhaps be the most proper course to begin the description of these facts with an analysis of speech processes. These have long been regarded as a function purely of the dominant (left) hemisphere, in which the nondominant (right) hemisphere evidently plays no part. A closer examination of recent findings and, in particular, the investigations of Simernitskaya and co-workers in our own laboratory, provides some concrete facts for the solution to this problem.

I shall begin by describing data relating to the analysis of *writing* and its disturbances in lesions of the nondominant (right) hemisphere.

In all the Indo-European languages using the phonetic principle of writing (analysis of the phonetic composition of speech and its subsequent conversion into sounds, i.e., phonemes into letters), both consonants and vowels are used in writing words. Consonants carry the maximal semantic information, whereas vowels have the apparent role of background components; the articulations of the tongue and lips, which lie at the basis of consonants, are far more informative than vowels, which are formed by other less informative components of articulations.

It is an interesting fact that in many ancient languages (e.g., Slavonic) and also in some modern languages whose manner of writing was established much earlier than others (Arabic, Hebrew), only consonants are represented in writing. Vowels are either completely omitted or are represented by punctuation below the line. All this suggests that two different levels must be distinguished in the process of writing: the most informative and meaningful (consonants) and the less informative, background component (vowels). This provides an approach to a closer analysis of the psychophysiological mechanisms of writing.

The first and most interesting data with respect to some of the central mechanisms of their organization have been obtained by the investigation of dichotic hearing. It is generally known that during the perception of the sounds of speech and of words the left hemisphere is as a rule dominant, and this is reflected in the dominant role of the right ear. But during perception of tones and musical melodies the right hemisphere is dominant, and this is reflected in the dominant role of the left ear. However, it is essential to note that similar dissociation has also been discovered in the perception and retention of consonants and vowels: a dominant role of the right ear (i.e., of the left hemisphere) has been distinctly identified in the perception and retention of consonants (whereas this dominant role of the right ear is not so clearly defined in the case of the perception and retention of vowels; the roles of the right and left ears are equalized (Shankweiler and Studdert-Kennedy, 1967; Milner, 1973).

These observations suggested that a lesion of homonymous regions of the left and right hemispheres (the "speech zones" of the left and analogous zones of the right hemisphere) disturbs the retention of consonants and vowels to different degrees. These findings were confirmed by Traugott (1973) and by Balonov and Deglin (1976), who showed that after inactivation of the nondominant hemisphere (by unilateral convulsive therapy) the discrimination and retention of vowels are affected more than after inactivation of the dominant (left) hemisphere.

However, the facts described by Simernitskaya (1972, 1974) are particularly interesting. Lesions of the speech areas of the dominant (left) hemisphere, especially of their temporal and postcentral zones, very often, if not always, lead to a disturbance of writing, generally known as agraphia. Closer analysis of the character of the disturbance of writing in these cases shows that it consists chiefly of the displacement of consonants (correlative or oppositional in milder cases and disjunctive in more severe cases), the impairment of analysis, the confluence of consonants (such as the "psk" in the word "Pskov" or the "rtn" in the word "portnoi") and, finally, a change in their order.

The much rarer cases of disturbance of writing observed in patients with lesions of the temporo-parietal region of the hemisphere nondominant for speech (right) are of a totally different character. In these cases the disorders of writing consist chiefly of the omission or replacement of the vowel (background) component of writing, whereas the principal component of the process, namely the writing of consonants, as a rule remains intact. Such patients may write the word "lisa" as "leso" or "lso"; the word "sobaka" as "sobaku" or "sabka"; the words "vot-vot" as "vat-vat." These are indeed typical mistakes made by them. In one case described by Simernitskaya, only 9 of 82 consonants were written incorrectly, whereas mistakes were made with 35 of 67 vowels, i.e., more than 50% of the cases. This could happen equally with the writing of unstressed and stressed vowels.

These results show that the process of writing includes principal and background components (represented in their most distinctive form by consonants and vowels), and that both hemispheres play a part in the writing of these components; one (the dominant) hemisphere is responsible for the retention of the principal (encoding) components of writing, whereas the other (nondominant) hemisphere contributes toward the writing of the background components. These findings are a first step in the study of this problem and, of course, they require confirmation and clarification.

Similar results have been obtained by investigating the role of the dominant (left) and nondominant (right) hemisphere in visual perception and in reading. Tachistoscopic studies of visual perception, excluding eye movements, have shown that verbal stimuli (letters, syllables, words) are distinguished more quickly when presented in the right visual field, whereas nonverbal stimuli (meaningless shapes, faces) are distinguished more rapidly when presented in the left field of vision.

This confirms that, as mentioned above, the left hemisphere has a dominant role in the perception of speech codes, whereas the nondominant (right) hemisphere plays the major part in the perception of nonverbal, visual patterns. These observations were completely confirmed by the experiments of Sperry and co-workers with division of the corpus callosum.

I pointed out earlier that in such cases, when joint participation of the two hemispheres connected by the commissures of the corpus callosum in the process of perception was ruled out, it was shown that the dominant (left) hemisphere, stimuli to which were directed into the right visual field, is clearly dominant in the perception of letters and of written words, whereas the nondominant (right) hemisphere is dominant in the perception of visual patterns not encoded in speech. An even more interesting finding is that the exclusion of the dominant (left) hemisphere leads to inability to name the patterns presented but does not at all prevent their identification or even their classification in a particular visual category. For instance, the patient perceiving a group of objects in the isolated left visual field (i.e., the occipital region of the right hemisphere only) is able to recognize objects concerned in the same visual action situation while disregarding cues of shape (e.g., grouping a cigarette with an ashtray, but not objects of similar shape, such as a pencil and a cigarette). These observations showed that the right hemisphere has its own generalizing functions, although the generalizations it is capable of are at a different level from the abstract generalizations carried out on the basis of language codes.

The phenomena I have just described lead us to a problem similar to that already mentioned above: Can we now assert that the nondominant (right) hemisphere can participate in a verbal function, namely *reading,* in which it has its own specific role that differs profoundly from that of the left hemisphere? Observations providing the answer to this question were made by Simernitskaya on patients with surgical injury to the posterior part of the corpus callosum resulting from the operative approach to a pathological focus (an aneurysm) in the region of the left side of the thalamus. Since such patients had right-sided homonymous hemianopia, they perceived visual stimuli only in the residual left half of the visual field, i.e., with the occipital region of the right hemisphere only. These observations yielded results of exceptional importance. One of these patients could not read a single word; however, she continued to grasp its general affective meaning. For example, when shown the word "tie" she said: "I don't know what it is . . . it is certainly something to do with a man. . . . Vo-lo-dya (a man's name) . . . no?" When shown the word "Natasha" (her daughter's name) she could not read it but said: "Something near to me, something related . . ."; when shown the word "north" she was also unable to read it, but said: "Something cold, but what it is I don't know. . . ."

Examples of the evaluation of the affective meaning of a word despite inability to read it were similar in character. "Water": "This is a little word something with which I am familiar . . . not a garden, something else . . .

when it is hot we take . . . and pour it from a watering can. . . . I can't say . . . a bath? No, not at all . . ." "Daughter": "Something I know but I can't say . . . what it is . . . somebody's head and face . . . it is familiar . . . like a child . . . but if this were a child's name it would start with a capital letter. . . ." "Vladimir": "This is something I know but I can't read it . . . it is certainly somebody's surname or Christian name. . . . I said it . . . a complete name, not a shortened form—not Kolya but Nikolai —a complete name. . . ." "Mother": "Something familiar but what it is I can't say . . . it is pleasant . . . certainly some sort of name. . . ."

All these facts are highly significant. They show that in reading also there are two different levels: a level of analysis of sounds and letters, leading to ability to read words, and a level of direct grasping of the appropriate meaning of words, which is evidently connected with the integral perception of words and which can be dissociated from the act of reading words letter by letter.

It is very interesting that whereas the first of these processes is connected with the dominant (left) hemisphere, the second can be a property of the nondominant (right) hemisphere, so that in this case also a complex act such as reading is performed with the participation of both hemispheres, each of which makes its own specific contribution to this complex process.

The principle expressed above, that each complex psychological function is performed by the combined activity of the two hemispheres, each of which makes its own specific contribution, is manifested not only in speech but in other forms of psychological activity.

Another example of this principle is *memory*. Psychologists are well aware that both the memorizing of material and its recall are not a simple process of imprinting and activation of traces. In fact, as will be pointed out below (Part III, Section 7) memory processes consist of complex mnestic activity, in which the ability to imprint and store traces constitutes the basic condition for "background," and the task of memorizing, retaining, and then recalling what was imprinted earlier constitutes the basic form of the process. It is thus possible to distinguish two main types of memorizing: involuntary (unpremeditated) and voluntary, the latter being a special form of conscious activity. Many investigations have shown that this last form of memory is closely connected with the incorporation of the material to be memorized in a certain system, and it takes place through the close participation of codes of language.

These observations raise the problem of what brain mechanisms are responsible for the process of memorizing, and they suggest that in this case it involves the close participation of both hemispheres; the dominant (left) hemisphere incorporates the process of memorizing into the system of voluntary activity which is intimately dependent on speech, whereas the nondominant (right) hemisphere caters to the "background" processes of memorizing and retention of traces, which take place without premeditation (involuntarily) and do not depend on a corresponding system of codes based on speech.

Soviet psychologists have developed special methods of investigating voluntary and involuntary memorizing. These have been described by Smirnov (1948, 1966) and by Zinchenko (1959). These workers used two different methods: one to study the course and capacity of voluntary memory, the other to study the course and capacity of involuntary memory.

To study voluntary memory, the usual well-known tests were carried out in which the subject was instructed to actively memorize a series of isolated words or numbers presented to him by ear or visually (a method firmly established in psychology ever since the classical studies of Ebbinghaus). To study the course and capacity of involuntary memory the subject was put into a different situation. He also was presented with a series of cards on which individual words were written, but instead of being asked to memorize these words, he was told to count the total number of letters in the word or to pick out all words which began with a certain letter (for example, the letter "K"). It will easily be seen that in the last case the problem of memorizing did not arise at all and was replaced by a completely different activity, and that any memorizing of the whole material that could be detected after the end of this test, if the subject was instructed to say what words in fact were written on the card, was involuntary in character and simply a "by-product" of the subject's activity.

Simernitskaya carried out both these series of tests on normal adult subjects, on patients with lesions of the parieto-temporal zones of the dominant (left) hemisphere, and on patients with lesions of the nondominant (right) hemisphere. Naturally, the patients with marked symptoms of aphasia and agnosia were excluded.

The results of these tests showed a significant difference between the three groups of subjects. In normal subjects the capacity of involuntary memory is considerably less than capacity of voluntary memory; the subject recalls on average 6 to 7 out of 10 words in the voluntary memory test but only 4 or 5 words in the involuntary memory test. In patients with lesions of the dominant (left) hemisphere the defect is much more severe: the capacity of voluntary recall was reduced by about 40%; these patients could recall only about 4 words, whereas the capacity of involuntary memory was reduced by a rather smaller degree. In the second series these patients recalled 3–3.5 words, representing a reduction in the productivity of recall by 30%.

The picture was completely different in patients with lesions of the corresponding zones of the nondominant (right) hemisphere. The productivity of voluntary memory was reduced in these patients by only 20–25% compared with normal patients, and they recalled 4 or 5 out of 10 words presented. However, in these patients the productivity of involuntary memory was reduced much more sharply: by 70% compared with normal subjects; they could recall only 1–1.5 words, and this number could be increased only negligibly after frequent repetitions.

As yet these results have been published only in a preliminary communication (Luria and Simernitskaya, 1977), but they show clearly that the role of the nondominant (right) hemisphere in memory activity is to provide the background (involuntary) components of memory, whereas the dominant (left) hemisphere, possibly because of its close connection with speech, is responsible for the active mnestic side of memory processes.

Subsequent investigations showed yet another series of symptoms distinguishing the process of memorizing in patients with lesions of the dominant (left) and nondominant (right) hemispheres. Analysis of memory disturbances arising in patients with lesions of the right and left hemispheres shows that the right hemisphere is more closely connected with the process of indirect consolidation of traces and that lesions of that hemisphere lead to a disturbance of direct imprinting and recall of stimuli, whereas in patients with lesions of the left hemisphere the memory defects are manifested chiefly in the delayed recall component (Kiyashchenko, Moskovichyute, and Simernitskaya, 1977).

The findings described above are still preliminary: the steps which have been made in the study of the role of the two hemispheres in memory processes are still very recent. Much more research is necessary. However, there is good reason to suppose that the principle expressed above, that complex psychological processes are not "localized" in any one hemisphere but are the result of interaction between the two hemispheres, each of which makes its own special contribution to the performance of a given function, is correct. It is hoped that future research will shed additional light on this difficult problem.

III

METHODS OF INVESTIGATING THE HIGHER CORTICAL FUNCTIONS IN LOCAL BRAIN LESIONS (SYNDROME ANALYSIS)

1. *Objects of Neuropsychological Investigation of Higher Cortical Functions in the Presence of Local Brain Lesions*

The principal objective of the study of the higher cortical function in the presence of local brain lesions is to describe the general pattern of change taking place in mental activity and, from this, to identify the fundamental defect, to determine the secondary systemic disturbances, and, in this way, to attempt to explain the syndrome resulting from the fundamental defect. Clinicopsychological investigation can thus assist in the topical diagnosis of brain lesions and forms an essential part of the general scheme of clinical investigation of the patient.

Let us now consider the methods that must be used for this purpose. The usual clinical examination of the patient includes a careful history, detailed observation of the patient's behavior while in the consulting room or hospital, analysis of the neurological symptoms, and a series of additional objective tests (otoneurological, ophthalmoneurological, roentgenological, electroencephalographic, and biochemical). By this means the foundations are laid for the topical diagnosis of a circumscribed brain lesion. However, these investigations are not enough.

The behaviorial changes observed with various circumscribed brain lesions are often very similar in character. In many cases, simple observation can only indicate some of the disturbances affecting the patient's general behavior and perceptual activity, but frequently it cannot establish the basic factors that are responsible for these disturbances or distinguish and evaluate symptoms that are due to various causes and that differ in their internal structure.

It is known, for example, that the overwhelming majority of patients with brain lesions (organic and functional) complain of "loss of memory." However, as has already been explained, this loss of memory may result from the most widely different disturbances. It is quite understandable, therefore, that special methods of investigation are required to establish the precise components and significance of a symptom, to describe a defect, and to differentiate its underlying factors. For this purpose, the patient must be studied under specially organized conditions whereby the defect can be demonstrated with the greatest possible clarity and whereby its structural features can be analyzed in the greatest detail. It is only under these conditions that the data essential for definition of the responsible factors can be obtained. These requirements are satisfied by neuropsychological (or, to be more precise, psychophysiological) methods of investigation.

The type of neuropsychological investigation that fulfills the aims of clinical diagnosis has certain special features and differs essentially from the usual investigation conducted in the psychological laboratory and from the "psychometric tests" frequently regarded in the foreign literature as the principal method of clinical psychological investigation.

The psychological or physiological laboratory investigation, aimed at solving general, theoretical problems, differs from the clinical psychological (or psychophysiological) investigation in two respects. The psychologist (or physiologist) occupied with a particular theoretical problem singles out a process that interests him, disregards all other processes, and studies it under specially created conditions. Neuropsychological investigation is organized quite differently. The neuropsychologist (or psychophysiologist) who has the task of diagnosing a patient's condition does not know which process or which aspect of the patient's mental activity should be the focal point for subsequent investigation. He must first make preliminary studies of the patient's mental processes, and from these preliminary results he must single out the crucial changes and then subject them to further scrutiny.

Unlike the psychologist or physiologist working in the laboratory, the neuropsychologist cannot allow his investigation to take too long, nor can he divide his study of the problem confronting him into a series of consecutive sessions. As a rule, his preliminary probes must be done in a relatively short time, usually one or two sessions; each of the sessions may not last longer than 30 to 40 minutes, for that is frequently the longest period of examination that the patient can tolerate.

If to this is added the fact that the neuropsychological investigation must, as a rule, be carried out at the patient's bedside, under circumstances in which the use of laboratory apparatus is highly restricted, some idea may be gained of the basic features of the neuropsychological (or psychophysiological) study.

From all the characteristics of the neuropsychological investigation as carried out under clinical conditions, it might appear that it bears a great resemblance to the short diagnostic tests, known as "psychometric tests," that have become widely adopted during recent decades outside the Soviet Union for grading children in special schools and neuropsychological investigation. This conclusion, however, is quite wrong. Many of the basic features of psychometric tests not only do not satisfy the demands made on the clinical psychological investigation of patients in general and of patients with circumscribed brain lesions in particular, but also may, on closer inspection, be seen to be entirely inappropriate.

Psychometric tests intended for the purpose of obtaining preliminary information on the psychological make-up of an individual for diagnostic purposes may, in principle, be divided into two different types. One type (exemplified by the Binet-Terman tests or any of their variants) utilizes a series of empirical problems, whose psychological significance is difficult to determine but which allows a quantitative evaluation of successful performance so that the subject can be graded in a particular population. However, these tests provide no basis for the qualitative analysis of the psychological abnormalities on which the subject's defects are based, and, accordingly even when used for such purposes as the detection of mental retardation in children and the differentiation of the various forms of disturbance of mental development, they are quite inadequate.* This is clearly apparent from the negative results obtained from attempts to use these tests for the differentiation of aphasias (Weisenburg and McBride, 1935) and lesions of the frontal lobes (Mettler, 1949; etc.).

The second type of psychometric test is designed for the study of particular mental functions; their objective is to reveal the degree of disturbance of each of these functions and to express this degree quantitatively. One example of this technique is Rossolimo's well-known psychometric scale, consisting of a series of tests for investigating such functions as "observation," "attention," "memory," "suggestibility," etc. To some extent, tests such as the Wechsler-Bellevue series (Wechsler, 1944), consisting of a selection of standard tests aimed at investigating a group of ideas, the understanding of arithmetical operations, memory, elementary formal logical operations, etc., belong to this group.

The well-known series of tests suggested originally by Halstead (1947) as a method of measuring "biological intelligence" has similar features. This series, widely different in character (the psychophysiological importance of some of them is still obscure), enables the investigator to obtain a general "index of lowering of biological intelligence." But at best these tests can provide only an overall picture compiled from the results of investigation of widely different processes; it is almost impossible to interpret the significance of these observations as a part of the concrete picture of the lesions.

Although these tests appear to be psychologically more highly differentiated

* Dul'nev and Luria (1960) and Luria (1960) give detailed analyses of psychometric tests and their uses.

than those of the first group, they are still unsuitable for the qualitative analysis of defects of the higher mental functions arising from circumscribed brain lesions. One important shortcoming of such tests is that they are based on a preconceived classification of "functions," in accordance with contemporary psychological ideas, that by no means always reflects the forms of disturbance of mental processes actually resulting from brain lesions. The second, and most important, shortcoming is that its purpose is not so much to analyze qualitatively the defects discovered as to evaluate them formally and quantitatively. Although this evaluation may indicate the degree of functional impairment in a particular subject, it is quite unsuited for determining the qualitative features of the disturbance and is even less suited for analyzing the fundamental defects responsible for the impairment. Naturally, therefore, the application of these tests to the diagnosis of circumscribed brain lesions has completely failed to justify the confidence placed in them, and even the most careful application of standard "batteries" of tests to the investigation of local brain lesions (as exemplified, for instance, by the work of Reitan and his colleagues, 1955, 1962, 1964, 1965) has yielded far fewer results than would be expected from such detailed and systematic studies.

The methods of neuropsychological investigation as applied to the clinical diagnosis of circumscribed brain lesions must therefore differ significantly not only from the usual methods of psychological laboratory investigation, but also from those in psychometric tests. They must satisfy other needs and must be applied in completely different forms.

Let us now consider the principal requirements of the methods of neuropsychological investigation as applied to the clinical diagnosis of local brain lesions. The neuropsychological (or psychophysiological) investigation in the consulting room or hospital is a component of the clinical neurological investigation of the patient. This means that, like any clinical investigation, it must be based on sound ideas of the possible types of disturbance that may be encountered in brain lesions and which must be brought to light during investigation of the patient.

For this reason, the neuropsychologist (psychophysiologist) engaged in the clinical investigation of local brain lesions must have a clear idea of the syndromes arising from brain lesions in various locations, and he must direct his investigation to the discovery of one of these syndromes. The investigation satisfying these requirements must include a *sufficiently wide range of absolutely definite tests* to act as a guide among the great variety of disturbances that may arise from local brain lesions. This pilot investigation must basically include a group of tests aimed at discovering the state of the subject's auditory, optic, kinesthetic, and motor analysis and synthesis. A disturbance of one or more of these processes may be the direct result of a lesion of a particular division(s) of the cerebral cortex.

The *investigation of the state of the individual analyzers* is only the beginning and by no means the whole of the preliminary study of the patient.

The result of the neuropsychological investigation must never be limited to the simple statement that a particular form of psychological activity is "impaired." It must always give a qualitative, structural analysis of the symptom observed and must indicate, as far as possible, the character of the observed defect and the causes or factors responsible for the appearance of this defect. The neuropsychological investigation is thus an important step toward what Vygotskii called the *qualification of the symptom* and an important stage along the path from its external description to its causal explanation.

The neuropsychological investigation must discern whether a particular defect is based on a disturbance of relatively more elementary components of the particular mental activity or whether it is due to a disturbance in organization at a more complex level of the activity; it must find out whether a particular symptom is the primary result of a disturbance of some special feature of the functional system under investigation or a secondary (systematic) consequence of some primary defect.

If a technique used in neuropsychological investigation permits a qualitative analysis to be made of an existing disturbance and if it enables the effect of this disturbance on the whole range of the patient's mental activity to be studied, the results obtained will be reliable and of diagnostic importance.

Neuropsychological investigation as applied to clinical practice must consist of a series of tests aimed at uncovering the complex pattern of mental activity and, at the same time, capable of subjecting that activity to systematic analysis. This requirement (like the one that the examination be of relatively short duration) can be met only if the study of patients with circumscribed brain lesions is not confined to special analytical tests on auditory, optic, kinesthetic, or motor analysis and synthesis but includes *integrated tests* for the examination of complex forms of activity, whose performance may be variously disturbed with different lesions.

The neuropsychological methods of patient examination must include tests on repetitive and spontaneous speech, writing, reading, comprehension of texts, and the solution of problems; each of these complex forms of mental activity is accomplished with the participation of a group of formations from the principal areas of the cerebral cortex and of the second signal system. However, given the right choice of problems and a proper analysis of the results, the difficulties experienced by the patient in the performance of these tests will reveal the particular type of disturbance of the activity in question; the diagnosis will depend on which factor essential for the performance of this activity is disturbed.

This brings us to the next requirement, which deals not only with the choice of adequate methods of investigation, but also with the manner in which the experiment is carried out and its results analyzed. The psychological investigation must be concerned not so much with whether a problem is solved as with the way in which it is solved. In other words, it calls for a careful qualitative analysis of the patient's activity, of the difficulties experienced, and of the mistakes made.

The qualitative analysis of the process under observation and the analysis of the factors underlying its disturbance necessitates the use of a series of supplementary methods, applicable to the investigation of the solution of any problem and facilitating the analysis of the changing structural pattern of the defect. In other words, these techniques allow for the *analysis of the structural dynamics*. In order to gain a better understanding of the nature of the defects interfering with the performance of a particular task and to identify as precisely as possible the factor(s) responsible for the difficulties, it is not enough to merely carry out a particular experiment in the standard manner. The experiment must be suitably modified so that the conditions from time to time making the performance of the test more difficult, as well as those enabling compensation to take place, can be taken into account.

The conduct of the investigation is made much more complicated by the analysis of the structural dynamics; much greater variability and flexibility are required, and any attempt to apply static standardized experimental psychological techniques must be entirely discouraged. Only if this condition is satisfied (which, to do so, requires great experience) will the clinical psychological investigation prove effective.

This principle of structural dynamics in neuropsychological investigations as applied to clinical practice introduces yet another condition to be taken into consideration if useful and reliable results are to be obtained. The disturbance of the higher cortical functions in the presence of brain lesions is always the result of the neurodynamic changes characteristically found in nerve tissue under pathological conditions. The neuropsychological investigation must therefore be so devised that the results obtained from it indicate not only the defect of the corresponding form of mental activity, but also the *neurodynamic changes* underlying the disturbance.

This last requirement is equally important in the investigation of disturbances caused by circumscribed (systematic) brain lesions and those caused by a pathological condition of the brain as a whole. The difference is that with lesions of the whole brain (increased intracranial pressure, hydrocephalus, concussion, tumors of the ventricles directly disturbing the function of the reticular formation) the pathological process leads to a generalized weakening of cortical activity, to a lowering of cortical tone, and to an increased liability to fatigue of the processes taking place within all analyzers. In contrast, with circumscribed brain lesions these defects are selective in character, usually either confined to one analyzer or disturbing only the highest levels of organization of the cortical processes.

In all these cases, as has been pointed out (Part I, Section 3), the neuropsychological investigation must not be limited to the demonstration of the loss of a particular mental function, but it must show, as far as possible, *what type of neurodynamic defect* underlies the disturbance affecting mental activity. A neuropsychological experiment must reveal the pathological weakness of nervous processes in one or several analyzers, disturbances in the integrative activity of the cerebral cortex, defects of internal inhibition and the attendant impulsiveness, pathological inertia of the nervous processes, and, finally, defects of afferent feedback systems leading to significant disturbances of behavior as a whole. In this way, much more than the psychological description of the defect can be obtained, and a giant step forward is made in the analysis of the fundamental pathophysiological disturbances leading to changes in mental activity. In satisfying this condition, an accurate topical diagnosis of the lesion can be made and much information about the pathophysiological nature of the disturbances can be gained. The latter aspect of such investigation is bound to become increasingly important in the future.

Neurodynamic analysis of the results demands that, as the patient performs the various tasks, the attention of the investigator be constantly directed to the nature of the disturbances observed. In so doing, certain experimental circumstances must also be taken into consideration so that supplementary methods utilizing this information can be used. Among the experimental situations with an important bearing on the neurodynamic changes being observed is the development of fatigue during the course of the experiment. The fact that fatigue does not develop uniformly in different types of activity (especially during activity associated with different analyzers) may be particularly important. In studying cerebral lesions attention must also be paid to the inhibitory effect of irrelevant stimuli, which may block an activity already begun and thus prevent the performance of the task. Among the special methods that may enhance the analysis of the neurodynamic defects are a change in the tempo of the experiment, presentation of the stimuli at a faster rate, or extension of the scope of the tasks—all of which may easily induce a protective inhibition. These variations may act as "sensitizing conditions" and, in so doing, may help the investigator pass from the simple description of the observed defect to the evaluation of the neurodynamic changes primarily responsible for it.

This concern with structural dynamics in the course of neuropsychological investigation is one of the more important conditions ensuring that the study of the patient will lead to the correct diagnostic conclusion. However, even if all the aforementioned requisites are observed, there remains one further requirement without which the results will not have the required significance: The results obtained must be sufficiently reliable.

This question of the reliability of the results is of fundamental importance in any psychological experiment. The results of the investigation may be subject to chance influences and may vary greatly from one experiment to another; it is always necessary, therefore, to know how constant and reliable the results actually are.

During psychological investigations in the laboratory the problem of the reliability of the results is usually solved by the number of experiments performed and the degree of consistency of the data; the results are considered reliable if the variability in the numerical values is relatively small. This statistical approach is impossible in neuropsychological investigations. Clinical diagnostic experiments are usually conducted only a few times, the number being limited by the short duration of the investigation and the need, in order to examine as many aspects of the patient's mental processes as possible, to carry out a large number of different tests in a short period. An additional factor limiting the number of possible tests performed in one session is the rapid development of fatigue in the patient, so that if the same experiment is repeated too long one begins to get different results. For these reasons, the results of each individual test during the neuropsychological investigation of a patient are highly questionable.

Neuropsychological investigations, therefore, are made reliable in a different way, namely, by the comparative analysis of the results of a group of assorted tests and the determination of general signs among these results, which are grouped together into a unified syndrome. Reliability of the results is thus ensured by *syndrome analysis*.

It was stated (Part I, Section 3, and Part II, Section 1) that each circumscribed lesion may give rise not only to primary disturbances, but also to a series of secondary, systematic disturbances whose component elements are integrated into a generalized type of defect. In the preceding analyses of the sydromes arising from the various local lesions, many findings illustrative of this statement were given.

Each neuropsychological investigation not only must distinguish the particular fundamental defect, but also must demonstrate how it manifests itself through changed activity by defining the complex system of disturbances that arises. Hence, if the results obtained by different methods are compared and a common type of disturbance affecting different forms of activity observed, the results of the investigation become reliable enough and acquire clinical significance. Syndrome analysis is thus not only the principal means of obtaining results adequate for clinical purposes, but it also gives the results the necessary reliability.

As a rule, before the neuropsychological investigation is begun, the *history of the present condition is obtained and a preliminary conversation is held* with the patient. The investigation begins with a *series of preliminary tests* with the aim of discovering the state of various aspects of the patient's mental activity and of obtaining preliminary information to provide a general background or description of the mental processes.

This series of tests must be relatively standardized in character and must include devices for ascertaining the state of the individual analyzers (optic, auditory, kinesthetic, motor) and for examining the various structural levels of the mental processes—the level of direct sensorimotor reactions, the level of the mnestic organization of activity, and the level of complex, mediated operations (in which a leading role is played by the connections of the speech system). This group of tests, which must reveal the various aspects of the patient's mental activity with the utmost clarity, must include only those known to be within the grasp of any normal (including a relatively uneducated) subject. However, the complexity of the tests must vary from patient to patient in keeping with the patient's "initial" (premorbid) level; it is recognized that the same tasks will not always be adequate for subjects with differing cultural levels. This first stage of investigation, which must include a relatively large number of tests for different purposes (although all of short duration), will already enable the investigator to identify some of the defective aspects of the patient's mental activity, as well as other aspects of his mental activity in which no such defects can be found.

The whole subsequent course of the investigation, constituting the second (selective) stage, must be devoted to more detailed investigation of the group of mental processes in which the preliminary tests have detected the presence of definite defects. In contrast, therefore, to the preliminary stage, the second stage of the investigation must be strictly *individualized*. It must be built up, firstly, on the basis of the results obtained in the first stage and, secondly, by taking into account the facts that are obtained in the course of the second phase of the investigation itself. It is clear, therefore, that the second stage of the neuropsychological investigation is the more complex, yields richer results, and calls for greater flexibility in the conduct of the experiments.

The primary objective of the second stage is to obtain additional facts pertaining to the patient's fundamental defect, to define its nature, and to discover the underlying factors. The secondary objective is to ascertain the extent to which this fundamental disturbance is manifested in various aspects of the patient's activity, forming the basis of the particular syndrome.

It is in this stage that the investigator must make all possible use of the sensitizing devices at his command and must try to elicit the functions that have remained intact. The investigator must determine what residual forms of analysis and synthesis are being used by the patient in order to perform a task that hitherto was impossible and how a patient reconstructs his disturbed activity by bringing into play surviving analyzers and by transferring the solution of the problem to a level (higher) where the processes are carried out with the closest participation of the system of speech connections. It is at this stage, too, that special methods for determining the neurodynamic features of the discovered defect must be used.

Experimental teaching of the patient has a specially important role in the investigation of the patient and the qualification of the defect. In many cases the identification of a defect discovered in a patient as the result of a single investigation does not enable the stability of the defect to be assessed or the factors causing it to be analyzed. In such cases these two questions can be answered only as a result of experimental retraining.

By suggesting to the patient that he use various aids in order to solve the problem presented to him, we can discover which components of the process studied are disturbed and which remain intact. A careful examination of the dynamics of the disturbed function in the course of retraining thus provides an approach to the true qualification of the defect and enables primary disturbances of function to be distinguished from various types of disturbances of functional systems.

Usually the neuropsychological investigation is carried out at the patient's bedside and no laboratory equipment is needed. However, quite naturally, to pursue the investigation deeper and clarify the physiological basis of the defects observed, special methods of instrumental neurophysiological investigation can be incorporated. I have already given many examples above of results obtained in this way (e.g., the results of precise recording of movements by mechanographic and electromyographic recording of motor responses, the results of a plethysmographic and psychogalvanic study of autonomic responses, and the use of electroencephalography). However, these observations have additional importance, for they serve to clarify the facts obtained during the initial neuropsychological investigation.

The third, and final, stage of the investigation is the formulation of a neuropsychological conclusion, based on the results obtained and their comparative analysis. It must identify the fundamental defect, describe how this defect is manifested in the various forms of mental activity, and as far as possible describe the defect and indicate the pathophysiological factor(s) underlying it. Only after some such analysis is made can one presume to suggest a possible local lesion as responsible for the observed phenomena, and only then can one begin to distinguish the relative importance of the general cerebral factors which are more or less associated with local lesions of the brain.

Thus formulated, this conclusion is incorporated into the general clinical evaluation of the case to permit a tentative diagnosis of the disease. If all the aforementioned conditions have been met, the neuropsychological conclusion will be an important component of the clinical conclusion and the neuropsychological analysis will have become an important part of the clinical investigation of the patient with a local brain lesion.

After these preliminary remarks, the techniques used to secure a topical diagnosis in patients with circumscribed brain lesions can be described. Only a few of the most adequate methods, which have proved themselves best in practice, will be discussed. The results that may be obtained with each method in patients with lesions in different parts of the brain will be mentioned. The preliminary conversation that precedes each patient's investigation will be dealt with first, and we shall then describe a series of techniques for the investigation of gnosis, praxis, speech, and intellectual processes that may be used for the topical diagnosis of circumscribed brain lesions. Individual laboratory methods of neurophysiological investigation will be omitted from the discussion, for only those techniques that can be used at the patient's bedside are considered pertinent to this account. Of course, the tests that will be considered herein may be supplemented by numerous other clinical psychological tests, but the latter lie outside the scope of this book.

2. The Preliminary Conversation

An investigation for the purpose of establishing the topical diagnosis of brain lesions must begin with a preliminary conversation with the patient. The more care and attention to detail paid during this conversation, the more precise and purposeful the subsequent clinical psychological investigation of the patient will be.

This preliminary conversation has a twofold purpose. First, it enables the investigator to form a general idea of the state of the patient's consciousness, of the level and peculiarities of his personality, of his attitude toward himself and his situation. Second, it brings to light the patient's principal complaints and exposes the group of pathological phenomena that may be of localizing significance and that must be studied with special care. As a rule, the basic hypotheses concerning the nature and, sometimes, the location of the pathological process are formed during this preliminary conversation with the patient, and the rest of the investigation serves to confirm, modify, or refute these hypotheses.

The conversation is begun with a series of questions aimed at discovering the general state of the patient's consciousness. The investigator must obtain a rough idea of the extent to which the patient can orient himself in space and time, of his ability to judge an external situation and other people, of the adequacy of his estimation of himself and his condition, of the astuteness of his perception of his defect, and of his emotional reaction to it.

At the same time that it reveals the general state of the patient's consciousness, the preliminary conversation must also help the investigator to form an opinion on the patient's general premorbid level. The level of the patient's intellectual development, the range of his ideas, the level of his knowledge and skills—these are all very important factors, for they help to determine what questions and problems may later be put to the patient to obviate misinterpretation of difficulties that may arise in the course of the subsequent investigation. Furthermore, knowledge of the patient's occupational training serves as a check on a seemingly successful performance that may, in fact, mask a defect that is present. For example, it is obvious that the highly automatized arithmetical operations that a mathematician or engineer habitually carries out enables such patients to do simple calculations that would be impossible for a patient with an identical lesion but different occupation. Knowledge of the patient's premorbid state frequently has a very important bearing on the evaluation of such behavioral manifestations as slowness or quickness of response and emotionality or restraint, for such manifestations may either be a sign of disease or indicate individual traits in the patient's make-up.

A matter of great importance in the elucidation of a case is the discovery of clear or latent signs of left-handedness; such a finding is often decisive in the evaluation of a wide range of symptoms and in the formulation of general conclusions. Sometimes omission of this important aspect of the investigation has led to the false conclusion that no lesion was present; the so-called absence of symptoms referable to the hemisphere presumed to be "dominant", left, was owing to the fact that the left hemisphere was not dominant.

• • •

The preliminary conversation with the patient usually begins with questions regarding his name and his native language (which may be important when considering speech disorders, if present), his place of residence, his family, where he is now, and how long he has not felt well. If the replies to these first questions indicate that the patient is inadequately oriented in space and time and if he fails to identify persons in his immediate environment, he may be given supplementary questions to ascertain if he can give the dates of well-known events, if he knows whether he ever met the examining doctor before, etc.

Even at this initial stage of the conversation valuable information may be obtained that gives a tentative idea of the principal features of the patient's condition. This may be based on general observations on how the patient behaved during the conversation, how he spoke, and how he reacted to his surroundings.

As a rule, patients with circumscribed brain lesions experience no particular difficulty in replying to the simple questions just cited. However, their replies may be either quick and lively or slow and listless. Slowness and inertia of response may indicate a general state of inertia or adynamia or an increased fatigability (which may be found with intracranial pressure as well as with certain lesions of the forebrain or with deep-seated pathological processes near the ventricles); however, these features may also indicate specific speech disorders. In the latter case, the investigator must, in turn, distinguish whether the general sluggishness of the response is an outgrowth of dynamic aphasia (Part II, Section 4G) or defects in the understanding of speech or in the retrieval or articulation of appropriate words, comprising symptoms of different forms of aphasia (Part II, Sections 2D and E, 3F, 4D and F). The investigator should suspect the presence of dynamic aphasia or generalized aspontaneity if the patient cannot reply fully and consecutively to the question unless the required reply is already included in the question or if he is profuse in echolalic repetition of the question.

Observations of the patient's facial expression and his posture during the conversation are very important. An unexpressive, mask-like face, an immobile gaze, and a monotonous voice in a patient, in the absence of any general "emotional depression," can give valuable indications of a lesion of the subcortical ganglia. They may lead the examiner to be on the lookout for a whole group of symptoms of which these local brain lesions closely resemble the phenomena observed in parkinsonism.

The increased tendency toward echopraxia, when the patient copies the facial expression of the physician examining him, responding with a smile when the physician smiles and immediately changing his facial expression as soon as the physician assumes a serious air; a tendency to reproduce the intonation of the physician speaking to him; and, finally, a tendency to repeat the physician's questions echolalically before starting to answer them—all these may indicate the characteristic passiveness of a patient with a frontal lobe lesion. Often the phenomena of euphoria characteristic of the frontal syndrome are attributable not only to a profound disturbance of the patient's emotional sphere and critical faculty, but also to echolalic repetition of the cheerful tone with which the physician converses with his patient.

It is also very important to observe how the patient's emotional tone varies during the conversation. Emotional immobility and rigidity observed in patients with lesions of the subcortical formations, the phenomena of forced laughter and grief which arise so readily in patients with lesions of the brain stem, and the easy switching from one emotional state to another without any features of lasting experiences and moods characteristic of patients with frontal lesions can provide valuable supporting evidence when results obtained during further investigation are assessed. Naturally, therefore, facts revealing how the patient reacts to questions that should induce natural anxiety in him (questions about his future ability to work, about an operation to be undergone) can give invaluable material with which to judge the state of his affective sphere and his critical attitude toward his own disease.

The foregoing applies to the evaluation of the manner in which the patient converses. The most important information, however, may be obtained from the content of the replies. The preliminary conversation can reveal how the patient is oriented in his environment and in space and time, how he generalizes events, and how he recognizes people around him and his attitude toward them; in short, the preliminary conversation can provide important information regarding the state of the patient's consciousness.

As a rule, patients with circumscribed lesions of the cerebral cortex uncomplicated by marked symptoms of increased intracranial pressure are properly oriented in space and time and can give adequate information on where they are, their home address, their occupation, and the members of their family. They may find it rather more difficult to give information on dates (today's date, the day of the week, month, and year); usually the answer to this question is given by means of a series of intermediate links (counting from some date that serves as a prop, comparing today's date with yesterday's, etc.) and it may present considerable difficulty.

In some patients questioning may reveal obvious defects. A clear distinction must be drawn between primary and secondary difficulties in replying to questions aimed at elucidating the patient's orientation in place and time. Primary difficulties, associated with true disturbances of orientation in place and time, are especially marked with diencephalic and frontodiencephalic (less often with temporodiencephalic) lesions. Secondary mistakes may be a sign of inactivity, of a disturbance in the discriminatory process, or of pathological inertia (in which the required answer is replaced by an inert stereotype). The latter condition is more often found in patients with a lesion of the frontal lobes (Part II, Section 5D) than with lesions at other sites.

Patients with diencephalic or frontodiencephalic lesions, whose state of consciousness is not normal (they are sometimes half asleep), often cannot tell where they are. Although they give their surnames and given names correctly, and sometimes the names of close relatives, they will say that they are "at work," "at their job," etc. Sometimes, while appreciating the details of their surroundings, e.g., the physicians' white gowns, they reach false conclusions from these fragments and say that they are "at the barber's," "at the baker's," or "at the baths." Such patients characteristically make gross mistakes in identifying the doctor conducting the conversation with him; when asked "Who am I?" or "Have you met me before?", they will confidently give the name of some other person whom they know well and the place where they met him before. As a rule, they are grossly disoriented in time; they cannot tell the date and the time of day and, if asked what they were doing an hour ago or yesterday, they will say that they have just come from the factory, that they were taking a walk, or that they were working.

Disorientation in place and, especially, in time may be present even if the disturbance of consciousness is not so conspicuous. Although such disorientation may not be apparent during the first stages of conversation, it begins to appear as soon as the patient's answers require perfect accuracy of the organized traces of previous experience. It is this accuracy that provides the basis of the unity of conscious activity, involving functions that are easily disturbed in pathological conditions of the brain associated with a general lowering of the cortical tone. Such patients know that they are in the hospital, but they often confuse the town in which the hospital is located with that of a hospital at which they have previously been treated. Sometimes they cannot give their correct address or the place where they work but, instead, substitute some close association (for example, when asked to state their address they give the wrong Moscow suburb, etc.). These phenomena indicate a considerable loss of selectivity in the system of connections. They may be found both in patients with a depression of mental activity resulting from lesions affecting the brain as a whole and in patients with frontal or frontotemporal lesions. However, similar symptoms may also be encountered in patients with various forms of amnesia or aphasia; in these conditions they constitute only one of the manifestations of the speech syndrome and by no means imply any clouding of the consciousness. The investigator must therefore distinguish between these various forms of disturbance, for they lead to different interpretations of the pathological process.

The signs of disturbed orientation in time are no less clear in patients with local brain lesions. One such sign is the inability to answer questions relating to the day of the week, the month, or the date of the patient's admission to the hospital. Appreciable disturbances are also sometimes observed when the patient is asked the time of day, whether or not he has had dinner, etc. In all these instances the defective orientation in time may be very conspicuous, with the patient confusing the date, the month, and the year, substituting another date with firmly established past associations, and sometimes displaying early signs of difficulty in the direct assessment of time.

In both types of cases a distinction should be drawn between the *primary disturbances of the "sense" of time* and *disturbances in the verbal evaluation of time* that result from speech disorders. The former, referred to in the literature as "chronognosia," are often seen in patients with deep-seated temporal and temporodiencephalic lesions. They sometimes accompany generalized brain lesions accompanied by significant lowering of cortical tone and general changes in the level of consciousness.* The second, known in the literature as defects of "chronology," may frequently be found as a symptom of discriminatory impairment of the connections of the second signal system. Each type of disturbance may arise in association with lesions affecting different parts of the brain. Therefore, before a correct conclusion may be reached on the nature and significance of disorientation in time, it is essential that a careful analysis be made of the nature of the disturbances and of the symptom-complex of which they are components.

This first part of the conversation, which yields general information on the state of the patient's consciousness, is followed by the main part, in which the objective is to explain the patient's principal complaints and to prepare the investigator for the analysis of the symptoms constituting the essential elements of the disease that must receive further study.

As in the first part of the conversation, the subsequent answers have a twofold significance: First, the answers themselves characterize the state of the patient's consciousness and, second, they reflect those defects with a direct bearing on the topical diagnosis.

The first point to which attention must be directed when the patient is

* Some authors claim that a disturbance of time sense is particularly evident in patients with a lesion of the right hemisphere, especially of the right temporal region. However, there is insufficient evidence to support such a claim.

interrogated about the pathological disturbances that trouble him concerns both the number of the complaints and their character. The subjective complaints of a patient with a local organic brain lesion may be very slight and vague but, as a rule, they are persistent and disclose a well-defined disturbance. Conversely, the presence of a considerable number of varied and fleeting complaints, or affirmative answers to any question regarding a possible disturbance, should make the investigator suspicious of increased emotional reactivity or of oversuggestibility and should not be regarded as evidence of the presence of a local brain lesion.

The absence of complaints is very significant. In the presence of objectively demonstrated defects in the patient's behavior it indicates that these defects are not reflected in the patient's speech system. Absence of complaints may be found both in patients with a general lowering of cerebral activity as a result of severe hypertensive states and in patients in which the frontal lobes are involved in the pathological process. One of the signs of a lesion of the frontal lobes is impaired awareness of one's own defects.

Particular attention must also be paid to the character of the statements that the patient may make regarding his complaints. Patients whose condition is relatively good usually describe their complaints actively and give a clear account of the reasons for coming to the hospital. The exception is the patient with a lesion of the frontal lobes, who is unaware of his defect and can neither state the reason for his admission to the hospital nor give a connected history of his illness. Other exceptions are patients with various types of delayed reactivity or aspontaneity or with speech disorders of the dynamic aphasia type, who cannot put their complaints into words but from whom the necessary information can be elicited by means of specific questions. The contrast between the paucity of the complaints described spontaneously by the patient and the multiplicity and substance of the complaints revealed by the answers to deliberate questions frequently is indicative of the presence of a characteristic form of aspontaneity of speech accompanying either disturbances of the brain as a whole or a lesion of the areas of the brain situated anteriorly to the speech zones of the left hemisphere (Part II, Section 4G). This paucity of spontaneous complaints of patients with a lesion of the forebrain contrasts sharply with the rich and well-defined complaints of patients with lesions of the posterior divisions of the hemispheres who have clear-cut defects of different analyzers. These patients are well aware of their malfunctioning.

The significance of the complaints made by patients with organic brain lesions are largely of two kinds. One group of complaints, although undoubtedly indicative of a lesion, has no topical relevance while the other at once directs the investigator's attention to symptoms referable to a particular site.

Prominent among the *first group of complaints* are those of *generalized headaches*, which may occur with lesions situated in any part of the brain,* and of *impaired*

* Strictly localized headaches may be of topical significance.

vision. Impairment of vision may result from lesions of widely separated parts of the brain; the investigator must therefore always determine accurately both the time of onset of the impairment (visual impairment developing before has a completely different significance from that developing after prolonged and increasing headaches) and whether it is accompanied by other manifestations of increased intracranial pressure or is a relatively isolated symptom in a more or less healthy subject. A similar approach must be taken to complaints of difficulty in hearing, general inertia, etc.

A particularly important and frequent complaint is *loss of memory*, for which a very wide range of different disturbances of mnestic processes may be responsible. If such a complaint is made, the investigator must therefore take pains to discover the exact type of defect—whether it is (1) of a general nature (a forgetting of events, items read, etc.), (2) confined to linguistic difficulties (forgetting of words, difficulty in finding the right word, and writing defects), or, finally, (3) manifested as a forgetting of intentions. In the latter case, a patient will leave the house and forget why he left, or go where he is not supposed to go, etc. The topical significance of these three forms of memory loss is very different. Whereas the first form may be a symptom of a general cerebral disturbance of cortical tone, the second may suggest specialized amnestic-aphasic disturbances; the third form is an early symptom of a disturbance in the processes of preliminary associations—processes which have a controlling effect on behavior—and is common, when severe, with lesions of the anterior divisions of the brain.

Among *complaints with direct topical significance* are psychosensory disorders, fits with a distinctive pattern of aura; defects in particular types of movement; and, finally, disturbances of speech, writing, reading, calculating, musical skill, etc.

Interrogation of the patient in order to bring to light essential information for the topical diagnosis of brain lesions must begin with a careful search for the presence of *psychosensory disorders* and, above all, for auditory and visual *hallucinations*. The side from which these hallucinations emanate and the degree to which they assume complex forms are particularly important pieces of information. Simple hallucinations (phosphenes, tinnitus, etc.) may develop as a result of stimulation of the peripheral receptors (the retina and the inner ear) or of the conducting tracts or projection zones in the cortex, whereas formed hallucinations (visual images, micropsia, macropsia, auditory hallucinations in the form of music, calling out, etc.) may have topical significance, indicating stimulation of particular divisions of the cortex or—in the case of complex "hallucinated scenes"—pathological processes affecting the deeper divisions of the temporodiencephalic region.

A detailed analysis must be made to explain psychosensory disorders having the character of disturbed body image. Episodic changes in the concept of body scheme (sensations of excessive growth of the hands and feet, of changes in the shape of the head, etc.) are valuable symptoms, pointing to the effect of a pathological process on the systems of the parietal cortical divisions. Similar in meaning are the paroxysmal changes in the perception of external objects, with distortion of their size and shape (micropsia, macropsia, and metamorphopsia). These symptoms usually indicate optic-spatial disturbances arising in association with a pathological process in the parieto-occipital region. Changes in auditory sensation (hyperacusia, sudden transformations of musical melodies into noise, paroxysmal disturbances of the understanding of speech) usually accompany a pathological condition of the temporal systems, and so on. Here can be included the diverse psychosensory phenomena of the hallucinated scenes—*déjà vu* and the paroxysmal visions of catastrophe and terror that contribute to the eschatological feelings—that indicate a pathological process situated in the depth of the temporal region. These phenomena, which sometimes arise as symptoms of temporal epilepsy, may be valuable evidence for the topical diagnosis of brain lesions. The rare complaints of a change in the direction of sounds or of their spatial dislocation, like the spatial displacement of visual perception (in which an object is perceived in the wrong position in space [optical allachesthesia]), can be an important sign of a lesion of the parieto-occipital cortical divisions.

Gustatory and olfactory hallucinations, like abnormalities in the perception of the taste of food and of smell, are also of great topical significance. Signs both of irritation in this sphere (increased sensitivity to smell and perversions of taste) and of depression (loss of the sense of smell and tastelessness of food) may be evidence of a lesion in the deep portions of the temporal or frontobasal region. If these disturbances are associated with affective disorders and symptoms related to the brain as a whole, their topical significance increases considerably. It should be noted, however, that these psychosensory disorders are not by any means invariably the direct results of a lesion of a circumscribed area of the brain; their localizing significance can be evaluated only by taking into account the whole syndrome of which they are a part.

During the interrogation of the patient special attention must be paid to vague hypochondriacal complaints bearing the character of dysesthesiae, for they (unless they have different sources) may indicate the influence of a pathological process in the deep, diencephalic divisions of the brain. This group includes the complaints, difficult to put into words, of vague and hardly localizable pains, sensations of cold, formication, or other paresthesias of uncertain location. These complaints sometimes have an emotional overlay or are accompanied by vague affective states of fear, alarm, or anxiety. In the presence of other signs indicating an organic local lesion, the appearance of unmotivated emotional change accompanied by sleep disturbances, sudden changes in general tone, increased thirst (polydipsia) or hunger (bulimia), metabolic disorders, and changes in sexual desire, calls for a careful search for additional symptoms indicative of a pathological process affecting the thalamic and hypothalamic regions.

Complaints of episodic occurrences become especially important if fits are part of the picture. The localizing significance of the aura preceding the epileptic fit and of the course of the fit itself is well known from the literature, starting from the first descriptions by Jackson and ending with the extensive investigations by Penfield and his collaborators. This aspect of patient interrogation therefore requires no special description. We shall only stress that visual, auditory, or sensory auras (phosphenes or the "appearance" of objects, music, or cries; sensations of "electricity" or paresthesias), as well as the appearance of focal convulsive movements (starting with a spasm of one muscle group and ending with adversive fits, with rotation of the eyes and head) are of great topical significance and must be carefully analyzed. Other fits of great topical importance are those associated with a sudden, sharp lowering of tone and those that induce an immediate and deep unconsciousness without an aura. Fits of this character suggest pathological processes involving the deep portions of the brain or the frontal lobes.

So far we have limited our description to that part of the history taking that relates to complaints of episodic symptoms. However, complaints pertaining to constant or gradually progressive symptoms are no less important. Besides progressive *changes in the sensory sphere* (a gradual loss of vision or hearing or a disturbance of cutaneous sensation), these include constant or increasing *motor dysfunction*. Among the complaints of considerable localizing significance are weakness or impaired precision of movements, motor awkwardness, handwriting changes and loss of writing fluency, and loss of previously acquired skilled movements (such as playing a musical instrument and typing). Complaints of loss of skilled movement without general loss of motor strength and without sensory disturbance may be indicative of the presence of a process impairing the function of the premotor cortex, and this may be confirmed by other signs of a lesion in this region. Other important complaints are those of irrepressible motor automatisms (for example, purposeless, continuous walking or turning in circles) or of unmotivated, impulsive actions, which, if no special explanation can be found for them, may be the result of a lesion of the forebrain.

The aforementioned symptoms are manifestations of disturbances of relatively simple functions, often associated with a lesion of specific, circumscribed area of the brain. During the preliminary conversation no less attention should be paid to phenomena suggesting a *disturbance of the higher cortical functions*. Such a disturbance may be signified by impairment of gnosis, praxis, and the complex cortical processes like speech, writing, reading, and calculation. Only occasionally will the preliminary conversation reveal the true nature of such disorders and identify them in sufficient detail. However, this conversation will bring these disturbances to light if they are present. Disturbances thus revealed must later be carefully studied.

Complaints of a disturbance in optic or acoustic gnosis are rarely sufficiently illuminating; usually they are masked by vague, general complaints of "poor eyesight" or "poor hearing." Sometimes, however, the patient will complain that he has begun to have difficulty in reading or in hearing what is said to him. In either case the investigator must clarify these complaints. In the first place, he must try to compare the phenomena described by the patient with objective findings—is there a general impairment of vision or hearing, a contraction of the visual fields, or a narrowing or instability of attention? Any of these conditions may lead to perceptual defects. Sometimes it is useful to apply very simple tests of visual acuity or hearing there and then, after which the significance of the patient's complaints may become clearer.

To uncover optic-spatial disorders, the patient must be asked if he has ever noticed that he makes mistakes in relation to space, i.e., takes the wrong turn, puts his arm into the wrong sleeve when putting on his coat, etc. Besides this type of impairment, writing and reading impairments, characterized by difficulty in writing the letters of the alphabet (particularly if asymmetrical in outline) and difficulty in recognizing letters, numbers, musical notation, etc., may come to light. The discovery of optic-spatial disorders of this type (especially if clearly defined) may be of considerable topical importance, for a lesion of the systems of the inferoparietal (or occipitoparietal) region of the cortex may give rise to them.

Possibly the most important part of the conversation is that devoted to the detection of signs of lingual deficiencies. These observations and questions include those relating to the understanding of unfamiliar speech, to the character of the patient's expressive speech, and to the patient's proficiency in writing and reading. Lingual disturbances will be specially described (Part III, Sections 7 to 9), so that here only those disturbances that should attract the investigator's attention during his interrogation of the patient will be mentioned.

It was mentioned that a disturbance in speech comprehension may come to light objectively in the course of the conversation by the patient's inability to hear the questions properly. The best way to detect these defects objectively is suddenly to change the content of a question, to exclude the possibility of understanding from context. It is also important to ask the patient if he has had any trouble understanding unfamiliar speech and if there have ever been times when he was unable (for a protracted period or episodically, while in good condition or before a fit) to understand what was said to him or when the sounds of speech seemed to be an unintelligible noise. Such questions, in the context of similar questions about changes in the perception of music, may immediately direct the investigator's attention to a series of phenomena of great importance to the topical diagnosis.

Observation of the patient's expressive speech is no less important. In the preliminary conversation it is possible to detect immediately such phenomena as general slowness of reaction, monotony, scanning or slurring of speech (indicating the subcortical or pseudobulbar character of the lesion), difficulty in articulation, disruption of the fluency and derangement of the grammatical structure of speech, and perseveration—all characteristic of motor aphasia (Part II, Section 4D and F). Finally, great importance should also be attached to a claim that finding the right word usually presents difficulties, a disorder that may be manifest both in the patient's continuous speech and in his answers to questions; it may be a symptom of the various forms of amnesia or aphasia that accompany a lesion of the left temporal (Part II, Section 2E), left parieto-occipital (Part II, Section 3F), or left postfrontal (Part II, Section 4G) regions. Sometimes clear signs of inactivity of the speech process may be detected in the course of the conversation, i.e., if the patient is unable to give a detailed description of his complaints and tends to answer questions with echolalic repetition (Part II, Section 5C).

Other important information may be obtained by asking the patient whether he has had difficulty in spontaneous speech and, if so, what the nature of the difficulty was (difficulty in pronunciation, "stumbling," difficulty in finding the necessary words, or obstructed flow of thought). Finally it must be ascertained whether his understanding of unfamiliar speech was preserved.

The order of appearance of these symptoms must be discovered. The interpretation of a case in which speech disorders were the earliest symptom, developing in an otherwise healthy person, will naturally differ from that in which they appeared comparatively late, in association with other, more general symptoms.

It is important to collect carefully all the information relating to writing disturbances if they are mentioned by the patient. A mere reference to writing difficulties rarely allows for interpretation of the phenomenon. However, a remark to the effect that one's handwriting has changed, that the writing has lost its fluidity, that one has forgotten how to write such and such a word, or that mistakes have begun to appear in his writing, (e.g., letters are omitted, etc.), may all be topically significant. Careful inquiry on the details of the writing disturbance may therefore prove to be of great help in the subsequent study of the patient.

The collection of information on the patient's reading difficulties is equally important. These complaints may differ in implication so that great attention must be paid to precise demarcation. Difficulty in reading may be due to a simple loss of visual acuity, to constriction of the visual field, or to simultaneous agnosia (Part II, Section 3C); in these disturbances the patient is compelled repeatedly to run his eye along a line where previously he could grasp a large part of it at once. A particularly clear type of reading defect occurs with left-sided fixed hemianopsia, in which the patient disregards the left half of a text and, consequently, has total disintegration of the act of reading. Finally, complaints of difficulty in reading may be manifestations of optic alexia, in which the patient can no longer recognize letters or integrate them into words. Since interrogation in and of itself cannot identify the nature of a reading defect in every case, the presence of such complaints should instigate a thorough and objective analysis of the process.

If they are alluded to, great attention must also be paid to disturbances in arithmetical operations. As in the preceding complaints, the simple statement that for some time the patient "has had trouble with figuring" is of no particular clinical psychological significance for the "trouble" may have ensued from a wide range of defects. Sometimes, however, these complaints do not form part of a symptom-complex of general inactivity or general loss of memory: instead, the patient will state that he frequently cannot understand a simple number called out to him, gets confused when calculating mentally, loses the order of the digits, and adds the tens together with the units or else that he can no longer do the more difficult calculations that he had formerly found easy. The investigator must verify these statements by objective experiments and correctly classify the defects responsible for the loss of arithmetical skill.

The objectives of the foregoing aspects of the preliminary conversation are to determine whether localizing signs of a lesion are present and to discover defects for subsequent objective investigation.

• • •

One further aspect of the preliminary interrogation remains to be considered. It is important in its own right and can benefit by subsequent testing only to a limited extent. This is the elucidation of the effect of the disease on the patient's personality and emotional reactions and of his attitude toward his illness.

If the patient is asked how he has changed recently, it is only rarely that his answers will be specific enough to be of any localizing value. Usually such a question prompts the patient to declare that "I have become irritable," "cannot control myself," "am emotionally upset," etc. These remarks can hardly be taken at face value, and, as a rule, they implicate no particular system in the cerebral cortex. As far as the patient's reaction to his disease is concerned, his answers can only suggest that he is still able to assess his disability and, therefore, they can only be regarded positively. A different conclusion may be drawn from the patient's statements that he is "losing interest in things," that he has "become apathetic and indifferent," that he has "difficulty in starting a job," that he has "become stagnant," that "no ideas come into my head," that he "begins something and then at once gets bogged down and can make no further progress," or that he has "become dull and indifferent." If no appropriate explanation of these complaints can be given and if they do not result from phenomena affecting the brain as a whole or from some general reaction to a disease, they may be indicative of a lesion of the anterior divisions of the brain and may be considered symptoms of a progressive akinetic-abulic syndrome (Part II, Section 5A and C).

At the beginning of this section attention was drawn to the very great importance of the absence of any complaint of personality change, especially if this is in sharp contrast to the objective findings of profound alterations in the patient's behavior. As has already been stated, unawareness of one's own defects is one of the clearest symptoms of a lesion of the frontal lobes. Whereas a patient with a lesion of the posterior divisions of the brain will immediately be aware of his defect, a patient with a frontal syndrome is often unaware of the changes taking place, even after his behavior has begun to undergo considerable change and his acquaintances notice an advanced degree of disintegration of his personality. For this reason, information obtained in this way concerning changes in the patient's personality, group behavior, and emotional state must always be checked with his friends and relatives. They may be able to describe new, pathological behavioral features before the patient himself can do so. The contrast between the patient's own sketchy account of personality changes and the wealth of detail on these changes obtained from friends and relatives provides a most significant lead and should prompt the investigator to pay careful attention to the possibility that the syndrome is due to a lesion of the frontal systems of the brain.

• • •

It was previously stated that the finding of latent left-handedness in a patient is of great importance to the topical evaluation of observed symptoms. Frequently a lesion of the temporal or fronto-parieto-temporal region of the left hemisphere in a right-handed individual may be unaccompanied by any noticeable speech disorders. In some cases the pathological focus (a tumor, for example) may extend outside the speech area (e.g., into the depth of the hemisphere) and, because of its location, the lesion does not necessarily cause disorders of speech activity. In other cases, the slow growth of a tumor lying within the speech areas disturbs their function only gradually, and the function can be transferred to the nondominant (right) hemisphere. Finally, in the third group of cases, the absence of symptoms from the focus is explained on the grounds that the left hemisphere is not dominant in such patients and that we are dealing with cases of latent ambidexterity or even of latent left-handedness. The experience of many investigators (Part II, Section 1) has shown that partial left-handedness or ambidexterity are far more common than is usually supposed (Zangwill, 1960). The presence of ill-defined signs of left-handedness and sometimes even a high incidence of left-handedness in the patient's family (Luria, 1947) may have great relevance in the evaluation of symptoms caused by circumscribed brain lesions. In such cases even extensive lesions of the left hemisphere may be unaccompanied by marked disturbances of the higher cortical functions and, conversely, a lesion of the "subordinate" right hemisphere may lead to "paradoxical" speech defects. If it is remembered that the tactics of the surgeon operating on the left hemisphere will be modified if he is firmly convinced that the right hemisphere is dominant, there will be no doubt about the diagnostic importance of knowledge of the degree of dominance of one or the other hemisphere.

Questioning the patient is the foremost means of uncovering suppressed or latent elements of left-handedness. Whether the patient was left-handed as a child, which hand is mainly used when he is working, throwing a ball, etc., which hand plays the active role when he claps, and how easily he uses his left hand when the right hand is busy doing something else all have special pertinence in this connection. Careful inquiry must be made to find out whether any members of the family are left-handed, and, if there are several such members, special attention must be paid to this fact.

Questions to discover signs of latent left-handedness may be supplemented by a series of tests that not only will supply objective information on such a possibility, but also will reveal the presence of partial left-handedness even when unsuspected by the patient himself.

Interlocking of the fingers is one such test (Fig. 110). In latent left-handedness the left hand plays the more active role, and the left thumb is placed uppermost. If the right thumb should chance to be uppermost, this position of the hands is described by the patient as "not as it should be." Determining the relative strength of the two hands, as with a simple dynamometer, is also valuable. Wrist bending when the hands are placed with their palmar surfaces together is also revealing, for, when a great effort is made with both hands, there is a differential in pressure, with the weaker hand subjected to the greater force and consequently bending more than the other (Fig. 110). Similar tests are the clapping test (a subject with latent left-handedness will clap actively with the left hand and passively with the right) or the "Napoleonic pose" test. In the latter, the arms are folded in front of the chest; if the subject has latent left-handedness the left arm will be uppermost (Fig. 110). Finally, latent left-handedness can be educed by comparing the width of the fingernails of both hands; the little fingers are best for this purpose. A wider nail on the left little finger is indicative of latent left-handedness.

Tests for eliciting partial left-handedness may also prove useful. The investigator should ascertain which leg plays the most active role in jumping, kneeling, etc.; which ear is used for listening (it is essential to exclude the factor of any difference in hearing acuity between the two ears); and which eye is used for looking through a tube. Reliable information about which eye is dominant can be obtained by asking the patient to keep both eyes open and to place a pencil, held vertically in his hand, in line with a point (or vertical line) on the opposite wall or window. If the pencil appears to move to the right when, without interrupting the experiment, the subject's right eye is covered, and if the pencil appears not to move when the left eye is covered, the right eye is dominant. The converse result (movement of the pencil to the left when the left eye is covered and absence of movement or a smaller movement to the right when the right eye is covered) demonstrates the dominant role of the left eye and allows for a diagnosis of partial left-handedness (Fig. 111).

Besides the above methods, which are only of limited importance, there are also the methods of injecting sodium amytal into the left or right carotid

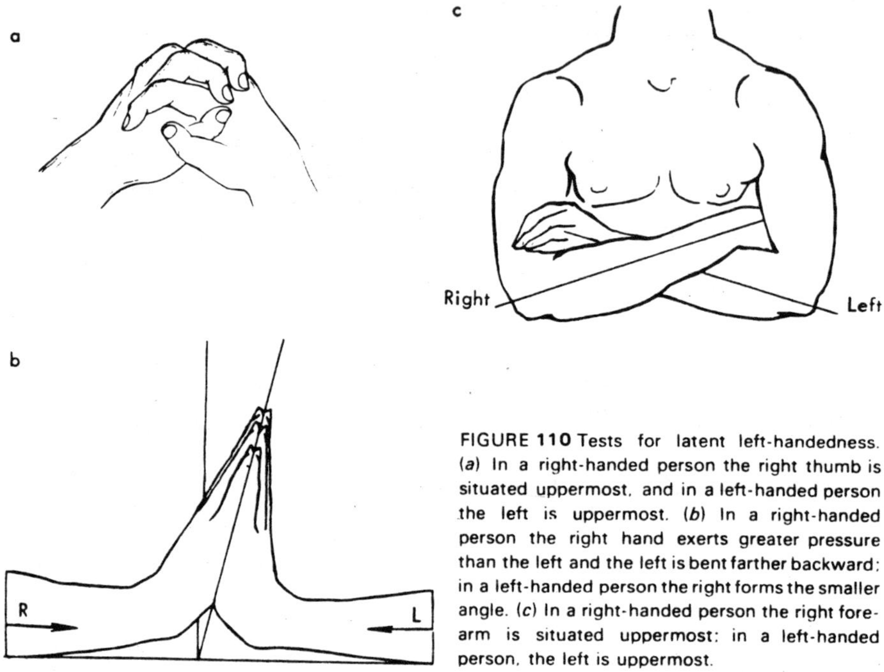

FIGURE 110 Tests for latent left-handedness. (*a*) In a right-handed person the right thumb is situated uppermost, and in a left-handed person the left is uppermost. (*b*) In a right-handed person the right hand exerts greater pressure than the left and the left is bent farther backward; in a left-handed person the right forms the smaller angle. (*c*) In a right-handed person the right fore-arm is situated uppermost; in a left-handed person, the left is uppermost.

artery, suggested by Wada, and the dichotic listening test suggested by Kimura. These methods, which are both very reliable, have been described above (Part I, Section 1B).

Evidence of overt or latent left-handedness gained in this manner may be decisive when the topical significance of the symptoms discovered in a patient is being assessed.

• • •

As well as supplying a history and offering an opportunity for general observation of the patient and supplementary interrogation of his friends and relatives, the preliminary conversation is the jumping off point for the systematic neuropsychological investigation of the patient's condition, undertaken in order to reach an accurate topical diagnosis of a brain lesion. Because of the information it yields on the state of the patient's consciousness and because it can bring to light certain specialized symptoms, the preliminary conversation can direct the subsequent experimental investigation into the proper channels and can clarify its findings. As stated earlier, this investigation begins with general screening tests and continues with more specialized tests, carrying the procedure further in the required direction.

Later in this section some of these tests will be considered in greater detail. Tests for the examination of the *motor, optic, and auditory functions;*

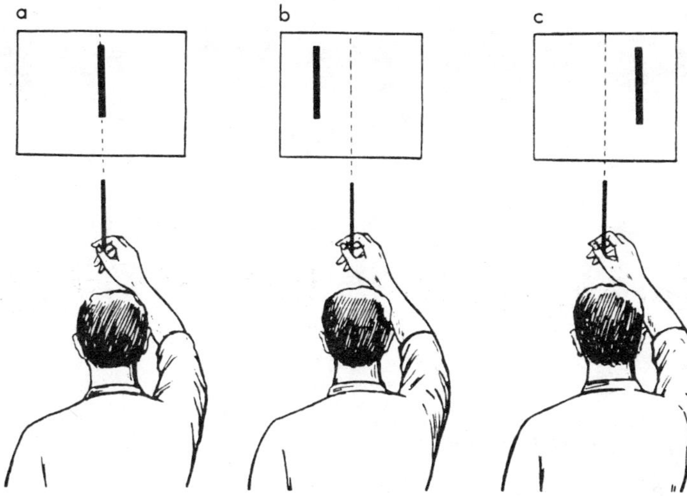

FIGURE 111 Depiction of an experiment to determine the dominant eye. (*a*) Initial procedure: A pencil is placed in vertical line with an object during eye fixation with both eyes open. (*b*) While this position is maintained the left eye is closed (the pencil appears to move to the left). (*c*) In the same manner the right eye is closed (the pencil moves to the right). If the right eye is dominant, the pencil moves as in example *c* and the movement shown in *b* does not take place. If the left eye is dominant, the movement is as in *b* and that in *c* does not take place.

speech, writing, and reading; arithmetical skill; and mnestic and intellectual processes will be dealt with. Naturally, we cannot describe all the possible tests. Therefore, the account will be limited to those tests that have proved their suitability for the topical diagnosis of a pathological process and to those with which we have had adequate experience.

3. *Investigation of Motor Functions*

A. PRELIMINARY REMARKS

Investigation of motor function for diagnostic localization involves an analysis of the complex forms of construction of voluntary movements known in clinical neurology as praxis. They may be disturbed by lesions of various divisions of the cerebral cortex. As mentioned (Part II, Section 4A and B), a disturbance of the complex forms of organization of the motor act cannot be sharply demarcated from a disturbance of the more elementary forms of movement. The investigation of motor functions should therefore begin with a short analysis of the state of the elementary components of the motor act with a view to ascertaining the degree to which they remain intact: this will facilitate the study of the more complex forms of voluntary movement.

Certain prerequisites must be met before any voluntary movement can be effectively carried out. The first of these requirements is adequate muscle strength and a consistently normal tone, without which precise coordination of voluntary movement is impossible (Bernshtein, 1947). The presence of adequate muscle power and tone is only one basic condition for the construction of a complex movement. The next condition to be satisfied is the preservation of the group of afferent systems within whose framework every goal-directed objective or locomotor movement is constructed.

Possibly the most important condition for the construction of a complex movement is the preservation of a flow of kinesthetic afferent impulses adequate to direct the motor efferent impulse to its proper destination and to maintain a constant control over the movements. The gross disturbances of motor activity caused by inadequacy of this afferent organization are well known (Part II, Section 4C). The normal performance of a complex motor act also demands an intact optic-spatial afferent system, for it is this system that ensures the correct construction of the movement within the coordinates of external space (up, down; right, left; near, far). This optic-spatial coordination is carried out by the occipitoparietal divisions of the cortex. It requires the precise differentiation of the signals received from the dominant (right) hand, so that disturbances in this process lead to loss of the correct disposition of the movements in external space and to the disintegration of the spatial scheme of the motor act (Part II, Section 3E).

The successful performance of complex movements, especially of those consisting of a chain of consecutive links, such as is found in skilled movements, requires continuous inhibition of one group of muscles and recruitment of other groups. In other words, it demands considerable mobility of those impulses that create the structure of movement. The organization of a motor act taking place over a period of time requires some degree of generalization of the motor innervations and their conversion into plastic kinetic melodies. As described above (Part II, Section 4E), an important role in this dynamic organization of movement is played by the premotor divisions of the cortex so that a lesion of this region causes a characteristic disturbance of skilled movement.

So far only the "technical" conditions necessary for the performance of a complex movement have been cited. We know, however, that every complex human voluntary movement has a definite goal and that this goal can be clearly expressed by a verbal command. It follows, therefore, that the capacity for selecting movements that correspond to the over-all goal and the capacity for subordinating the activity to the regulating influence of the verbal associations that indicate the purpose of the action and compare the results with the original intention must be maintained if complex motor acts are to be executed in normal fashion. The importance of the frontal lobe systems in the preservation of this discriminatory capacity and, as a corollary, the gross impairment of complex organizational activity with lesions of this part of the brain have already been pointed out (Part II, Section 5C and D).

Methods of investigating motor function must be so devised that they disclose both the extent to which each of the necessary components is preserved and the symptoms that have localizing significance. Because many of the methods used to investigate motor function were dealt with in the descriptions of the corresponding syndromes, they now will be described as succinctly as possible.

B. INVESTIGATION OF THE MOTOR FUNCTIONS OF THE HANDS

The special investigation of the patient is begun with an analysis of his motor functions. This is so for two reasons: It does not require spoken communication with the patient and the results prove useful during the subsequent analysis: The investigation usually starts with an analysis of possible changes in the power or accuracy of movement, disturbances of muscle tone, and manifestations of ataxia, hyperkineses, or pathological synkinesis.

This type of information is provided by the ordinary neurological examination, although it is useful to do special tests of the state of these basic elements of movement for the ancillary information may contribute to the evaluation of disturbances of complex motor acts that may come to light during subsequent investigation.

The patient is instructed to touch the fingers in turn with the thumb while counting them, to do these movements with both hands at the same time and as quickly as possible. The presence of paresis, a lack of precision, or of pathological dystonia and ataxia or tremor is clearly revealed by this test. Similar results may be obtained by instructing the patient to separate his fingers and bring them together or to alternately clench and relax the fingers of both hands for a long time. A difference between the performance of the movements by the two hands in these tests, especially an earlier onset of fatigue in one hand than in the other, may be valuable signs of a disturbance of the power, accuracy, speed, and coordination of the movements. This disturbance must be taken into consideration when subsequent findings pertaining to the disturbance of the complex structure of a motor act are evaluated.

In individual cases these motor defects may readily be recorded on a simple device utilizing pneumatic or pulley transmission; if greater accuracy is desired, an electromyograph should be used. Characteristic features of paretic or dystonic disturbances of movement may be obtained by recording the continuous tapping of the finger on a pneumatic receiver; this method will be described subsequently (Part III, Section 4C).

Further investigation of motor function must be carried out by means of a series of special tests, each of which, although complex in nature, is intended primarily for the investigation of the integrity of the required afferent systems. These tests may also be used to evaluate symptoms of topical significance.

Investigation of the integrity of the kinesthetic basis of movement construction should begin with an analysis of how the fingers experience deep sensation. This can be accomplished by ordinary neurological means. In some cases, however, more accurate methods of examination are required. The kinemometer, for example, serves this purpose. The patient's hand or finger is placed at a certain angle and he is instructed to reproduce this angle. The same apparatus may be used in a more complicated form, i.e., with his eyes closed the patient is instructed to place his left hand at the same angle at which his right hand had been positioned by the experimenter (or vice versa). An obviously poor performance of this test or the gradual appearance of mistakes as fatigue develops is evidence of a defect in kinesthetic analysis and suggests malfunctioning of the kinesthetic divisions of the cortex of the opposite hemisphere.

A valuable means of investigating the optic-kinesthetic organization of a complex movement is to ask the patient to reproduce the different finger positions demonstrated by the experimenter. In this test the patient is asked to reproduce one of the positions of the hand shown in Fig.112. Or, he is asked to place the index over the middle finger, etc. The patient should have as little visual control as possible over his movement; for this purpose, his hand may be passed through a hole in a screen.

A true disorder of the kinesthetic basis of movement will also be revealed by this test when the patient is not immediately able to achieve the necessary selection of movement (Part II, Section 4C). In such instances the movements will be diffuse in character; sometimes, instead of extending the index and little fingers the patient will continue to extend the middle and ring fingers, and sometimes, being unable to perform the test with the corresponding hand, he will try to help himself by bending the fingers with his other hand. All these disturbances, unaccompanied by paresis, may be clearly evident in the hand contralateral to the site of a circumscribed lesion, although sometimes they may also be present, in less marked form, in the ipsilateral hand. When thus presented they are indicative of a disturbance of the kinesthetic basis of action and of afferent (kinesthetic) apraxia.

Secondary defects during the performance of this test, unconnected with a disturbance of the kinesthetic basis of movement, are quite different in character and can easily be differentiated from the ones that have been described. Among these is mirror-image reversal of the movements, i.e., the patient, sitting face to face with the investigator, extends the little finger of his right hand when he should extend the index finger, tries to extend the ring and little fingers when he should extend the index and middle fingers, and generally fails to allow for the change in spatial relationships. Mistakes of this nature, which are easily corrected if the investigator sits side by side with the patient or if he sits face to face with him but asks him to reproduce with his left hand movements presented by the right hand, are manifestations of echopraxia, a condition most commonly seen in the passive states of patients with a frontal syndrome. This symptom sometimes also appears in association with the profound disintegration of the speech organization of movements observed in aphasia, and its topical significance naturally differs in the two cases.

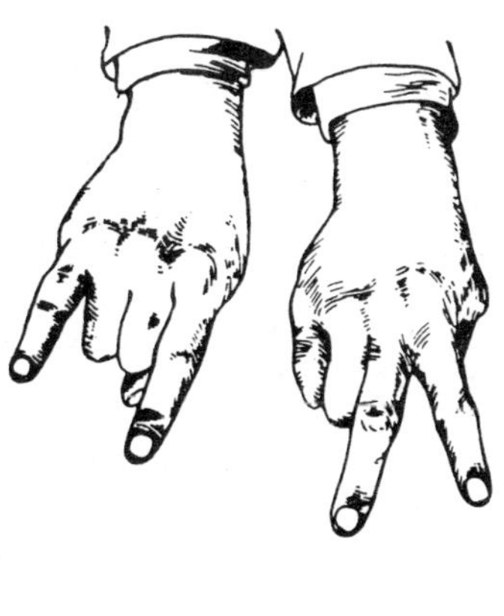

FIGURE 112 Test used to investigate postural praxis. The patient is asked to extend the index and little fingers or the index and middle fingers.

We may also see difficulties of inhibition of a movement once initiated, like perseveratory movements; the patient, once he has carried out a suitable movement, cannot transfer to a new one but continues to reproduce it inertly. These phenomena, however, have a different implication. This pathological inertia of motor acts, accompanied by preservation of the postural praxis, is usually a sign of a lesion of the anterior divisions of the cerebral cortex.

It is important to find out how well the patient can transfer the pose assumed by one hand to the other hand. This test is quite sensitive. The examiner places one of the patient's hands in a certain pose and requests that he reproduce the pose with the other hand while keeping his eyes shut. Defective kinesthetic afferentation of movement comes to light particularly well with this test. As a variant of this test, the patient is instructed to carry out a given movement, not by copying, but from a verbal command; this deprives the movement of its optic afferent organization and thus better defines the nature of the observed disturbances.

Whereas the primary purpose of these tests is to demonstrate defects in the kinesthetic basis of movement (although, as we have seen, the elicited disturbances may be due to other causes), the second group of tests is given to *detect defects in the optic-spatial organization of the motor act.*

This group also includes tests in which the patient is required to reproduce particular positions of the hands. They are as simple as possible in their kinesthetic aspect (they do not include differentiation in digit position), but they possess clearly defined spatial coordinates (horizontally, frontally, or sagittally). Figure 113 depicts some of these tests. As shown, one or both hands may be involved, the tests with both hands in different spatial planes naturally being more complex.

In the simpler variant of this test the investigator sits side by side with the patient (thus avoiding the necessity for mental transformation of the right and left hands); in the more complex (refined) variant, the investigator sits facing the patient. Under the latter condition, the patient must mentally transfer the position of the two hands and avoid a mirror-image reproduction of the required pose.

To demonstrate disturbances particularly clearly, the investigator gives the patient a pencil and asks him to place it in the horizontal, frontal, or sagittal planes, in conformity to the demonstrated position; kinesthetic factors concerned in placing the hand in the required pose are thereby completely excluded.

When evaluating the results of this test the investigator must pay attention to the disturbance of both the patient's ability to place the hand (or pencil) in the required position in space (for example, to change it from the sagittal to the frontal plane) and his ability to transpose the position of the hand (or pencil) in space mentally, an indispensable condition of the refined experiment. Lesions of the inferoparietal and parïeto-occipital cortical divisions (usually of the dominant hemisphere), without causing noticeable kinesthetic disturbances, may lead to appreciable difficulty in the performance of acts requiring integrity of the basic optic-spatial functions. These tests thereby acquire localizing significance.

A very similar test was devised by Head (1920): The investigator sits facing the patient and asks him to reproduce the position of his hand. When he raises his right hand, the patient must raise his own right hand; when the investigator raises his left hand, the patient must raise his own left hand (i.e., he must mentally recode the demonstrated image).

In simpler variants of this test the patient is requested to reproduce (frontally, horizontally, or sagittally) the position of one hand; in more complex variants, the patient must reproduce the position of one hand touching the ipsilateral (or contralateral) ear or eye. In still more complex variants, he must reproduce the position of two hands, with the right hand, for example, touching the nose and the left touching the right ear (Fig. 114). Naturally, with each of these trials the patient must mentally change the position of the hands to overcome the tendency to reproduce the pose in mirror-image fashion. In the course of the experiment the investigator may correct mistakes, at first by asking "Did you do it like this?" and later by explaining the patient's mistake. The investigator subsequently verifies the degree to which the patient has profited by his experience.

To exclude the influence of visual imagery, which allows the patient to reproduce the pose in mirror-image form, the experiment can be changed so that the movements are carried out in response to a spoken command ("Hold your left ear with your right hand" etc.). The significance of the result thereby becomes quite different. Inability

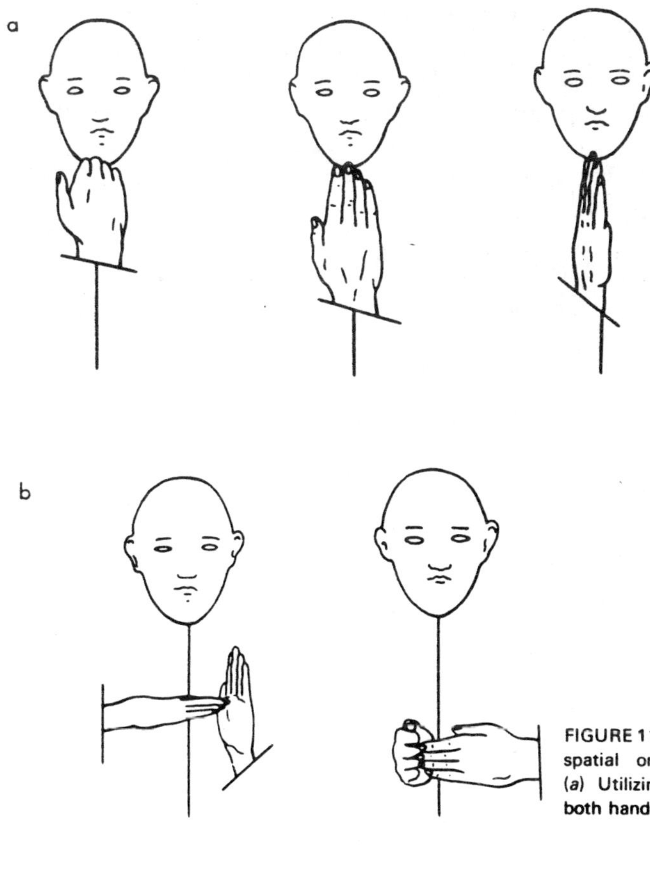

FIGURE 113 Test for assessing the spatial organization of movement. (*a*) Utilizing one hand. (*b*) Utilizing both hands.

to place the hand in the required position may indicate a disturbance in the optic-spatial constituent of the motor act. This difficulty in transposing a demonstrated pose while imitating it and this inability to overcome the tendency to mirror-image movement (which causes no difficulty in a healthy subject but is quite difficult for patients with brain lesions) may be a result of echopraxia (previously referred to), and thus indicative of a general lowering of activity, or, as some authorities believe, may represent a disturbance of the speech organization of action.

Like any other neuropsychological test, Head's test is complex in character and the disturbances revealed by its use may be the result of different pathological factors. As was stated above, primary defects of the performance of this test are the result of a disturbance of spatial synthesis and they arise in lesions of the parieto-occipital (or inferior parietal) zones of the left hemisphere. In these cases the patient actively seeks the position in which he should place his hands, often invoking verbal analysis of the task, but his attempts to find the correct spatial arrangement for them meet with considerable difficulty.

However, the characteristic defects in the performance of this test may be the result of the patient's general inactivity, typical of frontal brain lesions. The patient cannot set about the difficult analysis and recode the visual pattern shown to him; instead, he replaces this complex task by the simple echopraxic repetition of the position of the hands as he actually sees them. Because of this inactivity the patient performs Head's test in a mirror image version. His inactivity is manifested in two ways: he never perceives mistakes he has made; and corrections introduced by the examining physician as a rule do not result in any improvement in his performance.

Characteristically, in some cases of a relatively mild disturbance of frontal lobe function, the introduction of analysis spoken aloud (the patient is per-

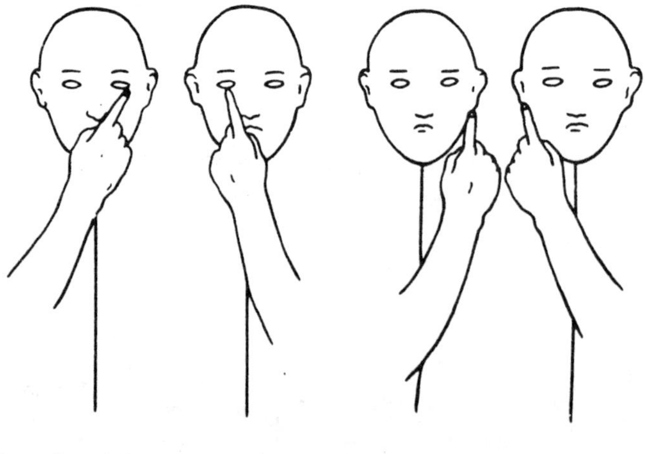

FIGURE 114 One of the variants of Head's test. See text for explanation.

mitted to analyze the assigned position of the hands aloud and then to repeat them himself) improves the performance of the test. However, prohibition of this extended verbal analysis once again causes the patient to obey his direct impression and reproduces a mirror image of the position of the physician's hands.

Although Head's test is an excellent method to elicit defects associated with brain lesions, the topical evaluation of these defects is a matter of great difficulty because of the complex character of the conditions involved.

The investigation of the optic-spatial basis of movement is carried out by a series of tests specially devised for the assessment of optic-spatial analysis and synthesis. These include tests of constructive praxis, which will be discussed in another context (Part III, Section 6C).

Of considerable importance to the establishment of an accurate topical diagnosis are methods of *investigating the dynamic organization of the motor act*, whose disturbance is clearly apparent with lesions of the premotor divisions of the brain (Part II, Section 4E). The most suitable tests for this purpose are those in which the patient is required to smoothly perform a simple series of movements, whose components follow in connected sequence.

This purpose is served by a test for assessing reciprocal coordination of the movements of both hands that was suggested by Ozeretskii (1930). In this test the patient is requested to place both hands in front of him, one with the fist clenched and the other with the fingers outstretched (Fig. 115). He is then asked to simultaneously change the positions of both hands, stretching the first and clenching the other. A patient with a lesion involving the kinesthetic element of the motor act will not evince any marked defects in this process. In contrast, a patient with a lesion of the premotor system (especially of the anterior divisions of the corpus callosum) is frequently unable to perform these movements quickly and smoothly. He either starts by carrying out each movement separately, so that, instead of a simultaneous change of position,

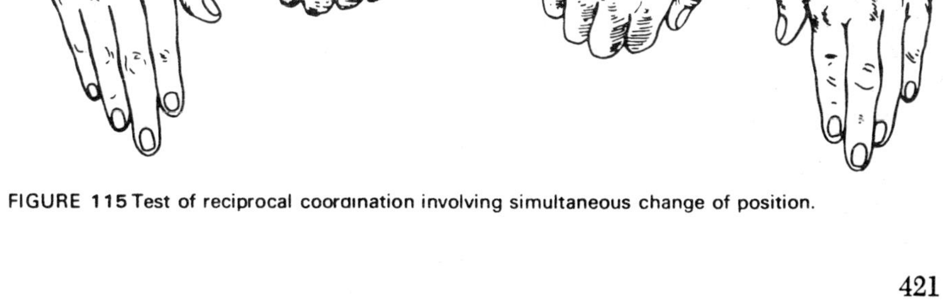

FIGURE 115 Test of reciprocal coordination involving simultaneous change of position.

consecutive, isolated movements are produced, or by performing similar movements with both hands, so that reciprocal coordination is replaced by equivalent coordination. Characteristically, in the presence of lesions of both the premotor and postcentral regions of one hemisphere, this test reveals that one hand (contralateral to the lesion) usually lags behind the other. With a parasagittal lesion, affecting the anterior divisions of the corpus callosum, reciprocal coordination of the two hands becomes completely impossible although the patient is still able to carry out movements of one hand that have a dynamic organization (which will be discussed subsequently).

Another variant of this test is equally important. The patient is requested to place both hands in front of him and to alternately tap twice with his right hand and once with his left hand, changing smoothly from one hand to the other. This test is conventionally recorded as $\begin{array}{l}R\\L\end{array}\left[\begin{array}{ccccc}\| & & \| & & \|\\ & | & & | & \end{array}\right.$. After this is executed the order of the taps is reversed. With lesions of the premotor divisions of the cortex the corresponding movements lose their smoothness and each tap is produced as an isolated phenomenon; the patient begins to make superfluous taps or performs identical movements with both hands, thus: $\begin{array}{l}R\\L\end{array}\left[\begin{array}{cccc}\| & & \| & \\ & \| & & \|\end{array}\right.$ or $\left[\begin{array}{ccccc}\| & & | & & |\\ & | & & | & \end{array}\right.$ The defects are particularly pronounced if the patient is requested to do this test quickly. Characteristically, patients with a premotor syndrome perform this test with insufficient smoothness but usually manage to correct the mistakes they make, while patients with a lesion involving the subcortical ganglia frequently begin to make a series of superfluous impulsive taps, which they cannot stop. Patients with lesions of the frontal lobes often simplify the program given to them, either by tapping out a rhythm alternately with both hands ($^{\prime}{}_{/}{}^{\prime}{}_{/}{}^{\prime}{}_{/}$), or they begin to tap haphazardly, without relating their movements to the problem set and without correcting their mistakes.

Other tests of similar significance in the study of the dynamic organization of movement are described by Ozeretskii (1930).

If one hand is affected by paresis, making bimanual testing impossible, tests for the dynamic organization of movements involving only one hand may be used. The easiest of these tests is the "fist-ring" test, in which the patient is instructed to thrust his hand forward with the fingers alternately making a fist and a ring (Fig. 116). A patient with a lesion of the premotor divisions of the cortex finds it difficult to perform this skilled movement; one movement does not merge smoothly with the next, so that one position of the hand becomes "fixed." The patient either thrusts his forearm forward without changing the position of the fingers or changes the position of the fingers but does not thrust the forearm forward. A similar test was suggested by Eidinova and Pravdina-Vinarskaya (1959): The patient has to concurrently extend the elbow and the fingers, with the latter initially clenched into a fist (Fig. 117). The patient with a premotor lesion cannot as a rule perform this activity smoothly. Particular difficulty arises when the instruction is changed, i.e., when the

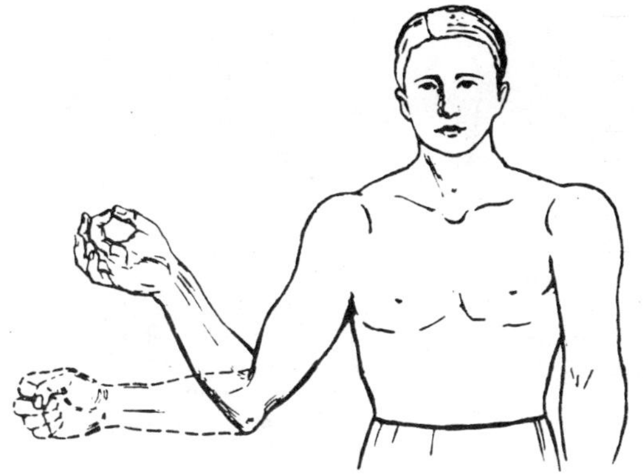

FIGURE 116 The "fist-ring" test. The patient must produce the positions alternately.

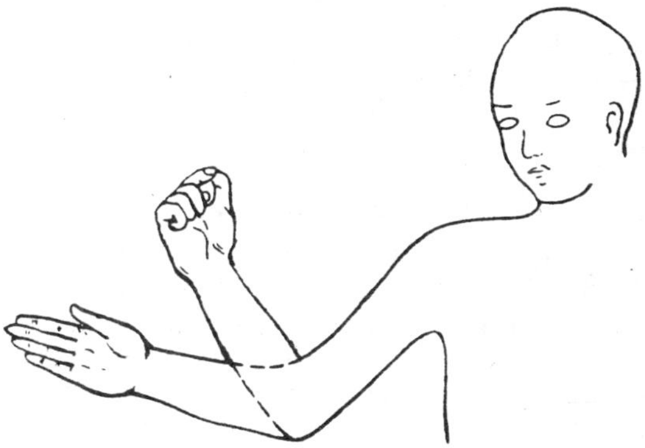

FIGURE 117 Test of the dynamic coordination of movement. (*From Éidinova and Pravdina-Vinarskaya 1959.*)

patient is requested to do this test in the opposite order (straightened fingers initially, converted to a fist when the elbow is extended).

The formation of a skilled movement involving three consecutive components is much more difficult. One such test is the "fist-edge-palm" test, in which the patient is requested to successively place his hand in three different positions: a fist, extended fingers with the "edge" of the hand showing (vertical palm), and the palm resting flat on a table (Fig. 118). Even a healthy subject may experience some difficulty in carrying out this sequence; therefore, the instructions should be verbally and visually repeated several times. Normally, learning this sequence does not take too much effort and the subject soon performs it faultlessly, slowly at first and then quickly and smoothly. In patients with brain lesions, however, no such kinetic melody can be established; the patient either loses the correct sequence of poses or continues to repeat the previous pose (for example, the fist) or the previous position in space (for example, a horizontal fist pose is followed by a horizontal palm pose) inertly. These defects are especially conspicuous in patients with lesions of the anterior cortical divisions; their performance of this sequence becomes increasingly nonautomatic in character.

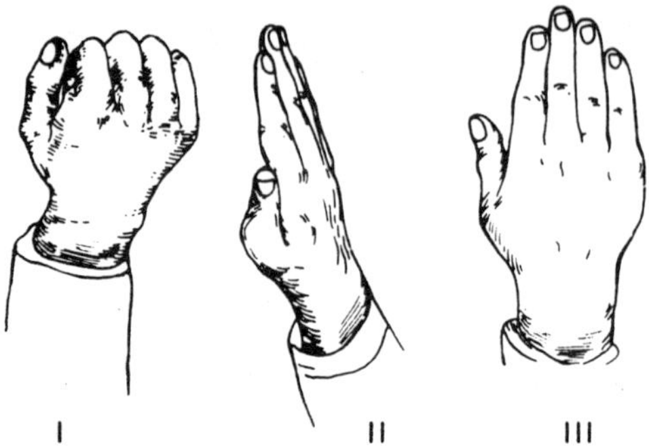

FIGURE 118 Test of a movement comprising three consecutive changes of the pose of the hand: "fist-edge-palm." The successive positions are shown.

Finally, this group includes the no less difficult test in which the patient is requested to place his hand on the table in the piano-playing position and to successively "play" with the thumb and the index finger (I, II) and the thumb and the other four fingers (I-V). Whereas a healthy subject can perform this task relatively smoothly after a short period of training, a patient with a brain lesion, especially one with a lesion of the forebrain, is usually unable to inhibit the movements once started, so that he continues to "play" in the same direction (I, II, III or I, II, V); he does not form the complex kinetic melody requiring inhibition of the series once begun and a return to the first movement.

The instituting of spoken commands rendered by the patient himself can greatly enhance the patient's performance of these three tests. If it is not possible for the patient to perform these tasks directly, the investigator may tell him to first give himself a spoken instruction (for example, "fist," "edge," "palm," etc., or "first," "second," "first," "fifth," etc.) and then to carry out the corresponding movements. A patient with a lesion of the premotor systems may find reinforcement by speech regulation in this manner effective with improvement in the execution of the required sequence. In contrast, in many patients with a frontal syndrome the regulating influence of speech is so weak (Part II, Section 5D) that, even though they may repeat the instruction correctly, they continue to perform the required action incorrectly.

During the investigation of the dynamic organization of movement considerable help may be obtained from graphic tests in which the patient is instructed to draw a design composed of two alternating components (for example, ПΛПΛПΛ). For the patient with a lesion of the premotor systems, this constant alternation of movement involving the performance of a single kinetic melody is very difficult. The execution of the task becomes nonautomatic in character and is sometimes replaced by perseverations of one element. These tests were described in detail in Part II, Section 4E.

All the tests that have been described are designed to analyze the individual elements of construction of the motor act (its kinesthetic, optic-spatial, and dynamic organization). However, observation of the patient's performance of complex, purposeful tasks (fastening a button, lacing a shoe, etc.) can also yield information regarding the patient's praxis. This type of test is common in clinical neurology. Although it does not have the qualities of analytical tests, it does provide a preliminary idea of the state of the patient's motor processes when confronted by complex acts and it shows how the defects that have been described can be manifested in complex, purposeful actions.

Tests of patient performance of an imaginary act, widely used in clinical neurology, are of special significance. The patient is instructed to carry out an action with objects that are not present (for example, to show how to pour and stir tea, to turn a coffee grinder, to thread a needle, or to cut with scissors). These tests, like those involving the performance of symbolic actions (e.g., to beckon with the finger, to threaten) are very sensitive indicators of the degree to which complex forms of praxis are preserved, but, because of the complexity of the action, they do not easily lend themselves to the topical diagnosis of the observed defects.

C. INVESTIGATION OF ORAL PRAXIS*

The object of the aforementioned tests was to determine the degree of preservation of those individual elements required for the successful accomplishment of hand movements. These movements demand a particularly fine cortical organization and are of utmost importance in human activity. No less important functions, however, are performed by the tongue, lips, and face, for they are instrumental in the construction of the speech act.

Besides aphasic disorders, the syndrome of impaired movement of the speech apparatus may also embrace paretic, dystonic, and hyperkinetic disturbances in those muscles participating in articulation. Sometimes these disturbances are so marked that we speak of a combination of aphasic and dysarthric defects of speech. In other cases, however, they are almost imperceptible and can be elicited only after special functional loading tests. However, the slightness of these symptoms does not mean that they do not contribute to the structure of the speech defect as a whole. Such disturbances must therefore be brought to light and analyzed for both diagnostic and corrective purposes.

Defective innervation of the mimic muscles may affect the articulation of labial sounds and may make speech insufficiently expressive and distinct. A symptom of such insufficiency is asymmetry of movement when showing the teeth, puffing the cheeks, wrinkling the brow, frowning, or screwing the eyes tightly. It is especially important to detect defects of muscle innervation of the lips and cheeks. If the patient can bare his teeth once and with one movement comparatively symmetrically, it is important to ask him to repeat

*Written in conjunction with E. N. Pravdina-Vinarskaya.

the movement many times over or to maintain the pose of bared teeth for a long period of time. This type of functional loading may also be used to detect defects of the other facial muscles.

Particular attention must be paid to the evaluation of the state of the tongue muscles. In mild cases, paresis of the tongue will be revealed by such tasks as placing the tip of the tongue on the upper lip, putting the tongue out as far as possible, and keeping it in this position. As the patient continues with his attempt to perform these tests, evidence of paresis is to be found in the diminished range of tongue movement, deviation of the tongue to one side, the onset of difficulty in the innervation of the movement, the high incidence of associated movement (synkineses), and the loss of smoothness of movement.

Increased tension of the tongue muscles and spasms developing during voluntary movement (frequently unilateral) indicate disturbed tone. Insufficient mobility of the tongue causes increased articulatory difficulties, for it interferes with the ability to sense the position of the tongue during articulation and makes pronunciation of complicated sounds impossible. Paresis of the muscles of the soft palate, which interferes with the regulation of air flow, also leads to loss of precision in pronunciation. Paretic or tonic disturbances affecting the muscles of voice production may make the patient's voice weak, easily fatigued, and incapable of adequate modulation.

These disturbances are all associated with a disorder of the peripheral innervation of the articulatory apparatus, and they must be sharply differentiated from aphasic changes in the speech act. However, defective articulation may also be encountered with lesions of those divisions of the cerebral cortex that are associated with the complex forms of organization of speech processes. In such cases they often have the character of apraxia of the speech apparatus (oral apraxia).

Elements of oral apraxia are observed with lesions of the inferior portion of the sensorimotor zone and of the adjacent parietotemporal areas of the cortex. Impaired oral praxis has a fundamental effect on the mechanisms responsible for certain forms of speech disorder.

The investigation of oral praxis must satisfy the requirements listed in connection with investigatory methods for motor disturbances of the hand. The essential difference is that optic-spatial afferent systems play an incomparably smaller role, and kinesthetic afferent systems a much larger one, in the organization of movements of the mouth. For this reason, when analyzing the state of oral praxis, the investigator must direct his attention principally toward the degree of preservation of the kinetic and dynamic organization of the corresponding movement.

It is important to note that many articulatory movements of the lips, tongue, and soft palate are determined by the phonetic system embodied in a particular language and are therefore closely connected with the auditory afferent system. Those forms of movement that are especially related to speech will be examined subsequently (Part III, Section 8B).

The investigation of oral praxis begins with a series of tests whose object is to *discover the simplest disturbances of lip and tongue movements* (pareses, dystonia, ataxia). For this purpose certain tests, well known in clinical neurology, are used: protracted extrusion of the tongue and observation for signs of tremor, deviation, or general inability to maintain this position; protrusion of the lips and consideration of the tone of the appropriate muscles; etc. The investigator must also try to detect such signs as tremor of the lips, paresis of the facial muscles, and salivation, for they will contribute to the evaluation of subsequent findings.

After this is done, the investigator may proceed with the main tests of oral praxis. The patient is requested to reproduce movements of the lips and tongue demonstrated by the investigator: to stretch the lips and bare the teeth, to extend the tongue flatly or to roll it up, to puff out the cheeks, to place the tongue between the teeth and the lower (or upper) lip, etc. As a rule, patients with signs of oral apraxia associated with a lesion of the inferior divisions of the postcentral region of the cortex and with a corresponding kinesthetic disturbance of movements of the oral cavity have difficulty in carrying out these movements; they make prolonged attempts to find the required movement and often substitute it with others or form inadequately differentiated movements. Often, these patients may have difficulty in switching from one movement to another and repeat the same movement over and over again. This is especially obvious in patients with a lesion of the anterior divisions in the region of the Sylvian fissure.

For a specific analysis of the dynamic organization of oral movements, the patient is instructed to reproduce two (or three) movements in succession—for example, to bare the teeth and then to extrude the tongue or to roll the tongue and then to place it between the teeth and the lower lip and to repeat these movements several times in succession. Rapid performance of the first movement followed by inability to switch to the second, or persistent fixation on one movement, suggests increased inertia in the motor system, which in some cases is a symptom of a lesion of the anterior divisions of the motor cortex.

Integrative tests of oral praxis have a special place in this study. The patient is asked to reproduce (whether from a demonstration or a spoken command) familiar movements such as chewing, kissing, spitting, and whistling. These tests do not allow for an analysis of the conditions responsible for disturbance of these movements, if present, but they do demonstrate even very slight disturbances of oral praxis.

It is important to compare the natural performance of an action with performance on request. Frequently, a patient who can easily chew food, blow away a piece of fluff from his hand, or spit is quite unable to rid his mouth of inedible material on command. This ability to act in a real situation but inability to carry out the equivalent movements on command may indicate a lowering of the level of organization of the action, such as is characteristically found with many brain lesions; however, as with other tests we have discussed involving analogous imaginary situations, it is difficult to evaluate its localizing significance. Methods for investigating the forms of oral praxis associated with the pronunciation of the sounds of speech will be considered subsequently (Part III, Section 9).

D. INVESTIGATION OF COMPLEX FORMS OF ORGANIZATION OF MOVEMENTS AND ACTIONS

So far I have described methods used to test elementary motor functions. In all such cases the patient was shown a movement which he had to copy, or he was given direct instructions which he had to convert into a motor act. Analysis of difficulties encountered by such patients reveals what lies at the basis of the observed defect and which aspect of his analytical and integrative activity is disturbed.

However, it is only rarely that human movements are copies of visually observed patterns or are performed in response to a direct command. The great majority of human movements are performed according to complex programs, and they are, as a rule, controlled by certain inner schemes which arise as a result of previous associations or preliminary recoding of information directly received. Such movements require the participation of the most complex forms of organization, and they are performed with the aid of the highest levels of brain activity.

Naturally the disturbance of these forms of organization of movements arises not so much through lesions of the cortical levels of particular analyzers as through lesions of the complex apparatus of organization of the motor act, which functions with the closest participation of external or internal speech.

The investigation of a patient's ability to perform a complex conditioned movement (or, in other words, a movement organized on the basis of a preliminary program) begins with the investigation of simple motor responses in accordance with a preliminary spoken instruction. The patient is told that whenever he hears a certain signal (e.g., a tap) he must raise his hand and immediately lower it. After the examiner has made sure that the patient has retained this spoken instruction, the test begins. If the examiner wishes to record the patient's motor response, raising the hand is replaced by pressing on a telegraphic key or a rubber balloon. The motor responses are recorded by means of a suitable electrical system or a Marey's tambour on moving tape.

As a rule, the performance of simple responses is rarely disturbed in patients with local brain lesions. Pathological changes are manifested only in the form of the motor response (which in patients with severe hypertensive states or with lesions of the anterior zones of the brain may assume a tonic character; the passive part of the movement, lowering the raised hand or relaxing the hand squeezing the rubber balloon, is omitted and the movement "freezes"). Frequently the lesion is manifested either by a progressive decrease in amplitude of the motor responses so that they soon disappear altogether (this is often found in easily exhausted patients with a general cerebral or frontal syndrome), or the patient begins to react prematurely, before receiving the conditioned stimulus, as a simple "reflex to time." In the clinical picture of local brain lesions this defect is seen most frequently in lesions of the anterior brain zones, associated with generalized disinhibition. Characteristically, patients with a marked frontal syndrome are unaware of their mistakes whereas patients with other brain lesions notice them and correct them.

The next stage of investigation of the organization of movements consists of tests evoking a response of choice to a spoken instruction. The patient is instructed to respond to one signal (e.g., one tap) by raising his hand, and in response to another signal (e.g., two taps) by refraining from moving; or to respond to one signal (e.g., one tap) by raising his right hand, and to another signal (e.g., two taps) by raising his left hand.* As soon as the patient can reproduce the spoken instruction the test begins.

As a rule it falls into two stages. To begin with, these signals are presented in random order, and the examiner determines whether the patient can carry out an instruction he has just repeated. In the next stage of the test the two signals are given in regular alternation (A-B-A-B-A-B), and the corresponding stereotype of motor responses is formed in the patient. In the third stage of the test this stereotype is suddenly broken, and one of

* Some writers, notably A. G. Ivanov-Smolenskii (1956), have proposed replacing the performance of a simple motor response or a response of choice by tests in which a conditioned motor response is formed with verbal reinforcement. For this purpose, a patient who has received no preliminary instruction is shown signals accompanied by "verbal reinforcement" (e.g., "squeeze" or "don't squeeze"). The examiner waits until a conditioned motor response is formed by the patient and he performs the appropriate movements without waiting for the verbal reinforcement. The test shows, however, that in such cases the gradual conditioning does not take place, and the subject begins to formulate quite quickly a rule to govern the course of his subsequent motor responses. The "formation of conditioned motor responses with verbal reinforcement" test is thus in fact converted into a test with the formation of motor responses to a verbal instruction, the only difference being that the instruction is formulated by the subject himself; the examiner cannot determine when it appears or what form it takes. For that reason tests involving "the formation of motor responses with verbal reinforcement" have been abandoned or their use has been restricted to other purposes (e.g., to analyze how complex action programs are formed under conditions when the subject himself has to find and formulate a hidden program).

the signals is presented unexpectedly out of order (e.g., A-B-A-B-A-B-B). In this way the examiner tests whether under these conditions the patient can still perform the movements in accordance with the instruction, or whether the movements no longer conform to the assigned program and the motor stereotype prevails over the instruction.

If the performance of motor responses by the patient is found to be disturbed, the examiner must ascertain whether the patient retains the instruction given to him. In special tests, which it is useful to employ whenever the patient continues to respond incorrectly, the examiner may ask the patient to respond verbally rather than by movements (e.g., to respond to the signals by the words "I must!" or "I must not!" or by the words "Right!" or "Left!" depending on the conditioned meaning of the stimulus). If the test shows that the patient's performance of verbal responses is better than that of the actual movements, the examiner can go on to the next type of test, in which verbal and motor responses are combined; the patient is told to give himself the necessary instruction ("I must!" or "I must not!" or "Right!" or "Left!") and perform the necessary movements at the same time. This test, suggested some time ago by Khomskaya (1956, 1958), can reveal to what extent the program of motor responses can be maintained provided that constant support is given through the verbal instruction of the patient himself. The next type of test, in order of increasing complexity, is the sensitized test. In this case a test involving a response of choice is used, but this time the patient has to carry out more precise differentiation of movement: e.g., in response to one signal he must give weak movements, and in response to the other signal strong movements of the same hand (e.g., in response to the different signals he must raise his hand gently and strongly, or squeeze a rubber balloon gently and strongly). This test, while retaining the psychological structure of those described above, requires far more precise differentiation of the motor responses themselves. To record the results of this test more accurately, the method of recording the intensity of motor responses on moving paper tape previously described can be used.

Tests requiring performance of simple motor responses or responses of choice in accordance with a preliminary verbal instruction usually present no great difficulty to patients with local brain lesions. Only if the patient fails to grasp the meaning of the verbal instruction or is unable to retain it firmly do difficulties arise; however, the repetition of the instruction with an appropriate gesture can easily overcome the difficulty.

Patients with a generalized hypertensive syndrome usually perform tests involving simple responses of choice quite successfully. Only under the most difficult conditions is the latent period of their motor responses appreciably increased, and they sometimes make mistakes, although they try to correct them. Reinforcement of the instruction, or the switch to tests with additional verbal self-stimulation, usually stabilizes the performance of the necessary program. The patient's performance begins to deteriorate, and the necessary responses are omitted or distorted only if the subject is fatigued. Characteristically, these patients as a rule notice their mistakes and try to correct them. Similar results are obtained in tests on patients with local lesions of the posterior zones of the hemispheres. Patients with lesions of the parietal (kinesthetic) zones of the cortex, it is important to note, can perform relatively simple tests perfectly well but they have poor control over the intensity of their movements, as is required in the last of the tests I have described; this loss of control is seen particularly clearly in the limb contralateral to the focus. However, as a rule these defects can be compensated by the introduction of additional verbal self-stimulation.

A completely different picture can be observed in patients with massive lesions of the frontal zones.

As was stated above (Part II, Section 5C, D), patients with massive lesions of the frontal lobes accompanied by increased intracranial pressure or by toxic manifestations are unable to perform tests with a simple motor response consistently well. Although they readily retain and repeat the instruction given to them, they can respond to it correctly only once or twice; later their responses become slower and less strong and soon they disappear completely, replaced by stereotyped repetition: "Yes, I must press . . ." or even "But I have already pressed. . . ." The introduction of self-stimulation by the subjects' own verbal responses causes little change in the performance of the test.

In patients with smaller frontal lesions but with a sufficiently well-marked frontal syndrome tests involving a simple motor response may proceed without noticeable difficulty; however, on the change to tests with a response of choice, abnormalities are quickly found.

These patients will often start to perform a test involving a response of choice correctly; however, the slightest increase in complexity of the conditions of the test immediately produces disturbances of movement. For instance, having performed the necessary alternation of movement in stereotyped order several times, they will no longer respond adequately when the stereotyped order of presentation of the stimuli is broken. In that case the patients often continue to give motor responses in rigid order, so that the connection between the responses and the actual stimuli applied is lost; sometimes they correct their mistakes, sometimes they do not perceive any defects in the performance of the instruction, and they continue to give a stereotyped series of responses. Neither statements by the examiner nor the introduction of the patients' own verbal responses (which in milder cases still remain correct, although in the case of a more severe frontal syndrome they are themselves deformed under the influence of the inner stereotype) renders the necessary assistance. The ease with which the patients' motor responses cease to be controlled by their assigned program is an essential symptom of frontal lobe lesions.

As was stated earlier, these disturbances are manifested with different degrees of severity, but the defect of the controlling function of speech always remains one of the most important symptoms pointing to a lesion of the frontal system of the brain.

• • •

The next series of methods in order of increasing complexity is devoted to investigation of the organization of actions when there is conflict between the direct meaning of the stimulus and its conditioned meaning.

It could be seen in some of the tests described above that certain groups of patients with local brain lesions exhibit a tendency to obey the direct meaning of the stimulus rather than the meaning attached to it by the instruction (its conditioned meaning). For instance, patients with massive frontal brain lesions, if instructed to raise the right hand in response to one tap and the left hand in response to two taps, will frequently modify the conditions of the test; in response to two taps they will lift their hand twice, thereby echopraxically reproducing the direct qualities of the stimulus as they receive it.

To investigate this tendency to subordinate actions to the direct meaning of the stimulus a special series of tests is used in which the conditioned meaning of the stimulus conflicts with its direct meaning. The simplest form of such a test is that in which the patient is instructed to lift his finger when the examiner raises his fist and to raise his fist when the examiner raises his finger. Some patients listen attentively and retain the instruction, but during its performance they replace the conflicting movement required by echopraxic repetition; in response to the examiner's raised fist they raise their own fist, and so on.

This tendency toward an echopraxic response (frequently persisting even after the patient instructs himself aloud in order to reinforce the instruction) brings to light a tendency for the complex recoding of information obtained from the stimulus to be eliminated and for the patient's own movements to be subordinated to its direct action. It is not found in patients with a syndrome of generalized increased intracranial pressure or in patients with lesions of the posterior zones of the hemispheres, but it is clearly manifested in patients with massive lesions of the frontal lobes.

Similar results can be obtained by testing the reaction of choice. In this case the patient is instructed to raise his hand twice in response to one tap and to raise it once in response to two taps, or to respond to a weak movement by a strong movement, and to a strong movement by a weak movement, or yet again, to give a short response to a long stimulus and a long response to a short stimulus. As the investigations of Khomskaya and Maruszewski (1966) I have already mentioned above showed, these tests can reveal pathological changes of behavior in patients with frontal lesions but, as a rule, they reveal no signs of disturbance in local lesions outside the frontal lobe.

• • •

Tests involving the performance of complex motor programs constitute a special series of investigations for the analysis of disturbances of complex forms of organization of movements and actions. These tests reveal the extent to which the patient can retain a complex action program given to him by means of a spoken instruction and the degree to which his performance is deformed under the influence of irrelevant factors.

If the patient is instructed to repeat a series of movements or actions described in an instruction, he forms a complex program which can be broken down into a series of consecutive subprograms. The performance of each of these subprograms necessitates inhibition of the tendency to inertly repeat the previous stage of the movement and the tendency to simplify the whole program by giving it a more elementary character. Naturally, in patients with brain lesions, this task may be difficult, and the irrelevant factors just mentioned may considerably disturb the performance of the required program. Tests involving the performance of complex motor programs can thus be an important step in the investigation of patients with local brain lesions.

Such a test in its simplest form involves the repetition of a series of consecutive alternating movements given either by visual demonstration or verbal explanation. Examples of such tests were given above (Part III, Section 3B) and are described as the "fist–edge–palm" or "1–2, 1–5" test. As was shown there, the spoken instruction was retained, but the actual simplification of the required program with perseveration of its individual stages was an essential symptom of the disturbance of organization of activity in patients with frontal brain lesions.

Even clearer results can be obtained by tests involving the performance of an "asymmetrical program": e.g., the patient is instructed to arrange a series of checkers in accordance with the scheme "one black and two white" or to draw a successive series of figures consisting of "two crosses and one circle."

Both these programs can be demonstrated visually (the investigator begins the appropriate series which the patient has to continue) or given as a spoken instruction, which the patient first repeats in his own words and then starts to perform. Both present a typical task which breaks up into a cycle of subprograms: the subject has to take note simultaneously of the meaning of the elements of the task (black and white checkers, cross and circle) and also the number of elements in the task, and at the proper time he must switch from one stage of the program to the next.

As the experiments of Lebedinskii (1966) described above (Part II, Section 5D) showed, patients with lesions of the posterior zones of the brain have no difficulty in carrying out this task, but patients with massive frontal lobe lesions experience considerable difficulty in its performance. Usually they start to carry out the test properly, but very soon they simplify the program, either switching to performance of the "symmetrical program" (arranging a series of two black and two white checkers or drawing two crosses and two circles, and so on), or replacing the performance of the required program by the perseverative repetition of the same element.

Characteristically, in the severest cases, patients with massive frontal lesions do not notice their mistakes, and even if they correctly repeat the instruction and give themselves the right instructions, they continue to perform the task wrongly. Tests which repeat "asymmetrical programs" constitute some of the most demonstrative aids in diagnosing massive frontal lesions.

• • •

The investigation of how the controlling action of complex programs is disturbed can be seen in its last form, which is very simple but at the same time of very great diagnostic value, namely in tests involving the drawing of figures in response to a visual pattern or to a spoken instruction. In practice this investigation is best begun by tests involving the copying of simple figures (circle, cross, square) that are presented separately to the patient. The patient may copy directly from the sample or from memory (in which case the shapes tend to deteriorate exponentially for some time and finally disappear altogether). If a gross disturbance of the regulatory role of a visual instruction is present (for example, in patients with severe lesions of the frontal lobes) the patient will be unable to carry out this simple action normally (Part II, Section 5C); having started to reproduce the figure, he either immediately loses the selectivity of his action (for example, he continues to draw a cross or a circle) or he quickly begins to perseverate in the reproduction of the previous figure.

If this test fails to reveal any major dysfunction of the selective basis of action, the investigator may make the problem more complicated and instruct the patient to reproduce a series of simple figures (for example, △ ○ ○ – or □ □ △ +) shown to him for a short period of time (from 20 to 30 seconds) and then withdrawn. The typical disturbance found in patients with a brain lesion is that they either forget the end of the series or (if a true disturbance of the regulatory role of the instruction is present, as seen most frequently in frontal lobe patients) they reproduce the first series relatively well but in the second series replace some of the elements with perseverative elements from the first series. Often, the longer they continue to perform this test, the more obvious the loss of the regulatory influence of the instruction becomes.

In order to gain more precise information about a disturbance that has been so found, the patient is instructed to reproduce single figures or a series of figures in response to a spoken command. The patient is requested to draw independently figures that are separately called out to him by name, e.g., "circle," "cross," "square," or to draw at one time a series of named figures, e.g.,: "two circles, a cross, and a dot" or "a triangle, two minus signs, and a cross." To make the conditions of the test still more complicated.

the series of figures called out may be increased to four (or, more rarely, five) elements. The disturbances that may be brought to light by these experiments are similar to those revealed by the preceding series, the only difference being that they are even more obvious.

As a rule, patients with disturbances of the frontal and frontotemporal systems find this series of experiments particularly difficult. In less severe cases of such lesions the patients may repeat both the new and the old instruction correctly, but instead of carrying out the second task after having completed the first, they repeat the elements of the first stereotype. In severe cases the defect of the regulatory function of speech becomes particularly obvious; in lesions of the frontotemporal divisions of the brain it is complicated by misconstruction of the meaning of words, so that the patient may retain the verbal instruction but will draw quite inappropriate figures and will inertly reproduce previous motor stereotypes. In patients with lesions of the temporal divisions of the cortex, this perseveratory tendency is not as pronounced, and we are more likely to see an inability to retain a complex verbal instruction and signs of misconstruction of word meanings. The methods of investigating these features will be subsequently discussed (Part III, Section 8C).

Essential material for the differentiation of these various types of dysfunction may be obtained by comparing the results of experiments involving the drawing of figures from sight with those from spoken instruction. A patient with a lesion of the frontal divisions of the brain will exhibit impaired selectivity of his actions and in either of these tests will tend to replace the adequate action by an inert repetition of a stereotype. A patient with a lesion of the temporal divisions of the brain, whose performance in response to a spoken instruction is poor, may proceed to perform the same series and to reproduce the figures faultlessly by sight.

An excellent method of determining the precise mechanism of the observed defect is to modify the experiment by instructing the patient to repeat the command aloud. As a rule, in cases in which the regulating function of speech is adequately preserved, this reinforcement of instruction makes the task much easier to perform; however, it has no significant effect if there is a primary disturbance of this function. Therefore, the introduction of this modification may considerably improve performance in patients with lesions affecting the brain as a whole or with lesions of the temporal divisions of the brain but often will not improve performance in patients with a severe frontal syndrome. Extension of this perseveratory tendency to speech, as evinced by changes in the verbal instruction itself, may indicate that the lesion is massive.

The information obtained from such tests, as well as from a series of auxiliary methods of investigating a disruption in speech regulation (in particular, the use of experiments involving motor reactions to spoken instructions), were discussed earlier (Part II, Section 5C and D) and therefore will not be repeated here.

4. *Investigation of Acoustic-Motor Coordination*

A. PRELIMINARY REMARKS

Hitherto we have dealt with the influence of optic and kinesthetic afferent systems on verbal instruction and on motor functioning. However, an important factor in the diagnosis of circumscribed lesions of the cerebral cortex is the state of audiomotor coordination, or, in other words, of simple motor acts dependent on the auditory afferent system; these acts have a precise serial organization, and, in their purest form, consist of "motor melodies" in which the sequence is based on time intervals. The investigation of this activity comprises two series of tests. One is aimed at the investigation of the perception and the reproduction of pitch relationships and musical melodies; the other, at the investigation of the perception and the reproduction of rhythmic structures. These two series of tests will be dealt with separately.

B. INVESTIGATION OF THE PERCEPTION AND THE REPRODUCTION OF PITCH RELATIONSHIPS

The investigation of the perception and reproduction of pitch relationships and musical melodies is an important part of the study of the pathology of the temporal and premotor divisions of the cerebral cortex and with some lesions (for example, lesions of the right temporal lobe) may bring to light what is perhaps the only symptom of a disturbance of the complex cortical functions.

Because of the very great variation of human musical ability (Teplov, 1947), the investigation of the perception and the reproduction of pitch relationships and musical melodies must not go beyond the use of simple tests; more complicated tests should be given only to patients whose degree of musical development is sufficiently high.

This investigation must begin with simple tests in which the patient is requested to estimate the pitch of two notes (sung or produced by an audiometer or musical instrument), each with a sufficiently different pitch (any investigation aimed at assessing subtle differentiation is of a more specialized character). One's estimate of the relative pitch of sounds can be rendered either verbally ("higher," "lower") or by "equalizing"; by the latter means the patient, after being presented with a pair of tones on the audiometer and repetition of the first tone, tries to reproduce the second tone by turning the handle of the regulator.

The simplest form of the test is that in which the examiner sings two pairs of tones, sometimes the same, sometimes different, and the subject has to state whether the pairs of tones are identical or different.

A variant of this test that can be used to evaluate the ability to differentiate between groups of pitch relationships is contained in the experiment in which two groups of sounds are made the conditioned stimuli for a particular motor reaction. For example, the patient may be requested by a verbal instruction or by the method of speech reinforcement (repeating the instruction himself) to raise his right hand in response to the group ♩♩♩ and to raise his left hand in response to the group ♩♩♩, or, alternatively, to raise his hand in response to the former and not to move in response to the latter. A careful analysis of the way in which the reaction is formed, how quickly it becomes stable, how easily it is modified, and under what conditions mistakes take place may give valuable information on the state of acoustic analysis and synthesis. There may be a profound derangement of this function with lesions of the temporal system.

It must be remembered, however, that the process of formation, stabilization, and modification of conditioned motor reactions may itself prove difficult for patients with brain lesions. Hence, the evaluation of defects arising from disturbances in the operation of the auditory analyzer may be justified only when similar tests with visual stimuli reveal a relatively intact capacity for the formation, stabilization, and modification of conditioned reactions. A special place in this investigation is occupied by the experiment in which groups containing two or three successively identical tones and forming an inverse and symmetrical sequence of tones in relation to each other are compared, for example, ♩♩♩♩𝅗𝅥 and ♩♩♩♩𝅗𝅥 or ♩♩♩𝅗𝅥 and ♩♩♩𝅗𝅥. A patient whose ability to discern pitch relationships is impaired may consider the two groups identical. A very poor showing in this test may indicate a lesion of the cortical divisions of the auditory analyzer. As various studies have shown (Feuchtwanger, 1930), significant impairment in perceiving pitch relationships may occur not only with lesions of the left, but also with those of the right temporal region.

Much more varied forms of disturbance may be revealed by tests involving

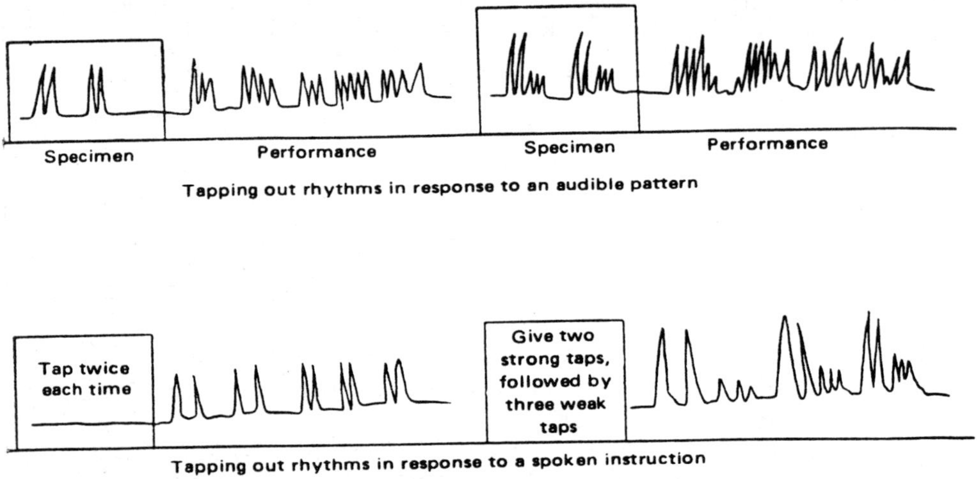

FIGURE 119 Tapping out rhythms by ear and in response to an instruction, by a patient with a left temporal lesion.

the reproduction of pitch relationships and musical melodies. In these tests, the patient is requested to listen to a series of tones and then to reproduce them by singing. The experiment usually begins with tests in which the patient sings series consisting of two, three, four, or sometimes five tones; particularly useful groups for presentation are those such as

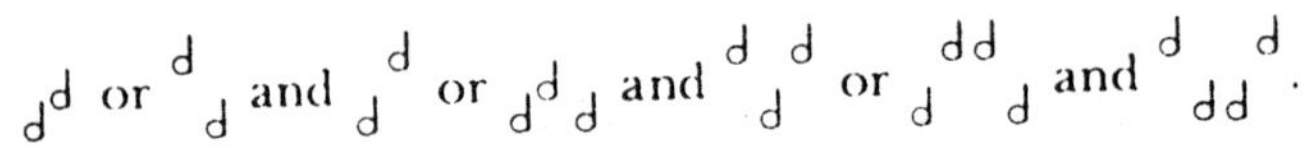

The groups consist of an equal number of tones presented in a different (sometimes a mirror-image) order. In more complicated tests, the patient is asked to repeat a familiar melody immediately after the investigator renders it or to reproduce it from memory.

Poor vocal reproduction of the presented tones may be the result either of a disturbance in acoustic analysis and synthesis arising from a lesion of the temporal divisions of the brain or of defects associated with pathology of the motor process of vocalization.

In the first instance the patient may have difficulty in assessing pitch relationships. He frequently is unable to retain a melody presented to him, and, although he has no difficulty in the act of phonation itself, he manifests a major disability in the differentiation and reproduction of pitch relationships and musical melodies. In cases of what is called "sensory amusia," arising as a result of lesions of the temporal region of the cortex, these disturbances may be particularly prominent.

Audiomotor coordination is disturbed in a quite different way in the presence of lesions of the various parts of the motor analyzer. With bilateral lesions of the anterior divisions of the sensorimotor zone (with that of the right hemisphere especially provocative), leading to pseudobulbar disorders, and with lesions of the basal ganglia, the act of phonation may itself be severely impaired. The patient cannot sing a note smoothly, but, instead, it becomes a series of intermittent, unmodulated vocal impulses. With lesions of the inferior divisions of the premotor zone associated with signs of pathological inertia in the motor analyzer, the process of switching from the reproduction of one sound to another is seriously deranged and motor perseverations develop; these are exhibited just as clearly in singing as in speaking. Finally, with kinetic dysfunction in phonation, as observed with extensive lesions of the postcentral region of the cortex that give rise to signs of kinesthetic apraxia, similar disorders in pitch differentiation may occur; they constitute the basis of the phenomena of "motor amusia."

The investigation of the perception and the reproduction of pitch relationships and musical melodies is a special but important aspect of the study of audiomotor coordination; it can yield valuable data for the topical diagnosis of certain cases.

C. INVESTIGATION OF THE PERCEPTION AND THE REPRODUCTION OF RHYTHMIC STRUCTURES

The investigation of the perception and reproduction of pitch relationships comprises only one phase of the study of audiomotor coordination. Another avenue of approach is the perception and reproduction of rhythmic structures. This aspect of the investigation has, unfortunately, been neglected in clinical practice, but it is of very great importance in the topical diagnosis of brain lesions.

The tapping out of rhythms to form an audible pattern in imitation of a given pattern is a complex activity composed of separate elements. It requires, in the first place, acoustic analysis of the rhythmic structure of the model, and it invariably becomes difficult whenever the possibility of acoustic analysis is restricted. Secondly, it requires the recoding of the perceived acoustic structure into a series of consecutive movements. Even if the ability to analyze sound is intact, the performance of this task will suffer if the serial organization of simple motor acts is deranged. The disturbance in this instance, though, will take a different form.

The test involving tapping rhythms usually starts with an analysis of the extent to which the patient can perceive and evaluate a group of acoustic signals presented to him. For this purpose, groups of rhythmic taps, following each other at 0.5- to 1.5-second intervals are presented. These taps are at first rendered in single groups of two or three taps (″ or ‴) and then as a series of these groups (″ ″ ″ ″ or ‴ ‴ ‴). In more complicated tests the rhythmic groups are further distinguished by accentuation, to form rhythmic complexes (∪ ∪ ∪ ′ or ∪ ∪ ′ or ″ ∪ ∪ ∪̣ or ∪ ∪ ∪ ″). The patient is instructed to *tell* how many taps are included in each group and, in the more complicated tests, to analyze the rhythmic structure of each group, pointing out the nature of the taps (strong or weak) of which it is composed.

In order to make the experiment more sensitive to flaws, the rhythmic groups may be presented either in quick succession (within a period of 1.0 to 1.5 seconds), which makes their acoustic analysis difficult, or more slowly (with intervals of 1.5 to 2.0 seconds between individual taps), which necessitates integration of the memory images of the sounds. In the latter variant, the patient's tongue must be gripped between the teeth to prevent counting aloud or articulatory analysis. In order to find out whether compensation for the defects discovered is possible, the task may be carried out with associated rhythmic movements or with simultaneous rhythmic counting aloud.

Healthy subjects perform this simple task without difficulty. Likewise, it presents no difficulty for patients with a circumscribed lesion situated outside the temporal and frontotemporal divisions of the brain. The situation is entirely different for patients with lesions of the cortical portion of a temporal lobe (usually the left but sometimes the right), for they may experience considerable difficulty in carrying out this test. Sometimes, no sooner is the rhythmic structure presented at a slightly faster rate or is rhythmic counting aloud forbidden, than the patient is unable to evaluate it, declaring that the taps are being presented too quickly and that he cannot keep up with them or overestimating the number of taps composing the rhythmic group. The latter phenomenon is usually most conspicuous when a slowly presented group of two taps is immediately followed by a faster presentation of the same group; in such instances, the last group is often judged to contain three taps.

Similar difficulties arise in these patients when a given rhythmic group is repeated many times (for example, ″ ″ ″ ″ ″ ″ ″). Although such repetition merely simplifies the evaluation for a healthy subject, by enabling prolonged comparison of one group with another, patients with disturbances affecting the auditory (and audiomotor) analyzer find the analysis much more difficult. The patient often exclaims that there are far too many taps and that he cannot identify the rhythm in which they are presented. Naturally, such patients have equal difficulty when confronted with complex accentuations; they find such rhythmic structures to be beyond their grasp.

No information is yet available to indicate how the perception of rhythm is disturbed by a lesion of the motor system. The important evaluative role played by the motor analysis of rhythms suggests that a lesion of the anterior divisions of the brain may also interfere with the proper evaluation of rhythmic structure. With lesions of the frontal lobes the evaluation of rhythmic structures is significantly impaired, but, as a rule, this disturbance is of the nature of inadequate analysis of the rhythmic structure; as a result, groups of rapidly presented rhythms are constantly overestimated and successively changing rhythmic structures (changing from groups of two to groups of three and vice versa) frequently give way to an inert stereotyped response ("two," "two," "two," etc.).

When spoken evaluation of the presented rhythms is difficult for some reason or other (as, for instance, in aphasia), it can be replaced by pointing to one's fingers to indicate the number of taps or by raising the hand at the appearance of particular rhythmic groups. In these experiments a group of two taps becomes the conditioned stimulus for raising the hand and a group of three taps the stimulus for not responding.

With all its advantages, however, this method has the disadvantage that possible disturbances of the interconnecting activity of the cortex, making the formation of a differential system of reactions especially difficult, are not precluded.

After it has been established that the auditory perception of rhythms is adequately preserved, the next step is to investigate the *motor performance* of rhythmic groups. In order for this activity to be analyzed with sufficient precision, the experiment should be carried out in two parts. In the first, the patient must reproduce the actual rhythms presented; in the second, he is instructed to reproduce rhythms that are described verbally. The first test investigates the state of audiomotor coordination, a process that may be disturbed either from defective acoustic analysis or from defective motor organization of the act. In the second test the need for acoustic analysis of the rhythm is no longer present, so that the integrity of the motor process in this activity is more patent.

As in the preceding tests, the required rhythms may be presented at different rates and may consist of groups differing in complexity; modification of established rhythms is another way of making the test more sensitive. As methods of compensation for the difficulties arising during the reproduction of the rhythms, it is possible to make use of visual or kinesthetic aids (by presenting auxiliary visual schemes of the given rhythms to the patient or allowing him to tap them out at different places on the table) and of articulatory analysis (by allowing the patient to count out loud). Yet another means of complicating the test, therefore, is revocation of the use of compensatory devices.

The rhythmic groups that the patient must reproduce are usually presented in a standard order, allowing consideration to be paid not only to disturbances associated with difficulty in the analysis of the presented patterns, but also to disturbances associated with defects of the mobility of the nervous processes. To recapitulate:

Series A. Reproduction of rhythms from a pattern presented acoustically:

(1) " " " " (2) "' "' "' "' (3) " " " " (4) " ∪ ∪ ∪ " ∪ ∪ ∪ " ∪ ∪ ∪
(5) ∪ ∪ ∪ " ∪ ∪ ∪ " ∪ ∪ ∪ " (6) " " " (7) "' "' "'

Series B. Reproduction of rhythms after verbal instruction:
(1) "Make a series of two taps." (2) "Make a series of three taps." (3) "Make a series of two taps." (4) "Make two strong taps and three weak taps." (5) "Make three weak taps and two strong taps." (6) "Make a series of two (or three) taps."

Series C. Reproduction of the rhythmic patterns presented in Series A and B but with verbal auto-reinforcement. The patient is told to say aloud every time: "one–two!" or "one–two–three!" and so on.

There are many advantages to be gained from carrying out the experiment in this way. First, it is possible to determine under what conditions the patient finds it especially difficult to perform tests based on rhythm. Do difficulties arise from defects in the analysis of acoustic images, defects in the regulatory role of verbal instruction, or defects in motor function in the narrow meaning of the term? Second, the transition from the reproduction of one rhythmic structure to another is an excellent test of the mobility of the nervous processes, revealing any signs of pathological inertia present.

As a rule, patients with lesions of the temporal divisions of the brain experience particular difficulty in reproducing rhythms from an acoustic pattern (especially when the rhythms are presented quickly and the patient is unable to count them out.). Often, such patients do not make the correct number of taps, merge separate groups into a single amorphous group, or tap chaotically without distinguishing between the individual rhythmic groups. They find the reproduction of groups of accentuated rhythms even more difficult. After unsuccessfully trying to discern the required rhythmic structure, they frequently abandon the attempt.

In sharp contrast to this state of affairs is the performance of the same group of patients when rhythms are detailed verbally. Usually verbal instruction greatly minimizes their difficulties, especially if they are permitted to vocalize the rhythms out loud, counting off the corresponding taps in their proper sequence. When prohibited from vocalizing, their reproduction of the rhythms is often much less satisfactory, and, deprived of the aid of speech, these patients will start to look for support based on the spatial organization of the process and will tap on different parts of the table. The cause of these disturbances is usually not confined to lesions of the left hemisphere; lesions of the right temporal lobe have a similar effect. However, a search for such differences is still required. It seems that patients with lesions of the right temporal region are less able to apprehend that they have performed the test incorrectly.

Disturbance of the reproduction of rhythms by lesions of the premotor region is quite different in character. As was mentioned (Part II, Section 4E), the characteristic consequence of these lesions is a disturbance of the system of higher automatisms, which makes smooth kinetic melodies impossible. In these patients, every tap forming part of a rhythmic pattern requires an isolated impulse, with no automatic rendition of the rhythmic pattern developing. Their difficulty in reproducing motor rhythms is further compounded with each attempt to increase the tempo; the inhibition of the rhythmic taps becomes more difficult, and superfluous taps appear. The patient is well aware that these taps are out of place, but he is not always able to suppress them. Sometimes, disturbance of the mobility of the nervous processes in the motor analyzer leads to considerable difficulty in the reproduction of accentuated rhythms, and their rendition is consequently distorted. As a result of this disturbance, the various elements composing a complex rhythm come to have the same number and strength of taps, so that the rhythm ″ ∪ ∪ ∪ begins to be reproduced as either ″ ″′ or ″ ″. Sometimes, it is difficult for the patient to change from one rhythmic group to another; after tapping the rhythm ″ ″ ″ he continues to tap out the same sequence rather than the new rhythm ″′″′. Characteristically, no difference between the reproduction of rhythms in imitation of an acoustic "image" and from verbal instruction can be observed in patients with lesions of the premotor divisions of the cerebral cortex. Figure 62, referred to previously, depicts characteristic motor rhythms of patients with lesions of the premotor cortex.

The reproduction of rhythms by patients with lesions of the frontal divisions of the brain has certain special attributes. Typically, because of the disruption of the regulatory function of speech that has been described, the reproduction of rhythms from the introduction of verbal instruction is not only not improved in these patients (in contradistinction to patients with temporal lesions) but is considerably worsened. They readily forget the rhythm described in the instruction or remember it for only a very short while, after which they readily fall under the influence of the inertia of previously formed impulses, and find it very difficult to switch from the old rhythm to the new.

Usually no distinction is made by a patient with a frontal syndrome between the required and the reproduced rhythm and he is unaware of his mistake. Often, he continues to tap out a series of two taps at a time when asked to tap it out in threes, or he continues to give an accented rhythm (″ ∪ ∪ ∪) even when instructed to change to a simpler, unaccented rhythm. This tendency toward perseveration of a previously formed stereotype and this inability to correct mistakes may often persist when rhythms are reproduced from an acoustic pattern. This indicates that the fundamental defect in the reproduction of rhythms by patients with a frontal syndrome is associated with a disturbance of the selective aspect of the motor act and of the regulatory influence of the instruction originating it.

In patients with lesions of the frontotemporal divisions of the cortex difficulties may arise that comprise those characteristic of both groups of patients. For this reason, incoordination of audiomotor rhythms may assume its most marked forms in these patients.

5. *Investigation of the Higher Cutaneous and Kinesthetic Functions*

A. PRELIMINARY REMARKS

The investigation of cutaneous and kinesthetic sensation is an essential component of every neurological examination. The methods used have been perfected in clinical practice, so that this part of the investigation can be described briefly.

This phase of the investigation of the patient usually falls into two independent parts. The first comprises the study of cutaneous sensation in the strict sense of the term, and the second deals with the investigation of muscle and joint sensation. Both parts are of fundamental importance in the evaluation of the state of the cutaneokinesthetic analyzer, and the abnormalities that they reveal may indicate a lesion of the postcentral or inferoparietal divisions of the cortex. This examination as a whole is rounded off by the investigation of stereognosis, the most complex form of cutaneokinesthetic function.

B. INVESTIGATION OF TACTILE (CUTANEOUS) SENSATION

The examination of the cutaneous and kinesthetic functions is accomplished by a wide range of techniques, some of which are devoted to the study of the most elementary indicators, i.e., the acuity of cutaneous sensations (nociceptive, thermesthetic, and tactile), while others are used to study the more complex forms of discriminative cutaneokinesthetic sensation, which Head (1920) called "epicritic sensibility." In all these tests the investigator attempts, as far as possible, to prevent any participation of the patient's kinesthetic and visual receptors; therefore, these investigations are usually carried out on the patient's immobilized limb and with vision excluded.

Investigation of the Higher Cutaneous and Kinesthetic Functions

The investigation of cutaneous sensation* begins with the study of the most elementary cutaneous functions, the sense of touch. For this purpose it is customary to use Frey's hairs, by means of which the acuity of the tactile sensation can be measured. The tactile stimuli are usually applied to the patient's fingers, palm, forearm, and shoulder, at first with very low pressure and then more strongly, to establish the threshold beyond which the hair is clearly felt. A diminution of sensitivity on one side of the body usually indicates a lesion of the postcentral divisions of the contralateral hemisphere or of the corresponding conducting tracts.

When investigating the thresholds of tactile sensation by means of these tests it must be remembered that the thresholds vary with the frequency of stimulation; it is customary, therefore, to apply stimuli at a frequency that makes allowance for the normal aftereffect period of tactile sensations. The intervals between the stimuli should be varied in order to avoid the pseudosensations that ensue from pathological inertia of each analyzer when the stimuli follow each other at regular intervals.

These tests are followed by experiments whose objective is to study the simplest forms of tactile discrimination. The patient's skin is touched with a pin, sometimes with the point, sometimes with the head, and he is asked to state which. As in the first test, the alternation of sharp and blunt applications must not follow a regular pattern, for stereotyped alternation may easily give rise to false decisions by patients with circumscribed brain lesions, suggesting not only changes in cutaneous sensation, but also a tendency to give inert, stereotyped responses. A similar phenomenon was observed by Pravdina-Vinarskaya (1957) during the study of oligophrenic children.

It must also be remembered that variations in a given patient's assessment may arise, due to the rate at which the stimuli are applied and the onset of fatigue. Therefore, incorrect replies do not constitute the only sign of a pathological process, for changes in their number as a result of an increased frequency of stimulus application and fatigue also may ensue from a cerebral lesion.

In a more sensitive variant of this test the patient is subjected to the action of three stimuli of different intensities that are applied in random order, and he must classify them by conventional signs (for example, the number "1" denoting the weakest and "3" the strongest stimulus). With higher frequencies or after prolongation of the test, ranking errors involving an affected upper extremity may indicate a pathological state of the cutaneous analyzer and provide a means of studying the progress of the lesion.

An essential part of the investigation of tactile sensation is the test for tactile localization. In this test, a sharp point is applied to the patient's arm and he is asked to indicate the part of the skin touched. If the tactile functions are disturbed, localization of touch may be affected and the patient may point to a spot far removed from the required one.

A still more sensitive version of this test may be used, in which the patient is requested to point, not to the part of the skin touched by the experimenter, but to the corresponding point on the opposite limb. This experiment demands not merely the preservation of the capacity for accurate tactile localization, but also requires the ability to identify the symmetrically opposite area of the skin. In both tests the defects observed may be measured in millimeters (or sometimes in centimeters)

*In this discussion the investigation of temperature sensation will be excluded, with attention confined to methods of investigating tactile functions.

on the basis of the distance between the point of application and that designated.

This experiment is followed by one testing the sense of spatial discrimination, or, more accurately, by a test to assess the patient's discernment of the number of stimuli applied simultaneously to different points of the skin. This experiment may be used for two distinct investigative purposes: (1) to estimate the thresholds of spatial discrimination of cutaneous stimuli and (2) to estimate the constriction of the field of sensory information that may be addressed at one and the same time to the cutaneous analyzer. For the first purpose, Weber's well-known touch-compass is used. The investigator, by gradually separating the arms of this instrument, establishes the threshold at which the patient begins to distinguish two-point sensation. In affected areas of the skin these thresholds are much higher.

The experiment is performed differently for the second purpose. The investigator simultaneously applies two stimuli to the patient's skin, touching areas so far apart from each other that the stimuli applied to them are well outside the thresholds of tactile discrimination. The phenomenon appearing in pathological conditions of the brain, studied in detail by several workers (Teuber, 1959; etc.), is as follows: Patients with a lesion of the parietal cortical region can distinguish only one tactile stimulus at a time; if two stimuli are applied simultaneously they disregard or fail to perceive the stimulus applied to the affected zone. Hence, patients with a lesion of the right hemisphere usually notice a tactile stimulus applied to the right side but fail to notice one applied to the left side of the body; however, if either of the stimuli is applied alone, it is easily discerned. Constriction of the field of tactile sensation thus elicited is a valuable and sensitive indicator of the degree to which cutaneous sensation has been minimized.

The last test used to study the tactile functions is that concerned with the identification of the direction of movement of an object touching the skin and the identification of numbers or letters traced on the patient's skin by the investigator. Both these processes are widely used in clinical practice and call for no special description.

It should be noted that all that has been stated in regard to the need to vary the rate of presentation of stimuli and to present them in random order also applies to this group of tests, for a change in adequate response may also be observed in this function and on the same bases as in the others—the rapidity of presentation rate leading to the onset of fatigue and realization that the stimuli are being applied in accordance with a definite stereotype.

It is also important to note that the accuracy of the replies (especially in the last of the aforementioned tests) is largely determined by the number of possible alternatives. If, therefore, the patient is forewarned that the investigator will trace only two figures (a circle and a cross) on his upper limb, their discrimination is much easier than would be if he does not receive this information beforehand. On this principle, the change from tracing geometrical shapes to tracing numbers may essentially reduce the accuracy of the patient's evaluations.

A disturbance of tactile function may accompany lesions in different parts of the brain. A primary disturbance of these functions, however, indicates a lesion of the postcentral or, sometimes, of the posterior parietal divisions of the cortex of the contralateral hemisphere. However, the latest findings of Teuber and his collaborators (Semmes, Weinstein, Ghent, and Teuber, 1960) indicate that a disturbance of various forms of cutaneous sensation may be a symptom of lesions in different locations. For instance, diminished acuity of tactile sensation in the right upper limb may indicate a lesion in either the sensorimotor or the postcentral region of the left hemisphere; cessation of two-point discrimination and misinterpretation of the direction of cutaneous passive movement may occur with lesions of either the postcentral or the posterior parietal region of the left hemisphere.

Another interesting phenomenon brought to light by these workers is that impairment in the tactile functioning of the right (dominant) upper limb is usually caused by the more highly localized lesions of the left hemisphere, usually not extending beyond the borders of the sensorimotor, postcentral, and posterior parietal region; in contrast, such impairment of the left upper limb may be caused by lesions of the right hemisphere extending beyond the confines of the zones cited, and in some cases they may even result from lesions of the ipsilateral (left) hemisphere. The fact that the cerebral localization of the higher tactile functions is more highly concentrated in the left (dominant) hemisphere is extremely interesting and demands further special investigation.

Lesions situated outside the sensorimotor, postcentral, and posterior parietal regions of the left hemisphere usually cause no disturbance of tactile sensation; mistakes in evaluative tests observed in such cases may be ascribed to the general inertia of previously formed stereotypes found in generalized cerebral disorders, which lowers the mobility of nervous processes; similar phenomena may sometimes result from distraction of attention.

These disturbances in the dynamics of tactile sensation, as manifested by changes in ranking values and instability of the orienting reflexes evoked by the stimuli (especially obvious after the prolonged application of threshold stimuli), are particularly interesting and may be used as dependable criteria of malfunction in the cutaneous analyzer. However, the facts at our disposal are insufficient to enable us to describe fully these phenomena.

C. INVESTIGATION OF DEEP (KINESTHETIC) SENSATION

The investigation of kinesthetic (muscle and joint) sensation is equally familiar in clinical neurological practice, and the techniques used have, in the course of time, been refined to the same extent as those used to investigate cutaneous sensation. They will therefore be only briefly described.

Examination of kinesthetic sensation of the upper extremity usually begins by placing the patient in a sitting position with his eyes covered and his arm, hand, and fingers in a certain position. The patient must then tell the investigator whether his arm, hand, or fingers are being moved upward, downward, or to the side. One widely used method is to tell the patient to reproduce independently a given position of the limb or, likewise, to place the opposite limb in the corresponding position.

A more complicated variant of this test is one in which the patient's forearm is passively flexed to a certain angle and then moved to another angle (for example, to angles of 40° and 20°). The patient is instructed to repeat these consecutive movements or to reproduce them with the opposite forearm. Finally, for more detailed investigation of deep (kinesthetic) sensation, the limb may be placed in two consecutive positions (with the elbow flexed to 40° or 20°) and the patient asked to say whether the two movements were the same or different. To avoid verbal assessment and to carry out the experiment under conditions permitting neurodynamic evaluation, each of these positions may be used as a conditioned stimulus for a specific positive or inhibitory reaction. For example, a bulb can be squeezed when the other forearm is flexed to 40° but not squeezed when it is flexed to 20°. Such a technique can be used to measure disturbances of kinesthetic sensation with a fair degree of accuracy.

Investigation of deep sensation provides the neurologist with important data, for the ability to perceive this form of sensation and the state of the postcentral and posterior parietal regions of the cortex of the opposite hemisphere are closely related. It is with lesions of these cortical divisions that marked disturbances of muscle and joint sensation may arise, especially in the distal segments of the upper limb; these disorders lead to a significant increase in the number of evaluative errors during the tests that have been described. Investigation (Korst and Fantalova, 1959) has shown that a pathological condition of the central ends of the kinesthetic analyzer may interfere with the ability to determine the position of the upper limb. In the presence of such a lesion it is more difficult to evoke differential motor reactions to these stimuli; in some cases, signs of a pathological inertia of the evoked excitation appear, in the form of incorrect evaluation and false sensations and manifesting features of inert stereotypes.

Lesions of the occipital and temporal regions of the brain do not lead to a disturbance in deep sensation.

In frontal lobe cases it may be hard to obtain correct evaluations in the aforementioned tests and especially hard to obtain correct differential motor reactions on a kinesthetic basis; these difficulties may be due to the effect of a pathological inertia, which displaces correct evaluations with inert stereotyped speech or motor responses.

Disturbances of kinesthetic sensation are mainly found in the contralateral upper limb, and they may serve as a reliable symptom for localization of a lesion in a particular hemisphere. It is only in those cases of pathological inertia just mentioned that we find similar defects of postural orientation in both upper limbs; for this reason these defects may be regarded as the result of totally different factors, unconnected with disturbance of deep sensation. But it is not only in the upper limb that a disturbance of deep sensation may be found. Cases in which the muscle sense of the tongue and lips is disturbed are of great importance in neurology. Such a disturbance may arise as the result of a lesion of the inferior divisions of the postcentral region (especially of the left hemisphere) and may lead to disturbances in oral praxis. A description of these phenomena and of the methods used to investigate them has already been given (Part III, Section 3C).

D. INVESTIGATION OF THE HIGHER TACTILE FUNCTIONS AND STEREOGNOSIS

A disturbance of tactile and kinesthetic sensation may lead to defects of the higher tactile functions and, in particular, to astereognosis, which may arise, as has been suggested, against a background of relative integrity of elementary tactile and kinesthetic sensation, yet in fact is always to some extent connected with defects of the cutaneokinesthetic analyzer.

The investigation of the state of the patient's stereognosis is an essential part of the neurological examination. The methods used are well known in clinical practice so that they will be summarized below as succinctly as possible.

The investigation begins as follows: The patient sits with his eyes covered, and a small object (a match box, key, or comb) is placed on the palm of his hand. His palm is then compressed passively and he is asked to name the object in his hand. Difficulty in naming the object correctly still does not mean that astereognosis is present. The next part of the test must be carried out to confirm the presence of this disturbance. The patient is instructed to actively palpate the object lying in his hand; attentive watch is kept on the accuracy of the movements of his fingers as they feel the object, and the appearance of clumsy movements, such as we sometimes see in this test, is noted. If the patient has difficulty in naming the object in his hand, the investigator may permit him to look at a few objects lying on a table, and ask him to select the one that previously was or still is in his hand.

In order to be as certain as possible that the inability to identify an object by touch is in fact a sign of astereognosis, the investigator places the same object in the patient's other hand. If the patient now recognizes the object without difficulty, when he could not do so before, it may be concluded that astereognosis is present.

It is characteristic of astereognosis that the patient can feel the object placed in his hand, can identify its separate qualities (size, texture, temperature) but has difficulty in integrating these signs and deciding the shape of the object. It is because of these defects that certain workers (for example, Denny-Brown *et al.*, 1952; Denny-Brown, 1958) believe that the phenomenon of amorphosynthesis can be pinpointed as the principal cause of astereognosis.

These investigations showed that the phenomena arising from astereognosis are closely associated with a disturbance in the dynamics of the higher cortical processes in the central ends of the cutaneokinesthetic analyzer. Hence, when studying astereognosis, it is essential, first, to pay constant attention to the fine disturbances of differentiation of elementary sensation, to changes in threshold, and to the loss of stability of the mental images of cutaneous and kinesthetic stimuli. This was pointed out by those workers who attempted to approach astereognosis physiologically (Delay, 1935; Bay, 1944; etc.). Second, the investigation of astereognosis must, therefore, be accompanied by analysis of those defects in fine movement that may interfere with the process of synthesis of the tactile image (Part III, Section 3).

The phenomena produced by astereognosis usually arise as a result of a lesion of the parietal regions of the cortex and are exhibited in the contralateral upper limb. Bilateral astereognosis is therefore very rarely encountered. Defective synthesis of the tactile image may also occur in association with disturbances of the motor segments of the sensorimotor region of the cortex and, perhaps, with lesions of the premotor cortex. However, little has yet been accomplished in the study of these phenomena so that they cannot at present be described with adequate clarity.

6. *Investigation of the Higher Visual Functions*

A. PRELIMINARY REMARKS

The investigation of higher visual function, in particular, of visual or optic gnosis, is an important part of the clinical psychological examination for the localization of brain lesions. Not only does it reveal the state of the cortical divisions of the optic analyzer, but in some cases it may also help to identify disturbances in other regions that affect the processes of visual analysis and synthesis.

The analysis of higher visual function must always be preceded by an extremely careful *investigation of the elementary aspects of vision*, such as its acuity, its color sense, the integrity of the visual fields, and the quality of visual adaptation. This neuro-ophthalmological investigation is necessary because (1) it can immediately detect the presence of visual defects and thus make it less likely that any visual defects that may be observed be mistakenly regarded as manifestations of optic agnosis and (2) because, as many investigations have shown (Part II, Section 3A), there is no clear-cut boundary between disturbances of the elementary and higher visual functions. Complex disturbances in visual perception are frequently based on such phenomena as visual asthenia, visual maladaptation, etc.

The fundamental visual functions are investigated by the *ordinary neuro-ophthalmological methods*, so that their investigation will not be considered further. However, a word of caution: It must be remembered that when these functions are investigated by the usual methods the results are based on the subject's spoken responses. It follows that both the patient's speech and his level of consciousness have a direct bearing on the judgment that he is required to exercise. Therefore, the results obtained during the investigation of the elementary visual functions, both in patients with severe disruption of attention (for example, pathological constriction or inertia of attention) and in patients with aspontaneity and manifestations of pathological inertia—not to mention patients with aphasia, alexia, etc., must be assessed with the utmost care. Attention must always be paid to the patient's behavior.

For this reason, *laboratory methods* of studying visual function sometimes assume great importance, for in them objective responses of the orienting reflex are used to demonstrate the patient's reactions to the application or modification of visual stimuli. In these tests the subject is given an appropriate visual signal, and recordings are made of the objective motor, autonomic and electrophysiological reactions—all components of the orienting reflex. These reactions may be absent when the intensity of the signal is lowered, and the graphic representation of them may be considered an objective indicator of sensitivity thresholds. If the same stimulus is repeated many times in succession, these reactions (contraction of the neck muscles, the psychogalvanic skin reflex, vasoconstriction, depression of the alpha-rhythm, etc.) may be suppressed, but they reappear when the stimulus is changed. This phenomenon can be made use of in the evaluation of differentials in reaction, in particular, the patient's discriminatory capacity in regard to the intensity of light and color. Finally, recordings of the components of the orienting reflex developing in response to illumination of a particular point on the retina by a thin pencil of light and consequent illumination of another retinal point can yield objective data for perimetry.

However, the application of these methods to the clinical investigation of patients with brain lesions is somewhat limited, first, because of their complexity and, second, because of the fact that the dynamics of the orienting reflex may be considerably upset by the process. We shall therefore do no more than mention these methods of investigation and refer the reader to the original sources for details, i.e., Sokolov, 1958, 1959.*

Of all the basic elements of higher visual function there are two of special interest: the visual fields and the eye movements.

In neuro-ophthalmological practice *the visual fields* are usually investigated by perimetry, whereby, with his gaze fixed on a fixed point, the subject must report the appearance of a stimulus at the periphery. This activity is dependent on the patient's ability to perceive two points simultaneously— the fixed point at the center and the point appearing at the periphery—and, as previously mentioned (Part II, Section 3C), certain conditions preclude it. In pathological conditions of the occipital lobe of the cortex the patient is usually able to perceive only one stimulus at a time (Balint, 1909; Luria, 1959; etc.), and this pathological narrowing of visual attention may interfere with the results of perimetry and lead to an incorrect assessment of the visual fields. This possibility must always be borne in mind during the neuro-ophthalmological examination of patients with local brain lesions.

If constriction of the visual fields is present, the degree to which this defect is realized and compensated for by the patient is an important consideration. Investigations conducted by Luria and Skorodumova (1950, etc.) have shown that right-sided hemianopsia, accompanying a lesion of the left hemisphere, is appreciated by the patient and compensated for by appropriate shifting of

* Similar methods can be used for the objective study of hearing and cutaneous sensitivity.

the gaze. In contrast, left-sided hemianopsia, associated with a lesion of the right hemisphere, is frequently embodied in the syndrome of anosognosia, so that it is not appreciated by the patient and therefore not compensated for by shifting of the eye toward the left; the gaze assumes a fixed character. The study of these two types of hemianopsia by perimetry is not sufficient. Other methods must be used, such as having the patient freely (i.e., without gaze fixation) count cards lying before him on a table or read a text written in large letters. In this test, the failure to notice the left side of the visual field, a characteristic feature of left-sided fixed hemianopsia, becomes quite obvious.

The second part of the neuro-ophthalmological investigation with which we are concerned is the *examination of eye movements* or, more precisely, the direction of the gaze. When complex forms are perceived with the eye, the gaze is not static; instead, the eyes continually move about and, as it were, palpate the object and establish its distinguishing signs. Therefore, investigation of these movements is an indispensable part of the study of visual functions.

The integrity of two types of eye movement must be carefully investigated in a patient with a circumscribed brain lesion, those conventionally known as *elementary (reflex)* and *complex (psychomotor)* movements. In the first type, it is a matter of the reflex fixation of the point to be perceived by a movement of the eye so that the projection of this point lies in the central visual field. This type of eye movement is the responsibility of the lower divisions of the brain (the brain stem) or of the posterior oculomotor centers of the cortex so that it is disturbed by lesions of these structures. The second type involves the direction of the gaze in response to a verbal instruction or in accordance with the patient's own intention; although reflex in character, it is much more complex. It requires the participation of the second signal system and is principally disturbed by a lesion of the anterior oculomotor centers or of those parts of the frontal lobe lying anteriorly to these centers. This type of regulation of eye movement is very important in the active examination of an object, so that careful investigation of eye movement may be extremely important (Luria and Khomskaya, 1962).

Simple methods are used to test eye movement *clinically*. To examine reflex-type eye movements, the examiner stands in front of the patient and shows him a bright object (for example, a lamp), first in the right and then in the left visual field, and notes how the patient fixes his attention on it. Alternatively, with the patient's gaze fixed on the examiner's finger (or lamp), the examiner gradually moves the object, first to the right and then to the left, and notes how the eyes follow it.

To examine optic psychomotor functioning, the examiner asks the patient to "look to the right" or "look to the left." In variants of the test the same instruction is given under more complicated conditions. For example, a bright or striking object is shown on one side; in order to obey the instruction to "look to the other side" the patient must suppress the reflexive tendency to look at the object.

If the eye movements are the same (in regard to speed, range, and steadiness) in both types of test, both of the aforementioned systems can be companied by disturbances (delay, low amplitude, and fatigability) (Fig. 120) or complete absence of psychomotor eye movements may indicate a considerable defect in the cortical apparatus associated with this higher level of visual regulation. In such an eventuality, the examiner should be on the lookout for disturbances in active inspection of an object and in visual perception.

Via special *laboratory methods* involving graphic recording, eye movements can be discerned with greater accuracy. Several methods are used for this purpose: (1) filming the eye movements (i.e., motion pictures) followed by automatic analysis of the results (Shakhnovich, 1964); (2) tracing the movements of a spot of light reflected from a mirror attached to the cornea (Yarbus, 1956, 1961); (3) oculography; (4) recording the movements of the pupil (Shakhnovich, 1961). The latter is accomplished by means of a system comprising a photoelectric cell and automatic transmission of the eye movements to a moving tape (Vladimirov and Khomskaya, 1961). Examples of the use of this method for the more precise recording of eye movements during examination of a complex picture by patients with frontal brain lesions have been given in an earlier part of this book (Part II, Section 5E). Offsetting their advantages, these laboratory methods require special technical apparatuses and are not always feasible in clinical practice.

B. INVESTIGATION OF THE VISUAL PERCEPTION OF OBJECTS AND PICTURES

The investigation of the perception of objects and their pictorial representation and the analysis of the phenomena arising on the basis of visual agnosia constitute one of the most important aspects of the study of the higher visual functions.

As has been pointed out (Part II, Section 3C), an object or pictorial representation of one usually constitutes a complex optic stimulus so that the process that leads to its proper visual perception incorporates several consecutive activities: examining the object, distinguishing its essential features, establishing the relationships between these features, and integrating them into patterns. Other essential components are the suppression of features that possess optical intensity but that are not essential signs and the correction of mistakes that may arise as a result of premature evaluation, i.e., evaluation before careful analysis and integration of individual features has taken place.

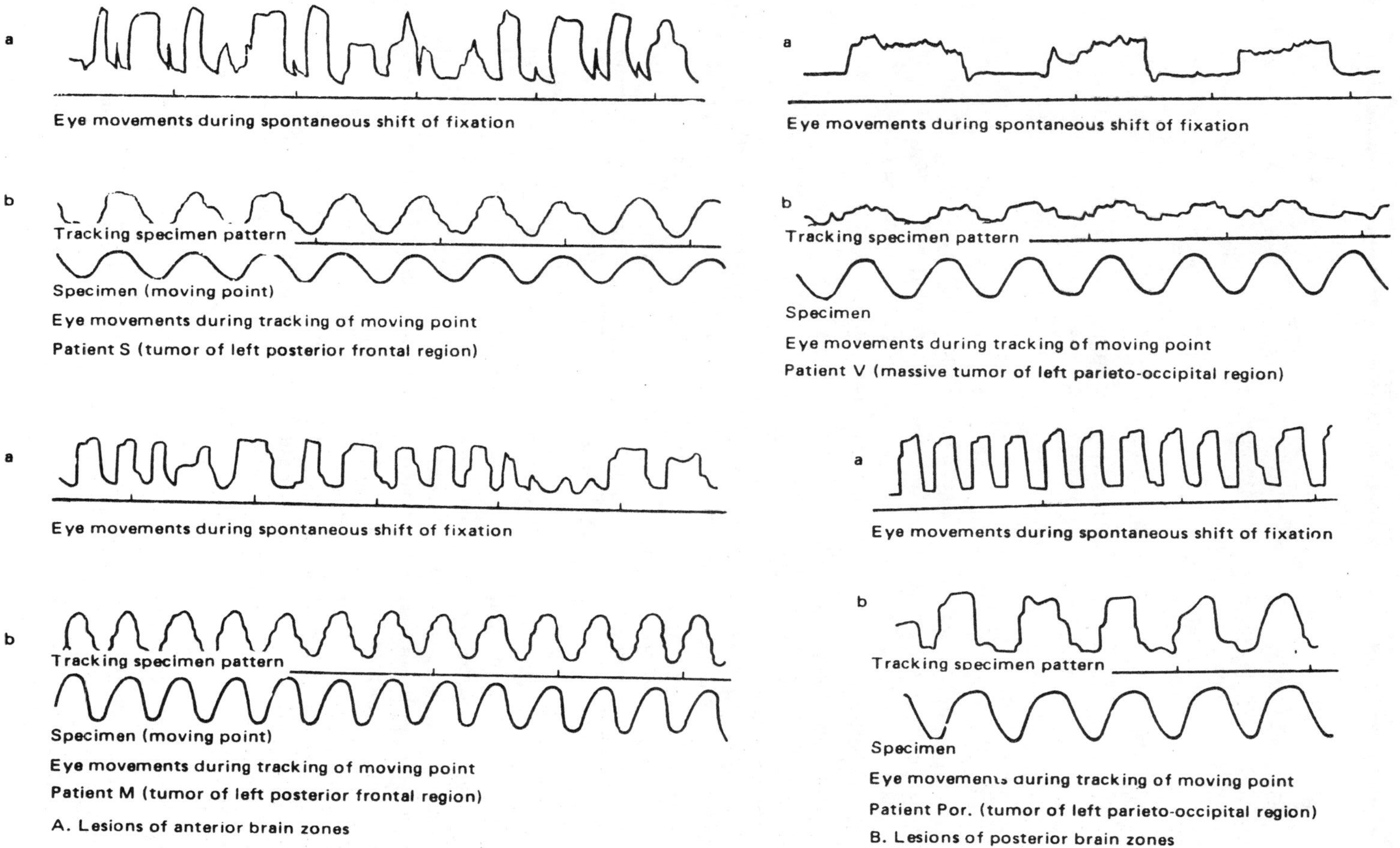

FIGURE 120 Eye movements (a) during a spontaneous shift of fixation, and (b) during tracking a spot of light with a rhythmic motion within a 30° sector by patients (A) with

The more complex the visual structure of an object or picture and the less familiar it is, the more complex and lengthy the process of visual analysis and integration required for its perception.

The visual evaluation of simple and familiar objects and pictures is easily achieved by a healthy individual, for the analysis of them is concise in character. Only in pathological conditions—disturbances in one of the component activities—is this process impaired, so that the analysis becomes protracted and auxiliary methods are brought into play (tracing of the outlines of the object with the finger, verbal musings on the possible nature of the object, etc.). Analysis of these auxiliary devices may provide information that can be very valuable in determining which step in the complex process of visual perception is disturbed.

As in other cortical functions, visual perception of a "complex" object may suffer if any one stage in the process is disturbed. Hence, each functional type of disturbance—defective active examination, defective recognition of the essential cues, defective visual integration of these cues, defective correction of premature conclusions, or defective evaluation of the information —may be reflected in different ways in the structure of visual perception of an object and may lead to the appearance of a group of symptoms with distinctive topical significance.

The investigation of how objects or pictures are perceived must therefore be so constructed that it yields results readily amenable to qualitative analysis. It usually begins with the presentation of objects or of clearly drawn pictures of objects to the patient, who is asked to examine them carefully (with no time limit) and to name them. If speech is disturbed, some method of nonverbal communication can be used by the patient to indicate the result of his appraisal.

If no disturbance is evinced by the first test, other attempts at detection must be made. In this spirit, the patient should be presented with complicated or indistinct pictures of objects. Suitable for this purpose are pictures lending themselves to many interpretations (e.g., those in which individual details are misleading and those that can be interpreted correctly only by careful integration of the principal parts), outline or silhouette drawings, or pictures composed of dots or incorporating intricate designs. These last two types may prove especially difficult to perceive and recognize. Outline drawings so constructed that they might easily be construed as a special form of handwriting are particularly suitable for this purpose. Other appropriate

lesions of the anterior, and (B) with lesions of the posterior zones of the brain (recorded by Vladimirov's photoelectric method). In patients with lesions of the anterior zones the act of spontaneous shift of fixation is most severely disturbed, but in patients with posterior brain lesions tracking movements of the eyes are mainly disturbed (after Khomskaya).

pictures are those used by Tonkonogii and Tsukkerman under conditions of "visual interference." These workers showed that the degree of "interference" with the picture can be graded and that tests involving the analysis of such pictures provide a sensitive method of investigating the finer forms of disturbance of visual perception.

The third stage of the investigation involves showing the patient pictures that are scribbled over or superimposed on one another, a method introduced by Poppelreuter (1917-1918). In these conditions visual perception of the object is made difficult by the need to pick out the required picture from the irrelevant elements in the background or to identify the outlines of the various superimposed figures. Examples of such pictures are shown in Figs. 121 and 122.

The last and most difficult task in the investigation of active visual perception consists of a problem in which the patient has to isolate a given shape from a more complicated unit. In one variant, he must identify a figure in a complex design (Fig. 123). Figures of this type were introduced into the field of psychological investigation by Gottschaldt. In another, he has to identify a given figure (a cross with a white or black center, a rectangle, etc.) from a background of uniform squares (e.g., a chessboard) (Fig. 124). In each form of the experiment, the patient has to trace the outline of the figure with his finger. To do so, he must first be able to form a clear idea of the figure.

In a special series of experiments of this type the patient must not only distinguish a definite visual structure, but also differentiate it from another; in certain variants he must also identify the principle of construction. An example of this type of investigation is Raven's (1939) well-known test. A structure from which a portion is missing is submitted to the patient. He must complete the structure by choosing from a series of offered insets the one that matches the particular structure. An element of difficulty is injected when the required inset must be differentiated from others bearing

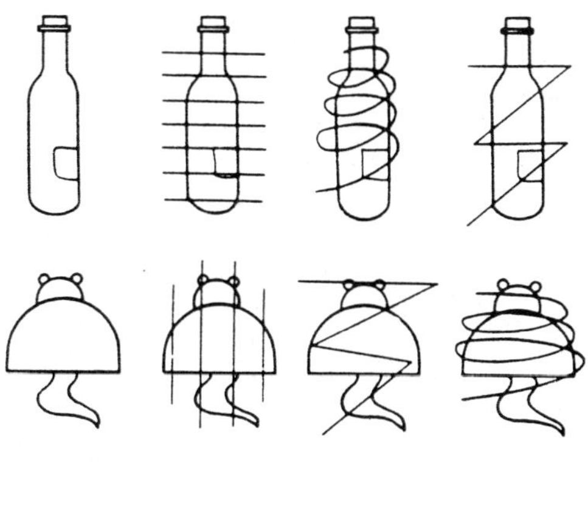

FIGURE 121 Outline drawings used in the investigation of visual perception. Note the scribblings on the objects.

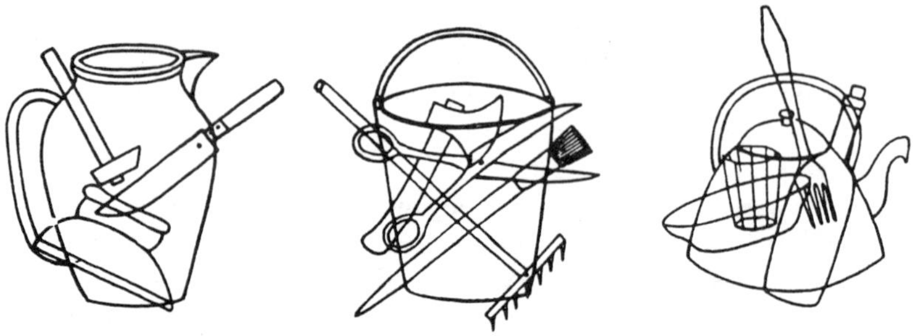

FIGURE 122 Superimposed figures used in the investigation of visual perception. (*Modified from Poppelreuter, 1917–1918.*)

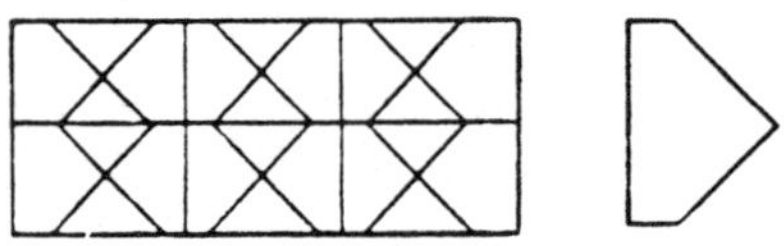

FIGURE 123 Hidden visual structures used in the investigation of visual perception. (*After Gottschaldt.*)

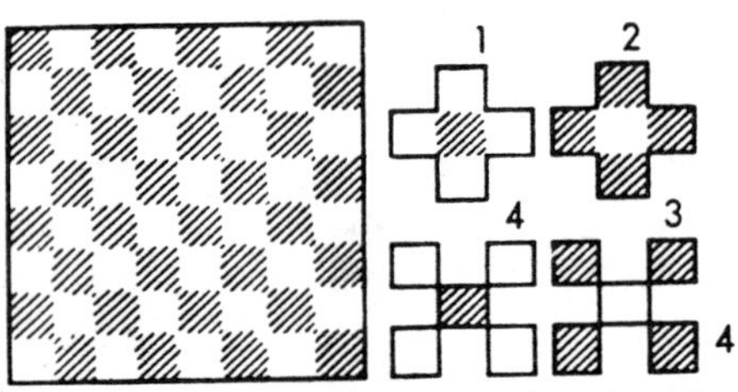

FIGURE 124 Distinguishing shapes on a chessboard—another test of visual perception.

a close visual resemblance to it but not possessing the full complement of suitable cues. The solution of this problem requires complex analytical and integrative ability, so that this test, besides being one of the most complex, offers the widest scope for analysis.

As a rule, no time limit is imposed. The patient may examine the figures for as long as he finds it necessary. Frequently, the actual process of examination of the figure, the feelers the patient puts out, and the conclusions he reaches all provide valuable insight into his perceptual capacity.

When an investigation of this type yields no positive findings, special, more sensitive methods may be used. In these variants, the figure may be available to the patient for only a short period of time (in some cases tachistoscopic presentation of the figure may be used for this purpose). Or, the figures or pictures may be presented in the wrong position; patients with defective optic gnosis are frequently utterly unable to recognize a figure that is upside down or they perceive it incorrectly.

In simplified forms of the tests the patient is instructed to trace the outlines of a figure with his finger; or, he may be given leading questions, some of which suggest the proper meaning of the figure; or, finally, the examiner may point to any one of the essential signs, thereby aiding the patient to find the correct meaning of the picture.

A special form of test to study the disturbance of optic gnosis is the recognition of portraits of familiar people or the identification of the picture of a familiar person among many that are unfamiliar. Such a test can reveal the finer disturbances of recognition of faces characteristic of patients with "agnosia for faces" described in the literature and which is most frequently found in patients with lesions of the occipito-parietal zones of the nondominant (right) hemisphere.

Experiments for the purpose of studying a patient's visual perception of objects and pictures reveal the nature of the changes affecting optic gnosis that accompany circumscribed brain lesions. Particularly demonstrative results may be obtained in patients with *lesions of the occipitoparietal divisions* of the cortex (especially if bilateral or on the left side) and optic agnosia (Part II, Section 3C). Patients of this group may manifest noticeable defects during identification and visual synthesis of the essential cues of a picture. As a rule, they grasp only one sign—the most prominent or conspicuous—but fail to correlate it with the other signs or to integrate the necessary group of signs visually; they draw premature conclusions regarding the meaning of the picture, guessing at it from the single fragment that they have perceived.

In the severest cases, patients cannot recognize even relatively simple objects or realistic pictures. For example, they may identify a pair of spectacles as "a bicycle" because they cannot synthesize two circles and a series of lines into the required image, or they may refer to a steamboat as "a factory" on the basis of the windows and chimney* (Part II, Section 3C). In less severe cases, difficulties of this sort emerge only during the visual recognition of pictures with a complex structure; the evaluation of such a structure requires identification of more than one sign, while their recognition demands the integration of several signs. It is in such cases that the picture of a sofa with a cushion lying at each end becomes an "automobile" (the cushions being mistaken for "headlights"), etc. In still less marked cases, the same defects may be brought to light only during the examination of outline or silhouette drawings, drawings with intricate designs, drawings on which a linear pattern of clear lines (forming spirals, angles, etc.), is superimposed or, finally, outline drawings superimposed on one another.

* Naturally, it is always easier to recognize objects than representations of them. This may be attributed to the fact that the kinesthetic components of the object play a far more important part in its recognition than the visual ones. Obviously, then, a patient with optic agnosia will easily recognize an object if he feels it.

It is characteristic of patients with *lesions of the occipital lobes* that they steadfastly persist in the active examination of pictures presented to them, shifting their attention and trying to select and correlate the necessary identification signs. Their speech, which abounds in guesses and, sometimes, in corrections, is equally active in character. Such patients hardly ever express confident opinions regarding the meanings of pictures that they have examined. Their conclusions constantly contain doubts, expressed, for example, in such phrases as "Of course it is a bicycle . . . , or perhaps it is something else . . ." accompanied by complaints of their "poor eyesight."

The disturbance in perception is highly distinctive in patients with symptoms of simultaneous agnosia (Part II, Section 3C). As a rule, such patients can perceive only one element (or one picture) at one time. Therefore, when they examine pictures, the results are unstable and variable. When they perceive the whole picture, they evaluate it properly. When, however, they begin to examine its details, they lose sight of the whole picture and perceive it only as isolated fragments. The fact that the examination of objects by these patients is accompanied by an obvious ataxia of gaze makes the diagnosis of this form of lesion considerably easier.

Patients with *frontal lobe lesions* may exhibit very characteristic disturbances during their efforts to perceive visually pictures. As previously discussed (Part II, Section 5E), the disturbances of visual perception observed in these patients (especially when combined with the general loss of visual acuity that is frequently encountered in these patients) may assume such marked forms that they can easily be confused with true optic agnosia.

The first means of clearly distinguishing patients with a frontal syndrome from patients with true optic agnosia is to take note of the way in which a picture presented to them is examined. As a rule, patients with frontal lobe lesions are incapable of true, active examination of a picture; they therefore "look" at it passively. They either look at it without changing the direction of their gaze, or they shift their gaze only very slightly from one part to another. They make little attempt to "seek out" the identifying signs and yet, as a rule, immediately reach a confident conclusion about what the picture represents. If the picture is simple enough, the conclusion will probably be right; if, though, it is complicated, reasoning from a particularly conspicuous single detail may lead to an incorrect conclusion, which the patient usually offers confidently and with no attempt at correction. No doubts arise regarding the correctness of the opinion given, even if the examiner requests that the picture be studied more carefully and that the description of it be more accurate.

When called upon to recognize pictures presented under more complicated conditions, such patients very often reach impulsive and incorrect conclusions. It is easy to see that defects in the perception of pictures in patients with frontal syndromes are associated with inactivity of perception. No sooner are they shown a picture upside down than this defect becomes quite obvious, for it is clear that they make no attempt to invert the picture mentally and to analyze its true meaning. As a rule, such patients evaluate pictures in the position in which they are presented; a picture of a cup and saucer shown upside down may be described as a "mushroom," and so on. The perception of crossed-out or superimposed figures naturally creates insuperable difficulties. The patient's general impression is one of chaos from which he can distinguish nothing, and he usually refuses to give any opinion on the picture.

The second characteristic of the visual perception of patients with frontal syndromes is its pathological inertia, a feature distinguishing their mental activity as a whole. This inertia may take the form of visual perseveration, in which a picture seen previously affects the subsequent perception of a modified picture (Figs. 104, 105). In other cases, the evaluation of a series of different pictures is itself characterized by perseveration, i.e., the different pictures begin to be interpreted in the same way. In the latter instance it may be a question of inertia of designation rather than a true perceptual inertia. Clearly, the active identification of a figure, a homogeneous background or, even more so, of a figure masked by other figures, is absolutely impossible for these patients (Part II, Section 5E).

These defects are among the most characteristic of disturbed perception from lesions of the frontal lobes. The pseudoagnostic disturbances of perception accompanying lesions of the frontal lobes sometimes assume forms so outwardly similar to the manifestations of true optic agnosia that only by careful observation of the passive character of the perceptual activity and of the presence of the syndrome of generalized inertia and lack of a critical attitude towards performance will these defects be correctly diagnosed.

C. INVESTIGATION OF SPATIAL ORIENTATION

Orientation in space is a function that must be investigated carefully before a topical diagnosis of brain lesions can be made. Being primarily concerned with direction in relation to such coordinates as up and down and right and left, orientation in space is a complex process. Besides simultaneous visual perception, with the participation of differential eye movements, it also involves vestibular analysis and synthesis (which largely provide its elementary physiological basis) and kinetic stimuli from the dominant (right) upper limb (which give that space comprising man's environment its asymmetry). Because of these components, spatial orientation can only loosely be regarded as one of the higher visual functions.

We know that perception of spatial relationships, with a clear distinction between right and left, appears comparatively late in childhood, is largely dependent on the identification of the dominant hand, causes difficulty in cases of ambidexterity or left-handedness that is latent (suppressed by training), and is disturbed by lesions of the inferoparietal and parieto-occipital regions of the cortex. Evaluation of the extent of residual orientation in space is therefore of considerable importance for the localization of brain lesions. Different avenues of approach may be used in this investigation.

When, earlier in this division of the book (Part III, Section 3B), we discussed the investigation of the motor functions of the hand, we described a series of tests that are used in the examination of spatial praxis. The investigation of orientation in space may include another group of tests, not involving motor functioning but, rather, on the visual-image plane. Finally, the investigation of orientation in space and its disturbances may also be undertaken from the point of view of operations taking place at the level of symbolic schemes, in whose construction orientation in space occupies a primary role.

When describing tests involving the perception of pictures presented upside down (Part III, Section 6B), we were, in fact, discussing a process relying on the preservation of the ability to carry out those operations that are necessary for orienting an object (or picture) in space. Defects in this function may be revealed by a patient's failure to recognize a deliberate error in the examiner's spatial positioning of a picture, such as when a series of picture cards is displayed in the wrong position, or by the patient's own, uncorrected errors in laying out a series of cards with pictures of objects. However, this type of defect can be seen only in the very severest disturbances, so that adequate investigation of the state of orientation in space calls for special and more highly sensitive methods.

Such methods include a series of graphic tests in which the subject has to analyze the spatial arrangement of the lines composing familiar figures and either to discover the resemblance and difference between lines and figures placed mirror-wise or to draw these figures or build them up from matches.

Figure 125 illustrates such a task. The patient is shown one of the figures and is asked to copy it, to construct with matches, or to say what differences he can detect between the figures forming a pair. In more sensitive variants he may be asked to draw these figures or build them with matches after inverting them mentally, so that the spatial position of the elements of the resulting figure corresponds to that of a figure in front of the examiner as he sits at a table opposite the patient.

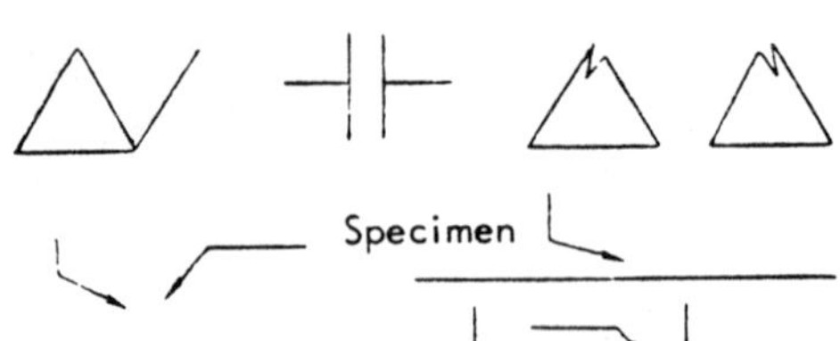

FIGURE 125 Tests involving the analysis of spatial relationships.

Significant impairment of performance of this test may be indicative of the presence of a primary disturbance of visual-spatial orientation which implies a lesion of the inferoparietal (or parieto-occipital) area of the brain. This conclusion can be drawn, however, only if, after active attempts to analyze the spatial arrangement of the elements of the figure, the patient finds that he cannot do so, i.e., he cannot distinguish between elements of a figure forming mirror images or he erroneously judges the direction of the lines composing the figure and fails to recognize their relationship to each other. In such instances, the disturbance forms part of a syndrome that includes other types of spatial disorientation (easily confusing right and left, losing the way in a building or street, symptoms of apractagnosia, etc.). This condition was discussed earlier in the book (Part II, Section 3E). Certain superficially similar defects, due to a syndrome of generalized inactivity and manifested as the impulsive mistaking of mirror-image relationships, must be given a totally different interpretation, for they suggest the disturbance of selective, active behavior characteristically found with lesions of the frontal lobes.

A similar test is one based on analyzing the positions of the hands of a clock (Fig. 126). In a variant, the patient is asked to arrange the hands of a model clock so as to indicate a particular time. Confusion between symmetrically situated numbers and mistakes in the positioning of the hands relative to one another indicate a similar disturbance of spatial orientation.

Similar difficulties may also arise in the course of an operation in which the patient has to match correctly placed letters or numbers with others drawn as mirror images (Fig. 127). Inability to distinguish an incorrectly composed letter or number ("they are both correct"), reference to the mirror image as the actual letter or number, or mirror-image writing (by the patient himself)—all this supplies valuable additional information for use in the evaluation of a disturbance of spatial orientation.

Other instructive tests used in the investigation of spatial orientation are those based on geographical relationships—recognizing geographical relationships on maps; drawing a plan of one's room or the ward; planning the route one would take to the doctor's office, to a nearby shop, etc. This technique was developed and used by Shemyakin (1940, 1954, 1959) and Kolodnaya (1949, 1954).

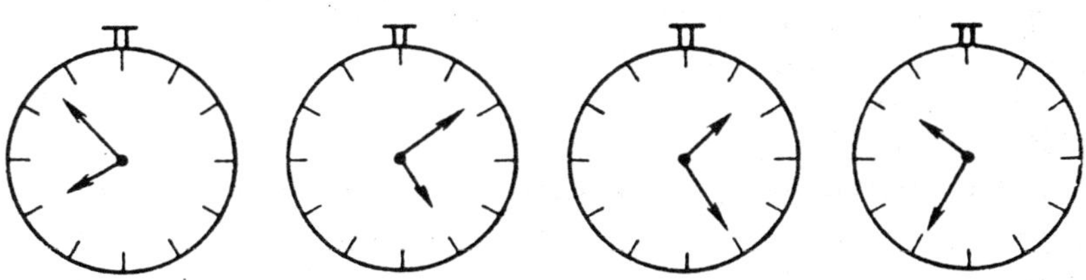

FIGURE 126 Test involving the evaluation of the position of the hands of a clock.

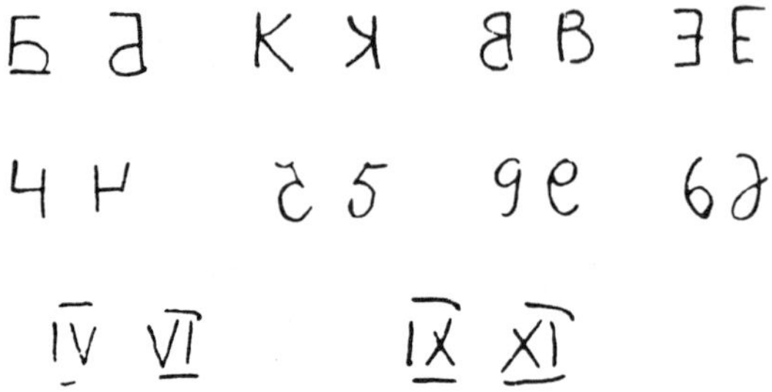

FIGURE 127 Test for the spatial analysis of letters and numbers.

As has been pointed out (Part II, Section 3E), reproducing the principal spatial coordinates of a map is especially difficult for patients with parieto-occipital lesions. Difficulty in the correct identification of east and west on these coordinates and in placing of towns, seas, etc., in relation to each other constitute one of the most important symptoms of this group of spatial disorientation. For this reason, the examiner should be particularly alert to mirror-image errors in the drawing of geographical schemes. Examples of defective performance in these tests were given earlier (Figs. 50 and 51).

D. INVESTIGATION OF INTELLECTUAL OPERATIONS IN SPACE

Tests of visual orientation with regard to spatial relationships bring one to a series of tests that go beyond the investigation of higher visual functions and are directed at spatial syntheses underlying complex constructive activity and intellectual operations in space. In these tests the patient is given a constructional task—to build a figure from wooden blocks, to build a cube from a series of specially shaped units, to analyze the scheme of a lever either practically or pictorially, etc. Naturally, such tasks can be performed adequately here only when spatial orientation and the appreciation of the principal spatial relationships have not been impaired.

Among the best-known tests, and one satisfying these essential requirements, is Kohs' test. In it, the patient is required to construct a particular pattern from blocks, with each side of the pattern diagonally divided into two differently colored halves. When assembling complex designs (Fig. 128), the patient has to break up optically homogeneous parts of the pattern into their component spatial elements. When the units of the visually perceived details of the pattern do not coincide with the edges of the individual blocks, the solution of the problem can present considerable difficulties for patients with visual-spatial defects.

In another of these tests, proposed by Rupp (Fig. 129), the patient is instructed to copy a pattern resembling a honeycomb. Patients with a disturbance of functions involved in complex spatial operations find it extremely difficult to copy this pattern, to avoid the simple and direct

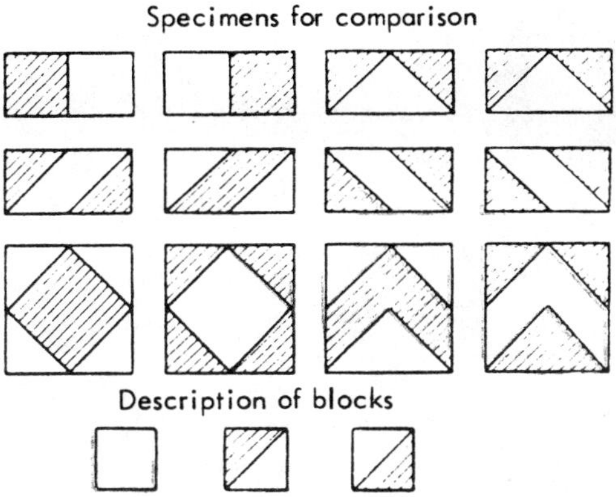

FIGURE 128 Kohs' test. See text for explanation.

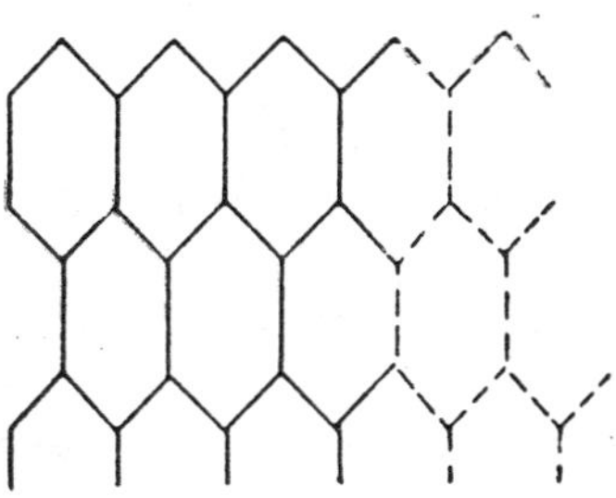

FIGURE 129 Rupp's test. A sample of a complex system of lines is presented to the patient; the broken lines indicate the expected continuation of the pattern.

reproduction of its component elements, and to maintain the required system of spatial relationships.

A similar test is one proposed by Yerkes. The patient is shown a diagram of a complex figure composed of blocks (Fig. 130). He has to work out the number of blocks used in its construction. The fact that not all the blocks composing the figure are visible in the figure adds to the difficulty of the task. Patients with an impairment in intellectual operations involving spatial orientation may reveal appreciable defects when performing this test. In similar, widely used tests, the patient is required mentally to change the position of a presented figure in order to establish that it is identical with a given specimen. Tests such as the parallelogram test or the hands test (Fig. 131) call for a particularly high degree of preservation of visual-spatial images and may be used to detect latent defects of these images.

It would not be forgotten that these tests are relatively difficult and are not always easily performed even by healthy subjects.

It would not be forgotten that these tests are relatively difficult and are not always easily performed even by healthy subjects. When they are used for clinical purposes, only the most elementary tests should therefore be

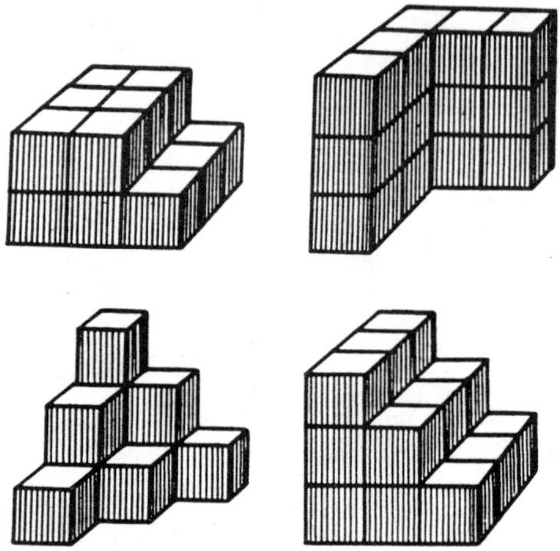

FIGURE 130 Yerkes' test. See text for explanation.

chosen and the types of difficulty which the patients experience when performing them must be carefully studied.

Special investigations (Tsvetkova, 1966) have shown that patients with lesions of the parieto-occipital zones of the cortex retain the task firmly but have difficulty in finding the necessary spatial relations between the individual elements of the structure. Conversely, patients with lesions of the frontal lobes have no difficulty in operations with spatial relations but usually find difficulty in making a careful analysis of the pattern shown: they readily deviate into performing the task according to their first impression, making no effort to analyze the conditions and readily abandoning the ultimate goal.

The true cause of the difficulties which these two groups of patients experience during the performance of these tests can therefore be clearly revealed if they are given different forms of help. The suggestion to use aids to facilitate spatial analysis of the elements will substantially assist patients with lesions of the parieto-occipital zones but will be of no benefit to patients with frontal lesions. Conversely, the consecutive program of the patients' behavior (look at the figure; pick out the first two; count the number of elements in it; pick out the first of them, and so on), while unnecessary for patients with lesions of the parieto-occipital zones of the brain, will enable patients with frontal lesions to compensate considerably for their defect.

All the tests so far described are wholly concerned with the investigation of visual perception and are only partially related to the study of intellectual activity involving spatial images which are included in the analysis of visually perceived structure.

Another widely used test in this type of examination utilizes the aforementioned Link's cube (Part II, Section 5G). In this test the subject is

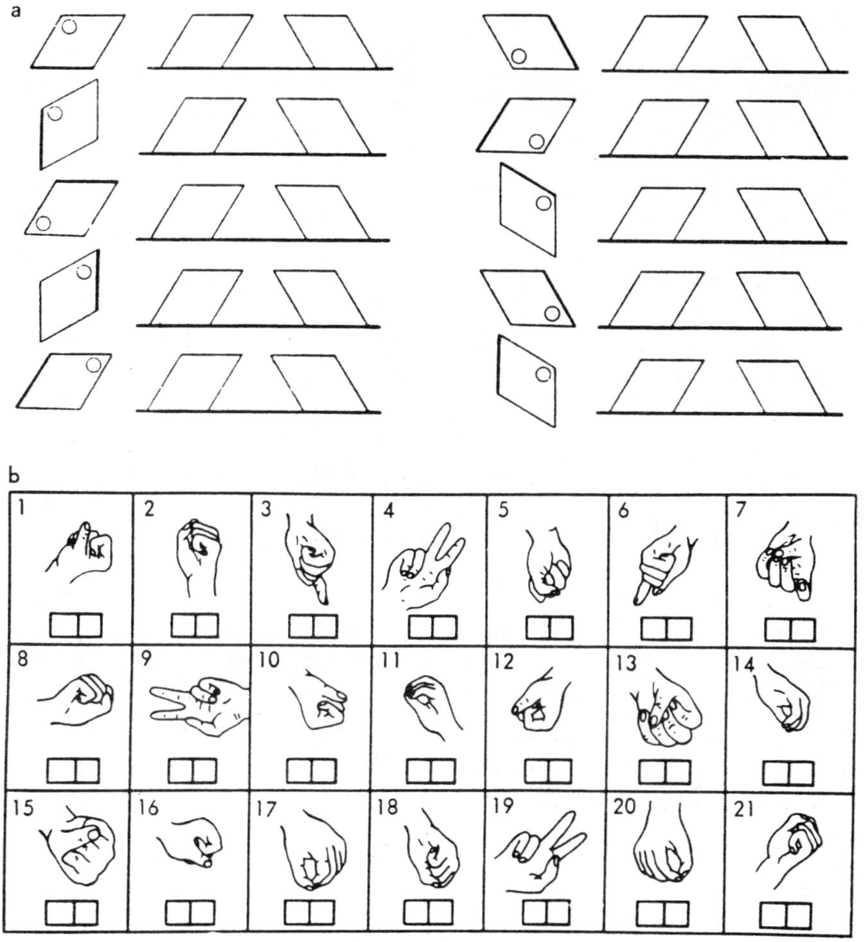

FIGURE 131 Tests based on analysis of a figure involving mental rotation. (*a*) The parallelogram test. The subject is instructed to place a circle in the appropriate corner of the parallelogram in order to obtain a figure identical with the picture on the left. (*b*) The hands test. The subject has to decide which hand—right or left—is illustrated in the drawing and to place a cross in the appropriate square.

given 27 small cubes whose sides are each painted a different color, and he is instructed to build a cube of a certain color (for example, yellow) with them. Since the 27 small cubes include four with three yellow sides, eight with two yellow sides, and one with none of its sides painted yellow, the subject has to work out a way of arranging the various small cubes in order to make the required large cube.

As was pointed out, healthy subjects begin solving this problem by forming a general scheme; by identifying the positions in which the cubes having three, two, or one yellow side must respectively be placed; and, having classified the cubes, by arranging them in accordance with the preliminary scheme.

Patients with impaired visual-spatial orientation but with intact goal-directed intellectual functioning can begin to perform this test by carefully following this plan of solution, but they run into difficulties because of the need to arrange the individual elements in relation to the appropriate spatial coordinates.

Patients with disturbances in selective, goal-directed activity, i.e., with frontal lobe lesions, show gross defects in their performance of this test. As was stated earlier (Part II, Section 5G), these patients are unable to construct a plan of action that includes all the necessary individual operations. Instead, they make random, impulsive attempts at solution, without appreciating the requirements for performance of the task with the available material. As a rule, they fail to arrive at a solution, not so much because of a disturbance of visual-spatial images as on account of the disintegration of their intellectual activity as a whole, so that their actions are no longer subordinated to a given plan.

All the tests that are aimed at the study of intellectual operations in relation to space are complex in character. Therefore, *their application to topical diagnosis is relatively limited;* their value lies not so much in the discovery that the patient is unable to arrive at a solution as in their *revelation of the types of difficulty* experienced by the patient in the course of searching for a solution and of *the manner of his performance*; these insights alone can provide an explanation of the mechanism of the disturbances that exist.

7. *Investigation of Mnestic Processes*

A. PRELIMINARY REMARKS

The investigation of mnestic processes is one of the most important sections of the neuropsychological investigation. Its purpose is to discover whether the patient has a disturbance of memory, and if he has, which forms it takes.

In psychology it is customary to distinguish between two main forms of memory. One form is connected with general orientation in place and time and is closely related to the investigation of states of consciousness. This form of memory may be disturbed in concussion and acute brain injuries, where it assumes the well-known forms of retrograde and anterograde amnesia. In patients with brain tumors it is more severely impaired if the lesions are in the brain stem, lowering general cortical tone and leading to a disturbance of wakefulness, to oneiroid states of consciousness, and to disorientation in place and time. It may be manifested as Korsakov's syndrome or closely allied pictures of memory disturbance. Sometimes it is associated with phenomena of confabulation, which can be seen most frequently in patients with fronto-diencephalic lesions, when a disturbance of trace imprinting is superposed against a background of a general depression of critical faculties and a disturbance of the selectivity of psychological processes.

Disturbances of this form of memory are best found during conversation with the patient (Part III, Section 2) and by a general psychopathological investigation.

Another form of memory is concerned with the complex activity of memorizing and recalling material presented (demonstrative or verbal). This form of memory, which is far more closely connected with the activity of individual analyzers and which may be modality-specific in character, involves imprinting, storing, and recalling (reproducing) the suggested material. In turn, it can be divided into two main types: direct memorizing (imprinting of traces without any special aids) and indirect (logical) memorizing (memorizing with special aids). Whereas the first type of memory is more closely connected with a process of perception and is the direct consolidation of impressions reaching the subject, the second type of memory is more closely connected with complex intellectual forms of activity.

Disturbances of this second form of memory can arise in patients with local lesions of various parts of the brain.

The object of the neuropsychological investigation of memory is to establish which form of memory is in fact disturbed. If it is memory as the active process of imprinting that is disturbed, what factors lie at the basis of its disturbance, and what forms of memory (visual, auditory, or kinesthetic, demonstrative or verbal) are affected most in the particular patient?

If a patient with a general disturbance of memory is investigated, the neuropsychological tests must attempt to discover what mechanisms lie at its basis. For that purpose they must establish under what conditions in that particular patient the disturbances of accurate imprinting of traces may arise, causing a state of confusion of his consciousness.

I shall accordingly examine the methods used for testing the direct imprinting of traces. I shall then analyze the processes of rote learning, and I shall go on to describe methods of investigating indirect (logical) memorizing.

B. INVESTIGATION OF THE DIRECT IMPRESSION OF TRACES

The study of the direct impression of traces, well-known in psychology and clinical practice as "Merkfahigkeit," occupies an important place in the investigation of the mnestic processes. Its object is to determine to what extent the patient is able to preserve direct traces left behind by various stimuli, i.e., to discover whether changes have occurred in the range and stability of the preservation of these traces and, if so, whether the disturbance is confined to any one sphere (visual, auditory, tactile). Confirmation of the latter has especial relevance in the clinical study of local brain lesions, for this type of manifestation is often a symptom of a *lesion affecting the cortical end of one of the analyzers*.

The investigation of the direct impression of traces may begin with the analysis of the effect of consecutive images; abnormal aftereffects were considered in relation to the pathology of the *occipital cortical divisions* (Part II, Section 3C). It is well known that every external stimulus evokes a process of excitation that continues for some time even after the stimulus itself has ceased to act. The immediate aftereffect of this stimulus may be investigated by means of a number of physiological and psychophysiological techniques, among which is the examination of what are known as afterimages.

The phenomenon of afterimages is best demonstrated in the *visual* sphere. If a subject is shown a bright red figure (a square or circle) superimposed on a homogeneous gray (or white) background for 15 to 20 seconds, he will continue to see a trace of this figure for a short time after the figure itself has been removed. As a rule, the trace of this figure is in the complementary color (in this case, greenish-blue). This image, appearing at a fixed point on a homogeneous background, is called the negative afterimage, to distinguish it from a positive afterimage.* As a rule, it retains well-defined outlines, which only gradually fade. The image persists for a short time and then gradually disappears, sometimes reappearing once or twice. In healthy subjects, the visual afterimage is present for between 15 and 30 seconds, after which it loses its definition and disappears. Its duration and intensity depend on the individual peculiarities of the subject, the brightness of the stimulus, and the duration of its fixation.

The investigation of visual afterimages may be of great importance to the study of general and local brain lesions. As various investigators have shown (Bogush, 1939; Kaplan, 1949; Balonov, 1950; etc.), the brightness and duration of afterimages may be considerably altered in pathological states of the brain, reflecting general changes in the excitability of the cerebral cortex. In patients inclined to hallucinations, the brightness and persistence of the afterimages may be enhanced (Bogush, 1939; Popov, 1941; etc.). A particularly interesting phenomenon was observed by Zislina (1955); he found that with *tumors of the occipital lobe* there is a decrease in the brightness and duration of the afterimages and sometimes total disappearance. Characteristically, in some such cases this phenomenon appears as one of the early symptoms of the presence of a lesion, long before any appreciable disturbance of direct visual perception has been demonstrated.

The investigation of visual afterimages is in a special category for it is limited to the study of the most elementary processes involved in the direct impression of traces and can be associated only with the visual analyzer. In contrast, the investigation of acoustic and tactile afterimages is more complex and cannot always be carried out under clinical conditions. Much greater value is attached to methods of investigating the effect of verbal stimuli inducing more complex processes; these methods are widely used in experimental psychological investigations in the clinic. They include, first, methods for measuring the range and duration of the direct retention of a series of concrete visual or verbal elements. These methods of measuring short-term memory were partially considered in another context (Part III, Section 10).

In order to investigate the direct retention of visual traces three or four visual images (simple geometrical figures) are presented for 5 to 10 seconds; after this period of time has elapsed the figures are covered and the subject is required to draw as

* The positive afterimage is characterized by the preservation of the actual color of the stimulus. It can easily be obtained by illuminating an object in a dark room, to which the eyes have become adapted, with a short flash of bright light. For a few seconds thereafter (sometimes for as much as 30 seconds) the subject is aware of a positive afterimage of this object.

many of them as he can remember. To investigate the retention of *acoustic* traces, a series of rhythmic beats or notes is presented for the subject to reproduce (Part III, Section 4). Likewise, to investigate *kinesthetic* memory, a series of positions of the hand is presented for the subject to reproduce (Part III, Section 3B). To investigate the stability of retention of *verbal* traces, the investigator dictates (or presents in writing) a series of three or four words or figures for immediate repetition (Part III, Section 9C).

In all these tests the range of elements that the subject is capable of retaining is ascertained by means of a successive increase in the number of stimuli in the group presented to him. The stability of direct retention is investigated by lengthening the interval between the presentation of the series of stimuli and the beginning of their reproduction up to a period of 10 to 15 seconds. In individual cases it is useful to introduce certain distractions, such as by filling the interval with irrelevant conversation; the inhibitory effect of this factor may significantly modify the reproduction of the material.

The test to study direct retention of verbal traces thus consists of three consecutive stages. In the first stage a series of three words, followed by one of four words and, finally, one of five words is read to the patient (or shown to him visually); he must listen to (or observe) them and repeat them immediately. In the second stage, a pause of 5 to 10 seconds is introduced between the reading of the series of words and their repetition, and by subsequent repetition of the series it is possible to discover how firmly the appropriate traces are retained. In the third stage the repetition of the series of words is separated from its presentation by a pause of 10 to 15 seconds, during which the patient is distracted by irrelevant conversation. This stage of the test is aimed at discovering how easily trace recall can be inhibited by irrelevant stimuli. In all the cases the patient is asked to repeat the words in the order in which they were presented.

To discover how easily the patient can switch from the recall of one series of words to the recall of another series, after the first test he is asked to reproduce the same series of words presented in a different order (e.g., the series "house, forest, table, cat") is followed by the series "table, forest, cat, house." As a result of pathological inertia the patient may be unable to switch to the new order and may still continue to repeat the series of words in the order in which they were presented to him the first time.

Experience has taught that the direct impression of traces may be severely impaired with both general and local brain damage. Whereas a normal subject can retain and reproduce a series of five or six elements (figures, words, numbers) without difficulty, a task of this range would be quite impossible for a patient with a pathological condition of the cerebral cortex, who may be able to retain a series of perhaps only three or four elements. Characteristically, frequent repetition often does not increase the number of elements that the patient can retain. A change from one series to another leads to perseveration, a phenomenon previously discussed; it is a sign of pathological inertia of the nervous processes, which is characteristically found in patients with *organic brain lesions*.

It is significant that patients with *general changes in cortical activity* demonstrated narrowing of the range and instability of the directly retained traces more or less uniformly in the different spheres, while patients with local brain lesions show these deficiencies predominantly in one system; that is why in the latter type of condition the analyzer whose function is most severely affected by the particular lesion can be pinpointed by these disturbances. For instance, in circumscribed lesions of the *left temporal lobe* a marked narrowing of the range and decrease in the stability of the traces are manifested in the response to the auditory presentation of a series of words, with visual presentation of shapes or figures not evoking such specific pathology. In contrast, in patients with *lesions in the occipital area* this narrowing of the range and instability of the traces are manifested in the response to visual stimuli and are compensated for if the speech system is brought into play.

It is characteristic that patients with a lesion of the left temporal region and with a weakness of audioverbal traces usually cannot repeat more than two, three, or four words and, significantly, they often lose the necessary order of their repetition.

In contrast, patients with a lesion of the anterior brain zones can repeat relatively easily a series of words (it does sometimes happen that they perseverate the same word twice; instead of repeating "house, forest, table, cat" they may repeat the series as "house, forest, table, house"). But they have greater difficulty in switching to a new series of words when they continue to reproduce the previous order inertly.

Certain tests aim to study how firmly differentiated groups of traces are retained, the extent to which they are mutually inhibitory, and whether under these circumstances the selectivity of each group stored in the memory is lost.

For these purposes it is convenient to use tests involving proactive and retroactive inhibition of traces. A group of three words (e.g., "table, forest, house") is read to the patient, and he is warned that he must keep this first group well fixed in his memory. After he has repeated it two or three times he is given a second group of three words (e.g., "bridge, night, cross"), and this he also repeats. He is then asked what words were in the first group and what words were in the second group.

The healthy subject can perform this test easily; a patient with a disturbance of memory is unable to do so and will either repeat the first group or will confuse (contaminate) the elements of both groups (e.g., by repeating "house, night, cross"). This test reproduces under experimental conditions the phenomena of disturbance of selectivity which, if the patient's condition becomes worse, may be manifested as mixing the elements of different events and as confabulation. The disturbances of performance of this test are particularly noticeable in patients with fronto-temporal or fronto-diencephalic lesions, when disturbances of the critical faculty are added to trace weakness.

Tests on the retelling of stories fall into a similar category. A simple story is read to the patient and he is asked to retell it. This is then repeated with a different story (but one which includes certain elements of the first). The examiner determines how completely the patient can relate the content of each story and whether he introduces additional associations into his narrative (i.e., whether the elements of the first and second stories are mixed by the patient and whether "contamination" arises).

After the patient has retold the second story, he is asked to recall the first. Inability to do this is evidence of increased retroactive inhibition; in its simplest form it establishes the phenomena which may arise in severe amnesia.

I usually use for this purpose two stories by L. N. Tolstoi.

I. "The Jackdaw and the Pigeon" A jackdaw heard that the pigeon had plenty of food. The jackdaw painted herself white and flew to the pigeon house. The pigeons thought that she also was a pigeon and took her in. But she could not restrain herself and cried like a jackdaw. The pigeons saw that she was a jackdaw and turned her out. She returned to her own kind but they did not recognize her and also refused to have her.

II. "The Ant and the Pigeon" An ant went down to a stream to drink. The water covered him and he started to drown. A pigeon flew passed. She threw the ant a twig. The ant climbed on the twig and was saved. Next day a hunter set a net to catch the pigeon. But when he took her from the net the ant climbed up and bit the hunter on his arm. The pigeon escaped and flew away.

Patients with general cerebral changes of higher cortical functions (a syndrome of increased intracranial pressure) perform this test with difficulty. The stories have to be read to them several times before they can retell them.

Patients with a lesion of the left temporal region and acoustic-mnestic defects, as has already been stated (Part II, Section 3E), are unable to retain the necessary material. They ask for it to be repeated, they omit individual details, and sometimes they replace certain words ("crow" instead of "jackdaw"; "mosquito" instead of "ant," and so on). Frequently these patients are unable to revert to the first story after the second has been read to them, and they declare that they have forgotten or that they remember only individual fragments of it.

Patients with lesions of the frontal (or fronto-temporal) zones, as was stated earlier (Part II, Section 5F), exhibit disturbances which differ from those just described. While repeating the very first story they often show a weakness in selectivity of trace retention. They mix irrelevant associations with elements of the story, wander off into the repetition of details not present in the story, and do not correct their mistakes. When turning to narrate the second story they confuse its elements. They exhibit typical "contamination," and frequently, instead of giving an organized narration of the story, they confuse the actions of persons figuring in it (e.g., instead of "hunter" they say "fisherman," or they say that "the pigeon bit the ant," and so on). As a rule, they find it very difficult to go back to narrate the first story. These disturbances of the selectivity of mnestic processes are an important symptom of a lesion of the anterior brain zones (Luria et al. 1969).

One further special method used in this investigation concerns the phenomenon of "fixed orientation" or "set," which has been studied in detail by Uznadze (1958). In fact, the Soviet psychological literature is replete with descriptions of it. It is illustrated by the following: If a subject is instructed to grasp different size spheres 10 to 15 times with both hands, each time taking the larger sphere in the right hand and the smaller in the left, and if then, in a control experiment, spheres of identical size are placed in both hands, the subject usually has an illusion of contrast, known as "Charpentier's illusion" (i.e., the sphere in the right hand seems smaller than that in the left). This illusion, a phenomenon of aftercontrast in the sphere of *cutaneous and kinesthetic sensation*, may persist for a considerable period of time. It is then gradually extinguished, the course of its extinction typically fluctuating so that it may sometimes be observed after considerable intervals of time (measured in hours or even in days) have elapsed. In some cases, the illusion may spread to other analyzers. Once an illusion has been formed in the tactile sphere, it may then be created in the visual sphere; for instance, if two equal circles are presented to the eye, the right appears smaller than the left.

Application of the examination of fixed orientation to the clinical study of patients with general and local brain lesions has resulted in the uncovering of important findings. Patients with epilepsy may show a sharp increase in the stability of their fixed orientation or set, whereas patients with other psychopathological manifestations (schizophrenia, hysteria) give different results (Bzhalava, 1958). Patients with severe *lesions of the temporal cerebral divisions* show signs of a loss of stability of set (Luria and Bzhalava, 1947). Finally, it is especially interesting to note that patients with diencephalic lesions (*tumors of the third ventricle*) and the associated *lowering of cortical tone* sometimes exhibit such gross instability of set that traces of tactile orientation can be observed only during one or two tests carried out immediately after its formation. Intervals of 3 to 5 seconds after the main experiment are enough to cause disappearance of the illusion created by the fixed environment (Konovalov and Filippycheva, unpublished data).

C. INVESTIGATION OF THE LEARNING PROCESS

The processes involved in learning and their modification by pathological states of the brain have also been the recipients of much attention in modern general and special psychology. The investigation of these processes may yield valuable results for the clinical study of local brain lesions. The most important aspect of this investigation is the analysis of the methods used in the process of learning, of the way in which the volume of retained material increases during the process, and of the patient's reaction to any mistakes he might make.

At first, the patient is presented with a series of completely unrelated words (or numbers) that is too long to memorize, usually ten to twelve words or eight to ten numbers. The subject is asked to memorize this series and to reproduce it in any order. After he has written down those elements he has retained, he is given the series again and the results are again recorded. This procedure is repeated eight to ten times. Each time, the results obtained are plotted on a memory curve to gain a better idea of the order of memorization; the investigator denotes each reproduced word by numbers corresponding to the order of their reproduction.

It is very useful to combine this experiment with investigation of the changing pattern of the level of aspiration made by the subject on his memorizing process and on the way in which these changes depend on the results obtained in the preceding experiment. For this purpose the subject, who has just memorized a certain number of words, is asked how many words he feels he will be able to memorize when the series is next repeated; he then proceeds to learn them again. If this method is adopted, the results are similar to those presented in Table 3.

Table 3

Results of a Learning Experiment

Serial No.	Level of aspiration	Actual result	House	Forest	Cat	Night	Table	Needle	Pie	Bell	Bridge	Cross
1	—	6	1	2	3	—	4	—	—	—	5	6
2	8	7	1	2	3	—	4	5	—	—	6	7
3	8	8	1	2	3	4	5	6	—	—	7	8
4	10	9	1	2	3	9	4	5	—	6	7	8
5	10	10	1	2	3	9	4	5	10	6	7	8

The results of each experiment are plotted on a learning curve, which, as a rule, shows a continuous rise at a varying rate.

A disturbance of the higher cortical functions in patients with local brain lesions may lead to significant changes in the process of learning, affecting both the quality and the character of the results obtained. Patients with *general cerebral changes in cortical activity*, like patients with circumscribed *lesions of the posterior divisions of the brain*,* evince the same qualitative features of the learning process characteristically found in normal subjects. When they tackle problems they take into consideration the results obtained in the preceding experiment and their level of aspiration usually lies rather higher than the number of elements they are capable of memorizing. They strive to learn the proffered words in a particular order, paying attention each time to the words that they could not

* Patients with aphasic speech disturbances naturally cannot take part in this experiment.

remember the last time. They make few mistakes and usually do not repeat the same mistake many times in succession. However, the duration of the process may differ significantly from that observed in healthy subjects. Very frequently, the patients' learning curves rise very slowly, the volume of material they are capable of learning being much smaller than in healthy subjects; many patients cannot memorize more than five or six words. A characteristic feature of this limited scope is the ability to reproduce a new group of presented words but, in so doing, leaving out the group previously memorized.

Many patients begin to experience fatigue in the course of the experiment so that the learning curve, having reached its peak at the fourth or fifth repetition, begins to decline and becomes dome-shaped. Examples of normal and pathological learning curves are shown in Fig. 132.

Different results are obtained during the investigation of patients with well-defined *frontal syndromes*. As mentioned (Part II, Section 5E), the distin-

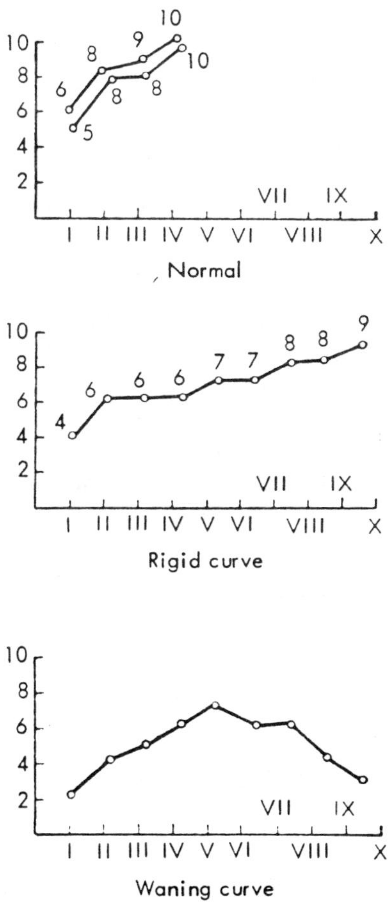

FIGURE 132 Normal and pathological learning curves. The abscissa denotes the experiment number; the ordinate, the number of words retained.

guishing features of such cases become apparent during the process of learning. For instance, many patients exhibit pathological features in their level of aspiration: In response to a request to predict how many elements of the next series they will memorize, they state any number without taking into account their real capabilities. Sometimes they will continue to repeat inertly a low number, even after they have demonstrated that their actual results are higher than this. In memorizing a series, they often reproduce the words in random order, without giving any special attention to the words they had not remembered the previous time; the series they passively continue to give may be either stereotyped or nonrepetitive. As a rule these patients continue to repeat a mistake once made, with no attempt at correction. Often, they repeat the same word twice in a series, again without correcting their mistake.

The learning curve of these patients often reflects an inactive character of the memorizing process, not rising above a certain limit so that it assumes the shape of a plateau (Part II, Section 5E).

The experiments herein enumerated not only enable the investigator to determine the limits of the patient's ability to memorize, but also yield valuable evidence on the processes of active mental function characteristically present in different groups of patients.

D. THE ROLE OF INTERFERENCE IN DISTURBANCES OF MNESTIC PROCESSES

The direct imprinting of material and its learning are only some of the basic phenomena of mnestic activity, and these two processes do not give a complete picture of the changes in mnestic processes which arise in pathological states of the brain. In the last decade phenomena have been discovered which reveal much more fully the mechanisms of these changes and which can form the basis of new techniques for their investigation.

All these phenomena stem from a single, paradoxical observation. Investigations carried out in the last 10 to 15 years have shown that neither the volume of direct imprinting nor the learning curves just described can reflect sufficiently completely the memory defects arising as a result of pathological lesions. Even patients with a gross disturbance of memory and a severe Korsakov's syndrome may show no sufficiently clear abnormality when tested by the two methods described above.

How can the phenomenon of loss of memory observed in most patients with local brain lesions be explained? What are the mechanisms lying at the basis of these defects, and what method can be used to discover these defects most clearly?

In the last two decades two theories attempting to explain the mechanisms of forgetting in both health and disease have been discussed in the literature. The first of these theories explains forgetting as the result of trace decay. The second considers that this explanation is inadequate, and that the basic mechanism of forgetting is the inhibitory effect of distracting, irrelevant processes. This last theory, known for a long time as the theory of proactive and retroactive inhibition, has more recently been referred to as the theory of the inhibitory effect of interfering factors.

According to the first theory memory defects are based on instability of imprinting; the second theory holds that forgetting is a defect of trace recall, that the traces themselves remain in a latent form but their ecphoria is disturbed by interfering factors.

There are many grounds for disputing the validity of the first theory: the well-known facts of reminiscence (an increase in the number of elements recalled after a certain time interval), an upsurge of apparently long-forgotten experiences and patterns after hypnotic action, and so on. These arguments compel the more careful examination of the second theory in order to discover whether the memory disturbances in pathological states of the brain can be reduced essentially to increased inhibitability of traces by interfering factors.

To test this theory a very simple method was used (a method which, as we found out later, had been suggested earlier by Petersen and Petersen [1962], although admittedly for a different purpose). In order to determine the degree of stability of imprinted traces during exposure to distracting or interfering factors, the subject was instructed to repeat two or three words: after a short pause (an "empty" pause, i.e., not filled with interfering activity), lasting from 30 sec to 1–2 min, the subjects were again instructed to recall the previously imprinted group of traces. As a rule in this test even the most seriously affected patients had no appreciable difficulty. The main series of tests was then carried out. These differed from the previous series in the fact that the pause after imprinting of the test elements was *filled with irrelevant (distracting) activity.* In some cases this activity was simple conversation with the patient on unconnected topics, in other cases the patient was given a simple arithmetical exercise, such as to count from 100 backward in 7's, to recite the names of the months in the reverse order, and so on (heterogeneous interference); in other cases subjects who had just retained a group of 2 or 3 words were instructed to recall and repeat a second group consisting of another 2 or 3 words (homogeneous interference), after which they were asked to recall which words formed the first group, the one they had reproduced previously.

There are several alternative forms of this test. Groups of words (numbers) of different size (consisting of 2, 3, or 4 elements) could be presented: the memorizing of words presented by ear could be followed by the memorizing of figures presented visually, and so on (so that the modality-specificity of the stability of recall of the material could be investigated). The group of isolated words could be replaced by whole organized semantic structures (short or long sentences), in order to test how the inhibitory effect of homogeneous or heterogeneous interference on the stability of the recalled material varies. Finally, the groups of words or sentences easily retained directly could be replaced by more difficult material (e.g., whole stories), repetition of the text of which goes far beyond the bounds of direct memory, but must also include the retention and recall of the basic theme or model of the story.

In all these cases the tests can be carried out under the two conditions specified above: by comparing the volume of direct recall with that of recall after an "empty" pause, and with material recalled after heterogeneous or homogeneous interference.

The results of the two basic series of tests carried out in the manner described above were found to differ profoundly (Kiyashchenko, 1973; Kiyashchenko et al., 1975; Luria, 1976). The recall of previously imprinted material after a short "empty" pause by patients with brain lesions did not differ significantly and the level of performance was the same by all patients (except patients with acoustic-mnestic aphasia, in whom traces of imprinted series of words were too unstable, and patients with optico-mnestic defects, in whom the recall of a series of visually presented figures also was too unstable). The second group of tests in which direct trace recall was accompanied by interfering activity gave totally different results. In this case the patients had no difficulty with direct recall of material but they were quite unable to recall the first series imprinted after performing some other (heterogeneous or homogeneous) interfering activity. Usually they stated that "they had already forgotten" the first series, or that "they could not recall" the first series of words given to them; they either repeated a very small part of the first test series of words or they mixed up the elements of the second and first groups, replacing correct repetition by contamination.

In the tests involving the recall of a series of isolated elements, definite defects (rarely observed in normal subjects) were found even in patients in whom clinical examination revealed no appreciable memory defects.

In some cases increased inhibitability of traces by interfering factors was modality-nonspecific in character and was manifested equally whether words, numbers, drawings, and so on, were recalled. In other cases the difficulties of recall were modality-specific and were manifested particularly clearly only in the recalling of audioverbal or visual traces; however, the general position regarding pathologically increased inhibitability of traces by interfering factors still held good.

Modality-nonspecific manifestations of increased trace inhibitability were observed in patients with deep brain lesions (pituitary tumors with parasellar spread, tumors of the third ventricle and the hippocampus); the manifestations of modality-specific increased trace inhibitability were clearly manifested in local lesions of the left temporal region with phenomena of acoustic-mnestic aphasia (in these cases the recall of previously imprinted word series after interfering factors was severely disturbed whereas the recall of previously imprinted visual patterns, e.g., geometrical shapes, remained relatively intact). The opposite state of affairs was observed in lesions of the parieto-occipital zones of the cortex when pathologically increased trace inhibitability by interfering factors was manifested more clearly in the recall of visual patterns whereas the recall of audioverbal traces was relatively intact.

Considerable differences also were found in the character of the disturbances revealed by these tests in patients with lesions in different situations: whereas patients with deep lesions or lesions of the systems of the left temporal region simply abandoned all attempts to recall elements of the first series presented in the test or mixed the elements of the first and second series (contamination), patients with lesions of the frontal zones showed quite different defects. Traces of the last series of words were so inert that the patients of this group could not leave them and return to the traces of the first group and, instead, they inertly perseverated the traces of the last group; when asked to recall which words formed the first series and which the second, they invariably repeated the words of the last group, and they were unaware of their mistakes.

Significant disturbances of recall were found in the patients of various groups when they changed from recall of a series of isolated elements (words) to the recall of organized structures (sentences).

In patients with relatively ill-defined pathology of deep brain zones this change from recall of isolated structures to recall of organized structures is followed by disappearance of the defect. Although they are unable to recall series of isolated words, they can easily recall the first of two sentences after recalling the second.

In patients with more severe lesions (massive deep brain tumors) the symptomatology is appreciably different: defects (forgetting, contamination) observed in tests involving the recall of series of isolated words continues to be manifested in tests involving the recall of complete sentences. For instance, having easily recalled the first sentence ("Apple trees grew in the garden behind the high fence"), followed by the second sentence ("The hunter killed a wolf at the edge of the forest"), the patient, when instructed to recall the first sentence again, could only say: "Oh, I have quite forgotten . . . what was it? . . . ," or, "In the garden . . . at the edge of the forest . . . and there was something else. . . ."

More serious defects still are found when these tests are carried out on patients with massive lesions of the frontal lobes. Having repeated both the first and second sentences correctly, these patients are then unable to recall the first sentence because of the pathological inertia of the second. When, therefore, they are asked to recall the first sentence, after some hesitation they will say: ". . . The hunter killed a wolf at the edge of the forest . . . ," and when asked to recall the second sentence, they will either say: ". . . also . . . the hunter killed a wolf at the edge of the forest," or they will make some partial changes in the stereotype, realize that something is wrong, and say: ". . . At the edge of the forest . . . the hunter killed . . . a hare!" It can easily be seen that in these cases pathological inertia of established stereotypes extends equally to the semantic organization of the material.

Some even more interesting results were obtained in tests of the recall of material outside the bounds of possible direct recall. Tests of this type include the recall of complex texts, either by direct repetition or repetition after intervening interference. The repetition of this material requires quite different forms of activity on the part of the subject from repetition of isolated words or sentences.

In order to recall a text the subject must analyze it, pick out its most essential semantic components and separate them from less essential components, and put together the general semantic scheme of the tests, thus creating a *closed semantic system,* which is to serve as the object of recall and to define its limits.

Disturbances arising in this form of mnestic activity differ widely in lesions of different parts of the brain. Patients with various forms of aphasia find it very difficult to recall the corresponding verbal components of the text (lexical, morphological, and syntagmatic); they may exhibit definite paraphasia (replacing the proper word by another or incorrectly recalling the acoustic structure of words); they may have difficulty in recalling the syntactic structure of the text (this is a particularly conspicuous feature of the "telegraphic style" syndrome); and they may have difficulty in grasping the meaning of logical-grammatical relations embodied in the text (this happens in patients with semantic aphasia). However, the *general meaning* of the text as a closed semantic system still remains intact and, in their attempts to recall it, these patients never transgress its limits.

The picture is quite different in patients with massive lesions of the frontal lobes. As a rule these patients do not take active steps to analyze the semantic structure of the text, they do not pick out its essential elements, and they do not make a choice from the many associations evoked by the text; for that reason a sufficiently stable *closed semantic system* of the text given to them is not created. The recall of a text, which likewise is not an active reconstruction of this system in these patients, thus ceases to be a goal-directed activity of recall, and it begins to resemble the recall of a system open to all irrelevant influences (direct impressions or associations).

For instance, when patients of this group attempt to recall the story "The Hen and the Golden Eggs," they easily slip into irrelevant associations established previously (such as: "Eggs. . . . the old man hit, hit—did not kill; the old man hit, hit—did not kill" * and so on), or they fall

* A reference to another Russian children's story.

under the influence of direct impressions and intersperse their narrative with elements of their immediate situation. When trying to tell the story "The Jackdaw and the Pigeons," they may say: "A jackdaw . . . painted herself white . . . like these gowns we are wearing . . . and went into the hospital . . ." and so on. Finally, the selective goal-directed repetition of a text given to them previously can easily be replaced by the inert, stereotyped, repetition of any one component of it (Part II, Section 5G).

Consequently, whereas in lesions of the posterior zones of the brain individual *mnestic operations* are disturbed, but goal-directed mnestic activity (active memorizing and recall) remains intact, in lesions of the frontal lobes the opposite picture is found and the disturbance of active, goal-directed mnestic activity makes it impossible for the patient to perform the test although the individual operations involved in that activity are preserved.

Thus disturbances of complex forms of mnestic activity of this kind (the recall of material exceeding the volume directly reproducible) are manifested equally in both ordinary tests and tests involving interference. The facts thus observed provide a deeper insight into some of the important characteristics of the pathological process with which we are concerned. A fuller description of the results of such investigations is documented elsewhere (Luria, 1976a, 1976b).

E. INVESTIGATION OF LOGICAL MEMORIZING

The investigation of logical, or indirect memorizing, a concept introduced into psychology by Vygotskii and developed by Leont'ev (1931), is a phase of the psychological investigation that relates equally to the study of memory and to the study of intellectual processes. Its purpose is to describe and define the active aids invoked in the memorizing of logical material and the intellectual activity concerned with this task.

The subject is first asked to memorize a series of 12 to 15 words by using appropriate cards as aids for each word; by glancing at an appropriate one he should be able to recall the required word. Such cards must not depict the direct meaning of the word but must be so chosen that the subject has to establish a chain of meaning between the word to be remembered and the pictorial representation. For instance, a picture of an umbrella is used for the word "rain," or a picture of a lock is used for the word "burglar;" in more complex tests, a picture of an overcoat is used for the word "summer" (the connection being that in summer it is warm and overcoats are not needed).

There are two variants to the test of logical memorizing. In the first of these each word in a given series corresponds to one picture, and this picture must be used as an aid in memorizing the word. In the second (or "free") variant a group of

15 or 20 picture cards is laid out before the subject, and he has to choose the one most suitable for memorizing a presented word. Each time, the subject is asked what chain of logic he uses to memorize the particular word. After the auxiliary picture for each word has been chosen, the group of selected pictures is shuffled and presented in random order. As each picture is presented the subject must recall the corresponding word. As special investigations (Leont'ev, 1931; Zankov, 1944; etc.) have shown, the process of using logical connections for memorizing begins to develop in children before they reach school age and is finally established at the beginning of the school period, after which it becomes progressively more complex.

Patients with local brain lesions but without general dementia show no noticeable abnormality in this process. As a rule, they eagerly take part in the experiment and readily make use of simple logical connections to help them compensate for their defects in direct memorizing. With the aid of a chosen picture they can recall comparatively easily the associated word. Only occasionally (especially when fatigue is present) will the patient have difficulty in matching the required word to the picture. Such aids are extensively and successfully utilized in re-education. It is only in patients with *severe forms of diencephalic syndrome* and *general disturbances of the mnestic processes* that this selective logical connection may be lost. If this happens they cannot use this method for the effective compensation of their defect.

Significantly different from this state of affairs are the disturbances observed in patients with *lesions of the frontal lobes*. Patients with marked frontal syndromes, as was pointed out (Part II, Section 5F), very frequently cannot select and use logical connections as aids to memorizing. The picture offered to the patient often gives rise to independent associations quite unconnected with the corresponding word. However, when the word and picture are joined by some form of common logical connection, this connection is not used for the subsequent reproduction of the word. When, therefore, pictures intended to be used as aids for the recollection of the required word are presented for a second time, they do not remind the patient of the word but continue to arouse independent associations and, consequently, are of no help to him. The inability to form a connection to be used as an "afferent feedback" in the process of active memorizing is therefore one of the most important symptoms of a disturbance of the higher mental processes associated with lesions of the frontal lobes.

One other variant remains to be mentioned. It was originally suggested by Vygotskii and was developed by several of his collaborators. This test, which has been called the "pictogram" method, is conducted as follows: The subject is asked to memorize a series of words or phrases; to enable him to do this, he is instructed to draw a certain sign or picture each time to help him to remember the particular word. The words or phrases used in the test are such that they cannot be drawn directly (for example, "a deaf old man" or "a hungry boy" or abstractions like "development" and "cause"). The patient must therefore choose some sign to serve as a pictogram.

After a series of words has been depicted in this way, the patient is shown the pictures he has drawn and from them he must reproduce the necessary words.

The results thus obtained during the examination of psychiatric patients and during the study of mentally retarded individuals reveal profound changes in the formation of logical associations. This method has been used only to a limited extent for the study of patients with local brain lesions; when so used its results were similar to those in connection with the other experiments on logical memorizing.

8. Investigation of Speech Functions. Receptive Speech

A. PRELIMINARY REMARKS

The investigation of speech functions comprises a very important part of the study of a patient with a defect in higher cortical functioning. This is true because a very large proportion of man's higher mental activities is formed and functions in close association with the second signal system and because speech has such an important function in human social intercourse and intellectual activity. Until this point in our discussion of investigative methodology, speech was considered only in relation to those operations in which it has a subsidiary role; in the present discussion, the state of the speech functions themselves will be of central interest.

Human verbal communication means the transmission of information by the use of the codes of language. The process of verbal communication begins with the motive which compels a person to communicate with another person (with a request, the transmission of information). It includes a certain formulation of a general idea (or plan) to be converted into speech, it then passes through the very important (and still inadequately studied) stage of "internal speech," in which the initial plan begins to assume the form of a verbal expression, and it ends with the expanded verbal communication.

During the understanding (decoding) of a verbal expression the process is reversed. It starts with the perception by the listener of the speaker's expanded speech, it then passes into a complex process of analysis of the essential components of the expression (which in some cases will be very easy but in others will require certain transformations, making the meaning of the expression more understandable), it again goes through the intermediate stage of "internal speech," which represents the most essential meaning of the communication in compressed form, and finally it is converted into the idea (or sense) of the communication received.

The whole of this complex path was described originally by Pick (1913), and the actual structure of formation of the verbal expression and its decoding was analyzed in detail by Vygotskii in his classical book *Thought and Speech* (1934).

This complex structure of verbal communication incorporates widely different psychological components. In patients with lesions of different parts of the brain the individual stages of this process may be differently affected.

In general, it can be said that a lesion of the frontal lobes leads primarily to a disturbance of stable motives, generating verbal communication, or (as in patients with lesions of the posterior frontal and fronto-temporal systems) it causes a disturbance of the "internal speech" component forming the plan of verbal communication. This invariably causes a disturbance of verbal communication as an active process, whereas the individual operations connected with the linguistic codes of language (the use of phonemes, lexics, syntactic structures) remain intact.

Lesions of the posterior parts of the speech areas of the cortex (the left temporal and left parieto-occipital regions) lead to the opposite effects. The motives lying at the basis of verbal communication in these cases are preserved whereas the individual operations (the use of the phonemic structures of speech, the stable isolation of the lexical, syntactic, or semantic components of the verbal expression) may be substantially impaired.

In a whole series of investigations carried out in the last decade, the fundamental structure of disturbances of verbal expression in patients with lesions of different parts of the brain has been described in detail (Luria, 1972, 1974a, 1974b, 1975, 1976).

This highly differential character of speech disturbances in lesions of different parts of the brain can be manifested both in the formation of verbal expression (expressive speech) and in its decoding (impressive or receptive speech). This must be borne in mind when we go on describing the methods by means of which speech activity is investigated.

There are two principal ways to investigate speech processes: First, the function of speech can be considered as comprising two broad categories—*receptive (impressive)* and *motor (expressive) speech*—with each form receiving special attention. Second, attention must also be paid to the *different levels* of disturbance of the speech processes, some more complex than others. As recent investigations by Chistovich have shown, the elementary level of perception of the sounds of speech is the level of simple acoustic recognition (which can be discovered by the simplest imitation of sounds), whereas the more complex level of the perception of sound is linked with its categorization, as revealed by completely different tests. Although both of these approaches find a place in every investigation of speech they will be considered separately in the present discussion.

It is generally accepted that the speech functions fall into two clearly defined categories—receptive and motor. The former usually refers to the perception of the sounds of speech, the understanding of the meaning of words and phrases, and, ultimately, the understanding of consecutive speech. Reading is a particular form of receptive speech. Expressive speech refers to the articulation of the sounds of speech, the pronunciation of words or phrases, and, ultimately, execution of spontaneous, consecutive speech. Writing is a particular form of expressive speech.

Despite the fact that these two aspects of speech are indisputably independent, the distinction between them is rather arbitrary. It is well known that pronunciation depends on the perception of unfamiliar speech and on its acoustic analysis and synthesis. One has to recollect the grossly defective pronunciation in persons deaf since birth or who have become deaf in early life to appreciate the role of acoustic analysis in articulation. On the other hand, it is also well known that phonemic hearing is itself formed in close association with articulation, just as musical hearing is formed in close association with singing movements (Part I, Section 3; Leont'ev, 1959). The fact that acoustic analysis is abnormal in stutterers with an anatomical defect of their articulatory apparatus is quite significant. For these reasons, every investigation of speech must be concerned with both aspects—comprehension of unfamiliar speech with preservation of its acoustic composition and pronunciation of spoken sounds and words.

For didactic reasons, as well as because of the fact that primary disturbances of the impressive and expressive aspects of speech are completely different in topical significance, they will be considered separately. It must be remembered, however, that in practice both aspects of speech are investigated at the same time and sometimes by the same methods. It should also be borne in mind that the superior temporal divisions of the left hemisphere, comprising the principal apparatus for the analysis and synthesis of speech sounds, work in close association with the sensorimotor divisions, which are responsible for articulation (Part II, Sections 2C–D and 4D). A disturbance in phonemic hearing must inevitably, therefore, lead to a secondary disturbance in speech articulation and expressive speech, while a disturbance of the articulatory processes and of internal speech must also inevitably affect impressive processes, e.g., the perception of the sounds of speech and the understanding of the meaning of speech. Therefore, although described separately, awareness of the intimate interrelationship between receptive and expressive speech will always be in the background and attention will be directed toward the determination of which disturbances of these aspects of speech are primary and which secondary or systemic.

The speech functions may also be studied from the point of view of their levels of construction. It is well known that speech activity may be constructed at different levels and may consequently differ in complexity. For instance, a simple exclamation expressive of an emotional state is the simplest form of expressive speech; the naming of a familiar object or the answer to a simple question, although habitual in its form, is much more complex in structure. The naming of an unfamiliar object, the pronunciation of a phrase, and, still more, spontaneous, highly developed speech are even more complex processes. All these forms of expressive speech incorporate systems of connections of different degrees of complexity and stability and at different functional levels. If the numerous references Jackson, Goldstein, and others made to the "low" (emotional or habitual) and the "high" (voluntary or intellectual) forms of speech are recalled, the differentials involved in speech construction will be appreciated.

The same applies to the impressive aspect of speech. Whereas the grasping of the emotional tone of speech or of well-established forms of address or words is simple enough and may remain unimpaired even in the presence of gross cortical lesions, the understanding of the nominative aspect of speech (its objective categorization) is a far more complex process. The understanding of complex categorical systems of associations, represented by words, is still more complex, while the analysis of logical-grammatical constructions (like the understanding of the meaning of a short text or of the "general sense" of a fragment) requires activity organized at a far higher level.

All these forms of expressive and impressive speech naturally include systems of associations organized at different developmental levels and requiring different physiological systems for their performance. Many eminent neurologists and psychologists (Jackson, 1884; Head, 1926; Pick, 1931; Goldstein, 1948; Ombredane, 1951; etc.) have therefore insisted that whenever the character of impressive and expressive speech is studied, a careful investigation be made of the level at which disturbance occurs. Some of these workers have considered this principle so important that they have used it as a basis for the differentiation of motor aphasia from dysarthria or of "central" aphasia from its "peripheral" forms (Goldstein, 1948).

Both these aspects of the study of speech functions must be taken into consideration when the technique of investigation is being formulated; although a primary disturbance of the impressive or expressive aspect of speech may directly indicate a circumscribed lesion and hence may be of direct topical significance, analysis of the patient's level of speech may provide important information concerning the complexity of the systems involved in the pathological process and the extent of the brain damage. In the discussions on disturbances of receptive and expressive speech, we shall describe the tests we use in such a way that, so far as possible, the various levels of speech construction are examined.

The investigation of speech functions is usually undertaken after a preliminary investigation has been made of the state of the "nonspeech" processes. The whole of the subsequent investigation of speech must, naturally, be based on the composite findings, taking into account the previously discerned abnormalities in the sensory and motor functions and in the general behavior of the patient.

B. INVESTIGATION OF PHONEMIC HEARING

It was mentioned earlier in this book (Part II, Section 2C) that investigation of speech sound differentiation, a fundamental factor both in phonemic hearing and in the development of phonetic speech, must be preceded by a careful investigation of the auditory functions as a whole.

We know that a relatively slight decrease in auditory acuity in early childhood is an impediment to the differentiation of speech sounds and, hence, to speech development (Boskis, 1953), with inadequate clarity of pronunciation (Rau, 1954; Bel'tyukov, 1960; Neiman, 1960). The presence of *adequate auditory acuity* is therefore a basic condition for differentiation of the sounds of speech. The examiner must be satisfied that hearing is intact before starting to make a special investigation of the receptive aspect of speech. This is accomplished by the ordinary methods used in otoneurology, with emphasis on the information obtained by means of ordinary tuning forks or the audiometer and whispering.

Valuable results may be obtained by investigating the ability to differentiate sounds not only in relation to simple attributes (pitch, intensity, timbre), but also to more complex qualities, having signal value and pertaining to groups of sounds (chords and, in particular, sound sequences). This latter type of investigation may be especially germane for it leads directly to the study of those aspects of the differentiation of sound groups that when impaired give rise to the phenomena of sensory aphasia. Some of the methods used to evaluate the differentiation of sounds and groups of sounds have already been described (Part III, Section 4B) so that they will be omitted from the present account.

Usually, relatively simple methods are used to appraise the integrity of phonemic hearing. The patient is asked to repeat simple, isolated sounds ("b," "p," "m," "d," "k," "s," "sh") or to repeat (and distinguish) pairs of sounds, including sharply differing (disjunctive) phonemes (e.g., "m–p," "p–s," "b–n") and similar sounding (oppositional or correlating) phonemes ("b–p" and "p–b," "d–t" and "t–d," "k–g" and "g–k," "r–l" and "l–r"). To make this test more difficult, the patient may be given a series of three sounds or simple syllables, incorporating either disjunctive phonemes (e.g., "a–o–u," "u–a–i," "b–r–k," "m–s–d") or correlating phonemes (e.g., "b–p–b," "p–b–p," "d–t–d," "t–d–d"). Whereas the first test is solely directed toward appraising the differentiation of the sounds of speech, the second test also examines the retention of phonoarticulatory traces.

As was explained, the testing of discrimination of speech sounds by having the patient repeat sounds encompasses both phonetic auditory discrimination and the pronunciation of the corresponding sounds. Clearly, this test will yield uniform results only when the act of pronunciation itself remains undisturbed, or, in other words, when the pronunciation of a sound is not beset by articulatory difficulties or by pathological inertia within the motor system. Therefore, for control purposes, the discrimination of speech sounds must be tested by means of other indicators. This is particularly important in those cases in which the integrity of the motor aspect of speech is in doubt.

Such tests may include the one in which writing substitutes for vocal repetition. (The much greater distinction between "b" and "p" and between "d" and "t" when written than when pronounced avoids the difficulties that arise in the finer discrimination between the corresponding articulemes.) Another method is to ask the patient to point to those letters placed before him that designate the sounds presented to him. Finally, the patient may simply be instructed to give an opinion on pairs of either identical or of different sounds presented to him (e.g., "b–p" or "p–p," "d–t" or "t–t").

To conduct these tests in a sufficiently pure form, the patient must not be permitted to pronounce the sounds aloud (a stipulation that imposes a considerable handicap with this form of discrimination) or, at least, to compare the results obtained with and without such pronunciation. A control device for this purpose is having the patient hold his tongue between his teeth or his mouth closed while the experiment is being conducted.

In certain cases, the sound discriminatory capacity may be studied by utilizing the conditioned-reflex principle. The patient is instructed to raise his right hand during the pronunciation of one sound (e.g., "b") and to raise his left hand when another, similar sound is pronounced (e.g., "p"), or else the first sound is made the positive signal for raising the hand and the second becomes the inhibitory signal requiring the hand to be left as it was.

A more sensitive variant of this test introduces additional complications: Different sounds (e.g., "b" and "p," "d" and "t") are pronounced at the same pitch, and identical sounds (e.g., "b" and "b") at different pitches. This variant can be used to discover which component—the phonemic sign or an accidental phonetic one (not essential for the phoneme)—allows for the discrimination of the speech sounds.

Incorporation of conditioned reflexes into this study, notwithstanding all its advantages, has the drawback of a lack of specificity. An incorrect response may ensue not only from defective sound discrimination, but also from other neurodynamic defects (weakened stimulatory and inhibitory processes, disturbed mobility of these processes in the motor analyzer, etc.). These possibilities therefore have to be ruled out. This can be accomplished only by comparing the differentiation of phonemes, nonspeech sounds, and visual signals as indicated by this means.

A very valuable method of investigating the highest levels of perception of the sounds of speech is by relating a given sound (phoneme) to its corresponding letter (grapheme). For this test, the patient is given a few letters (e.g., D, T, K), and he has to show which phoneme the examiner is speaking. A disturbance of the complex process of categorization of the sounds of speech can be expressed as pointing to the wrong letter. In that case it will be clear whether the difficulties observed are based on confusion between similar "opposition" phonemes (for example, "D" and "T") or whether the disturbance is deeper in character and is connected with the fact that the patient distinguishes one of the elementary qualities (e.g., plosiveness) and begins to confuse phonemes such as "T" and "K."

Disturbances in phonemic hearing, constituting the fundamental symptom of a lesion of the *posterosuperior cortical region of the temporal lobe of the dominant (left) hemisphere* (Part II, Section 2D), are exposed by these tests by the obvious difficulties patients have in differentiating speech sounds. Patients with extensive lesions in this area are unable to differentiate clearly even strikingly different (disjunctive) phonemes. In less severe cases the patient may still be able to differentiate between disjunctive phonemes but cannot clearly discriminate between similar (correlating or oppositional) phonemes.

When presented with pairs of sounds like "b" and "p" or "t" and "d," the patient declares that he can hear two identical or barely distinguishable sounds, and often he cannot put into words the difference that he detects. As a rule, such patients can neither repeat these sounds clearly nor write them down correctly; they are not even able to point to the corresponding letters. Even in the test utilizing conditioned motor reactions to different sounds of speech, these patients give vague responses; they readily confuse essential (phonemic) and unessential (tonal) differences, (so far as language is concerned) in the pronunciation of these sounds. Naturally, the more complicated tasks (e.g., repetition or differentiation of a series of three sounds) are completely beyond the power of such patients. Characteristically, they persist in giving insufficiently confident reactions, for they cannot grasp or retain the notion that the presented sounds can be categorized in clearly defined phonemic groups.

Patients with a *disturbance in the kinesthetic component* of speech activity (Part II, Section 4D) may also evince marked defects in response to this test. However, there are two essential differences between these groups of patients: First, the disturbance in phonemic hearing may be less marked in the latter; second, the latter may also show obvious difficulties in the discrimination of speech sounds with quite different acoustic characteristics yet similar methods of articulation (for example, the sounds "b" and "m," "d" and "n"). In patients with *efferent (kinetic) motor aphasia* (Part II, Section 4F), just as in patients with gross lesions of the premotor systems, no obvious primary disturbance in discrimination between correlating phonemes may be present, yet they readily display signs of diminished mobility of the nervous processes in the acoustic-articulatory sphere. During the performance of these tests, these patients may experience difficulty in switching from one phoneme to another and show signs of perseveration, the latter interfering with the assessment of the true nature of the observed defect. Especially marked disturbances are found in these patients when they attempt to reproduce a series of three identical consonants with changing vowels. They are unable to repeat the series of sounds "bi–ba–bo" (they perseverate them as "bi–bo–bo" or "bo–bo–bo"); nor are they able to change from one series to another (e.g., from "bi–ba–bo" to "bo–bi–ba"), but tend to produce an inert repetition of their first series of responses. All these disturbances are typical of patients of this group.

Marked difficulties associated with disruption of the organization of a relatively long sound sequence, with signs of changes in the order in which a series of sounds are pronounced, also appear in patients with *malfunctioning of the frontotemporal systems of the left hemisphere*. Defects in the reproduction of rhythms are often found in patients with *a lesion of the right temporal lobe*, but their ability to discriminate between speech sounds is preserved; the latter distinguishes this group from patients with a lesion of the left temporal lobe or with a syndrome of sensory (acoustic) aphasia. It is interesting to note that in these patients impaired phonemic hearing often exists with considerable preservation of musical hearing, and that they experience only slight difficulty in reproducing rhythmic structures (Part III, Section 4C).

The subsequent investigation of the degree to which discrimination between the sounds of speech is present is undertaken by means of tests to study the phonetic analysis and synthesis of words and syllables presented to the patient; these tests will be considered in connection with the investigation of writing (Part III, Section 10A).

C. INVESTIGATION OF WORD COMPREHENSION

The second stage in the investigation of the receptive aspect of speech is the investigation of word comprehension. As was stated (Part II, Section 2D and E), to understand words there must be, first, adequately precise and stable phonemic hearing and, second, adequate association between these groups of sounds and the objects, qualities, actions, or relationships denoted by them. Therefore, words can be misinterpreted both by patients with defective phonemic hearing (Part II, Section 2D) and by those with temporo-occipital lesions (Part II, Section 2E), in whom the cortical structure of words may remain intact but the system of sound traces or associations of sound groups is disturbed.

To investigate word comprehension, or the nominative function, the examiner presents individual words that the patient must define either verbally or by pointing to the objects represented by them. As a rule, this investigation starts by showing the patient the objects to be named. Sometimes objects are named that are not directly visible and that the patient must "find" (for example, he may be asked to point to "the eye," "the nose," "the ear"); in other instances the patient may have to identify the objects portrayed in pictures placed before him (for example, representations of a glass, a pencil, a knife). While the first of these tests requires active, kinesthetic identification of the named object and is somewhat more difficult, the second, in which the named object can be compared directly with its visual image, provides easier conditions.

A more sensitive means of studying word comprehension is frequent repetition of the same words (for example, "show eyes"–"ear"–"nose"–"ear"–"eyes"–"nose" or "point to a glass"–"pencil"–"knife"–"glass," etc.). This frequent return to the same word is liable to "estrange" its meaning as the reader can verify by repeating the same series of words over and over again.

Another sensitive method is the presentation of two or three words at once; the patient must point to the corresponding parts of the face or to the objects ("show me an eye and a nose," "an ear and an eye," "an eye and an ear," "a glass and a knife," "a pencil and a glass," etc.; or, "show me an eye, a nose, and an ear" or "a glass, a knife, and a pencil," etc.). In this test the subject must not only perceive these words, but must also remember their order in the series and utilize memory traces for comprehension. This widening of the scope of the problem is one of the most important ways to increase the sensitivity of a test.

In another variant of the preceding experiment the patient is asked to identify a picture whose title he is given from among three, five, or seven pictures placed on the table. Since the ease with which the patient discovers the meaning of the word and points to the appropriate picture largely depends on the number of alternatives available to him, the number of pictures from which he has to select the one named has a direct effect on his performance. Therefore, a patient, with a disturbance of word comprehension may be able to choose satisfactorily from two or three pictures the one corresponding to the title given by the examiner but may be utterly unable to make the proper selection from a greater number of pictures. In other sensitive experiments the patient may be given more complicated and less familiar words (for example, he may be asked to point to his "knee," "heel," "cheekbone," or "fingernail" or to state the meaning of the words "caterpillar," "centipede," "magnolia," etc.) or a group of words differing from one another only on the basis of one phoneme (for example, "temple," "sample," "dimple"). Confusing the meaning of such words is one sign of a disturbance of phonemic hearing and of instability of word meanings.

Among the special methods used to investigate the understanding of words and their "semantic fields" is a group of tests which requires special laboratory investigation and which provides objective evidence on the basis of which it can be established which groups of words occupy the same common semantic field. One form of this test was described elsewhere (Luria and Vinogradova, 1951); for the objective study of "semantic fields" the vascular component of the orienting reflex is recorded.

A glass thimble is placed on the subject's finger so that changes in the volume of the finger resulting from constriction and dilatation of its blood vessels can be recorded by a special instrument. Any orienting reflex is known to be reflected in constriction of the blood vessels at the periphery of the body (Sokolov, 1958, 1959), and vasoconstriction is known to continue until the orienting reflex is extinguished. Such vasoconstriction of the finger also is exhibited in response to the presentation of different words. If this response to different words is extinguished through repeated presentation of them, and as soon as the autonomic responses to them have ceased, if one word is made the "test" word (e.g., if the subject is instructed to press with his other hand on a key or to count these words in response to this particular word), the vascular response to the "test" word will be restored and will continue for some time.

Characteristically, however, this response begins to be evoked not only by a given "test" word, but also by a whole group of words occupying the same "semantic field" as the test word. Investigation has shown that in normal subjects this vascular response can be evoked by words of similar meaning to the "test" word, whereas words of similar sounds as the test word but not closely related to it in meaning (e.g., "skripka" (violin) and "skrepka" (clip) do not evoke such responses). In some groups of patients (e.g., in oligophrenics) the opposite results are obtained.

The objective investigation of semantic fields, by using other methods also, can be successfully used for a fuller study of the changes in word meaning and in cases of local brain lesions.

This series of experiments is usually sufficient not only to reveal the presence of a disturbance or instability of word meanings, but also to establish the responsible factor.

When performing this test, patients with a *lesion of the left temporal lobe and a syndrome of sensory (acoustic) aphasia* manifest obvious extinction of word meaning. Either they fail to perceive the presented word and its constituent sounds clearly enough, so that they cannot understand its precise meaning, or they quickly lose the meaning of the words after a few repetitions of the word series presented to them. The extinction of word meaning developing with increases in the number of words presented at any one time is particularly symptomatic of a lesion of the middle portions of the left temporal region, associated with the syndrome of acoustic-mnestic aphasia. The mutual inhibition induced by the simultaneously presented words is so great that these patients either fail to retain the whole series of words or quickly lose the power to understand their meaning. Although their appraisal of individual words is fair, they begin to exhibit extinction of meaning as soon as words are presented to them in groups. These phenomena were described earlier (Part II, Section 2D and E) and they will therefore not be considered further.

Patients with the *afferent (kinesthetic) form of motor aphasia* (Part II, Section 4D) usually do not exhibit primary extinction of word meaning but may have difficulty in understanding words if they attempt to pronounce them aloud in order to clarify their phonetic composition, for they may articulate the component sounds incorrectly. Patients with the *efferent (kinetic) form of motor aphasia* (Part II, Section 4F) also may comprehend individual words providing articulatory difficulties do not arise and pathological inertia in the sphere of speech is not given an opportunity to manifest itself. As has been stressed, this inertia interferes with the swift and smooth transfer from one verbal form to another. The limitations in word comprehension in the various forms of motor aphasia require further study, and the suggestion, most probably true, that a disturbance of the motor aspect of speech must inevitably affect its receptor aspect also must be subjected to further analysis.

The gross disturbances taking place in patients with *frontal and*, in particular, *frontotemporal syndromes* significantly differ from those in the aforementioned groups of patients. As a rule, these patients adequately understand individual words presented individually, but experience difficulty when considering one word after another. Frequently, they keep inertly to the same meaning when different words are presented to them in succession. They cannot inhibit this tendency, so that when presented with the next word they respond with characteristic "paragnoses," i.e., they continue to give it the same meaning as the preceding word. This perseveratory type of extinction of word meaning may be found in patients with extensive lesions of either frontal lobe and, especially, in patients with lesions of the frontotemporal systems. In the latter, this phenomenon is revealed in its clearest form in the test involving the drawing of separate figures (or series of figures) from a spoken command (Part III, Section 3D), because the manifestations of pathological inertia in the motor (and speech-motor) analyzer are supplemented by manifestations of instability of word traces and of extinction of meaning.

It would be wrong to assume that the extinction of word meaning in the various forms of aphasia means no more than that words completely lose their meaning and are transformed into empty, senseless groups of sounds. Careful investigation shows that these disturbances, which are especially marked in sensory aphasia, may cover a wide range of phenomena, extending from relatively slight defects to the total disintegration of comprehension.

There are some forms of vagueness or diffuseness of word meanings that are particularly interesting. In these forms the direct objective categorization of particular words (in other words, their association with a clearly defined objective pattern) is lost, and the patient begins to define or *interpret the words* afresh. For example, he may interpret the word "zausenitsa" (the root of the fingernail) as "something that crawls," confusing it with "gusenitsa" (a caterpillar). These cases are specially pertinent to the analysis of the system of irrelevant associations into which words become introduced and that are inhibited in the normal course of conscious mental activity. These are naturally particularly important in patholinguistic analysis.

Another distinctive form is limitation in the range and plasticity of word meanings. Various investigators (Zeigarnik, 1961; Kogan, 1947, 1961; etc.) have shown that this limitation develops in patients with generalized cerebral disturbances and in certain cases of circumscribed brain lesions. The meaning becomes narrowed, and the varied systems of associations resting upon it are lost; words come to be understood only in a narrow, rigid context or only in the presence of the corresponding visual image, with metaphorical word meanings completely ceasing to be understood. These defects arise in relation to the selective meaning of words expressing spatial relationships ("beneath," "above," "before," "after") and complex prepositions and conjunctions.

This is a characteristic feature of patients with *lesions of the parieto-occipital region and a syndrome of semantic aphasia* (Part II, Section 3F). However, the localizing significance of these disturbances (other than in the last one) is still far from clear. There is reason to suppose that they may indicate a lowering of the general level of cortical analysis and synthesis, leading to generalized defects in the second signal system, rather than any particular circumscribed lesion.

D. INVESTIGATION OF THE UNDERSTANDING OF SIMPLE SENTENCES

The next step in the study of the impressive aspect of speech is to investigate the patient's comprehension of simple sentences which, according to many philologists (Potebnya, 1862, 1888; etc.) and neurologists (Jackson, 1884; etc.), comprise the fundamental unit of speech.

To understand sentences (or, in other words, complete expressions) one must understand individual words, but this is not all. Besides appreciation of the fundamental grammatical structures uniting words into sentences, the ability to retain traces of word series forming sentences in memory and the ability to inhibit premature conclusions regarding the meaning of an expression drawn from only one fragment of the whole phrase are also necessary. If the last condition cannot be satisfied, true understanding of an expression is replaced by a simple guess at its meaning.

The complex character of the process involved in understanding sentences explains why derangement can result from the most widely different lesions of the brain. For this reason it is not enough merely to state that these disturbances may occur; they must be subjected to a minute analysis.

As has been specified (Part III, Section 2), to investigate sentence comprehension the examiner begins by asking the patient a series of questions and noting his answers. The stage of investigating his true understanding is reached when, among the other questions, the patient is asked some that are unrelated to the preceding ones in context and that can be understood only by perception of the constituent words and syntactic connections creating the unity of the sentence.

The investigation of the understanding of simple sentences (methods of investigating the understanding of complex logical grammatical structures of speech are given below in Part III, Section 8E) usually continues by giving the patient a series of simple phrases and asking him to find, after each presentation, a picture illustrating the event described by the phrase. Another widely used method in clinical practice involves the giving of verbal instructions encompassing a wider range of phrases, as in Marie's well-known three-action test, in which three successive actions for execution are detailed in a single sentence (for example, "Take the book, put it over by the window, and give me the plate."). This method may be used as a sensitive gage of the patient's readily available range of information. Defects in the understanding of individual, isolated actions and "contamination" of individual parts with distortion of the meaning of the whole expression are typical signs of a disturbance of the integrative activity of the cortex at the level of the second signal system.

An important feature of the investigation is ascertaining the understanding of constructions whose meaning is not limited to objects mentioned in them. Also, the command contained in them requires preliminary analysis of the corresponding speech structures for execution: "Show me whose pencil this is"; or "Whose spectacles are these?"; or "Show me what is used to start the fire" (pictures illustrating a stove, firewood, and matches are shown). If the patient has a tendency to follow this instruction without analysis he may fail to perceive that the words are joined into a whole phrase and will understand them as isolated words. In the first two tasks he points to the pencil or spectacles mentioned in the sentence (and not to their owners); in the last one he points to the fire mentioned in the sentence, an action indicating his fragmentary perception of the meaning of the expression.

Also in this group of tests are those containing "conflicting" instructions: "If it is night now, place a cross in the white square, and if it is day now, place a cross in the black square." Inability to overcome the well-established, direct association (night–black, day–white) and to carry out the instruction properly may be a symptom of the defects just mentioned.

Comprehension of a simple sentence with no complex governing forms usually presents little difficulty to patients with brain lesions. The fact that the simple sentence is the commonest and the most firmly established unit of conversational speech means that the patient retains the ability to understand it reasonably well. Even when the patient can no longer understand the meaning of individual words, he often can be made to do so again by including the particular words in familiar sentences.

However, the understanding of sentences may be limited. One factor making the understanding of a sentence more difficult is an increase in its scope. Patients with lesions of the *temporal divisions of the cortex* (the cortical termination of the auditory analyzer, notably of that part of it concerned with speech) may experience appreciable difficulty after even a slight increase in the range of a sentence rendered as a spoken command. Individual constituent words are lost, the sentence is no longer perceived as a whole, and the patient shows a tendency to react to isolated words taken out of context. Hence, the fragmentary forms of understanding referred to previously may often be observed in patients with severe lesions of the temporal cortical divisions.

The second complicating factor is related to the need for inhibiting guesses at the meaning of a sentence prompted by individual words in the sentence. The chance of substituting a guess for true appreciation of the meaning of a sentence is particularly great if the meaning is contrary to that to which the patient is accustomed; its individual fragments then evoke habitual associations not in agreement with the context of the whole sentence.

Impulsive responses of this kind may be encountered both in patients with *generalized brain disturbances* and in patients with specific *frontal or frontotemporal syndromes*. The abnormalities arising in this group of patients during the solution of such problems have already been described (Part II, Section 5G). Because of these abnormalities, tests of this type are very useful in studying patients with anterior cortical lesions: In essence they involve the understanding of sentences of simple construction which conflict with customary associations arising from the perception of a sentence fragment.

Disturbances of the understanding of simple sentences by patients with motor aphasia is a matter of special interest. Hitherto it was considered that the understanding of simple sentences remains intact in such patients, and that there is a sharp dissociation between disturbance of the syntactic and prosodic aspects of speech in such patients, whose understanding of the sentence is preserved.

This situation still holds good. However, when passing from the understanding of the semantic structure of sentences (which remains intact in the patients of this group) to the understanding of the syntactic structure of sentences, these patients may have serious difficulties. For instance, they frequently consider that the sentence "Parokhod idët po vodoi" (The steamship goes * along the water) is quite correct, and if they are told that the sentence is in fact incorrect and they are asked to discover the mistake and correct it, they make semantic changes and not formal syntactic changes to the sentence, offering to replace it by another sentence, such as "Parokhod idët po moryu" ("The steamship goes along the sea). Inability to detect features of syntactic structure of expression while preserving the understanding of its semantic structure is evidently an important feature of the patients of this group (Jakobson, 1971; Luria, 1973).

The last factor hindering adequate understanding of the meaning of whole expressions is complex logical-grammatical structure. This condition was excluded from the experiments just described. However, it is so important that it merits special examination.

E. INVESTIGATION OF THE UNDERSTANDING OF LOGICAL-GRAMMATICAL STRUCTURES

Elsewhere (Luria, 1947) attention was drawn to the fact that at a certain stage of lingual development grammatical forms appear that reflect not only isolated objects, actions, or qualities, but also the complex relationships between them. In a developed language, such relationships are denoted by familiar methods, such as the system of inflections, the order of the words in the sentence, and the various auxiliary words (prepositions, conjunctions),

* The word "idët" in Russian is restricted to animate objects; the correct word to be used with "Parokhod" would be "edet."

that act as special devices for the transmission of relationships. These factors form the directive system underlying lingual syntax.

In some constructions it happens that these auxiliary devices conflict with the simpler function of the direct connotation of objects and actions. These cases are of particular interest here. For example, in the expression "the father's brother" we are not concerned with either person mentioned, but with a third person not directly mentioned in this situation—the "uncle." In the sentences "the dress caught on the oar" and "the oar caught on the dress," the same objects and actions are directly mentioned, but the arrangement of the words gives the sentences different meanings. Finally, in the construction "a circle beneath a square" it is not just two objects that are mentioned, but also the spatial relationship between them.

In some language constructions, a system of connections expressed by means of certain grammatical devices may come into conflict with the order of the actions directly presumed from the order of the words in the sentence. This can be easily seen, for example, in the command "Point to the comb with the pencil." When carrying out this task, the subject must not follow the order of the words given in the sentence, but must inhibit the tendency to start by giving his attention to the last-mentioned object in the sentence, thus performing the action not in direct, but in reverse, order. This is the manner by which any inverted construction is understood. Comprehension of all the aforementioned logical-grammatical constructions involves a highly complex process.

It was stated earlier (Part II, Section 3F) that, to grasp the meaning of such a grammatical construction it is essential not only to understand the meaning of the separate words, but also to combine these words into unified structures expressing these relationships. We have already discussed how this operation requires a special form of synthesis of the individual elements, in which the consecutive scrutiny of these elements is transformed into a simultaneous operation.

In the investigation of logical-grammatical appreciation it is useless to employ long phrases with a complex structure. The understanding of such phrases requires memorization of their elements, and this makes the investigation difficult. For the analysis of the degree to which the patient can still understand logical-grammatical relationships, we therefore use constructions consisting of the minimal number of words expressing a given relationship. Moreover, the meaning of these constructions can be understood on the basis of well-established past associations.

This investigation usually begins with an experiment devised to assess the understanding of simple inflective constructions. Three objects are placed in front of the patient (e.g., a pencil, a key, and a comb), and he is in turn given three variants of instruction, using the same operative words but in different logical grammatical relationships:

1. The patient is asked to point to two objects in turn by name: "pencil–key," "key–comb," "comb–pencil," ect. It is easy to see that this (affective) construction is composed of two isolated words and has no special significance beyond the names of the isolated objects.

2. The patient is next given an instruction incorporating the same words, but placed in special relationship to each other by means of instrumental prepositions: "Point with the key toward the pencil," "with the pencil toward the comb," etc. This construction now extends beyond the simple nominative function of words, and the patient has to orient himself not only to the objects denoted by the corresponding words, but also to the relationships expressed by these prepositions.

3. In the third variant the instruction is further complicated by requiring analysis of the word order and inversion of the action: "Point to the pencil with the comb," "to the key with the pencil," etc. Before the patient can carry out this instruction correctly, he must first inhibit the tendency to carry out the action in the order in which the objects are named and then invert that order. Naturally, these conditions require that the patient completely suppress echopraxia and allow his actions to be directed by a system of logical-grammatical associations.

Patients with different types of brain lesion experience various degrees of difficulty in carrying out the instructions just described. A patient with a *lesion of the temporal division of the left hemisphere and manifestations of acoustic aphasia* is frequently unable to perform even the first of these tests. Since he easily loses the meaning of the words presented to him, he is unable to repeat them; rather, he points to objects that do not correspond to the words. Extinction of the meaning of words is also, of course, a considerable handicap in the performance of the other and grammatically more complex variants of the instruction. We have repeatedly observed patients with elements of temporal aphasia grasp an inflective relationship expressed in the ablative case ("point with the pencil to the key") but point to other objects because of the instability of word comprehension (for example, pointing with the comb to the key). Presentation of complicated variants is therefore meaningless in such cases.

Patients with *lesions of the parieto-occipital systems of the left hemisphere* do not exhibit extinction of word meanings and easily perform the first of these tests, but because of the defective simultaneous synthesis and spatial orientation previously described (Part II, Section 3F), they often cannot manage the second, inflective, variant. The construction "with the pencil–key" is perceived just as agrammatically as the construction "pencil–key"; as before, they continue to point separately to the two named objects, paying no attention to the relationships established between them by the inflective structure of this syntagma. However, a defect of this type develops only from relatively severe lesions of this region; those with less severe lesions understand this instruction reasonably well.

Patients with lesions of the anterior divisions of the brain (or with a generalized syndrome of increased intracranial pressure and secondary loss of spontaneity) usually are able to carry out the first two variants of the instruction but frequently have difficulty with the third, inverted variant ("point to the key with the pencil"). The echopraxic tendency to follow the order of the words in the sentence and the omission of preliminary analysis of the associations contained in the instruction result in a lack of awareness of the need for inversion; the patient continues to carry out mechanically the instruction in conformity to the order in which the objects are named, changing the inverted construction into a direct one ("point with the key to the pencil"). Often, this echopraxic performance proves so persistent that even after suitable explanation is given the patient continues to follow inertly the direct order of the words. These tests are relatively complex in character, and their performance involves a number of processes, making analysis of their results difficult. For this reason, when trying to detect such disturbances these complicating factors must be reduced to a minimum. In contrast, the difficulties characteristically encountered by a patient with *receptive agrammatism* (as occurs with semantic aphasia) must be intensified. These are accomplished by presenting constructions whose understanding demands specialized operations of simultaneous synthesis. These constructions utilize the attributive genitive case, prepositional constructions, and certain comparative constructions. These will be discussed briefly because the reasons for their selection were fully described elsewhere (Part II, Section 3F; Luria, 1945, 1947).

The first of these tests is concerned with the understanding of constructions using the attributive genitive case.

The patient is given a picture of a woman and a girl and is asked to point to the "daughter's mother" or the "mother's daughter." For patients with more pronounced cases of semantic aphasia this may be formulated more simply "Where is the daughter's mother?" or "Where is the mother's daughter?" In another variant the patient is asked to state the meaning of "the father's brother" and "the brother's father," "the foreman's brother" and "the brother's foreman," etc., and to state whether or not these paired expressions mean the same thing.

Patients with a disruption in simultaneous synthesis and with manifestations of receptive agrammatism are usually unable to grasp this construction as a single conceptual entity. In response to the first test they frequently point to two pictures in succession, saying "Here is the daughter, and here is the mother." In their attempt to analyze the second construction they become greatly confused and finally conclude that the pairs of expressions have the same meaning. Attempts to obtain a precise definition of the meaning of the corresponding constructions are very often unsuccessful because of the difficulties experienced by these patients as soon as they try to reach beyond the nominative function of words and to proceed to the synthesis of relationships designated by special constructions.

Equally valuable tests are those designed to study the understanding of prepositional constructions, especially those involving spatial or similar relationships.

In these tests the patient is asked to place "a cross beneath a circle," "a circle beneath a cross," "a dot beneath a triangle," etc. (to make this test more sensitive the patient may be asked to do the drawing from top to bottom) or to "place a circle on the right of a cross," or "a cross on the right of a circle," etc. In a variant, the patient is asked to state which is correct: "Spring comes before summer" or "Summer comes before spring." In a more complicated form the patient is asked to "place a cross on the right of a circle but on the left of a triangle." The correct analysis of such a construction is beyond the capacity of most patients; it can therefore be used for specificity only in individual cases.

As a rule, patients with manifestations of semantic aphasia experience great difficulty in the performance of these tests and point out that the analysis of constructions expressing spatial relationships is particularly complex for them. They usually exhibit well-defined symptoms of receptive agrammatism, grasping the meaning of individual words but understanding the instruction "Place a cross beneath a circle" to mean "Place a cross, and a circle beneath it," whereupon they draw these figures in the order in which they were called out. Because of these difficulties, comparing such constructions as "a cross beneath a circle" and "a circle beneath a cross" is almost impossible. In answer to the question whether the two statements mean the same thing, they reply that the two constructions differ only in the order of the words but that essentially they are the same. Similar responses may be obtained when these patients are asked to decide which particular drawing relates to a given grammatical construction. Their attempts to analyze these constructions usually end in failure—the patient insists that he of course understands that this is a question of different relationships, but what they denote is not clear to him. When the patient tries to perform the other tests he has similar difficulties combining two elements of a construction into a single entity and understanding the relationship expressed in the construction.

Other types of patients experience completely different difficulties in performing these tests. Patients with *lesions of the temporal systems and with extinction of the meaning of words* may understand the necessary logical-grammatical relationships but they lose the correct meaning of the shapes when carrying out the operations; they frequently substitute the wrong shape, thus disturbing the objective basis of the problem.

Patients with *lesions of the anterior divisions of the brain*, with a tendency to form inert stereotypes, may quite easily grasp the necessary logical-grammatical relationship but are unable to solve the problem after its modification, even if it is made easier. For instance, having successfully completed two or three tests of the type "place a cross beneath a circle," they are quite unable to "place a cross above a circle," but continue to reproduce the established inversion (Luria and Khomskaya, unpublished investigation). In general, patients with a *marked frontal syndrome* cannot grasp the essence of the problem; they either draw both figures inertly at the same place or repeat the same figure over and over again, perfectly satisfied with their performance.

Testing comprehension of comparative constructions is done in a similar manner. Statements like "John is taller than Peter" and "Peter is taller than John" are presented. The patient is asked to compare them or to state which boy for instance, is shorter. This requires not only comprehension, but also mental inversion. In a variant the patient is asked to state which of the two constructions "a fly is bigger than an elephant" and "an elephant is bigger than a fly" is correct. Alternatively, two pieces of paper of different colors are placed before him and he is asked to say which is "lighter," "darker," "less light," and "less dark." If the two pieces of paper differ in size as well as in color, it will be apparent that the patient cannot combine the two qualities named into a single conceptual system and, instead of pointing to the "less dark" paper, points to the smaller dark paper.

The most difficult variant of this series, not by any means applicable to all cases, is Burt's well-known test in which the patient is told that "Olga is lighter than Kate but darker than Sonia"; he is asked to state which girl is lightest. Even if the receptive agrammatism is only latent, this task is beyond his capacity. Having grasped the significance of the relationship "Olga is lighter than Kate," the patient is unable to perform the necessary logical inversion and usually interprets the last part of the construction "but darker than Sonia" as a direct assertion that Sonia is darker. In these cases not even the arrangement of cards with pictures of three girls with different hair color or of cards with girls' names written on them improves the performance, and the combination of this complex construction into a single system of values remains impossible. The aspects I have just described have been the subject of special analysis by the author during the last decade (Luria, 1972c, 1976).

Similar tests are designed to examine the understanding of inverted grammatical constructions. Some of these structures have as their characteristic feature the fact that the order of the words does not correspond to the order of the actions designated, so that they have to be inverted or recoded mentally before they can be understood. An example of such a construction is: "Peter struck John. Who was the victim?" Sentences using the passive voice also belong to this group. ("The sun lights up the earth" is more likely to be understood correctly from its direct impact than "The earth is lit up by the sun".) Or, the patient is told "I had breakfast after I had sawed the wood" and is then asked "What did I do first?" The double negative construction is also used in this context: "I am unaccustomed to disobeying rules" followed by the question "Is this the remark of a disciplined or an undisciplined person?"

Such constructions, which cannot be understood correctly from their direct impact and which therefore require preliminary recoding, sensitively expose the difficulties associated with faulty analysis and synthesis of complex logical-grammatical constructions. Like many other tests, however, they can be used only when the other requisites for this process (ability to understand word meaning, ability to engage in goal-directed activity) are present.

Experiments used to analyze phrases with a complex grammatical structure, including subordinate constructions, distant (separated by intervening parts of speech) phrases etc., will not be dealt with in detail. Examples of how relationships expressed by this means ("The woman who worked at the factory came to the school where Dora studied to give a talk") are comprehended were given previously (Part II, Section 3F).

The use of the enumerated tests is of the utmost importance in the detection of latent manifestations of receptive agrammatism, true forms of which occur with lesions of the left inferior temporal and parieto-occipital regions. This disorder leads to the syndrome of semantic aphasia.

An important factor in ensuring the correct evaluation of the results is the preliminary experimental training of the patient, which provides him with various means of separating a particular construction into its component elements and thus enables him to draw conclusions regarding its meaning. These methods are fully described elsewhere (Luria, 1947, 1948; Bubnova, 1946).

By means of these suggested methods, the patient is often able to reach a logical solution of the problem (to determine the meaning of the construction) but remains unable to grasp its significance directly. This indicates that he reached the correct conclusion only as a result of a formal exercise and not as a result of "experiencing" the relationships as he should. Further, this conclusively demonstrates that the defect is based on receptive agrammatism and not on any other disturbance.

The investigation of the receptive, or impressive, aspect of speech is concluded by analyzing the patient's ability to understand complete texts. However, these tests are primarily concerned with the intellectual aspects of speech, so that they will be considered separately (Part III, Section 12B).

9. *Investigation of Speech Functions. Expressive Speech*

A. PRELIMINARY REMARKS

Expressive (or motor) speech is a complex process incorporating many different components and occurring at different levels. The pronunciation of speech sounds and their combinations, i.e., the articulatory structure of words, takes place on the basis of phonemic hearing; however, the articulation of sounds itself plays an active role in the formation of phonemic hearing. The pronunciation of the sounds of speech calls for precision in motor activity, which is possible only when impulses of considerable mobility are accurately directed to their destinations. The pronunciation of words requires a well-established serial organization of consecutive articulations, with adequate inhibition of previous movements and smooth transition to those following; these processes must be accompanied by adequate plasticity in modifying the articulation of a particular sound to conform to its position in the word. The evolution from pronunciation of a word to pronunciation of a whole phrase, and then of a whole sentence, requires, in addition, retention of the general scheme of the phrase or sentence and integrity of the whole of the complex path from the thought to the serially constructed spoken expression; the importance of such integrity has been recognized by many writers (Jackson, 1884; Pick, 1913, 1931; etc.). We know that internal speech contributes to this process (Vygotskii, 1934, 1956), although the exact nature of its participation has not been adequately studied.

As was stated previously, expressive speech may be formed at different levels, starting from simple ejaculations or affective exclamations (which may be possible even for patients with the most extensive lesions of the cerebral cortex) and ending with the most highly organized forms of developed speech, as exemplified by monologues.

These facts illustrate the breadth of expressive speech and the complexity of the task confronting the examiner who would study it. We shall therefore describe those methods of investigating expressive speech that are designed to elicit possible disturbances of its constituent elements and, at the same time, designed to permit a judgment on the constructive level of the disturbance.

B. INVESTIGATION OF THE ARTICULATION OF SPEECH SOUNDS

The study of how sounds are articulated must be preceded by the study of *the state of the muscular apparatus of the tongue, lips, and soft palate*; special attention must be paid to the power and range, as well as to the precision, rate, and mobility, of these motor components. This may be accomplished by well-known neurological methods, aimed at detecting asymmetry, paresis, dystonia, hyperkineses, ataxias, and the fatigability of movement. All these elements may be involved in the higher forms of speech disorder. Gross changes in the condition of the muscular apparatuses of this region, characteristically found, for example, with bulbar and pseudobulbar disturbances, may lead to dysarthric or dystonic manifestations and may thus be quite different in nature.

When the ordinary clinical methods prove inadequate, they may be supplemented by electromyography or by pneumographic or oscillographic recordings of the air pressure changes during the various articulations. Electromyographic recording of the activity of the vocal muscles, for which electrodes are placed on the larynx, the lower lip, or the tongue (the technique has been described by Bassin and Bein, 1957; Novikova, 1955; etc.) may reveal paretic signs, i.e., imprecise "addressing" of impulses and tardy inhibition of motor acts, that otherwise remained hidden. Likewise, diffuseness, dystonia, hyperkineses, and a tendency to fatigability may be first brought to light by this method. Both pneumographic recording of the changes in air pressure during articulation and the more advanced oscillographic technique facilitate a more detailed analysis of those movements of the oral cavity directly concerned with articulation and the associated air movement. By means of these methods accurate assessments can be made of the coordination between these fine movements, their strength, and their smoothness; early signs of muscle fatigue can be detected, and corroboration may be obtained of the presence of paretic, dystonic, and ataxic elements. A valuable auxiliary method proposed by Zhinkin (1958) is roentgenological analysis and filming of the movements of the tongue, the epiglottis, and the diaphragm, parts of the articulatory apparatus that are inaccessible to direct observation. Detection of changes in their dynamics by this means is therefore a valuable contribution to the general investigation.

The next step is *the examination of oral praxis*. This directly precedes the study of the articulatory movements themselves and may bring to light the presence of ataxia and pathological inertia in the complex forms of movements in this sphere. The methods used to test oral praxis were previously described above (Part III, Section 3C).

The articulation of speech sounds is usually investigated by instructing the patient to repeat sounds, as during the study of acoustic sound discrimination (Part III, Section 7B). The only difference between these tests is that in the present case the patient is not presented with closely similar (correlating or oppositional) sounds, which are difficult to differentiate by ear, but is told to pronounce the principal vowel and consonant sounds in turn, with those sounds of different articulatory complexity identified separately. The pronunciation of sounds such as "m," "b," "p" or "d," "n," "l" or "s," "sh," "zh" or "k," "kh," "g" is therefore of especial interest. The clarity of the patient's pronunciation of these sounds, its intensity, the ease of transition from one articulation to another, and, finally, the presence of the vocal component normally accompanying each articulation are essential features that require especial attention.

The patient may be asked to repeat sounds presented to him singly, in pairs, or in groups of three. In certain cases, the articulation of open and closed syllables or groups of several consonants ("tpru," "str," etc.) is studied, for in their execution any signs of inertia of the motor stereotypes of speech that may be present may be revealed. Special analytical methods may be invaluable in bringing to light the exact component(s) of the articulatory act that is disturbed, as well as those that remain intact. For this purpose, after the sound-repetition experiment solely utilizes aural representation, the patient is allowed to use other afferent systems as aids. He may examine his articulation in a mirror, the scheme of the articulation of a particular sound may be explained to him (using the pictures in a speech-training manual), other aids may be invoked (e.g., allowing him to touch the larynx of a person speaking to analyze the vibrations), articulations may be incorporated into practical actions (blowing away pieces of fluff, blowing out candles), or imitation of conventional lip movements may be used (pipe smoking for the articulation "oo," making a circle of surprise for "o," smiling for "ee," etc.). These methods can also help to determine how an existing defect may be compensated for. And, the nature of the underlying lesion can be clarified.

The nature of the articulatory defects that are thus brought to light may differ, depending on the nature of the local lesions responsible for them. Poor acoustic analysis of sound accompanying a *lesion of the left temporal lobe,* may lead to confusion between similar-sounding (and in the most severe cases, easily distinguishable) phonemes, although the act of articulation itself remains relatively intact. When purity of pronunciation of individual sounds exists in association with poor differentiation of phonemes and relative ease of compensation, on the basis of visual analysis of the articulatory act, the central divisions of the acoustic analyzer are implicated. A disturbance in the kinesthetic basis of articulation, resulting from a lesion of the *inferior portion of the sensorimotor region and the postcentral divisions*, causes the most marked articulatory disorders: loss of precise addressing of motor impulses and confusion between similar-sounding articulemes (Part II, Section 4D). Auxiliary (visual) aids are helpful in such cases, but the defect can be compensated for only with much difficulty. *Lesions of the premotor divisions of the speech area* do not cause primary articulatory difficulties, but they invariably lead to difficulty in switching from one articulation to another (Part II, Section 4F). This is revealed by the pathological inertia of the developing articulatory stereotypes, comprising the principal mechanism of the disorders observed in such cases. For this reason, resort to auxiliary methods may be beneficial only if the inhibition of one articuleme and its replacement by another (for example, the introduction of two successive articulations into different conceptual systems) is involved.

These tests clearly reveal disturbances in the working of the speech muscles that are unrelated to and clearly distinguishable from aphasia—paresis, dystonia, ataxia, dysphonia, etc.—and indicating bulbar or pseudobulbar lesions.

C. INVESTIGATION OF REFLECTED (REPETITIVE) SPEECH

The investigation of reflected (repetitive) speech has two objectives: First, it is a means of testing the clarity of the pronunciation of words, series of words, and phrases; second, it allows us to judge the stability of the traces that form the foundations of expressive speech and thus establish the neurodynamic conditions under which speech becomes diffuse and deformed.

Repetition is the hallmark of this investigation—repetition of words, repetition of series of words and, finally, repetition of phrases. The following factors may make repetition more difficult: presentation of more complex and less firmly established words, a lengthening of the time interval between pronunciation and repetition of the word, and an increase in the range of presented words (repetition of two, three, or more long series of words or repetition of long phrases and groups of phrases).

Tests involving repetitive speech must naturally draw the attention of the examiner not only to the quality of the articulated words, but also, and especially, to the degree of preservation of the acoustic and conceptual complexes and of their sequence. In this respect, repetitive speech constitutes the principal means of investigating complex speech disorders.

The investigation of repetitive speech begins with the repetition of single words, both simple in their phonetic composition and firmly established in past experience (e.g., "cat," "dog," "man") and more complicated (e.g., "table," "house," "apple") or possessing greater phonetic complexity and less familiarity (e.g., "rhinoceros," "screwdriver," "hairbrush"). These words may differ from one another only in one phonemic sign (e.g., "temple," "sample," "dimple"), a factor that makes for convenience of analysis of disturbances of the phonemic basis of repetitive speech. Finally, they may be complex in their phonetic composition and totally unfamiliar ("streptomycin," "arachnoidendothelioma," etc.). Experiments involving the repetition of this group of words may be used to define more accurately the quality of the differentiation of articulatory movements.

These experiments may be carried out under two conditions: The patient must pronounce the words either immediately (without a pause) or after a pause of 3, 5, 10 seconds, during which time nothing may happen or an irrelevant conversation may proceed. The last variant of the experiment reveals the stability of the traces left by the presented word and may be used as a sensitive indicator.

Next, experiments involving the repetition of series of words are conducted. Their purpose is the study of the integrity of the system responsible for word order and the range of traces retainable and perceivable by the patient. These tests already described above (Part III, Section 8), are particularly instructive, for they may reveal such pathological changes as weakening of acoustic traces, disordering of the serial organization of speech processes, and pathological inertia of developing stereotypes. Usually an increasing series of two, three, four, and, more rarely, five simple words or numbers are presented in intervals of 1 or 2 seconds, for the patient to repeat. These words must be simple in their phonetic composition and unrelated in meaning (e.g., "hat," "sun," "dog" or "hat," "sun," "dog," "bell"); and the same tone of voice must be used for each word. The patient must repeat them either at once or after a pause of 5 to 10 seconds. In a more complicated version, designed to reveal the stability of the traces, irrelevant conversation acting as a factor of external inhibition may ensue in the interim.

The series is then presented in a different order (for example, "hat," "sun," "dog," "bell" is replaced by "hat," "bell," "dog," "sun"), and the patient must strictly keep to the new order of the words. This constitutes a very sensitive test of the retentive ability and of the mobility of the nervous processes in the auditory and motor systems of speech. This test can, of course, also be applied with longer intervals between presentation and repetition of the word series.

As a special variant, the rate of presentation of some of the words may be altered; a faster rate imposes increased demands on the auditory and motor differentiation of the series; a slower rate facilitates the task but imposes greater demands on the stability of the traces. This test may therefore be used for analytical purposes. Similar tests may be carried out with the repetition of numbers and of nonsense syllables. To discover the contribution of the state of acoustic traces to the difficulty experienced by the patient in repeating series of words, the same elements (words or numbers) may be presented visually. However, this method can be used only if the patient is still able to read.

This aspect of the investigation ends with experiments on the repetition of phrases or groups of phrases. These experiments are designed to analyze the integrity of speech traces in more complicated conditions and to determine the extent to which the structure of the whole sentence is retained by the patient. The subject is asked to repeat a short sentence ("The weather is fine today") or a long sentence ("The apple trees grew in the garden behind a high fence" or "The hunter killed the wolf on the edge of the forest"), to be followed by a series of three short sentences ("The house is on fire—the moon is shining—the broom is sweeping"). When necessary, the mobility of the speech processes may be specially investigated by imposing more difficult conditions, e.g., by changing the order of presentation of these three sentences. Defective sequential reproduction or "contamination" may be indicative of a disturbance in the system responsible for the precise serial organization of complex traces or may reveal pathological inertia of the developing stereotypes. Naturally, this series of experiments also may be conducted either with immediate reproduction of the sentences or with an interval between presentation and repetition.

The investigation of repetitive speech may give valuable information for the identification of the large group of speech function disturbances arising from lesions of different parts of the brain. A lesion of the *left temporal lobe*, causing a disturbance in the complex forms of acoustic analysis and synthesis

(Part II, Section 2D), leads to an extremely poor performance. With the severest lesions of this region, accompanied by manifestations of sensory (acoustic) aphasia, the patient often cannot repeat even words of the simplest phonetic composition. However, this disturbance is based on acoustic, rather than articulatory, difficulties. The patient listens intently to the word presented, attempts to analyze its sounds, pronounces the word with paraphasias, sometimes fails to grasp its meaning, and never exhibits sufficient confidence in the correctness of his pronunciation. Sometimes, having discovered the meaning of a word but being unable to retain its phonetic composition, the patient replaces it by a verbal paraphasia, which may itself be mispronounced. Characteristically, while he finds difficulty in repeating the required word, the patient may be able to pronounce accessory words, retorts ("What does it mean? . . . I can't do a thing!"), or exclamations. Obviously, the precise repetition of meaningless combinations of sounds and words is completely impossible for such a patient.

Patients with more latent forms of temporal (acoustic) aphasia may repeat simple words relatively freely yet have great difficulty as soon as one of the aforementioned complications is introduced. For instance, although immediate repetition of a word is possible, difficulty arises as soon as a delay is introduced between presentation and repetition. Sometimes the instability of the acoustic traces of the word is so marked that a delay of 3 – 5 seconds is enough to make the patient forget it. If an irrelevant conversation is introduced between the presentation of the word and its repetition, the performance is even more adversely affected.

Patients in this group experience great difficulty in reproducing series of words or phrases. In some cases of a lesion of the temporal systems (including lesions situated in the middle and, sometimes, the inferior temporal gyrus of the left hemisphere), repetition of individual words is still possible but the change to series of words immediately evokes great difficulty. The patient repeats only one or two words and then exclaims that he has forgotten the rest and asks helplessly "What next?" This state of affairs is often accompanied by loss of the sequence of words forming a given series, the perseveration of words previously presented after changing to a new series, or the contamination of individual words forming the given series. The narrowing of the range of retainable words and the induced inhibition exerted by one word on another may be so marked that the number of words that the patient is capable of repeating is reduced to one or two.

The difficulties facing the patients of this group are particularly great in experiments involving the repetition of whole sentences. Although they sometimes grasp the general meaning of the sentence, they are unable to retain the words composing it; such patients begin to reproduce only part of the sentence or to reproduce it with paraphasias and contaminations or actually to replace it with other words. For example, instead of "The weather is fine today," they will say "The sun is out today," instead of "The apple trees grew in the garden behind a high fence," they will say "behind the fence . . . in the forest . . . there were pears." Such responses are typical for the patients of this group. These patients have the greatest difficulty in repeating short sentences. The repetition of the three sentences given previously ("The house is on fire—the broom is sweeping—the moon is shining") as "The house is on fire—the broom is shining . . . and something else . . . " typifies their difficulty.

There are considerable differences between the difficulties found during the investigation of repetitive speech in afferent (kinesthetic) and efferent (kinetic) motor aphasia. In *afferent (kinesthetic) motor aphasia* (Part II, Section 4D) marked difficulties arise even in the repetition of isolated sounds and individual words (especially difficult because of their articulatory composition). In these patients the processes of analyzing the presented sounds and discovering the required articulemes are so defective that sometimes the patient can name the object or answer the question correctly (this happens when the particular speech reaction takes place automatically and requires no special analysis of articulations) but cannot repeat the given word accurately (since this requires analysis of its phonetic and articulatory composition). The existence of these difficulties has led certain authors to speak of "conduction aphasia" (a form that has not received anatomical confirmation) in reference to these cases. A symptom specific for underlying kinesthetic *involvement* is the confusion, often found in these patients, between similar sounding articulemes ("khalat" - "khadat" or "stol" - "snol" - "ston"). Characteristically, the change from the repetition of one word to the repetition of a series of words or of a phrase does not create any additional difficulties for these patients.

Patients with the *efferent (kinetic) form of motor aphasia* (Part II, Section 4F) show a completely different picture during the investigation of repetitive speech. Although they easily repeat separate sounds, they frequently cannot reproduce a whole word; this defect is primarily due to pathological inertia of the articulatory analyzer. Consequently, the switching from one articulation to another presents considerable difficulty. Repetition of the word "mukha" as "mu. . . m. . . ma. . ." is typical of patients with the severest forms of this lesion. However, even patients of this group who have no difficulty in repeating individual words begin to experience difficulty when repeating series of words. In the absence of primary disturbances in the ability to retain a presented series, they may have great difficulty when passing from one word to another or from a given series of words into a revised arrangement of the same words. The appearance of marked signs of inertia of the developing stereotype is a particularly characteristic symptom of this group of patients.

Distinctive disturbances of repetitive speech occur in patients with *lesions of the left frontotemporal divisions* and with the so-called *frontotemporal syndrome*. These patients have no difficulty in repeating individual words (often even those with the most complex phonetic composition), but have great difficulty whenever they are required to repeat a series of words. The serial organization of the group is deranged and sometimes there are signs of increased inertia of the developing stereotype. The attempt to learn the required order by heart and by frequent repetition of the series usually fails to have the desired effect, with the words persistently rendered in a different order.

A disturbance of repetitive speech while fluent independent speech remains relatively intact has often been described by neurologists as "conduction aphasia."

I deliberately do not use this term, which is closely connected with simplified schemes and which interprets the aphasia as the result of disturbance of connections between the sensory and motor speech "centers." Recently I have given a more detailed analysis of this picture from the neuropsychological standpoint and have emphasized that the difficulty of repeating a given word is closely connected with the fact that in this case the patient is performing a special (and quite artificial) form of speech activity, concerned not with the expression of thought, but with a special analysis of audioverbal structure (Luria, 1976). However, this by no means exhausts the phenomenon known as "conduction aphasia," as was discussed by Goldstein (1948) some time ago. This problem still requires further careful study.

These facts show what a wealth of information may be obtained by the investigation of repetitive speech and what valuable data for localization is yielded by these tests.

D. INVESTIGATION OF THE NOMINATIVE FUNCTION OF SPEECH

When turning to the investigation of the nominative function of speech, we come up against one of the fundamental problems in the analysis of speech pathology. The naming of objects, their designation by words, comprises one of the basic functions of language, one that is specific for many of the operations carried out at the level of the second signal system and that is highly complex in structure.

To refer to objects, actions, or qualities by a particular word demands, first, the integrity of the phonetic composition of the word, a stable association between it and the object that it denotes, and the ability to find easily the required word on presentation of the corresponding visual image. However, the nominative function of speech is also associated with far more complex processes. It assumes that, of all the possible qualities of an object, its special, essential properties will be denoted by a word, i.e., that this object will be analyzed and placed in a particular category. It is therefore quite correct to stipulate that "every word is a generalization" (Lenin) and that "abstraction, together with generalization of innumberable signals" (Pavlov) is the fundamental function of the word as the principal "cell" of the second signal system. It is these definitions that have lain at the basis of the popular clinical assertion that the naming of an object (and, still more, of an action, quality, or relationship) is by no means a simple act but may, with complete justification, be regarded as a manifestation of complex mental processes.

The naming of an object has one further special feature that must be taken into consideration during the investigation of the pathology of the nominative function of speech. It would be wrong to imagine that the naming of an object results from the simple manifestation of the established association between the image and the particular unique name. As a rule, when we see an object (especially if we are not very familiar with it), not just a single name comes to mind, but a whole series of associations in which the particular object is enveloped. When we name an object we must select from these possible alternatives one association, inhibit all the rest, and thus, in fact, carry out an operation analogous to that taking place during differentiation.

If one of the requirements is not met, the process of naming of an object may naturally be affected. It is for this reason that the investigation of the nominative function of speech has occupied so important a part in the study of the higher cortical functions of patients with local brain lesions.

A series of special tests is used for this purpose. The simplest of these involves showing the patient objects or pictures of objects and asking him to name them. A sensitive variant is the exhibition of pictures of objects or parts of the body with names that are not particularly familiar (for example, a mortal, a bookcase, a poker, an elbow, a chin, a collarbone). Another sensitive test has been widely incorporated in clinical practice. The patient is asked to name not one object or picture, but two or three presented at the same time. With the number of possible alternatives increased, the name of one object may inhibit that of another by induction and any conspicuous weakness of the nervous processes concerned in the particular activity will lead to a marked disturbance of performance.

A second group of tests is based on the naming of an object from its description; this test can be used, however, only if speech is comprehended. In this test the patient is asked to answer the question: "What do you call the thing with which you comb your hair?", "What do you call the thing that tells the time?", etc. This test differs from the one previous in that the patient cannot see the object to be named and must first evoke the corresponding image before he can name it.

The last method used to test the nominative function of speech is based on the determination of categorical names. For this purpose the patient is shown a series of objects or pictures of objects (a table, chair, bed, sofa or a plate, bowl, cup, and saucer) and asked to give a general name to describe them ("furniture," "dishes"). The contrast between the easy naming of individual objects and the difficulty in producing suitable generic names suggests the presence of complex disturbances of the generalizing function of speech and a disturbance of the nominative function at a high level.

If the process of naming an object proves unusually difficult, a group of methods may be used to facilitate the discovery of the required word and, at the same time, to extend the analysis of the factors responsible for these difficulties. Prompting—the consecutive presentation of one or several of the initial sounds of the desired word—is one important method. If the prompting is quickly taken up, this means that the main difficulty does not involve distortion of the phonetic pattern of the word. If, on the other hand, prompting does not help the patient to recollect the required word, or if, paradoxically, he cannot remember the word even after nearly continuous prompting, it can be concluded that the nominative disturbance is closely connected with disintegration or instability of the sound structure of the word. A second method is the introduction of the word being sought into a conceptual context. If the patient has difficulty in finding, for example, the word "comb," he is given the sentence "I am attending to my hair," or if he has forgotten the word "fingernail," he is given the sentence "I have had a manicure."

The difficulty of naming (designating by speech) an object may be based on both general and special factors. The naming of an object is not just the simple association of the form of an object with a particular word.

As many psychologists have already shown, the object perceived may have many different aspects, it may be included in different situations, and it may belong to several different logical categories. As a result, during the perception or recall of any pattern and its designation by an appropriate word it is always necessary to make a choice from many alternatives which spring up involuntarily. The word which the subject chooses must be distinguished from other words of similar sound and similar morphological structure: he must pick out the essential characteristics of the particular object and must inhibit patterns, which spring up involuntarily, of other situations in which the given object may be found, or the designation of other objects belonging to the same category (e.g., when distinguishing the word "koshka" (cat), the subject has to inhibit words of similar sound, e.g., "kroshka" and "kryshka," associated words such as "moloko" (milk) and "mysh" (mouse), or words belonging to the same category, such as "sobaka" (dog), "tigr" (tiger), and so on). Clearly, therefore, the process of finding the necessary name is in fact a process of *choosing from many alternatives.*

In the simplest cases this choice is easy enough; in more difficult cases (the recalling of an insufficiently consolidated word, the name of a complex or unfamiliar object, the recalling of a personal name which does not fit into any clear semantic system), the matter may be much more complicated. It is in these cases that searching for a necessary word and its replacement by words similar in sound, in association, or in category may be complex. These phenomena as observed normally have been described by Brown and McNeill (1966); in disease the difficulties of choosing the right word from a number of possible alternatives are more conspicuous.

There is reason to suppose that these phenomena in pathological states may also have their physiological explanation. Selectivity of cortical activity is possible provided that what Pavlov calls the "law of strength" still applies. Under normal conditions, as he showed, a strong (or biologically important) stimulus evokes a strong response, whereas a weak (or unimportant) stimulus evokes a weak response. It is this which is responsible for the "selectivity" of function of the cerebral cortex that lies at the basis of normal behavior.

It is a quite different matter in inhibitory states or when pathological changes have affected the working of the brain.

In such cases the "law of strength" may cease to apply, and the normal phase may be followed by an "equalizing" phase in which both strong (meaningful) and weak (meaningless) stimuli evoke responses of equal strength. Under these conditions the selectivity of action of the cortex is disturbed, and the process of choosing the necessary response from many alternatives becomes impaired.

These pathological states of the cortex can be either general or regional in character, and in the latter cases they are restricted to the zone of the lesion and surrounding areas of the cortex. If such a pathological state affects the speech areas of the cortex and, in particular, the most complex "tertiary" zones (the parieto-occipito-temporal zones of the cortex of the left hemisphere), so that their mode of working is switched to that of the "inhibitory" or "equalizing" phase, naturally the traces of connections excited by each pattern or word will appear with equal probability, and choosing the right word (name) will be much more difficult.

This is what happens in patients described in clinical practice as cases of "pure" amnestic aphasia or "anomia."

Attempts to name objects are made difficult in such cases by the fact that different connections—and, consequently, the words reflecting them—spring up with equal probability, and the patient begins to exhibit phenomena of extended searching and "verbal paraphasia." Such a patient, when trying to recall the word "bol'nitsa" (hospital) as the name of an institution is just as likely to say "militsiya" (Police—a name of another institution and a word of similar morphological structure—or "shkola" (school)—by analogy: doctors—patients, teachers—pupils—or "Red Army" (through the association "Red Cross"), and so on. This "tip of the tongue phenomenon," is complicated in this case by irrepressible associations, and choice of the right word from all the possible alternatives is particularly difficult.

In the cases I have just described these difficulties of naming an object (or recalling a name) are of a general character, and they are not confined to any particular modality.

It is a different matter when lesions of the cortex spread to secondary zones of a modality-specific area (temporal—auditory, occipital—visual, postcentral—tactile). The "equalizing phase" in the cases I am describing may be confined to one modality, and both the difficulties in choosing the necessary word from any alternatives and the character of the resulting paraphasia may consequently assume a limited, modality-specific character. In such cases we therefore speak of the acoustic-gnostic sources of difficulty in word naming, of "optical" or "tactile" aphasia.

Recently the mechanisms of these difficulties of naming objects have been studied by Tsvetkova (1975). Her observations have shown that patients who have difficulty in finding the name of an object have at the same time defects in the *visual identification* of the object. They are unable to pick out the leading cues of the object and they cannot recognize stylistic pictures (e.g., they hesitate between calling an animal a hare or a cat when shown a stylistic drawing), they are unable to complete an outline drawing of an animal's body with its characteristic details, and so on. The basis of the difficulty of object naming in such cases is a defect of visual gnosis, in the identification of the essential picture of the object, the "diffuseness" of visual perception (Tsvetkova, 1975).

The nature of the difficulty in naming objects observed in patients with *lesions of the frontal lobes* (especially the postfrontal areas of the left hemisphere) is very different. As a rule, these patients are able to name concrete objects, but no sooner does the patient change to spontaneous production of complete sentences than marked difficulties arise in recall of the necessary words. Sometimes the defect is so serious that spontaneous speech is almost completely impossible. The mechanism of this remarkable symptom has not been adequately explained. It may be suggested that fluent spontaneous speech that stems from an appropriate plan and is not based on a ready-made assortment of visual images requires rather active attempts to find the necessary words as well as an inhibition of irrelevant words that involuntarily spring up. That is why patients with particularly severe lesions of the frontal lobes who attempt to find a particular word required in active speech have so weakened a process of inhibition that they are unable to suppress irrelevant associations and resort to paraphasias on a wide scale, reproducing words of similar sound but inappropriate meaning. These disturbances usually disappear or become much less frequent if the object or picture presented to the patient strengthens one of the possible associations and inhibits the rest. The mechanism of these remarkable amnestic-aphasic symptoms, so conspicuously affecting the spontaneous speech of these patients, requires further study.

Disturbances of the nominative function of speech with *lesions of the left frontotemporal divisions* are associated with the defective mechanisms of both regions and are therefore especially difficult to overcome. Diminished word traces and difficulty in object naming may also occur with *lesions affecting the brain as a whole*; they are particularly apparent with lesions of the diencephalon, for lesions in this area lead to a generalized loss of cortical tone. In such cases, however, these symptoms are superimposed on a general syndrome of rapid fatigue and depression of mnestic functions, and they thus lose their specificity.

A special section of the investigation of relatively simple forms of active speech is the study of verbal differences between the nominative and predicative forms of speech.

In its simplest form it is a test in which the patient is asked in the course of a minute to name objects (the nominative form of speech) and to name actions (the predicative form of speech).

As Tsvetkova's observations have shown, the normal subject performs both tasks equally easily, whereas a patient with a lesion of the anterior zones of the speech area and a syndrome of dynamic aphasia (Part II, Section 4G) chooses the names of objects three to four times quicker than the names of actions. There is reason to suppose that in these patients this feature is directly connected with the disturbance of the predicative function of speech.

E. INVESTIGATION OF NARRATIVE SPEECH

In conjunction with the investigation of the nominative function of speech, the investigation of narrative speech constitutes a vital part of the study of the most complex functions of expressive speech activity.

Every verbal expression made (including narrative speech) is a process of verbal communication using the codes of language. It begins with the motive, plan, or general intent and, as was said above, having passed through the stage of condensed "internal" speech, it is formulated as an expanded verbal expression.

This process clearly is dual in character and incorporates at least two basic components. One of them is the dynamic act of fluent expression, based on the connection between two words (primarily between subject and object), whereby a thought is transformed into an extended communication. This aspect of speech, usually known as its "*syntagmatic structure*," is manifested primarily as a communication of an event (Svedelius, 1897); it is based on the observation that every word of a language usually cannot exist alone but requires connections with other words, so that a simple expression is formed. In modern linguistics these connections are described as "lexical functions," or speech connections formed by a single word, which may differ in complexity from "monovalent" connections (e.g., "gun"— What does it do?), to complex polyvalent lexical function (e.g., "bought"-- Who? From whom? For how much?), and "owed" (Who?, To whom?, How much?, For how long?). The above forms have been described by Apresyan, 1974; Mel'chuk, 1977. These syntactic structures have also been studied by many linguists and psychologists (Chomsky, 1956, 1957; Miller, 1962, 1967 et al.).

In its simplest form the expression consists of subject and predicate (S → P) or subject, predicate, and object (S → P → O), and it describes a certain event. In more complicated cases it may consist of a chain of mutually subordinated, separate statements, sometimes highly differentiated in character, in which various methods are employed for the control of one system of words by another. Historically, language developed from the use of forms of co-ordination (parataxis) to the use of complex forms of subordination (hypotaxis) and from the simplest forms of contact suggestion to complex forms of distant suggestion (in which the continuity of thought is broken by inserted elements or clauses). These facts illustrate the complex path along which narrative speech has traveled. The presence in some languages of various forms of inversion, in which the order of the words differs sharply from the order of the actions designated by them—for instance constructions with reversal of word order, as in "Petyu udaril Vanya"* (= O ← P ← S)—is only one example of the independence that may be attained by the grammatical devices of fully developed narrative speech.

This complex structure of language corresponds to the complexity of the forms of speech development and to the complexity of the psychological processes by means of which this speech is brought about. Predicative expressions begin when the child's speech consists of a single word; however, with full justification, psychologists assert that this stage is really the stage of the "one-word sentence," for it is usually characterized by word denotation of the subject (for example, "ball"), whereas the predicate is expressed by an action or gesture (such as "give ball"). It is not until the next stage that the relationship of subject and predicate begins to be introduced into speech itself. This development takes place in the form of a dialogue, in which the complete syntagma (the relationship between subject and predicate) is often shared between two people: the sentence starts off with a question asked by an adult and is finished by the child's reply. It is only in the last stage of development that dialogic speech ceases to be the only form of speech and monologic (narrative) speech in the true sense of the term begins to be formed.

The characteristic feature of this monologic (and, later, of discursive) speech is the nature of the signal prompting its appearance. This signal is no longer a question asked by an interlocutor. It may be either a situation that is perceived and analyzed or a system of pre-existing speech associations formed in his memory as condensed traces and capable of expanding into a monologic expression when a particular situation or intention arises. We do not yet know the physiological mechanism of the "thought" that subsequently expands into an independent expression or of the "intention" that, under certain conditions,

*Translator's note: "Petyu" is the accusative case of "Petya"; "Vanya" is nominative. The sentence is translated as "Vanya (John) struck Petya (Peter)."

may be embodied in this thought. We know very little, too, about the mechanisms of the internal speech, which, according to Vygotskii (1934, 1956), possesses a predicative function and enables the original thought to be transformed into the fully developed expression.

All I have written above applies to only one of the two components of extended (narrative) speech, namely its syntagmatic structure. However, this aspect, which is clearly manifested in the "communication of an event," is only one part of the structure of expression.

The structure of expression includes the learning of complex logical-grammatical codes of language, which combine the "lexical functions" and syntagmatic structure of language I have described and also constructions expressing *relationships* (the "communication of relationships" of Svedelius). Typical features of this aspect of the organization of extended expression are complex structures expressed by inflections (of the type *"brat ottsa"*—the father's brother),* structures expressed by means of prepositions (such as *"krug pod kvadratom"*—a circle under a square),** and so on. All these structures, by contrast with syntagmatic structures, are usually termed "paradigmatic" (Jakobson, 1942, 1971), and ability to use them is the second important condition for both the understanding and the formulation of complex verbal expressions.

The complexity of structure of the extended verbal expression, embracing both its syntagmatic and its paradigmatic organization, is the reason for the complex pattern of the disturbances of verbal expression that may arise in patients with lesions of different parts of the brain.

As a whole series of investigations published in the last decade (Benson, 1967; Kerschensteiner, Poeck, and Brunner, 1972; Luria, 1975, 1976) has shown, there are two basic forms of aphasia—nonfluent and fluent.

The most characteristic feature of nonfluent aphasia, found in lesions of the anterior zones of the speech areas, is that fluent speech (the smooth transition from thought to extended expression), the lexical functions, and the syntagmatic structure of speech are grossly disturbed, whereas operations with the codes of language (its paradigmatic structure) remain basically intact. I have already given examples of such speech disorders when I described the picture of "efferent" and "afferent" motor aphasia and the phenomenon of the "telegraphic style" (Part II, Section 4).

The other basic form of speech disorder, fluent aphasia, is characterized by the opposite picture. The lexical functions and syntagmatic structure of speech are intact in these patients, and they continue to speak fluently, preserving isolated fragments of fluent verbal expression. However, their operations with complex (phonemic, lexical, or semantic) codes of language

* *brat*, nominative singular, brother; *ottsa*, genitive singular of *otets*, of the father.

** *krug*, nominative singular, circle; *pod*, preposition, under; *kvadratom*, prepositional case, singular, of *kvadrat*, square (translator).

and the paradigmatic organization of speech are profoundly disturbed; the concrete forms of these disturbances differ in character depending on the location of the lesion.

These observations provide a new approach to disturbances of narrative speech in patients with local brain lesions. It will be clear from the foregoing that expanded predicative speech, in its narrative or discursive form, is one of the structurally most complex processes of speech and that the investigator must not forget for one minute the extent of its complexity.

• • •

The complexity of the structure of spontaneous predicative speech also accounts for the complex character of its possible disturbances. Like all the other functions of speech, the expanded predicative (narrative) form of speech may be disturbed as a result of instability of word traces and extinction of word meaning; it may also be disturbed if the grammatical constructions forming the framework of the sentence cannot be used. However, these disturbances may ensue from other causes, which have not yet been considered. Narrative speech may be impaired when the intention itself is not formed or when the systems of traces of previous speech associations lose their regulating importance. This could happen when internal speech is disturbed and when the plan cannot be translated into speech and expanded into a predicative expression. Finally, a disturbance in predicative speech may appear as a symptom of loss of the higher automatisms, making the smooth performance of skilled movements impossible in whatever sphere may be affected. This multiplicity of causes of possible disturbances of predicative speech does not mean, however, that their complex mechanisms cannot be analyzed or that they cannot be used for diagnostic localization. As in all the other types of disturbance a thorough analysis is required of the forms in which these disturbances are manifested and the factors responsible for them must be brought to light.

Before proceeding with this investigation, a series of tests must be applied to study *the state of any form of fluent, automatized speech that is not predicative from any point of view, but whose integrity is an essential condition for the production of smooth sustained expression.* Methods widely known in clinical practice are used for these purposes; the patient is asked to recite a natural series of numbers (1, 2, 3, 4, 5, etc.) or an equally familiar series (days of the week, months of the year, etc.).

Inability to recite these highly automatized series fluently often indicates the disintegration of the corresponding established systems. This may occur with instability of the systems of speech traces associated with different forms of aphasia. In these cases the patient will omit the names of some of the days or months, or will give them in the wrong order. However, inability to perform this test may also indicate a general disturbance of highly automatized processes; in such cases the recitation of the series loses its fluidity and each word begins to require a special impulse. Such disturbances were discussed in connection with the syndrome associated with lesions of the premotor systems (Part II, Section 4E and F). Diminished ability to reproduce an automatized series smoothly may also be revealed by passive repetition of the group of words given by the investigator (for example, 1, 2, 3, 4 . . . 1, 2, 3, 4 . . . or January, February . . . January, February . . . January, February . . .), as in echolalia. Also, it exists if the patient cannot continue the series unaided or (as happens in latent cases) keeps to the rhythm used by the investigator when presenting the series and continues to recite it in the form of "inert groupings" (1, 2, 3, 4 . . . 5, 6, 7, 8 . . . 9, 10, 11, 12 . . . or January, February . . . March, April . . . May, June . . . etc.). This type of deautomatization is frequently observed in disintegration of the dynamics of speech activity accompanying certain *lesions of the anterior divisions of the brain* (Part II, Section 4G).

Experiments involving the reproduction of an automatized series may, however, be used for other purposes, in particular, to analyze the extent to which the patient can overcome firmly established speech stereotypes. The patient is asked to recite the same series (numbers, days of the week, months) backward. If, as is frequently found, the patient cannot perform this test correctly although he can reproduce the direct series automatically, a considerable inertia of established stereotypes is present. Inability to reproduce an established series in reverse order is particularly evident with *lesions of the frontal lobes*. However, other factors enter into the performance of this test (ability to retain series of word traces, ability to operate consciously with a system of associations, etc.). Poor reproduction of an established series backward may thus result from many different causes and may be found with many types of cerebral lesions.

These tests do not, however, constitute part of the investigatory procedures used in the study of narrative speech but merely serve to analyze certain factors that should be considered before the main problem is tackled.

The *investigation of predicative speech* is based on a series of simple tests that are widely used in clinical practice. It begins with the analysis of dialogic speech, in which the patient is asked a series of questions; one of these embodies the answer and can therefore be answered in a simplified form ("Have you had lunch today?" "Yes, I have") while the others require the formation of new associations before they can be answered ("Where do you work?" or "What did you have for lunch today?"). Attention is paid to the speed with which the answers are given, the presence or absence of echolalic repetition of the question, and the ability to change easily from the first (passive) to the second (active) type of answer. This test is followed by the principal part of the investigation of the predicative function of speech: The patient is given a simple picture and he must describe what it is about, or he is told a short story that he must reproduce in narrative form. This part of the test may be called the investigation of the reproductive form of narrative speech.

In evaluating the results, the investigator must pay attention to the fluidity of the patient's account of the picture or short story, his ability to reproduce the required narrative spontaneously, whether or not the speech is purely nominative in character (in which case development of the subject is replaced by a listing of individual objective details), and, finally, the extent to which the account is relevant to the subject matter of the picture or story. If the patient cannot give a coherent account, the investigator must give control questions, breaking up the topic into separate details.

Inability to narrate the gist of it and ability to do so in the form of answers to individual questions indicates a profound defect in spontaneous narrative speech and demonstrates that the patient's functions can operate only in a "reactive" form.

Subsequent experiments are devoted to the *investigation of spontaneous, productive, narrative speech.* For this purpose, the patient is asked to tell the story of a well-known theatrical production (*Eugene Onegin, The Queen of Spades*), or, as the most difficult test of narrative speech, he is required to make a speech on a certain topic (for example, on the theme of "The North"). The ability to reproduce coherently a familiar story coupled with the inability to give even a short discourse on a selected topic by one's own efforts or with limitation of the spontaneous development of the topic to a few stereotyped remarks is an important sign of general inactivity or lack of spontaneity and constitutes valuable evidence for the diagnosis of several types of lesions.

The last group of tests used for investigating narrative speech is more specialized in character, being concerned with the extent to which the patient can operate with *complex systems of grammatical expressions.* This group contains two principal tests. In the first of these the patient is given a written sentence that is broken off at a certain point or that contains a missing link, and he is asked to make good the omission (Ebbinghaus' test). Sometimes the sentence is interrupted at a point where completion is fairly easy; if expanded grammatical stereotypes ("language sense") are preserved, the test is easily performed ("Winter is very . . ." or "I went to the . . . to buy some bread."). At other times the task is made more difficult, i.e., the omission is made at a place where its replacement requires analysis of the whole phrase and synthesis of its available elements. Such tests include sentences in which the missing words are substantives ("The autumn wind was like a wild . . .") or essential auxiliary parts of speech ("The airplane came down . . . [although] its engine was working properly"). And sometimes the patient is asked to choose one of several words to make good the omission. These words are so selected that one is correct and the others, which may bear some resemblance to it at first glance, are found to be unsuitable after the sentence has been analyzed.

In the second of these tests the patient is given three isolated words (for example, "automobile – wood – garage") from which he must construct a complete sentence by adding suitable words. In another variant, a complete sentence is given, but its component words are disarranged (for example, "forest went – and – into – woodcutter – the – some – got – a – wood"), and the patient is asked to rearrange them in the proper order. In this experiment the individual words may be written in the form of a continuous text and the whole process of reconstructing the phrase may be done entirely by speaking aloud. In an easier variant, the words composing the sentence may be presented on separate cards, which the patient must lay out in front of him and rearrange in their proper order.

All these tests require conscious operations with phrases and special analysis and synthesis of the component parts of the sentence; they can therefore be performed only if the grammatical structure of the sentence is appreciated. For this reason, these tests can be used successfully for the analysis of latent grammatical disturbances.

Patients with lesions of different types and in different parts of the brain may vary in the difficulty they experience when performing these tests. Frequently, a patient with a *lesion of the temporal systems* and in the presence of *sensory or acoustic-mnestic aphasia*, can reproduce automatized series of words but has appreciable difficulty reciting the days of the week or the months of the year. In these instances individual names may be omitted or paraphasia of contamination may be present, so that there is difficulty in understanding the series as it is rendered. These difficulties naturally become particularly severe when attempts are made to recite an automatized series in reverse order.

Similar difficulties arise during dialogic speech because of the unstable verbal traces and extinction of word meaning. There is no noticeable difficulty in answering a question—the decisive feature is the absence of the necessary words and their replacement by others that just happen to come to mind; the answers to the questions thus often begin to be characterized by attempts to look for words, by exclamations expressing confusion, and by excessive paraphasia. The disturbances take on a particularly severe form when these patients attempt to produce sustained narrative speech. Although the pattern of intonation is intact, the vocabulary is grossly inadequate. Substantives are particularly impaired, being for the most part omitted or replaced by paraphasias. In its intonation and melodic structure, the sentence as a whole has the character of a complete expression despite its lacking of substantives; however, its meaning can be divined only if the general context of what the patient wants to say is known. In the presence of a latent syndrome of temporal aphasia, this structure of the expression may be replaced by sentences exhibiting a high degree of paraphasia and contamination but the general scheme of the expression remains unchanged. It will be clear that patients of this group will have equal difficulty in both reproductive and productive forms of narrative speech. Tests involving more complex operations with sentences are frequently impossible to perform because of the instability of the word traces and extinction of meaning.

It will thus be clear that the fluent syntagmatic organization of speech in these patients is primarily intact, whereas the lexical components of speech may be lost or unstable. A similar picture can be observed in patients with lesions of the parieto-occipital zones of the left hemisphere and in the phenomena of amnestic and semantic aphasia.

As I stated earlier, the main difficulty observed in these patients is that they lose the selective recall of necessary words and, instead, the process of word recall becomes expanded in character and is accompanied by frequent verbal paraphasia, which cannot be inhibited. Because of this difficulty (and not because of any primary disturbance of the syntagmatic organization of speech), fluent verbal expression is interrupted by searching for the necessary words and becomes substantially impaired.

Perhaps the most noticeable characteristic is that the patients of this group often attempt to use their residual fragments of fluent speech in order to surmount their difficulties. For example, when they have difficulty in naming an object (e.g., a comb) they try to get around the difficulty by resorting to their intact syntagmatic formation and say: "And so I took it . . . the thing I comb my hair with. . . ." Strikingly, in some cases the patients of this group will try to surmount their difficulties by an original method: in their narrative speech they resort to *"prose in rhythm,"* and on this basis they try to get around their speech difficulties.

For instance, one patient of this group, whom I have described in full elsewhere (Luria, 1972), when having difficulty with expanded narrative speech, the fluency of which was interrupted by word seeking, began to use this "prose in rhythm," and her narrative speech (especially written) became something like this: "And so—I want to tell you about my friend—how they treated me here for such a long time . . . the woman doctor was so important and so good-looking that you immediately felt confidence in her. . . ." and so on. I have described this curious way of obtaining support from the intact fluent syntagmatically organized speech elsewhere (Luria, 1975) and will not dwell on it further.

The disturbance of narrative speech associated with *lesions of the anterior divisions of the brain* is totally different in nature. Patients with lesions of the premotor systems accompanied by gross disturbance of complex skilled movements (Part II, Section 4E), may exhibit disintegration of the higher, more highly organized forms of activity and of speech processes. They experience considerable difficulty in reciting highly automatized series, as revealed by the slowness and unevenness of their speech. It may be concluded from the de-automatized character of their performance that the dynamics involved in sequential operations is profoundly deranged and that this disintegration is responsible for these symptoms.

When a lesion of the premotor systems leads to efferent (kinetic) motor aphasia (Part II, Section 4F), smooth narrative speech is impossible. Although the patient can easily point to separate objects and repeat isolated words, he cannot conduct a fully developed dialogue; he answers questions very briefly, exhibiting great difficulty when, because the wording of the answer is not formulated in the question, a new system of associations has to be developed. Expanded predicative speech is of course absolutely impossible. The preservation of nominative speech alone, combined with a total inability to produce spontaneous narrative speech, comprise the basic diagnostic feature of these disturbances.

Characteristically, the same profound impairment of predicative speech continues to be manifested in the latter stages of resolution of efferent (kinetic) aphasia. A typical finding is expressions consisting almost entirely of nominative words, referred to in the literature as the telegraphic style ("Here . . . head . . . operation . . . here . . . speech . . . none . . . talking . . . what . . . illness").

Rather different from this form is the disturbance of narrative speech found in patients with *lesions of the left frontal lobe*, not extending to the premotor systems and Broca's area. It is difficult to detect any defects in the speech construction of these patients: Phonetically their speech remains pure and there are no appreciable articulatory difficulties; it may also remain grammatically quite intact. Nevertheless, the speech activity of these patients is grossly abnormal. The peculiarity of their speech is revealed during simple tests involving the reproduction of automatized and well-established series. At first, such patients refuse to perform even the simplest test—for example, to recite the days of the week or the months of the year. Then, if the investigator himself starts the series, the patients repeat what he has said in echolalic fashion, but they still cannot continue the series by themselves; a further stimulus from the investigator is required every time. When, finally, they begin to recite the elements of the series, it is clear that they are passively reproducing the rhythm in which the beginning of the series was given to them. If the investigator started off the series with three numbers (1, 2, 3 . . .), the patient subsequently will passively continue with similar groups of three numbers, expecting additional stimulation every time in the form of questions like "What next?" or "Any more?"

Still more obvious defects are apparent in the dialogic and, in particular, in the narrative speech of such a patient. As a rule, questions put to him will evoke nothing more than echolalic repetition. Sometimes, especially if the answer is embodied in the question, the patient will give the answer; when, however, the answer requires the formation of new associations, the process does not get beyond the echolalic repetition of the question.

The narrative speech of such a patient is particularly affected. Even after attentively examining a picture or listening to a story, he cannot give a coherent or fluent version of the subject matter; he either simply states that he cannot tell anything about it or produces only an isolated fragment of an expression, usually declaring that he has forgotten it all. If, however, immediately after this test the subject matter to be grasped by the patient is broken up into separate sections and the investigator asks a series of consecutive questions, it becomes clear not only that the patient did retain the subject matter of the picture or story, but also that he can easily reproduce it in the form of separate answers to these questions. This test convincingly demonstrates that the principal defect in such a patient is associated with a profound disturbance of active expression and that his ability to recode the general subject matter into expanded narrative speech is severely impaired. Productive narrative speech (such as making a speech on a given topic) is completely beyond the ability of these patients. During our analysis of the forms of this dynamic aphasia (Part II, Section 4G) we showed that the whole productive speech of the patient is nothing more than the blurting out of ready-made stereotypes. We do not yet know the underlying mechanisms of these disturbances. There is reason to suppose, however, that further investigation of the internal speech of these patients, with its loss of predicative function, will lead to a considerable deepening of our understanding of this syndrome.

The description of the disturbance of active narrative speech found in patients with a marked frontal syndrome will be postponed until we reach the section devoted to the investigation of intellectual activity.

Even in its more elementary forms, the syndrome of afferent motor aphasia (Part II, Section 4D) gives rise to obvious speech defects. It is inevitable that such motor disturbances create difficulties in the investigation of narrative speech. In these cases, narrative speech is not affected by any new defects. Distinctive but not primary disturbances of expanded narrative speech, associated with disturbance of the systems of logical-grammatical connections and the amnestic-aphasic syndrome, may also arise in patients with semantic aphasia (Part II, Section 3E). Nonspecific disturbances of active narrative speech, associated with increased susceptibility to fatigue and, not infrequently, with instability of the mnestic traces, may also occur in *general cerebral disorders* as a result of the effects of hydrocephalus and increased intracranial pressure.

Taken as a whole, the study of defects of the nominative and predicative functions of speech, sometimes occurring together but equally often dissociated, is one of the most important aspects of the investigation of the defects of the higher cortical function resulting from local brain injuries.

The investigation of the principal forms of speech activity, the basic syndromes of speech disorders, and ways of restoring these disturbed functions are described in two other books by the present author (1947, 1948).

10. *Investigation of Writing and Reading*

A. PRELIMINARY REMARKS

The investigation of writing and reading is a phase of the study of the higher cortical processes that is of considerable importance to the topical diagnosis of brain lesions. As special forms of speech activity, writing, and reading differ essentially from spoken speech both in their genesis and psychophysiological structure and in their functional properties. Whereas spoken speech is formed in the early stages of the child's development in the course of direct association with other people, written speech does not appear until much later and is the result of special training. In contrast to spoken speech, which usually proceeds automatically and without the conscious analysis of its phonetic composition, from the very beginning written speech is a voluntary, organized activity with the conscious analysis of its constituent sounds.

The stage-by-stage character of this activity persists for a long time, and not until the later stages of its formation is writing converted into a complex, automatized skill. The psychophysiological structure of writing and reading is particularly characteristic and differs essentially from that of spoken speech (Luria, 1950).

In the great majority of languages both writing from dictation and spontaneous writing begin with the analysis of the phonetic complex that goes to form the pronounced word. This phonetic complex can be broken up into component parts, and the fundamental units composing the word—the phonemes—can be distinguished within the smooth sequence of sounds. Under acoustically simple conditions the discrimination of phonemes is not a particularly complex process. Under acoustically complicated conditions—including unstressed vowels, consonants modified acoustically because of their position, and elision of consonants—this process is transformed into a complex activity, involving the isolation of sounds from irrelevant acoustic signs and the recognition of stable phonetic units. The phonemes identified as a result of such activity must be arranged in a certain order and recoded into the corresponding optic structures—graphemes—possessing their own visual-spatial properties; in the final stage, the graphemes must again be recoded into a system of motor acts. This complex process is undertaken by means of a complex mechanism, the various components of which stand out clearly in the initial stages of the formation of the writing skill, when writing is still deliberate and extended and has not yet become automatized. It is only later that this process becomes condensed and acquires the character of the highly automatized skill easily observed in adult's writing.

Analysis of the phonetic composition of speech, the starting point of any form of writing, naturally requires adequate preservation of phonetic hearing. However, investigations on the initial stages of the writing skill have shown that articulation plays an essential role in the task of precise definition of the phonetic composition of words; in an elementary, expanded form, articulation is used by children during the first years of their learning to write. At that stage, it consists of speaking the words aloud, which is the motor component of their phonetic analysis. Observations on the writing of individuals who are deaf or with articulatory disturbances (Boskis and Levina, 1936; Boskis, 1953; Levina, 1940; etc.) have shown that both a disturbance of hearing and a disturbance of articulation may severely impair the differentiation of the required phonemes, a fundamental constituent of writing. Similar difficulties in phonetic analysis and, consequently, in the process of writing in the initial stages of education of the normal child may be brought about by blocking the articulatory components; this can be accomplished by instructing the child, for example, to write with the mouth open. A special investigation conducted by Nazarova (1952) showed that the number of mistakes during writing is increased manyfold when this is done.

In writing it is important to preserve the correct sound sequence; this demands analysis of the consecutive sound series in every word and inhibition of the strong components of this series if they are not in crucial positions. The complexity of this neurodynamic process has been sufficiently illuminated by the numerous investigations dealing with the process of elaborating the corresponding differentiation. Observation has shown that this process is easily disturbed by any diminution of active inhibition (Pevzner, 1960).

The second stage in writing, no less complex in nature, is concerned with the recoding of the identified phonetic elements (phonemes) into optic elements (graphemes) and with rendering them in writing. Every grapheme has its own particular visual-spatial structure, whose realization requires complex spatial analysis. The difficulties in understanding graphemes that arise with weakened visual differentiation, especially if associated with defective spatial analysis (associated with impairment in right-left distinction), are generally appreciated. The phenomenon of mirror-image writing, more commonly found when lateralization is inadequate (for example, before the dominant role of the right hand has been established and in left-handedness), is familiar to all.

Investigations have revealed the complex path the motor organization of writing travels in the successive educative stages. Gur'yanov (1940) and Pantina (1954) have shown that when one is beginning to acquire the writing skill every graphic element requires a special impulse and that in the subsequent stages generalization of the elements of the skilled movement with their combination into a single kinetic melody occurs by degree; eventually, the object of conscious performance is no longer the separate strokes of each letter, but the writing of the whole word or sometimes even of a whole short phrase.

The foregoing stressed the complexity and the systematic nature of the writing process. This helps to explain the variety of writing disorders found in conjunction with lesions of those cerebral divisions essentially concerned with this highly complex skill. At the same time, two further conclusions of considerable theoretical importance are possible.

The first of these conclusions is related to the evaluation of changes in the act of writing taking place in the successive stages of its development, and the second with the profound differences in the structure of writing in the various language systems. We have drawn attention to the expanded, stage-by-stage manner by which writing is carried out in the early stages of its formation. It is clear from what has been said, however, that in the later stages completely different and much more direct methods are used. The process of articulation (speaking aloud), which plays a decisive role in the early stages of education, has little to do with the highly automatized form of writing. A person capable of writing in this highly automatized manner can, therefore, do so even when articulation is excluded. We also know that the writing of familiar words, which has become a highly automatized action (the most obvious example of this is one's own signature), no longer requires acoustic analysis but is performed as a complex motor stereotype. This all suggests that in the different stages of writing development changes take place in its psychophysiological composition, so that *the part played by cortical systems in this activity does not always remain the same.*

The second conclusion refers to the psychophysiological structure of the process of writing in different language systems. All that has been said was in reference to language systems utilizing phonetic recording. In some languages, however, writing is not phonetic but ideographic, so that a difference in principle exists between the structures of the psychophysiological processes used in its performance. Written Chinese has, generally speaking, rid itself of the need for phonemic analysis of words. Its conventional signs do not record the phonetic composition of words but, instead, denote ideas. It is therefore easy to understand that the process of phonetic analysis and synthesis, the basis of phonetic writing, is not present here and that the process of visual (and symbolic) analysis of ideograms is much more complex. Similar (although less obvious) differences are found among the European languages. The purely phonetic writing in the Russian, German, or Italian languages differs essentially in its mechanisms from writing in French or English, in which writing components of conventional, rather than phonetic, nature occur far more frequently.

It is natural, therefore, that *the different bases for writing in different languages must entail a different cortical organization.* Therefore, analysis of the various writing mechanisms is essential to the understanding of the defects in this skilled activity that arise from various circumscribed lesions of the cerebral cortex (Luria, 1947, 1960).

• • •

The process that will be examined in conjunction with writing, i.e., reading, is equally complex in character. The initial process of acquiring the reading skill is so drawn out that its complexity is apparent. In languages written phonetically, the process of reading begins with perception of letters and analysis of their conventional phonetic value. This is followed by a very complex process, causing the most obvious difficulty in education—the process of fusion of the phonetic letters into words. The difficulty here is that the separate phonemes are bound to lose their isolated meaning; some of their characteristics are lost while others are modified by the influence of the position of the sound in the phoneme (a "t" before an "i" sounds quite differently from one before an "o"). It is only as a result of this modification that the sounds can be merged into a single syllable. Once this recoding of the isolated phonetic sounds into complete syllables has been done, the second stage—their combination into whole words—does not present any fundamental difficulty. The subsequent development of the reading skill consists of consecutive automatization, in the course of which the detailed cycle of operations directed toward the analysis and synthesis of individual phonetic letters is gradually contracted and simplified and is eventually transformed into the direct recognition of words by sight that is characteristic of fully developed reading skill and that endows it with its apparent simplicity.

One of the most important features of the reading process, and one displayed much more fully than in writing, comprises the radical changes in the psychophysiological components of the act of reading that occur in the course of its development and automatization. Whereas in the first educative stages a decisive role is played by the analysis of phonetic letters and the fusion of the isolated values of the letters into a single syllable (with all the complex recoding of values of individual graphemes), in the subsequent stages the process becomes transformed into the visual recognition of words and no longer depends exclusively on the analysis and synthesis of phonetic letters. This type of reading has approximately the same nature as the comprehension of the meaning of ideograms, although it still remains capable of expansion to the detailed mechanism required of phonetic analysis if need be. Therefore, what was said regarding the changing composition of the dynamic mosaic of the cortical zones responsible for the process of writing at its different stages applies with even greater force to reading. The recognition of such well-established symbols as USSR or USA or of words like "Moscow" or "Pravda" takes a totally different psychological course from that of the true-reading of words like "shipbuilding" and "disorganization." It bears repeating that in different languages reading may be based on different psychophysiological mechanisms. Recognition of Chinese characters involves a process utterly different in nature from that of reading a text written in a language utilizing phonetic transcription.

There is, however, yet another special feature of the process of reading that must not be forgotten. In contrast to writing—which follows the path of thoughts to words—reading follows the course of words to thoughts. It begins with the analysis of a ready-made, written word that, after the aforementioned stages, is transformed into the meaning of the object or action denoted by it or, in respect to a whole text, into the thought formulated therein. However, this transformation of words into thoughts is by no means always a one-way activity. Usually it has two aspects—afferent and efferent. The reader grasps the meaning of a certain group of letters and, sometimes, of words or groups of words that evoke in him a particular system of associations, or a sort of hypothesis. This "hypothesis" creates a certain orientation or "apperception" and makes the subsequent reading an active process in which the search for the desired meaning and the discernment of agreements or disagreements with the expected meaning begin to assume an almost exclusive role. Under normal conditions this process of comparing the expected meaning with the meaning actually expressed in a word (or text) proceeds rapidly and adaptively, so that a hypothesis that does not correspond to the true meaning of a word is at once inhibited and corrected. However, should the suggested word give rise to an excessively stable stereotype, or should the process of inhibition of the developing associations be weakened, the hypothesis may fail to be corrected. Most people, seeing a notice "Smoking Probited" where there was a fire hazard, would read it as "Smoking Prohibited" without noticing that a mistake had been made. It is well-known that most misreadings are constructed on the same basis. These specific aspects of reading have received special scrutiny by Khodzhava (1957).

Imperfect corrections may also be introduced into the process of reading under other conditions. A series of special investigations has shown that the initial formative stages of the reading skill cannot be considered simply as comprising the analysis and synthesis of letters with phonetic values. The mere fact that the child has grasped its first letter group is usually sufficient to cause it to make active guesses, which become even more firmly established if the word is illustrated by some form of picture. In this way, the child develops "guessing reading," which becomes predominant at times of weakened inhibition during the execution of this complex activity; acquisition of this ability marks a distinct period in the development of the child's reading skill (Egorov, 1953; etc.). The guessing aspect of reading is often difficult to overcome when weakening of the inhibitory processes occurs for any reason with pathological conditions of the brain or with fatigue; this is the principal difficulty encountered in the teaching of oligophrenic children of the excitable type to read (Pevzner, 1960). This peculiarity of the reading process is one of its most important properties. When studying the disturbances in reading that occur with pathological conditions of the brain, it must not be forgotten that this process of reading inevitably reflects the general features of the abnormal neurodynamics of the patient.

The foregoing amounts to the fact that writing and reading are functional systems of complex composition that may undergo various types of dysfunction as a result of the loss of individual components and, consequently, as a result of local lesions of different parts of the brain. The foregoing also disclosed how the psychophysiological composition of these acts changes in the successive developmental stages and in the different language systems, a factor that must be borne in mind when reading defects are investigated. Finally, the foregoing emphasized the complexity of the dynamic processes underlying writing and, in particular, reading. It is evident, then, that our investigation of the course of these processes must go beyond the study of particular techniques and must consider them in the light of general neurodynamic features.

B. INVESTIGATION OF THE PHONETIC ANALYSIS AND SYNTHESIS OF WORDS

The investigation of writing processes must be preceded by the study of the state of the patient's analysis and synthesis of sounds, for without adequacy of these processes writing is impossible. This investigation must establish whether or not the patient can still single out the component parts in the acoustic continuity of spoken speech, abstract and identify definite phonemes from the general pattern of sound signs not having the importance of signals, maintain the proper order of these phonemes, and, finally, integrate them into phonemic groups.

During the discussion of receptive speech (Part III, Section 8B), experiments directed toward the analysis of phonemic hearing were detailed. The experiments that will now be described continue this aspect of the investigation, the only difference being that the comprehension of the meaning of a whole word and the ability to perform complex operations involving the elements of its phonetic composition will now be scrutinized.

The experiments used to investigate phonetic analysis and synthesis are very simple and may be divided into several groups. The patient is given a certain word (at first phonetically simple, and later more complex) and is asked to tell how many sounds (letters) are in it (how many letters in the word "cat," "trap," "banana," etc.). Special attention is paid to the patient's ability to distinguish consonants and vowels (whose pronunciation is associated with fewer kinesthetic signals from the tongue, palate, and lips) and to select sounds from a complex group (for example, when consonants are elided). In order to discover how easily the patient can accomplish these tasks and what method of phonetic analysis he employs, the investigator keeps careful watch on whether the patient carries out the required analysis immediately "in his head" or by a piecemeal process of speaking the word out loud and "feeling" the articulation of its elements.

In order to more accurately discern the role of articulation in phonetic analysis the patient may be asked to carry out the same activity when articulation is not possible. For example, he may be required to tell the number of letters in a word while keeping his tongue clenched between his teeth or keeping his mouth open. Subtle disturbances in the mechanisms of acoustic analysis, compelling the patient to seek the aid of articulation even in the simplest cases, are clearly disclosed by this test. Of course, this symptom can be evaluated only if patients with well-established writing skill are investigated.

After assessment of the number of sounds in a word has been tested, the identification of individual sounds within a word is studied. For this purpose the patient is asked to name the second sound (letter) in the word "cat," the third sound in the word "most," etc. He is first given words with a simple phonetic composition and later words with elided consonants; finally, he is given words with unstressed vowels or with consonants that are difficult to distinguish (for example, "Wednesday"). As in the first test, the investigator studies the means the patient uses to carry out the task and the extent to which he makes use of articulatory analysis.

To make the test more difficult, articulation is excluded; to make it easier, the given word is pronounced clearly with each component sound pronounced separately. Correct appraisal of the number of sounds in a word whose qualitative analysis proves to be difficult would indicate the presence of defective acoustic-articulatory sound perception.

A special means of investigating phonetic analysis and synthesis is to evaluate the patient's discernment of the position of sounds in a word. For this purpose, the patient is asked to state which sound (letter) in the word "stop" comes after the "o" or before the "t" or which sound in the word "bridges" comes before the "g" or after the "d," etc. This task, which requires not only the separation of a sound from the whole word, but also the correct evaluation of the position of sounds in relation to each other, is an important element of the writing process and may be substantially disturbed in any type of defect that impairs the analysis of the phonetic structure of words or the recognition of the consecutive scheme of the sounds of which they are composed. Naturally, this test can be used only when the patient retains the concepts of "before" and "after" and, consequently, cannot be used for patients with semantic aphasia.

The last test is aimed at appraising the phonetic synthesis of the syllable or word, and it is of great importance in the analysis of the conditions essential for writing and, in particular, for reading. In this test a whole syllable or word (for example, "p-r-o," "c-a-t," or "s-t-o-p") is pronounced letter by letter, and the patient is asked to say what syllable or word these sounds make. In order to avoid the direct acoustic integration of these sounds and to ensure that secondary synthesis is possible, the sounds are separated by an intermediate word as they are pronounced. The problem is presented to the patient in the following form: "What word am I saying: C, then A, then T?" (or, alternatively, "S, then T, then O, then P?"). To analyze the difficulties that may arise, this test, like the preceding ones, may be conducted with or without the possibility of articulation (speaking aloud) by the patient. To make the test easier, the patient may be allowed to watch carefully the movements of the investigator's lips as he pronounces the given word.

Disturbances of phonetic analysis and synthesis may arise in association with lesions in different parts of the left hemisphere; however, as we saw during the analysis of the pathology of the other functional systems, the character of the disturbance may be different in each instance.

A lesion of the *left temporal divisions of the cortex*, giving rise to *impairment of acoustic-gnostic processes* (Part II, Section 2D), invariably leads to difficulty in phonetic analysis and synthesis. In the most severe cases the patient may even be unable to understand the problem that he must solve or may be unable to set about distinguishing the sounds from a phonetic group. Words are perceived by such patients as an indivisible noise, from which it may only occasionally be possible to select some fragment possessing the strongest acoustic or articulatory qualities. Hence, the patient can neither tell what sounds make up a particular word, nor, still less, can he identify the individual sounds and analyze their relationship to each other.

In less severe cases of a lesion of the left temporal lobe the picture may be essentially different. Although the patient can grasp the individual words and understand their meaning relatively easily, he continues to have obvious difficulty in analyzing their phonetic composition. These difficulties are apparent when the patient begins phonetic analysis of words containing unstressed vowels or elided consonants, for, although he can easily pick out the individual sounds in acoustically simple words, increased fusion of these units creates confusion. In these instances he invariably turns to articulation for help, by carefully saying the word aloud and basing his analysis of the sounds not so much on acoustic as on kinesthetic signals. Nevertheless, this type of aid is often inadequate, and the inability to detect sounds whose articulation is not absolutely precise continues. During the qualitative analysis of sounds, the already described difficulties are further compounded by difficulty in discriminating between closely related phonemes and difficulty in evaluating the relative position of sounds in a word. In the last instance, a confrontation with a complete group of sounds, not isolated ones, makes analysis particularly difficult; the patient omits first one, and then another, component. He readily loses the correct sound sequence and thus shows that he cannot solve the problem even with the aid of articulation. It follows that if articulation is out of the question, the patient is totally unable to perform the test. Patients of this group have equal difficulty performing tests involving the acoustic synthesis of words. Their powers of retaining a series of sounds are so limited and their traces are so unstable that they usually either refuse to carry out the assignment or retain only one fragment of the presented structure and guess what word this fragment might come from. Such disturbances are characteristic of those patients in whom the formations of the temporal divisions of the speech zone of the cerebral cortex are involved by the pathological process. Lesions of the middle and lower divisions of the cortex of the left temporal lobe, like lesions of the temporal pole, do not lead to the aforementioned disturbances.

Different types of defects in phonetic analysis and synthesis occur with a *lesion of the posterior divisions of the left sensorimotor region accompanied by a disturbance of the kinesthetic basis of the speech act* (Part II, Section 4D). In these cases the damaged link is articulation, an integral part of the analysis of speech sounds. Thus, the performance of these tests becomes difficult for other reasons. According to the experimental evidence, these patients can analyze the number of sounds forming a word more easily than patients with acoustic-gnostic disorders (with the sole exception of the identification of weakly articulated sounds—unstressed vowels and elements of complex consonants). However, appreciable difficulties arise here during the qualitative analysis of the sounds forming a word. In an attempt to identify these sounds precisely, the patient either omits certain sounds and selects only those components of the phonetic complex with the strongest articulation or he articulates them wrongly and, thus makes a wrong evaluation of the phonetic components of the word. The mistakes that were detailed (Part II, Section 4D; Part III, Section 8B), such as identifying the sound "n" as "l" or "d" and the sound "b" as "m," are typically associated with defective articulatory analysis of sounds. It is natural, therefore, that patients of this group, who receive no help from articulatory analysis, should have recourse to the analysis of the shape of the mouth (by watching the face of the person who is speaking or following the movements of their own lips in a mirror). The aforementioned defects prevent such patients from determining the position of sounds in a word and from synthesizing words from individual sounds. In the latter activity, one articuleme may be substituted for another closely related one, and this may lead to the drawing of wrong conclusions, e.g., evaluating the series "s – t – o – n – e" as "stole".

The disturbance of phonetic analysis and synthesis assumes a particularly serious form in patients with *lesions of the inferior portions of the premotor area of the left hemisphere*, giving rise to *efferent (kinetic) motor aphasia*. In the severest forms of this lesion the analysis of the phonetic composition of words is made difficult by derangement of the dynamic stereotypes of the changing sounds composing a word and by the pathological inertia of the nervous processes in the motor analyzer (Part II, Section 4F). Because of these defects, patients often cannot distinguish, still less articulate, a series of sounds composing a word (differentiation of vowel sounds is particularly difficult), and they find discernment of the order of the sounds in a word particularly trying. In this form of disturbance, therefore, mistakes are frequently made when the necessary order of the sounds in a word or syllable is disturbed and the most strongly articulated component of the group of sounds becomes dominant. In the word "match," for example, the sound "tch" is identified as the "first."

The disturbance of the analysis of the order of sounds, as expressed by inability to determine which sound follows or precedes a given sound, may be clearly apparent even in relatively slight or latent forms of efferent motor aphasia. Because of this, the synthesis of a word from its individual sounds may be grossly impaired. In typical cases, the Russian word "k – o – t" (cat) is evaluated as "kto" (who) or "tok" (current).

Similar forms of defective phonetic analysis and synthesis are encountered in patients with *lesions of the left frontal and frontotemporal divisions*. Instability of phonetic traces is combined with difficulty in perceiving the correct order and serial organization of sounds. Gross mistakes in the evaluation of the position of sounds in a word and in the synthesis of a whole word from its component sounds may occur and are often associated with impulsive guesses at the meanings of presented series of sounds. This impulsive behavior is based on weakness of the inhibitory processes and inadequate verification of the results of the patient's own actions (Part II, Section 5E).

The possibility of serious defects in phonetic analysis and synthesis, even when hearing and articulating are completely preserved, must be borne in mind. For instance, position analysis and, in particular, synthesis of individual sounds may prove exceedingly difficult for patients with lesions of the *inferoparietal (or parietotemporal-occipital) divisions of the left hemisphere*. The impairment of simultaneous synthesis associated with these lesions may result in the patient's difficulty in "surveying" the whole system of presented sounds. Although such a patient may reveal no defects in phonemic hearing or articulation, he may have considerable difficulty evaluating the position of the sounds in a whole word or in assembling a consecutive series of sounds into a single structure capable of being perceived simultaneously. However, the disturbances associated with such cases are of a different nature and are manifested in a different syndrome.

C. INVESTIGATION OF WRITING

The investigation of writing is conducted with a series of tests designed to analyze the state of the various elementary components and levels of writing. It immediately follows the investigation of phonetic analysis and synthesis of words. It begins with the writing of individual letters, syllables, and words and it ends with the investigation of complex forms of written speech.

The examination starts with the copying of letters and words presented to the patient visually. This series of tests is especially important in the evaluation of visual-gnostic and motor disorders, and it yields significant results in cases where the dominant symptom is depression of activity associated with echopraxic actions. The purpose of these tests is to find out whether the patient can perceive a letter and how precisely, whether he can grasp the essential (i.e., having signal value) elements of words, whether, instead of true copying of letters, he substitutes a slavish reproduction of their strokes, and whether he has any difficulty with the actual movements of writing.

For these purposes the patient is asked to copy letters (words or syllables), in handwriting or printing and in ordinary or intricate scripts. To test the patient's powers of visual perception and motor reproduction, he is asked to copy suitable signs from a visual specimen. To test the stability of the memory traces left behind by an object, the method of "visual dictation" is used in which the written word is shown for only a short period (3 to 5 seconds) and the patient is asked to reproduce it from memory. In analyzing results in this test, the investigator should note the ease with which the patient performs the task; he should note whether instead of transcribing the letters, he simply draws them, e.g., a printed version is not translated into handwriting but is simply copied and the inessential details of an intricate script are reproduced with the same care and attention as the essential elements. Special attention must be paid to spatial distortion of letters, or elements drawn without the necessary connections between them or as mirror images. These signs of visual-spatial agraphia (Part II, Section 3E) must be noted with the same care as are the lack of fluency in copying movements and the presence of superfluous strokes and perseveratory movements, which indicate a disturbance in the motor sphere (Part II, Section 4D and E).

To determine the extent to which the patient's ability to perform the fine movements used in writing is preserved, the patient is asked to write a certain word that had been converted, long ago, into a motor stereotype, such as his own signature. In this test the investigator's attention is directed toward finding out whether the patient is still capable of executing complex kinetic melodies or whether the skilled writing movements are replaced by the isolated delineation of individual letters with signs of perseveration typically associated with *lesions of the premotor zone of the cortex*.

If none of these defects are present and if neither simple copying nor ordinary writing is disturbed, the investigation may be continued in the usual way. If the technique of writing individual letters is found to be wanting, the study takes another turn, with the examination of the more complex forms of writing assuming special forms. Words may be built up from the letters of a cut-out alphabet, so that the principal problem of discovering the correct letters and placing them together remains while the difficulties arising during the copying of letters are surmounted.

The first test of writing proper involves the writing of individual letters of the alphabet from dictation. This investigation may be carried out under different conditions, starting with the dictation of clear phonemes and ending with the dictation of imprecisely pronounced sounds, so that the patient has to recode the sound he has heard into a particular phoneme; difficulty in this recoding indicates defects in acoustic or acoustic-articulatory analysis and synthesis. In testing the writing of single letters from dictation, the investigator must rule out any possibility of visual presentation of the pronounced sound (for example, by covering the written specimen with a sheet of paper). Difficulty in writing the required letter under these conditions also may indicate defects of the acoustic analysis of the sound. The investigator must pay attention to both the character of the writing process (the patient may perform the task immediately or he may search for a long time for the required sign, invoking the aid of speaking aloud) and the difficulties encountered and mistakes made in the course of the test. Difficulty in finding the configuration of the required grapheme and mistakes in putting it on paper indicate disturbances of visual-spatial synthesis associated with a *lesion of the temporo-occipital or occipitoparietal cortical divisions* and are symptomatic of optic agraphia, or a disturbance in constructional spatial synthesis (Part II, Section 3E). Finally, we must consider the response to dictation of individual sounds (e.g., "t," "n") in which the patient does not distinguish the required phonemes precisely enough and in writing them adds the supplementary sound present in the syllable that it forms ("te," "ne"). These signs may be indicative of a defect in the mechanism responsible for precise acoustic analysis of the sounds of speech.

Next, the patient's performance in writing syllables and words from dictation is evaluated. Simple open and closed syllables (e.g., "pa," "ba," "ot," "an"), syllables with elision of the consonants (e.g., "cro," "pre," "sti"), phonetically simple and complicated words (e.g., "cat," "match," "district," "antarctic," "contemporary"), or, finally, complicated and unfamiliar words (e.g., "Popocatepetl," "hepaticogastrostomy") are dictated to the patient and he is asked to write them down. The difference between the first and second parts of the experiment lies in the nature of the analysis: Whereas in the first part the analysis is purely acoustic (or combined acoustic and articulatory), because of the meaningless combinations of sounds, during the dictation of words the memory images of the visual form of the written word, and sometimes firmly established engrams, can be called into play. Also, the patient can memorize words more easily than nonsense combinations and can therefore return to them time and time again to analyze their sounds. It follows that, although defects of acoustic analysis and synthesis are easily revealed by both tests, they are brought to light in a much purer form in the writing of meaningless sound combinations.

As in the preceding tests, the investigator may vary the conditions under which the dictated words are written. For instance, the patient can be permitted to articulate the presented words or syllables or can be prohibited from doing so. Or, he may be allowed to use the shape of the mouth during pronunciation of the sound as a guide, by observing the investigator or watching his own lip movements in a mirror. To investigate processes specific to the writing of syllables and words, associated with the discrimination of sounds from complex groups and retention of their proper order, the method of building syllables and words from cut-out letters may be used. In these cases we circumvent the difficulties involved in first searching out and then writing down a grapheme, so that the processes of analysis and synthesis of the phonetic components are tested in purer form.

In the course of these tests the investigator not only observes the quality of the patient's writing from dictation (whether he performs the task immediately or with the aid of preliminary articulation and gradual identification of the precise phonetic composition of the syllable or word) but also notes the distinguishing features of the actual writing process. In evaluating the results it is important to note mistakes in the phonetic composition of a word (omission or substitution of letters) and changes in the order of the letters in a word, which sometimes may be especially marked in experiments involving writing words from dictation. Other factors to be considered are signs of repetition of individual letters or syllables and the presence of superfluous strokes, which are particularly common during the writing of letters consisting of several similar elements (such as "u" and "w" or "n" and "m").

Whereas the first group of symptoms indicates a disturbance of combined acoustic and articulatory analysis and synthesis, the second group indicates pathological inertia in the central portions of the motor analyzer.

Tests involving the writing of syllables and words from dictation are followed by tests in which the patient writes series of words and phrases from dictation. The series of tests for repetition of word series or sentences (Part III, Section 8C) are repeated. The only difference is that this test involves the more complex recoding of spoken speech into writing so that additional difficulties arise in connection with the technique of writing. These more difficult conditions may easily lead to inability to retain the word order required by the instructions and to perseveration, which often arises as a result of disintegration of an established series of memory traces. This has been discussed previously. Hence, the defects that are conspicuously present with *frontal and frontotemporal lesions* (Part II, Section 5D–F) may be particularly obvious during the performance of this test.

The last group of tests in this series involves the investigation of the patient's written speech in the true meaning of this word. For this purpose, the patient is asked to write down the name of a particular object, to write down the answer to a question, or to write a statement conveying a particular meaning. These tests are basically similar to those used in the investigation of nominative and narrative speech (Part III, Section 9D and E). They not only require the preservation of the capacity for acoustic analysis and synthesis of words, but also the preservation of the capacity to plan for the selective character of what is written. The only way in which these processes differ from the processes involved in narrative speech is the specially constructed operations, outside the ordinary everyday pattern of events, required in writing; they are complicated by the necessity for maintaining a deliberate plan for a long period of time and for recoding internal speech into a system of written signs. This series of tests, which is of particular interest to the study of active forms of speech, goes beyond the bounds of the investigation of writing and is used for the study of complex forms of expanded speech activity.

The various forms of writing disorder have already been discussed in relation to the syndromes arising from different local lesions of the cerebral cortex. We need therefore return only briefly to these symptoms and confine our attention to a comparison of the writing defects characteristically found in association with lesions of various localizations.

Lesions of the left temporal region, accompanied by a *disturbance in phonemic hearing and sensory aphasia*, lead to the well-defined and distinctive disturbances of writing that were described (Part II, Section 2D). Although patients in this group are able to copy (and not merely mechanical copying of a text) and although well-established motor stereotypes (for example, the signature) are adequately preserved, they manifest gross disturbances in writing from dictation and in spontaneous writing. They are often unable to write single letters from dictation, and they struggle helplessly to identify the sound they have heard. Their difficulties are even greater when they attempt to write syllables, especially if the acoustic structure is complex. In these cases all attempts to distinguish the phonetic elements of the syllable are unavailing, and the imperfect articulations that the patient resorts to afford only negligible help.

Similar disturbances are revealed in the writing of words. As long as the patient sticks to very familiar words he may have some success, but even this usually amounts to no more than a few fragments of the word. The attempt to write a slightly less familiar word on the basis of its phonetic analysis is usually unsuccessful. In such cases we find: omission of sounds or substitution of sounds with closely related (and sometimes with different) phonetic properties, inability to distinguish individual sounds from a flow of consonants, transposition of sounds, etc. All this completes the picture of a typical writing disturbance in a patient with temporal (acoustic) aphasia and is difficult to confuse with other writing disturbances.

It is naturally quite impossible for these patients to write a series of words or phrases. During attempts to carry out this task, the patient may reveal not only the aforementioned disturbances, but also fragmentary reproduction of the words contained in the phrases or verbal paraphasia. Figure 29 illustrates this type of writing disturbance. The disturbance can be compensated for only after prolonged retraining based on the visual analysis of the appropriate articulations.

Different forms of writing disturbances may occur in patients with *lesions affecting the kinesthetic basis of speech*, which produce the syndrome of *afferent (kinesthetic) motor aphasia* (Part II, Section 4D). As was pointed out, it is often extremely difficult for these patients to write even single letters. The patient with severe articulatory defects cannot use this means to determine the exact nature of the sounds composing a word. If he tries to produce the sounds aloud, he frequently emits diffuse incorrect articulations, and these further hamper the process of writing. Such a patient may refuse to write down a sound pronounced by the investigator, will fail to distinguish the sounds forming a word, and will introduce articulatory substitutions (writing "d" instead of "n" or "l," "m" instead of "b," etc.) when these symptoms are encountered, it can be confidently concluded that the patient is suffering from a disturbance of the kinesthetic basis of the act of writing and these defects can be used to localize the lesion.

It is characteristic that the principal difficulties in writing experienced by a patient with afferent motor aphasia are manifested when he tries to identify the sound that he must write. For this reason, phenomena like the transposition of the letters in a word are not as typical of this group of patients as of patients with temporal or efferent motor aphasia. It is also characteristic that observation of the shape and movements of the mouth (for example, when writing with visual control of the articulations by means of a mirror) may be very helpful in compensating for the defect and may sometimes completely change the writing structure. Examples of this form of disturbance of writing are given in Figs. 58 and 59.

Obvious defects in writing may also be exhibited by patients with milder forms of these disturbances. The difference here is that gross forms of kinesthetic differentiation (for example, with the aid of speaking every sound aloud) may remain intact whereas differentiation based only on memory traces of kinesthetic impulses, as when writing in silence, are defective. That is why if external articulations are prohibited, writing disintegrates almost completely (Fig. 60).

Very different writing defects are exhibited by patients with *efferent (kinetic) motor aphasia*, arising from *lesions of the inferior portions of the premotor zone of the left hemisphere*. As has been described (Part II, Section 4F), these patients characteristically have no particular trouble finding the required letter (since the capacity for acoustic and kinesthetic sound analysis is intact) but do have trouble switching from one articulation to another, reflecting a disturbance in the maintenance of smooth kinetic melodies; they also manifest signs of marked inertia in the motor analyzer. These same defects are also obvious in writing: The patient can write letters dictated separately but cannot write a complex syllable or word. This is so because he cannot keep the letters in their necessary order and replaces the required series of letters by perseverative repetitions, a typical finding in patients with disturbances of this kind. Figure 63 clearly illustrates this type of writing defect.

Writing impairments accompanying lesions of the *occipital, occipitotemporal, and occipitoparietal divisions of the left hemisphere* are of a totally different nature. As stated (Part II, Section 3E), because the acoustic and articulatory basis of writing is intact, these patients can carry out the phonetic analysis and synthesis of words easily enough. Difficulties arise in another link—during the recoding of the identified phonemes into graphemes.

In some cases (according to the results of some investigations, when the lesion is mainly situated in the left occipitotemporal divisions), a patient who knows exactly what sound he has to write is unable to find the grapheme corresponding to this sound. The system of optic-acoustic connections is so unstable that often the sort of grapheme that the patient tries to write does not bear the remotest resemblance to the required letter. However, these cases of optic agraphia, described by Kaufman (1947) are relatively rare. It is much easier to find patients who have great difficulty selecting the necessary letter because of individual visual-spatial disturbances; the individual elements of a letter are placed in the wrong spatial relationships, letters are written as mirror images, etc. These defects are naturally seen both in copying and in writing from dictation, and this is valuable corroborative evidence for diagnostic localization. Examples of such disturbances are shown in Fig. 50.

All that I said above applies to languages written on the basis of acoustic and literal analysis (as is entirely the case with Russian, German, and Spanish and partly with French and English).

It is completely different with languages using hieroglyphic writing rather than analysis of sounds and letters. In these languages (e.g., Chinese) the characters denote actual concepts, and the stage of acoustic and literal analysis of the word is dispensed with. A lesion of the left temporal zone (the cortical apparatus of the audioverbal analyzer) in this case does not cause a disturbance of writing, whereas lesions of the occipito-parietal zones of the cortex (the cortical apparatus of visuospatial analysis) make the patient completely unable to write.

It is even more interesting in the case of languages that are written partly as sounds (syllables) and partly heiroglyphically. An example of this is Japanese, in which there are two systems of writing: syllabic (Katakana) and hieroglyphic (Kanji). In lesions of the temporal zones of the brain the former (Katakana) is disturbed, whereas the latter (Kanji) remains intact. The opposite situation is found in lesions of the parieto-occipital zones of the brain, in which the hieroglyphic system (Kanji) is disturbed whereas the acoustic, syllabic form (Katakana) remains intact. Several papers confirming this state of affairs have been published in the last decade.

It now only remains to consider briefly the writing defects found in patients with *lesions of the frontal divisions of the brain*. Usually the defects are not primarily writing disorders, and they are therefore not specific. However, all the various forms of disintegration of the higher mental functions arising in the frontal syndrome are clearly reflected in the act of writing.

The considerable inertia of these patients and the ease with which they become fatigued may lead to a sharp loss of tone in the motor analyzer and, in turn, to the phenomena of "initial writing" and "micrographia." The patient, having started to write the required word, either comes to an abrupt halt or writes progressively smaller and smaller letters with the end of the word completely illegible. The inertia and weakness of the regulatory role of the plan or intention characteristic of patients with frontal syndromes (Part II, Section 5) are usually also reflected in their writing. Because of the loss of the over-all plan, the patient is often quite unable to perform the test; perseverations are much in evidence, making the script unintelligible. Even when the writing of single words causes no particular difficulty, as soon as the patient attempts to put his thoughts to paper these defects are clearly revealed. When he starts to write a letter, the patient keeps repeating the first phrase over and over again, so that it finally reads something like the following: "Dear Professor, I want to tell you that I want to tell you to tell you . . ." and so on. This is typical of these forms of disturbance of active mental function. However, these defects lie outside the scope of writing disturbances in the strict sense of the term and must be approached in a different context.

D. INVESTIGATION OF READING

Together with the investigation of writing, the investigation of reading constitutes one of the more important aspects of the study of the state of cortical functioning and it is of great importance in the localization of focal lesions.

As has been pointed out, the reading process runs counter to the writing process. Whereas in writing the thought leads to the phonetic analysis of a word, which in turn leads to construction of a grapheme, reading starts with the visual perception and analysis of a grapheme, passes on to the recoding of graphemes into the corresponding phonetic structures, and ends with comprehension of the meaning of what has been written. The fundamental distinguishing feature of reading, as already indicated, is the vast differences in its operational composition in the various developmental stages. Although in the initial stages reading is a piecemeal activity, incorporating all the enumerated operations, in the later stages it is transformed into a direct, highly automatized process, making hardly any use of phonetic analysis and synthesis and based on the direct recognition of the meaning of written words and sometimes of whole phrases.

The investigation of the reading skill is preceded by *preliminary examination* of visual acuity, range, and movement (Part III, Section 6A). Insofar as these tests rely on reading, they also serve to give us some preliminary information on the state of the reading skill (for example, forming words from cut-out letters or analyzing one's own writing). The *actual investigation* of reading begins with the analysis of the perception of letters and continues with experiments to determine the ability to read words and, finally, to read texts. As a rule, the testing method takes two forms: reading aloud (i.e., with the reader reciting) and internal reading (i.e., the reader reading to himself). In internal reading, recitation is excluded, and the patient has to grasp the meaning of a presented word directly and indicate his conclusion either by pointing to the appropriate picture or answering a question. As in the investigation of writing, reading tests may be made more difficult by shortening the time of exposure to the material or by making the material itself more complicated and may be made easier by the use of measures designed to help the patient sidestep the obstacles in his way. The various phases of the investigation will be examined separately.

The investigation of reading begins with a test for evaluating the *recognition of individual letters*. The patient is shown a series of isolated letters, either printed or written freehand, and he is asked either to name them or (if this is difficult because of speech defects) to point to the same letter written in a different script. Sometimes, in order to make sure that the patient has, in fact, perceived a particular letter, he is asked to give a word with which this letter is customarily associated (for example, if shown the letters "b," "j," and "s" he has to say which stands for "John," "Sue," or "Betty"). To uncover defects of visual recognition of letters, some are written in an intricate script, some appear as mirror images (which calls for recognition of the correctly written letter), or some are hatched over with additional lines (which makes the visual identification of the latter against the background more difficult). To simplify the process of recognition of a letter, the patient may be permitted to trace its outline with his finger, to analyze it by copying it, or to feel its shape when cut out of suitable material.

In this experiment the investigator must note whether the patient recognizes a particular letter at once and must observe the character of any difficulties that may arise. The latter is easily done by comparing the results obtained when different types of delineation of the same letter are presented with the performance during successive introductions of visual difficulties. Signs of literal visual agnosia, associated with a *lesion of the occipital lobes of the brain*, are clearly demonstrated by this experiment.

The principal phase of the investigation comprises experiments involving the *reading of syllables and words*. As a first step in the investigation of analytic-synthetic reading, the patient is asked to read a series of simple and complex syllables ("po," "cor," "an," "os" or "tro," "cra," "stro"). The investigator keeps a careful watch on the manner in which the patient reads these syllables to detect any narrowing of visual perception involving, at the least, a single letter; if such constriction has occurred, the patient cannot perceive the whole group at once. If the patient perceives the whole group quite well, the investigator must be alert to possible difficulties in recoding it into a system of sounds or in finding the proper sounds and combining them into syllables. Particular attention must be paid to the rendering of a meaningless combination of letters as a word with a meaning (for example, reading "prot" as "port"), for this symptom suggests the presence of a profound disturbance in the analytic-synthetic process of reading, extending beyond the limits of specialized defects of optic gnosis.

The next step is concerned with the *reading of whole words*. For this purpose, the patient is asked to read simple and familiar words ("Moscow," "truth," "bread,") or less familiar words with a more complex meaning ("bonfire," "cloakroom," "fertilizer"). A special place is occupied by the reading of words that have become so firmly established that they have been transformed into directly perceived ideograms (the patient's given name or surname, USA, USSR) and of words with a highly complex structure (insubordination, indistinguishable) or that are totally unfamiliar ("astrocytoma," "hemopoiesis").

As was pointed out, this experiment may be carried out with the patient either reading aloud or to himself. The investigator may find it appropriate to allow the patient to point to a pictorial representation of what he has read; or, the investigator may want to gage the patient's response to questions, orally posed, about the meaning of the word. In a sensitive variant of this test the patient is shown words rendered in letters of different styles or words on which additional lines are superimposed. Since the optic conditions for recognition of the word are thus made more difficult, latent defects in visual perception may be brought to light. In other sensitive versions a word is presented for a very short period of time (for example, in a tachistoscope or by covering it with the hand immediately upon presentation). These experiments preclude eye movements and thus may uncover a narrowing of visual attention or signs of simultaneous agnosia. A special variant is devoted to the patient's discernment of incorrectly written words: The patient must find the mistake in a word in which certain letters have been omitted or transposed but which is still recognizable.

The investigator must be particularly careful to distinguish between true reading of a word and its direct recognition by total impact. In true reading, the patient pronounces the word easily and sometimes recognizes and corrects his mistakes but often delays saying it because of articulatory difficulties. In direct recognition, the patient understands the meaning of a word and can write it down correctly or point to a corresponding illustration, but he cannot pronounce the word or any part of it or, still less, discover any mistake made in his writing of it. The reading of unfamiliar words is naturally quite impossible in such cases. This distinction between true analytic-synthetic reading and the direct ideographic recognition of a word may be of great diagnostic importance.

During the investigation of word reading serious attention must be paid to all symptoms indicative of a breakdown in simultaneous perception of the whole visual word structure, especially to the narrowing of word perception to one or two letters. Such is the case if the patient is unable to perceive the whole word at once but is obliged to put even the simplest words together letter by letter. The syndrome indicates a *lesion of the parieto-occipital divisions* of the brain and is among the most valuable of diagnostic signs.

The investigation of reading ends with *the reading of phrases and a whole text*. At first, the patient is asked to read aloud a whole phrase consisting of a few words. In order to assess the patient's capacity for true reading of a phrase, and to discern whether or not it is replaced by guesses at the meaning, the patient is given a sentence not conforming to its anticipated meaning (for example, "my leg aches very much" [instead of "head"] or "I am lying in Ward Eight" [instead of nine]). When the process of true reading is insufficiently stable and is easily replaced by impulsive, guesswork reading, accurate reading of phrases becomes impossible.

In the second part of this investigation the patient is asked to read a three-line passage from a clearly printed text. In the course of this test the investigator must be particularly sensitive to the quality of the patient's eye movements as he scans the lines and should also note the ease with which he moves from one line to the next. It is especially important to note the cases where the patient can easily read separate words but cannot read a continuous text, for this may mean that he loses his place in text and therefore picks out odd words at random. These disturbances, frequently found in cases of *simultaneous agnosia and optic ataxia* (Part II, Section 3C), should be carefully recorded.

A patient's disregard of half (usually the left half) of a text is another important finding, for it is indicative of left, fixed hemianopsia (Part III, Section 6A). Such a patient begins reading in the middle of the line instead of at the beginning and reads only the part of the text that lies in the right visual field, often exclaiming that the text, which he only partially perceives, does not make sense. There are also cases in which the patient starts to read a text fairly well but then suddenly changes to guessing reading and, in fact, interjects uncontrolled and irrelevant associations. Findings such as these, together with other signs of loss of selectivity of action, may frequently be encountered in patients with a *marked frontal syndrome*.

A disturbance in the reading of letters and words—literal and verbal alexia—has for a long time been regarded as a visual disorder and classed among the symptoms of a lesion in the occipital lobes of the brain. This is still true in the sense that primary reading disturbances are, in fact, associated with defective visual analysis and synthesis. However, to class alexia simply as a visual disorder and to claim that it can only develop in patients with a lesion of the occipital lobes, would be to ignore the vast complexity and the myriad manifestations of these disturbances. *Optic alexia*, constituting the principal form of reading disorder in patients with *lesions of the occipital divisions* of the brain, may occur in two main variants. In cases of *literal alexia*, the integrated perception of graphemes and the visual differentiation of those of their signs with cue value are so disrupted that either the letters lose their meaning altogether, or their identification becomes highly unstable. Letters that are similar in outline are confused ("m" is read as "n," "k" as "x," etc.). In latent forms of this disturbance the patient continues to recognize clearly printed letters, but a letter written in an ornate hand, or a crossed-out one, or one contained in a syllable can no longer be analyzed or, ultimately, distinguished. Since this condition is a variant of optic agnosia (associated here with the functional system of speech), tracing the outline of the letter with the finger may sometimes considerably help the patient identify it. This was originally pointed out by Gelb and Goldstein (1920). It constitutes the diagnostic and rehabilitative basis for patients with these disorders.

The second form of an optic defect in reading is the widely known condition of *verbal alexia.* Patients with this disturbance may easily recognize individual letters but they cannot grasp whole words; when confronted with whole words, they must resort to putting them together letter by letter before they are able to identify them. Characteristically, familiar, as well as relatively unfamiliar, words cannot be usually recognized. Even words so closely resembling ideograms as the patient's surname or symbols like "USA" are not perceived; the most the patient can do is decipher them slowly, letter by letter. Verbal alexia is itself a variant of simultaneous agnosia primarily associated with the speech system (Part II, Section 3C). This defect is based on the unique phenomenon of a pathological narrowing of visual perception, in which the capacity of the weakened visual cortex becomes so limited that it can deal with one point of excitation at a time. Verbal alexia is often found in conjunction with characteristic signs of a disturbance in gaze, in which the patient easily loses the line and picks out individual elements from a word and individual fragments from different lines. Some of the mechanisms of this association between simultaneous agnosia and optic ataxia were previously enumerated (Part II, Section 3C and D).

A special form of reading disorder is the condition known as left, fixed hemianopsia, whose distinguishing feature, as already noted, is loss of the left field of vision. Furthermore, the patient is not aware of his defect and therefore makes no attempt to compensate for it; such a patient may ignore the entire left side of a text presented to him and may regard the entire text as meaningless. In some patients this phenomenon also arises during the reading of individual words, i.e., the patient perceives only the right half of the word and can only guess at the meaning of the whole word. The testing of such a patient can be made quite specific: If the patient has no difficulty reading a word arranged vertically, the presence of hemianopsia is corroborated. The syndrome is usually found with *lesions of the parieto-occipital (or temporoparietal-occipital) divisions* of the brain, particularly when both hemispheres are implicated.

These forms of optic alexia greatly differ from *reading disturbances resulting from speech disorders*; in the latter forms the alexia may be regarded as an offshoot of more widespread aphasic disorders. Among these cases are, first, *reading disturbances accompanied by manifestations of sensory aphasia*; these ensue from *lesions of the left temporal region*. The nature of the reading disturbances in such cases is very distinctive. A patient with this form of alexia easily perceives and recognizes the meaning of whole, well-established words. Quite apart from the aforementioned optic ideograms, these patients have no difficulty recognizing the import of such words as "Moscow," "Pravda," "London," "Volga." The paradoxical feature is that the patient recognizes the meaning of these words at sight but is unable to read them aloud or even to read individual segments or letters of which they are composed. This amounts to the fact that the aptitude for direct recognition of familiar words is preserved but that complex processes of phonetic and literal analysis are severely hampered. Therefore, despite easy recognition of familiar words deprivation of the support of their phonetic values renders less familiar words meaningless—as nothing more than a series of signs. Examples of this type of reading disturbance are given in Fig. 133. In latent forms of temporal aphasia the recognition of individual words may be intact but the process of consecutive reading of whole sentences and, more especially, the process of analyzing the phonetic and literal content of a word may be profoundly disturbed. It stands to reason that in these patients reading aloud is more vulnerable than simple visual recognition of words.

Reading disturbances occurring in association with a defect in the kinesthetic basis of the speech act leading to afferent (kinesthetic) motor aphasia, are similar in nature to the preceding forms but differ essentially in details. As in cases of sensory aphasia, the direct recognition of well-established words may not be affected; however, the true analytic-synthetic process of reading is severely deranged. This disturbance often assumes other guises. For instance, when vainly trying to execute a necessary articulation with the required precision, such a patient frequently complicates the recognizing process. As was pointed out, the articulation of the palatoglossal "l" as "d" or of the labial "b" as "m" may cause the patient to read "Nina" as "Dina," "guba" as "guma," "babushka" as "mamushka," etc. Similar and still more marked defects arise when these patients attempt to read isolated words. An example of this form of reading disturbance is given in Fig. 134.

Patients with efferent (kinetic) motor aphasia evince different reading disturbances from those just described, the main difference residing in the fact that patients with kinetic motor aphasia can recognize, and sometimes pronounce, individual letters without difficulty but are confounded by the simplest fusion of letter sounds into syllables. The patient cannot modify the initial sound of a particular phoneme to conform to its position in a syllable and usually cannot elide sounds to form a syllable but, instead continues to read the syllable as a series of separate letters. However, contrary to simultaneous agnosia and verbal alexia, this defect is not due to

PHONETIC READING:

a	s	m	n	(bread) khleb	(palm) kist'
А	С	М	Н	ХЛЕБ	КИСТЬ
"a"	Gives up	"S?"	Gives up	"Les?" "No. I didn't recognize it"	"No. I don't know"

IDEOGRAPHIC READING:

Afonin (Patient's surname)	Sasha (Another name)
АФОНИН	САША
Recognized at once	+

Patient Af. Lesion of the left temporal region. Sensory aphasia.

PHONETIC READING:

o	s	(crack) tresk
О	С	ТРЕСК
"I don't know"	"This isn't a sound"	"No, I don't know. Certainly not"

IDEOGRAPHIC READING:

London	Volga
ЛОНДОН	ВОЛГА
"I know...I know...A town... A large town... The first city..."	"A large waterway... Our own river... Volga...ours... The first!..."

Patient L. Lesion of the left temporal region.

FIGURE 133 Reading disturbances in two patients with sensory aphasia, due to gunshot wounds of the left temporal regions.

the optic constriction of the field reading. Rather, its mechanism is associated with a breakdown in kinetic synthesis, found to some degree with all lesions of the premotor cortex (Part II, Section 4E) but manifested here in the functional system of speech. It is because of such defects that the reading of whole words is particularly disturbed. Although the patient can perceive the whole word letter by letter, he cannot perform the necessary kinetic syntheses; he very often abandons this impossible task and substitutes guesses at the meaning of words, on the basis of individual fragments, for true reading. An example of this form of reading disturbance is given in Fig. 135.

In these patients, the changeover to guesswork reading is perhaps induced by the difficulties encountered in joining the letter sounds into syllables. With

OPTIC RECOGNITION OF GRAPHEMES:

(Patient underlines identical letters, missing two lower-case d's in the first line) — Д Р D х g м н м ∂ в / Г р н г п п Б Т з т

READING LETTERS ALOUD:	sh	r	l
	Ш	Р	Л
	"o...s...no"	"s, no, r"	"t...t...s... l...n...l"

RECOGNITION OF LETTERS:	d	p
	Д	П
	"Is it m? No... k? No. r? No. d? e...e... (I'm not sure)."	"Is it s? No. Is it v? No. I don't know. (I'm not sure)...Is it m? Yes...No (I'm not sure). Is it p? p...yes...it's p (I'm not sure)."

READING WORDS:	(fly)	(skis)	(duck)	(cat)
	mukha	lyzhi	utka	kot
	МУХА	ЛЫЖИ	УТКА	КОТ
	Gives up	Gives up	Gives up	kon'ki (skates)?

	(a name)	(field)	(cart)
	Nina	pole	telega
	НИНА	ПОЛЕ	ТЕЛЕГА
	"Di-na, Ni-na. Ti-na."	"mu...mu... li?"	"Te...le...kha... te...nika (I don't understand). Te... ni...kha (I'm not sure)."

READING LETTERS:	b	l	t
	Б	Л	Т
	"I don't know...is it m? I don't know. Is it s? Don't know. Is it v? d? Don't know."	"p...n... s...l!"	"s...m...t"

READING WORDS:	(lip)	(sieve)	(grandmother)
	guba	sito	babushka
	ГУБА	СИТО	БАБУШКА
	"Gu...ma... guma?"	"S...si... lo...silo?... Si...l...l... silo?!"	"Ma...mushka?... Ma...bushka... babushka?..."

FIGURE 134 Reading disturbances in a patient (Patient G.) with afferent motor aphasia due to a gunshot wound of the left postcentral region.

lesions of the frontal lobes it may be a byproduct of the fundamental defect—derangement of the selective character of all speech-regulated processes and failure to compare the result of an action with the original plan, an important

READING LETTERS: No Difficulty

	ro	ko	so	pro
READING SYLLABLES:	РО	КО	СО	ПРО
	"R...o... together? rogo"	"K...no no...k...o"	"S...to? s...t... o?"	"P...r...o... together? poroda (breed)?"

	(onion)	(snow)	(window)
	luk	sneg	okno
READING WORDS:	ЛУК	СНЕГ	ОКНО
	"L, u, k, together? I don't know"	Gives up	"Kino (movies)? okino?"

(carp)	(Mitya has a puppy)
karas'	u Miti shchenok
КАРАСЬ	У МИТИ ЩЕНОК
"Ka...r...a...s. Together? Krasnyi (red)?"	"U mamy shchuka (mother has a pike)..."

FIGURE 135 Reading disturbances in a patient (Patient Kh.) with efferent motor aphasia due to a gunshot wound of the inferior divisions of the left premotor region.

precondition for the performance of a goal-directed act. It is on account of this defect that the reading of a text may be transformed into an uncontrollable pattern of guesses, random associations, and perseverations. However expressed, this defect is not the activity of reading in the narrow sense of the term so that disturbed reading must be regarded as one manifestation of a more generalized disorder.

• • •

In describing the individual forms of writing and reading disturbances that are present with different speech disorders and in stressing the dominant signs for each case, we deliberately undertook to describe them rather schematically, a policy which is justifiable on didactic grounds. It should be remembered, however, that all these forms of writing and reading disturbance are manifestations of a disturbance of the functional system of speech as a whole; in dealing with the disturbances of writing and reading associated with various forms of aphasia, these primary symptoms are in actual practice most frequently found in a complex and not in a pure form. Therefore, the investigator analyzing speech, writing, and reading disturbances must always be prepared to encounter the basic symptoms specified herein in various combinations. The differentiation of the dominant signs and their correct topical interpretation will depend on the skill and experience which the investigator brings to bear on the analysis of the syndrome as a whole. At the same time, it should be mentioned that the character of the symptoms observed is largely dependent both on the differing level of the premorbid development of skilled activity (speech, writing, and reading) and on the differing structure of the writing and reading functions in patients with different degrees of automatization of these processes; since the psychophysiological makeup thus varies from case to case, this variation is inevitably reflected in the symptoms as they arise.

Finally, it should be remembered that these processes may be sharply modified by the fatigue developing in the course of the examination and that their course may differ with changes in the general tone of cortical activity. Hence, while maintaining a systematic approach to the analysis of the symptoms, attention must be paid to the neurodynamic conditions appertaining to the processes under investigation, for they leave their imprint on the clinical symptomatology.

11. *Investigation of Arithmetical Skill*

A. PRELIMINARY REMARKS

The investigation of arithmetical skill comprises part of the basic program for studying disturbances of higher mental processes in the presence of local brain lesions, for it may shed light on certain important aspects of these disturbances. The reason for this is that arithmetical operations are based on spatial relationships that, in the early stages of mathematical development, were expressed in three-dimensional form in surveying and mensuration. Mathematics only gradually acquired the character of abstract, symbolic processes; despite this fact, however, it maintained its genetic connection with these spatial operations. These special features are evident during the analysis of the psychological processes underlying the ideal of number and arithmetical operations and may easily be studied by examining their formation in childhood. The work of Piaget (1950), Ingel'der (1960), Gal'perin (1959), Talyzina (1957), Davydov (1957), Nepomnyashchaya (1956), and others has shed new light on the stages through which the preschool child passes in developing number concepts, starting with material operations with objects arranged in space, passing through a phase of actions "materialized" with the hand and gaze, and ending with the formation of tabular calculation, the basis of the true concept of number and of the mental activities fundamental to fully developed arithmetical operations.

The notion of number always rests, to a greater or lesser extent, on some system of spatial coordinates, which may be linear in character or arranged in a tabular system. On this spatial grid the complex system of relationships determined by the decimal system is erected, and it thus provides the true basis of the concept of number and of the operations carried out with its use. It follows that this fundamental feature may be applied to the analysis of arithmetical operations.

During addition (14 + 3) or of the symmetrical but opposite operation of subtraction (14 − 3), we always act within a definite internal spatial field. If this operation necessitates carrying over from units to tens or vice versa (for example, 31 − 4 or 28 + 5), the process becomes incomparably more complex. Although it retains its spatial organization, it begins to operate within the framework of a system of graded categories; this adds considerably to the difficulty of the mnestic tasks confronting the person carrying out this operation. The person performing the arithmetical operation must break up the number concerned in order to make it possible to carry out the operation within a single series of ten; only when this has been done can he proceed with the second part of the operation—adding on the remainder. Initially, this operation is inevitably performed stage by stage—breaking up the numbers concerned and subsequently adding the remainder while maintaining the correct spatial orientation of the operation. Not until later stages do these operations take on a shortened, direct character; finally, an experienced person performs them automatically.

Although they are based on spatially oriented schemes, the different arithmetical operations differ in the degree to which they retain their association with such schemes. Whereas simple addition and subtraction exhibit this association to the full extent, the simple operations of multiplication and division, based on the multiplication table learned at school, begin to acquire a verbal character and to rest on established verbal stereotypes. The spatial components are relegated to the background and now become obvious only when the process is made more complex and ceases to be automatic in character. This arises, for example, if a number containing one digit is multiplied by one containing two digits (still more, if both contain two digits) and in most of the nonautomatized operations of division.

These preliminary remarks concerning the psychological features of the idea of number and of arithmetical operations will serve as the starting point for the subsequent analysis of disturbances of these operations. These matters have been examined in greater detail by the author elsewhere (1945) and by Rudenko (1953).

B. INVESTIGATION OF THE COMPREHENSION OF NUMBER STRUCTURE

The objective of the investigation of the comprehension of the structure of numbers in patients with local brain lesions is to discover to what extent their complex categorial structure is appreciated.

The investigation begins with experiments in which the patient is asked to write down or to read *numbers of one digit*. Provided that the patient's speech processes are adequate, he can do this by simply repeating what has been dictated. If the speech processes are impaired, the patient may be asked to write the numeral denoting the number of fingers shown to him or he may be shown a numeral and asked to point out how many fingers (or matches) it represents. If the patient has difficulty in writing or reading isolated figures, a natural series of numbers (1, 2, 3, 4 . . .) may be dictated to him (or given to him in writing) for him to write or read. During this experiment the investigator must analyze the patient's difficulties: Does he have difficulty in understanding the verbal name given to a number, or in writing the figures down, or, finally, in visually recognizing the figures shown to him.

A special and fundamental aspect of the investigation is the writing and reading of Roman numerals. These, of course, incorporate the spatial arrangement of elements, with the value of the number determined by its composition, and thus provide a very convenient means of examining the extent to which the patient is spatially oriented. For this purpose, the patient is asked to write or read visually complementary numbers such as IV and VI or IX and XI. Of equal significance is the task of specifying complementary Arabic numbers (17 and 71, 69 and 96). Spatial disorientation is clearly revealed by this test.

A vital part of this investigative phase is taken by experiments involving the writing and reading of *more than one-digit numbers*. The central objective of these experiments is to uncover the extent to which the categorical structure of number is comprehended. A series of upgraded tests, starting with simple ones in which the patient has to write (or read out) numbers with two or more digits and ending with more complicated variants, serves this purpose. First, the patient is asked to write (or read out) simple numbers (27, 34, 158, 396, etc.). Special consideration is given to numbers that are not written the way they are spoken, for example, two-digit numbers whose units digit precedes the tens digit in Russian and English, (e.g., 14, 17, 19). Also included are multidigit numbers in which some digits have the value of zero and, consequently, are not spoken (e.g., 109, 1023). In such instances the number must be recoded from its spoken form into the system of categorical names, and any distortion in perception of the firmly established categorical structure of number may lead to the echolalic writing of a spoken number (17 as 71, 104 as 100 and 4, 1023 as 1000 and 23 or 123, etc.).

Similarly, this experiment can be made more difficult by presenting multidigit numbers whose digits are arranged in an unusual manner. For instance, the patient may be forewarned that a number composed of several digits will be presented vertically. The number 326, for example, may be presented as

3
2
6

There is no room in this experiment for habitual stereotypes, and the patient is forced to show openly and purely by consciously applying the categorical scheme to the numbers arranged in this unusual way his appreciation of the categorical structure of number. The most important test in this experiment is the one in which the patient has to identify each category—the thousands, the hundreds, the tens, and the units—of a multidigit number written horizontally or vertically, either by calling each out consecutively or in response to the examiner's pointing to a particular digit. Failure to recognize the categorical structure of a number or the disintegration of their nominative value into a series of individual digital signs constitute important diagnostic signs.

The last part of the investigation consists of an experiment to evaluate the patient's ability to grasp the numerical difference between multidigit numbers. Its objective is to establish whether the assessment of the numerical value of multidigit numbers continues to take place in terms of the categorical structure or whether this gives way to direct evaluation of the component digits. For this purpose, the patient is first asked to state which of two stated or written numbers (e.g., 17 and 68, 23 and 56, 123 and 489) is larger. Then an element of conflict is introduced whereby the numerically smaller number of a pair contains higher digits in all categories below the highest (e.g., 189 and 201, 1967 and 3002). Any difficulty in the assessment of the over-all value of the written number or any tendency to be guided by the individual digits composing it may constitute additional evidence that categorical comprehension of number has disintegrated.

The analysis of the results obtained during investigation of ideas of number in patients with local brain lesions is not particularly difficult. When one-digit numbers are not easily identified, certain specific basic defects may be present. In some cases, this symptom arises from *extinction of the direct meaning of words*, such as occurs in *sensory aphasia*. Such a patient, although unable to understand a number when pronounced, can readily recognize it when written and can easily perform operations with it. In other cases, the symptom may be based on the phenomena of *optic alexia and agraphia* contributing to an *occipital syndrome*. Such a patient can neither write nor read out a written number but can indicate comparatively easily how many fingers correspond to a given number or can call out the number of fingers shown to him.

The specific distinctive features of miscomprehension of the categorical structure of number comes to light clearly in the *syndrome of visual-spatial disorders* arising in patients with *lesions of the inferoparietal and parietal and parieto-occipital divisions* of the cerebral cortex (predominantly of the left hemisphere) in which manifestations of *constructive apraxia and semantic aphasia* are present. Disturbances in the ability to comprehend the structure of number become apparent during tests involving the recognition and writing of Roman numbers. A patient who cannot differentiate between right and left cannot distinguish between symmetrically written (i.e., visually complementary) numbers and, consequently, confuses such numbers when writing them. The evaluation of numbers composed of several digits makes these disturbances even more apparent, for the categorical significance of number is then disregarded; the patient omits the categories not referred to by name when writing numbers, cannot read out a multidigit number, and gives wrong categorical values to individual digits.

In the most severe cases these defects may be apparent even during relatively simple tests. Latent cases, on the other hand, may require tests of greater sensitivity to be detected, such as asking the patient to read out numbers written vertically and to evaluate their categories. Marked deficiencies in the evaluation of multidigit numbers may also appear in these patients. A number of this type composed of high-value subsidiary digits (e.g., 1869) is frequently stated to be larger than a number composed of low-value subsidiary digits (e.g., 2012). All these disturbances are usually combined into one syndrome, as has been described (Part II, Section 3D-F), that presents no localizing difficulties.

A disturbance of the complex system of numerical concepts may also occur in patients with *lesions of the frontal lobes*, but in these cases it comprises part of the general syndrome of inactivity and loss of spontaneity. It may take the form of echopraxis in the writing and reading of numbers whose names do not coincide with their categorical structure, but these mistakes, such as writing 17 as 71 or 1023 as 1000 23, have nothing to do with a disturbance of the categorical comprehension of number and therefore do not form part of the syndrome under discussion.

C. INVESTIGATION OF ARITHMETICAL OPERATIONS

The investigation of arithmetical operations directly follows that comprehension of number structure. Its objective is to study the patient's ability to utilize the categorical structure of number for the performance of various arithmetical operations.

The investigation of arithmetical operations includes a series of tests of varying complexity that reflect processes taking place at different levels. In the simplest of these (for example, addition or subtraction of single digits or the very similar operation of addition by columns), the arithmetical operations comprise nothing more than well-established skills and relatively simple processes. With addition and subtraction outside the range of ten, which require intermediate operations (breaking up the numbers to be added into groups, operations with round numbers, and subsequent addition of the remainder), the process is much more complex in character. In still more complicated operations (addition or subtraction of multidigit numbers with repeated carrying over into the next column, compound multiplication and division carried out mentally) the process becomes even more difficult, for the proportion of the operations undertaken at the mnestic level is further increased. Finally, this process reaches its maximal complexity in operations involving fractions, in which the visual components are relegated to the background and the core of the operation is composed of abstract, verbal-logical operations.

The investigation of arithmetical operations begins with tests of *simple, automatized calculations*, such as multiplying on the basis of the multiplication table and adding and subtracting numbers no higher than ten. The patient must carry out these operations orally or in writing; however, if speech disturbances are present the result of these simple operations may be indicated by the fingers. Tests involving simple, well-established arithmetical operations can usually be used only to detect the severest forms of aphasic disorders and the most marked conceptual disintegration of number, associated with particularly massive lesions. Therefore, experiments comprising complex arithmetical operations occupy a central place in this investigation. In this phase, the patient is asked to do mental addition and subtraction involving carrying over from units to tens or vice versa (for example, 27 + 8; 31 − 7; 41 − 14). The patient is asked to carry out the operation aloud, reciting all parts of the process.

In control experiments the operation may be made more difficult. For example, the patient may be asked to perform an arithmetical operation solely mentally, giving only the answer. Or, it may be made easier by allowing the patient to arrive at a solution in writing. To facilitate assessment of the results, this operation of written calculation is requested in two forms: first, horizontally, which, although not requiring mental retention of all the elements, necessitates intermediate mental operations; second, vertically, which removes all mnestic conditions and reduces the whole operation to addition and subtraction of single digits with the automatic achievement of a more complex final result. The investigator must carefully watch how the operation is being performed, noting whether the categorical structure of number is appreciated, whether mistakes in the spatial organization are made, whether certain stages of the process are omitted, and, finally, whether written or verbal aids are invoked and, if so, to what extent.

To specially study the extent to which the patient continues to carry out arithmetical operations firmly within the system of the categorical structure of number, the same tests may be applied in a more complicated form. The patient may be given adding and subtracting tasks in which the numbers are not arranged in the usual, established form, but either as vertically arranged groups (A) or (for subtraction) in such a way that the number to be taken away is placed above the first number (B).

A	B
1	
7	18
+ 2	− 24
4	

Categorical impairment is obvious if the operation disintegrates into addition of digits from different columns or subtraction of the smaller digit from the larger one irrespective of its position, for this occurs when well-established stereotypes no longer come to the fore. To make a special study of the degree to which arithmetical operations are carried out at the conscious level, tests are used that evaluate the patient's attitude toward the arithmetical sign, or awareness of the nature of the operation. The patient is shown mathematical examples that include the answer but omit the sign (such as 10 . . . 2 = 8; 10 . . . 2 = 5; 10 . . . 2 = 12; 10 . . . 2 = 20) or include the sign but omit one number (such as 12 − . . . = 8; 12 + . . . = 16) and the patient has to fill in the missing item. These tests rule out the possibility of automatized performance, for they demand conscious awareness of the type of operation to be performed and of its component parts. Dissociation, characterized by the ability to perform practical operations (as revealed in prior tests) but inability to realize what is being performed, is an important symptom for the defining of the patients intellectual defects.

Serial arithmetical operations occupy a special place in the investigation of arithmetical operations, for these tests are used when it is necessary to determine whether the patient retains sufficiently stable traces of the various operative stages, or whether the performance is hindered by perseveration. For this purpose, three components (such as 12 + 9 − 6 or 32 − 4 + 9) are used, requiring the memorized retention of part of the operation. Any mnestic impairment will result in inhibition of the last part of the operation by the first part. Having completed the first part, the patient repeats, "12 + 6 = 18 . . . and then what?" or perseverates the last figure of the given example.

There is one variant which has become very important for the diagnosis of many cases. This is the performance of a series of consecutive arithmetical operations, for example counting backward from 100 in 7's or in 13's. This test makes particularly high demands on the mobility of the nervous processes at the level of the second signal system. Having done the subtraction, the patient must immediately convert the difference into the starting point for further subtraction and repeat this process over and over again. All these operations must be carried out by memory traces, with constant carrying over from tens to units and intermediate breaking down of numbers, addition of remainders, and so on.

For many patients, even if the categorical structure of the numbers is fully comprehended, this operation is impossible because it requires great stability, high selectivity, and mobility of the processes concerned. A patient with categorical comprehension begins the operation correctly but soon ceases to cope with it adequately, omitting certain stages or substituting perseveration of one operation (100–93–83–73–63 . . .) for true calculation. As we shall see below, this type of response is especially characteristic of patients whose higher nervous processes are inactive and inert.

Primary arithmetical disturbances or manifestations of *primary acalculia* occur in patients with *lesions of the left inferoparietal (or parieto-occipital) divisions*. In these patients, disintegration of visual-spatial synthesis may directly lead to marked arithmetical malfunctioning. The categorical structure of number easily loses its significance and the patient begins to have great difficulty in performing calculations.

Even those lesions of the parieto-occipital systems giving rise to comparatively few clinical manifestations become so unstable that they cause disintegration of precise, categorically organized arithmetical operations at the introduction of even a slight complication. This is so because processes requiring a firmly established system of categories have lost all stability. The patient loses proper control over the intermediate calculations, is unable to retain the integrated whole in the course of the arithmetical operation, and readily transforms the operation into a series of isolated fragments. Since the syndrome of primary acalculia has already been described in detail (Part II, Section 3G), it will not receive further consideration here.

Other local brain lesions may give rise to secondary arithmetical disturbances. Patients with *lesions of the left temporal region* and a syndrome of *acoustic aphasia* may still be able to perform arithmetical operations if they can do so on paper, for, with no obvious primary disturbance of spatially oriented operations, these patients retain both the meaning of individual figures and the categorical structure of number. However, they begin to experience difficulty as soon as they try to calculate aloud or to perform complex arithmetical operations in which individual stages must be carried out mentally and must rely on speech processes. These cases are characterized by marked instability of the traces of the verbal designations as well as by extinction of the meaning of figures or signs given verbally. Therefore, gross defects come to light whenever these patients calculate aloud; they also have difficulty with written arithmetical calculations requiring carrying over from different categorical units and other intermediate operations. Although they easily solve problems arranged in vertical units, they find it difficult to solve those arranged horizontally or in single vertical file. The solution of serial problems, i.e., with three components, invariably confounds them. Hence, even patients with forms of acoustic-mnestic aphasia giving rise to relatively few clinical manifestations immediately run into insuperable difficulties once they reach the last part of the operation; this is so even if they have successfully contended with the previous ones.

Important but much less fully studied arithmetical defects may also arise in association with *motor aphasia*. These defects are related to the profound impairment of internal speech. Under these conditions the mental performance of complex arithmetical operations and the transfer from one group of numbers to another may lead to difficulties. These patients often evince a tendency to simplify forward or backward counting by doing so in units rather than on the basis of tables; frequently, they will use this method even if they still retain the categorical structure of number.

The arithmetical disturbances occurring with the various forms of aphasia have been described by the author in greater detail elsewhere (1947) and by Rudenko (1953).

The nature of the arithmetical disturbances in patients with *lesions of the frontal lobes* is very specialized. In these cases both the categorical concept of number and elementary arithmetical operations may remain intact (except in the most severe frontal syndromes); nevertheless, because of the discriminatory disturbances and the breakdown in the regulatory role of the system of verbal associations (Part II, Section 5D–G), the determining role of the problem itself may be so weakened that the performance of the necessary arithmetical operations is severely hampered. The latter is replaced by a burst of irrelevant associations and by isolated fragmentary calculations, correct in themselves but completely irrelevant to the conditions of the problem.

Patients with frontal syndromes show particularly obvious defects when performing serial arithmetical operations, especially when they are given the task of counting backward from 100 in 7's. In fact, in these tests patients often perform the operation of counting backward from 100 in 7's only partially. For example, instead of facilitating the operation of carrying over the 10's by subtracting from the minuend three components of the number 7, so rounding off the minuend (e.g., converting the operation $93-7$ into the operation $93-3-4$), they perform only the first part of the operation ($93-3=90$), carry over the 10, and do not subtract the remainder but simply transfer it to the next 10 (so obtaining 84 instead of 86). Sometimes the patients perseverate the number in the 10's column, saying 96 instead of 86. Finally, patients with a particularly severe frontal syndrome may actually abandon this task midstream or replace it by an inert stereotype (e.g., 100—93—83—73—63 . . .), as previously stated.

Arithmetical operations may be appreciably disturbed in patients with *general cerebral disturbances* (e.g., hypertensive syndrome, generalized weakening of the cortical processes). These disturbances may be complex and may fluctuate in intensity, being especially marked in the phase of exhaustion. The results of a detailed investigation of disturbances of counting in local brain lesions have been published by Tsvetkova (1972).

12. Investigation of Intellectual Processes

A. PRELIMINARY REMARKS

The investigation of the intellectual activity of patients with brain lesions is one of the most complex of the clinical psychological tools. The importance of data on the integrity of intellectual processes is by no means the same in the various branches of clinical medicine. In clinical psychiatry, when the object is to study the general forms of change affecting a patient's conscious activity, this type of investigation is of prime importance; the results must lend themselves to psychological descriptions of the various types of disturbance of this activity. In the clinical study of local brain lesions, which is entirely devoted to the elucidation of the location of these lesions, attention is concentrated on the neurophysiological and psychophysiological analysis of the more specialized processes, with the aim of bringing to light the factors underlying the local lesions. The study of intellectual processes, which are highly complex in character, cannot therefore occupy a central place in the psychological investigation. However, lesions in different cerebral locations may produce completely different forms of intellectual disturbance. For this reason, the use of methods enabling a more accurate assessment of the various forms of intellectual change may also be of considerable help in the clinical study of local brain lesions.

As has been repeatedly mentioned (Part II, Section 5G), intellectual activity is a particularly complex form of mental activity, taking place only when the problem demands preliminary analysis and synthesis of the situation and special auxiliary operations by means of which it can be solved.

As a result of this analysis of the situation or, as is usually said in psychology, of this creation of a preliminary basic plan of the complex action, the subject picks out the most important elements in the conditions of the task and creates a hypothesis of the basic ways it can be solved. This hypothesis, or general scheme of the intellectual action, at once alters the probability with which the different connections may arise: some connections compatible with the hypothesis become most probable and are put into effect; other connections not corresponding to the hypothesis become less probable and are inhibited. As a result of this preparatory work, each intellectual process becomes organized, and the subsequent selection of the necessary intellectual methods or operations becomes planned and selective in character.

It may naturally be expected that a disturbance of intellectual processes would arise in patients with lesions of widely different parts of the brain, eliminating any of several factors necessary for the normal course of the intellectual act.

As I said above, for intellectual processes to run their proper course it is essential to distinguish the *goal,* which must be firmly maintained throughout the whole of the subsequent activity and must determine the subject's basic set. All premature impulsive attempts to respond to the task must be inhibited, and the subject must apply his energies to a preliminary scrutiny of the conditions of the task. This preliminary scrutiny must also lead to the formation of a certain hypothesis, or a scheme of action, which would make the appearance of certain essential connections more probable, inhibit other irrelevant connections, and would endow the subsequent process with a selective character. The subject must be able to choose and use the correct operation. Finally, at each stage of the intellectual process the results so far obtained must be compared with the initial conditions of the task, so that any irrelevant connections which have arisen can be inhibited and any inadequate solutions corrected.

Investigations have shown (Vygotskii, 1934; Leont'ev, 1959; Zaporozhets, 1960; Gal'perin, 1959, 1966) that this complex process is formed during prolonged development of the child. Initially it is extended and actively demonstrative in character and rests on external material or materialized support; in the next stage it can be performed with the aid of extended, external speech; only in the last stage, with the development of internal speech, is it gradually condensed so that it assumes the character of a contracted "intellectual" action which distinguishes the intellectual processes of the adult human being.

After all that was said in the previous sections of this book it will be clear that this process will be affected differently in patients with lesions of different parts of the brain.

A lesion of the frontal zones, causing substantial disturbances of the stability of plans, will lead to disturbance of the inhibition of direct and perseverative connections, and will easily cause a disturbance of the whole structure of intellectual activity. As a result of these defects the preliminary basic plan of action will be lost or reduced. The formation of a stable hypothesis, to determine the strategy of the intellectual act, will be disturbed, and the system of connections which arises will lose its goal-directed and selective character. The comparison of the results of the action with the original plan, essential for every intellectual act, is substantially disturbed and the subject is no longer aware of mistakes he makes and no longer corrects them. Naturally, therefore, the disturbance of intellectual activity in the patients of this group is particularly severe in form, despite the fact that habitual skills, whereby individual special operations can be performed, may remain intact.

The disturbance of intellectual activity is distinguished by totally different features in patients with lesions of the posterior (temporo-parieto and parieto-occipital) regions of the dominant hemisphere. Patients with such lesions can easily grasp and firmly retain a problem presented to them. They easily prepare stable plans, they work hard on them in order to understand the conditions of the problem; they create the necessary hypothesis, and they carefully compare each step of their argument with the original conditions of the task given to them.

The disturbances arising in this group of patients are totally different in character. As a rule they are connected with the fact that, although these patients retain the general "strategy" of the intellectual act, they are unable to carry it out adequately. Patients with lesions of the temporal zones experience considerable difficulties associated with a disturbance of the system of speech connections and the instability of their memory traces, which seriously impairs their ability to retain the necessary operations and to perform them on an internal "intellectual" plane.

Patients with lesions of the parieto-occipital zones of the left hemisphere have appreciable difficulty when, in the course of their task, they have to compare some elements of their action with others, and when their operations must be supported by "simultaneous syntheses." These difficulties are particularly great when in the course of problem solving they have to analyze certain grammatical structures or numerical relations. In such cases, although the patients firmly retain the necessary plan and work diligently to carry it out, they are unable to perform the necessary operations smoothly and automatically; the whole process of intellectual activity is severely disturbed, but this time at completely different levels.

Naturally, therefore, methods of investigation of intellectual activity must be so constructed that the character of the disturbance of intellectual activity is accessible for detailed analysis. Only if these conditions are satisfied can the investigation of intellectual activity be used for the topical diagnosis of brain lesions.

The investigation of intellectual activity as used in neuropsychology may proceed by analysis of the patient's constructive activity (Part III, Section 6D); it can use the analysis of understanding of thematic pictures or fragments of texts; finally, it can use analysis of the process of problem solving, in which all the distinguishing features of intellectual activity are expressed in a particularly clear form and which constitute convenient models of intellectual activity.

In all these cases the person investigating intellectual activity must pay particular attention not so much to the result or solution of the particular problem as to the analysis of the course of the intellectual process, and the identification of the difficulties which the patient experiences when solving the problem. Three groups of tests will be considered: investigation of the understanding of a subject, investigation of ideas, and investigation of the solution of problems demanding a sequence of independent intellectual processes.

B. INVESTIGATION OF THE UNDERSTANDING OF THEMATIC PICTURES AND TEXTS

The investigation of a patient's understanding of a subject expressed pictorially or verbally has for a long time been one of the most widely used clinical methods for the study of intellectual processes; it has been used extensively in psychiatric practice and under certain conditions may also be used for the topical diagnosis of local brain lesions. In this test the patient is shown a picture (or series of pictures) illustrating a certain subject or is instructed to read a short story (or fable) dealing with some general theme. Despite their different forms (pictorial versus verbal), both tasks require analysis of the subject, identification of its essential elements, and synthesis of these elements in such a way that the basic theme of the picture or story is brought out. To keep this process of comprehension from deteriorating into mere direct recognition of familiar material, the picture or story must be of a kind that the patient cannot interpret directly or by guessing from any one fragment. The theme of the pictures or stories used in these tests must therefore be relatively complex, with the meaning becoming clear only as a result of special analytic-synthetic activity.

Accordingly, the patient is shown a picture (or series of pictures) depicting a certain event. Besides relatively simple pictures depicting all the details of the event, pictures are shown that can be interpreted only after synthesis of a series of details and after certain deductions have been made. The same principle applies to the presentation of texts; first, very simple fragments directly describing an event and, finally, stories or fables simple in grammatical structure but complex in theme are offered. The gist of the latter type of narrative becomes clear only after careful analysis of the text and its internal relationships.

If the preliminary basic plan of the activity follows its normal course the subject will pick out the basic connections contained in the thematic picture or text, whereupon some hypotheses regarding their content will become more probable and others less probable. If the preliminary basic plan of activity is disturbed, the correct process of analysis is upset, and the subject may make random premature guesses which do not correspond to the meaning of the pictures or fragments of texts presented. In all these tests the patient is not given any time limit (sometimes being allowed to examine the material over and over again). The investigator attentively watches the course the analysis takes, the difficulties experienced by the patient, and the methods used to compensate for defects (if any exist).

Of course, experiments involving complex pictorial themes can be carried out only if the patient's powers of visual perception are preserved and experiments involving textual themes are possible only when the patient is still able to understand the meaning of words and grammatical structures. Some of both types of test will now be considered.

To test *comprehension of thematic pictures* the patient is first shown pictures with simple or rather complicated themes. He is instructed to examine them carefully and to describe the message or story they convey. The experiment begins with simple thematic pictures, examples of which can be found in any child's ABC book or reading primer (such as "The family," "Going for a walk in the forest," "The farmyard"), and continues with the examination and analysis of complex thematic pictures illustrative of some event whose meaning becomes completely clear only after careful scrutiny of the picture and synthesis of its details. Excellent material for the investigation is also provided by highly complex artistic works (for example, Klodt's *The Last Supper* and Fedotov's *The Major's Courtship*), for the general theme can be understood only by appraisal of the various minor themes and emotional background.

To enable him to evaluate the patient's ability to perceive the theme of the picture, the investigator must carefully watch how the patient analyzes it—whether he examines all its details and tries to find their essential connection or whether, on the other hand, he at once jumps to impulsive conclusions about its general meaning from a study of a single fragment. It is imperative to determine whether his conclusions are influenced by individual details, triggering off irrelevant associations, and whether they are made without confidence, with the patient expressing doubts about his comprehension as soon as the investigator raises the question.

A special place in this investigation is occupied by series of thematic pictures. In this type of test the patient is given not one, but a series of pictures illustrating the development of a certain event. Such series have been used in books on speech development and also by clinical psychologists (Bernshtein, 1921; etc.). The individual pictures are presented in no particular order. He must arrange them in the correct order and then state their unifying theme. In a simplified variant the pictures of the series are given in the correct order and the patient has only to understand the sequence of events depicted by them. The investigator keeps careful watch to see whether the patient understands that the various pictures simply illustrate stages of an event, noting whether he undertakes the necessary task of arranging them in a single thematic series or whether on the other hand, he describes each picture separately and is unable to progress from this to the synthesis of the evolving theme. Particular attention must be paid to the limitations preventing the patient from perceiving the series of successive events depicted in the series. The investigator must find out whether the patient makes use of repeated figures. He must discern whether the implied (i.e., by changes in the depicted scene) passage of time between the various occurrences hinder the patient in his evaluation of the single general theme. He must assess the effect of the necessity of understanding the motives of the persons taking part in the story. In other words, all possible factors must be taken into account.

These tests can produce evidence, familiar in abnormal psychology, of a general intellectual deterioration and also of defects that reflect specific disturbances of the higher cortical functions in local brain lesions.

Patients with latent forms of *visual agnosia* (especially simultaneous agnosia), arising in association with *lesions of the occipital divisions*, may experience considerable difficulty in understanding thematic pictures even in the absence of any true intellectual deterioration. These difficulties take the form of inability to grasp the whole situation illustrated in the picture at a glance and inability to carry out visual synthesis (Part II, Section 3C and E). Such patients may thus be unable to see at once all the persons shown in the picture or to establish the associations depicted visually; consequently, they are compelled to make tentative suggestions and guesses about the theme. The symptoms observed may be interpreted correctly if consideration is given to their specific character and if the examiner determines that other forms of activity unconnected with visual analysis are intact and that the patient can make normal critical appraisals through these other channels. Another characteristic of these patients is the type of behavior they display when they attempt to carry out the task—the numerous suggestions and guesses they make and, in particular, their lack of confidence in their conclusions.

A special form of disturbance in comprehension of a thematic picture is seen in patients who are able visually to synthesize the details of a picture but, as a fundamental difficulty, cannot correctly evaluate the theme as a whole, relating the story content, for example, to an inappropriate category of experience (such as the patient's own life). Such cases are sometimes encountered with lesions of the right hemisphere, but their precise nature has not yet been clarified.

Patients with various *aphasic disorders* also usually have difficulty in comprehending thematic pictures or series of pictures and often, although they understand the general meaning of these pictures, they are unable to express it in the proper way, but constantly ask themselves: "Well, let me see . . . how can I . . . I can't!"

However, these difficulties are sometimes of a more serious character.

The findings reported in the literature (Ombredane, 1951) suggest that the understanding of pictorial situations, even in series of pictures, is not necessarily primarily involved in these cases for the ability to grasp the unity of the theme and the emotional background may be quite well preserved. If the difficulties associated with the verbal formulation of the theme *

* The necessity for making a strict distinction between the direct perception of the theme of pictures and the verbal formulation of this theme was pointed out by Vygotskii (1934, 1956). He showed that the stages in the perception of a thematic picture described by Stern (1927) merely reflect stages in the development of speech, which passes from a nominative designation of an object to the subsequent designation of actions and attitudes.

are circumvented, noticeable difficulties may be observed only when the patient is given no guidance in discovering the nature of the theme (he can be guided, for example, by a suitable arrangement of the cards). In cases where the patient has to perform the operation mentally, with the aid of his defective internal speech, he can be helped simply by denoting the order of the series of pictures by numbers (Ombredane, 1951, pp. 355–356).

Gross disturbances in the comprehension of thematic pictures may be found in patients with *frontal lobe lesions* (Part II, Section 5G). The source of these disturbances is the fundamental defect in active, selective activity that is present in these patients, which makes it impossible for them to carry out the systematic preliminary survey of the picture and the subsequent analysis and synthesis of its details. Because of this defect, examination of the picture and attempts to understand its theme are replaced by impulsive conclusions, based solely on the basis of those direct impressions which the patient experiences during the perception of fragments in the picture. A characteristic feature of many patients with frontal lobe lesions is their inability to correctly comprehend those elements of works of art expressing emotion. A patient with this type of disturbance is completely incapable of evaluating the mimic gestures and the pantomimic means of expressing the various emotional states and of correctly identifying the emotional background of the picture.

Experience shows that patients with a severe frontal syndrome no longer examine the details of the picture attentively, correlate them with each other, or attempt to pick out the features that give the basic information on the general meaning of the picture. Often they inertly fix one detail and deduce from it a direct conclusion about the meaning of the picture as a whole (this type of defect is seen if the patients' eye movements are investigated, for they lose their active searching character). Frequently such patients impulsively pick out one detail of the picture and immediately formulate an hypothesis about the general meaning, never changing it or revising it, so that it becomes inert through all these patients' subsequent "arguments." For instance, having seen the sick girl's white dress in Klodt's picture "The Last Spring," one patient at once says: "A Wedding, she is soon going to be married"; having seen the figure of a soldier in the picture "The Hole in the Ice," he says: "Obviously a war!" or, having seen the notice "Danger!" he at once concludes: "An infected area!" or "High Voltage Cables!" and makes no further attempt to revise this inert hypothesis.

The distinguishing feature of these patients is the confidence with which conclusions are reached and the difficulty we have in making them doubt their false evaluations. This is one of the important signs of a disturbance in the assessment of the effect of a personal action and of the profound disintegration of the process of comparison of intent and result, a characteristic feature of the frontal syndrome.

Tests aimed at discerning *the understanding of a text* are similar in nature and importance to the preceding group of tests. The patient is given a passage of text and is required to analyze its meaning. The fragment selected usually contains both essential and inessential details, so that the subject is faced with the task of identifying the essential parts, synthesizing them, and thus reaching an understanding of the principal theme. As in the experiments on the understanding of thematic pictures, disturbance of the preliminary basic plan of action and inability to inhibit irrelevant associations invariably result in the appearance of impulsive, inadequate conclusions, incorrectly reflecting the meaning of the fragment. The distinguishing feature of the present group of tests is the fact that they are conducted entirely on the verbal plane. The subject must concern himself either with traces of verbal associations remaining from the fragment that has been read to him or with a written text if he is still capable of reading it himself.

This examination may be conducted in a number of stages. Usually these experiments begin with analysis of the patient's ability to understand logical-grammatical constructions and to grasp the meaning of metaphors. The methods of analyzing comprehension of logical-grammatical constructions have already been described (Part III, Section 8D and E) so that the present account will be confined to the investigation of metaphorical comprehension.

The understanding of metaphors is particularly significant, for it signifies that the subject has passed beyond the limits of the simple nominative function of speech and can grasp the subtle meaning a certain expression may acquire in a certain situation. This type of investigation has therefore always justifiably been regarded as one of the fundamental means of studying of mental activity (Vygotskii, 1934, 1956; Zeigarnik, 1961; Vasilevskaya, 1960; etc.). Every disturbance at the level of the system of associations must be reflected in the ability to understand metaphors.

This investigation usually begins by giving the patient a series of well-known metaphors (such as, "stony heart," "iron hand," "green thumb") or proverbs ("all that glitters is not gold," "don't count your chickens before they are hatched"), and he is asked to explain their meaning. If the patient finds difficulty in deciding the meaning of the metaphors or proverbs, leading questions are posed. He may be asked to tell whether the corresponding metaphor can be applied to a person with particular qualities or whether a proverb can be applied to an object or person not directly referred to in the expression. A special method allowing for deeper penetration of the nature of the intellectual processes associated with metaphor appreciation comprises concomitant presentation of a proverb and several phrases, some of which contain similar-sounding words to those of the proverb but having a different meaning, while the others express the meaning of the proverb by means of different words; the subject has to choose the phrase closest in meaning to the proverb. The following combinations may serve as examples:

Proverbs	*Phrases*
Strike while the iron is hot.	The blacksmith worked all day. Gold is heavier than iron. Don't delay until it is too late.

Still waters run deep.	A quiet person can be very bright. Pour oil on troubled waters. He found himself getting into deep water.

If the patient cannot solve the problem by his unaided efforts, the investigator helps him by explaining the corresponding meaning in one example; the patient is tested to find out if he can transfer the principle thus demonstrated to another expression. Particular attention must be paid to the speed and confidence with which the patient performs the test and to detecting whether he tries to find the internal meaning of the metaphor or proverb or whether he does not go beyond its narrow, concrete meaning, whether he transfers the newly explained principle to the new example, and how critical he is toward the mistakes he makes.

This series of experiments is followed by tests of the patient's understanding of the meaning of texts, especially passages culled from the works of famous authors. Relatively short extracts simple in grammatical structure but subtle in meaning are usually used for this purpose. The subject is thus required to identify the essential components of the text, to synthesize them, to inhibit premature conclusions, and, on the basis of this analytic-synthetic operation, to deduce the general meaning of the fragment.

To reiterate what was said previously, examples of this type of fragment are the "stories" contained in Tolstoi's book for beginners in reading, such as "The Hen and the Golden Eggs" and "The Crow and the Doves," respectively: A man had a hen which laid golden eggs. Wishing to obtain more gold without having to wait for it, he killed the hen. But he found nothing inside it, for it was just like any other hen.

A crow heard that the doves had plenty to eat. He colored himself white and flew tc the dovecote. The doves thought he was one of them, and took him in. However, he could not help cawing like a crow. The doves then realized that he was a crow and threw him out. He went back to rejoin the crows, but they did not recognize him and would not accept him.

Passages such as these are either read out loud several times or (if the patient is still able to read) given to him in printed form. The patient then has to repeat the fragment and to tell what it means. To this end, a series of additional questions are posed: In connection with the first Tolstoi "story": "What did the man do? Did he do right? What is the moral of the story?" In connection with the second story: "Why did the crow color himself? Why did the doves throw him out? What does the story as a whole mean? Can it be applied to man?" The investigator watches to see if the patient can grasp the passage easily and reproduce it coherently, if he breaks it up into fragments, if he can integrate the details into a single entity, if he understands the metaphorical meaning, and if he can easily make use of any assistance given to him.

Sometimes excerpts are used containing details whose meaning becomes clear only if the hidden meaning is discerned.

"The Lion and the Fox" is an example: A lion had grown old and could no longer hunt game. And so he decided to live by cunning. He lay in his den and pretended to be ill. The wild animals came to see him, but the lion seized and ate every one that came into his den. One day a fox came up to the entrance to his den and asked: "How are you?" "Not so well. Why don't you come inside?" But the fox replied: "I can see footprints. Many animals have gone into your den but none has come out again."

In order to understand the import of the last sentence, it is not enough to understand the sentence itself, but the general theme of the whole extract has to be appreciated.

In isolated cases the patient is given more sophisticated (educational or scientific) texts requiring identification of cause-and-effect relationships. Finally, the patient's ability to select essential connections and to inhibit irrelevant associations may be ascertained by asking him to give an account of the plot of a well-known play, opera, etc. (for example, *Eugene Onegin, The Queen of Spades*).

A valuable method which can give important additional information is that in which the patient is instructed to retell a story told to him or made up by him, and to form a plan for that operation: by this method it is possible to discover whether the patient can pick out the essential logical scheme of the text and follow this scheme during the subsequent narration. As we shall see below, the results obtained may be of definite diagnostic value.

As mentioned, the ability to relate the theme of a literary passage requires detailed analysis and integration of its components, with identification of the dominant pattern of associations and generalization of the fundamental theme. In pathological states of the brain, therefore, it is natural that this process should suffer and the patient should often be unable to understand the theme of the passage in adequate depth.

Patients with *generalized organic defects* of the brain (diffuse manifestations of arteriosclerosis, atrophic processes, oligophrenia, etc.) cannot carry out the necessary analysis of the associations contained in a text, nor can they do more than understand the meaning of each separate fragment. As a rule, therefore, they merely relate these individual fragments without showing appreciation of the general theme (Zeigarnik, 1959, 1961; Vasilevskaya, 1960).

Similar disturbances are encountered in patients with general brain lesions giving rise to an acute hypertensive-hydrocephalic syndrome; however, in contrast to the types of organic depression of intellectual activity just described, these patients do not exhibit a fixed lowering of the level of their intellectual processes. Frequently, they have difficulty retaining any type of material, a defect that becomes increasingly prominent as the passage to be read is lengthened; the systematic analysis of the contents of a longer passage and integration of its elements poses greater difficulties. None of these disturbances are fixed; they are less noticeable when short passages are presented and much more severe when the patient is tired.

Considerable difficulties in textual understanding may be experienced both by patients with *semantic aphasia* and by patients with *other forms of amnestic-aphasic disorders*. In the former, the limitations to understanding are naturally determined by the size of the passage, the number of details it contains, and the complexity of the logical-grammatical relationships implicated in these details. Hence, in the presence of a limited range of operation or of difficulties in grasping logical and grammatical relationships, the patient is unable to grasp the fundamental theme of the text. As a rule, however, these patients attempt to compensate for their difficulties by making a prolonged and systematic analysis of the text. Since they have no primary difficulty in understanding metaphors, this analytical work is not in vain—they are thereby enabled to understand the general theme of the passage as well as any subsidiary themes. Because complex logical-grammatical relationships present insuperable obstacles to these patients (Part II, Section 3F), difficulties arise if the text contains such constructions.

With amnestic-aphasic disturbances the difficulties in relating the components of any long passage are aggravated by defects in the understanding of words (in cases of temporal acoustic-mnestic disorders) or by a general inability to retain a long series of phrases. Attempts to understand a given text can be successful only if the patient uses auxiliary devices (writes down odd details of the story and puts them together on paper) and thus compensates for his fundamental defect. In both cases, however, the process of analysis of the text becomes a prolonged and systematic attempt to find the required theme. The patient, though, retains his selective capacity so that it often happens that, although he cannot retain the individual details, he can grasp the general theme (sometimes even an abstract one) of a text or its emotional tone. As experiments by Tsvetkova (1966) have shown, although such a patient is unable to relate the text of a story fluently, he does know what he is speaking about and he can form a plan for stating it.

The process of understanding a text is altogether different in patients with frontal lobe lesions. As was pointed out (Part II, Section 5G), the fundamental and essential precondition for the performance of this task is disturbed in these patients: They are incapable of sustained activity involving analysis of the content of a text, synthesis of its details, and verification of provisional hypotheses. In fact, a patient with a marked frontal syndrome replaces the systematic analysis of a text with impulsive guesses, an activity that comes easily to him because of his ability to grasp isolated fragments. Frequently, uncontrollable irrelevant associations and inert stereotypes produced in the course of previous operations are superimposed upon these conjectures. Because of these conditions, a nonselective series of fragmentary and irrelevant associations and perseverations replace selective analysis of the passage, often making adequate understanding of the passage completely impossible. Such patients naturally can understand a metaphor only if the corresponding associations are so firmly established by past experience that there is no need to distinguish them actively from the stronger, direct associations. As frequently happens, metaphorical meanings (especially when a proverb has to be compared with several statements presented in conjunction with it) cannot be discerned by these patients; the direct meaning of the verbal structures, consolidated by previous experience, is what comes to the fore. It is equally difficult for such patients to grasp the general theme of a passage; often, they can put it into words, but it is immediately superseded by irrelevant associations or stereotypes.

Distinctive disturbances of narration of a story are found in patients with lesions of the posterior frontal brain zones and with a general syndrome of inactivity.

Such patients are unable to relate the theme of a story unaided, they state that nothing will come into their head, and they usually do no more than echolalically repeat the same sentence. If, however, they are asked questions about the story, it is clear that they have grasped its theme and, although unable to relate it coherently, they can easily and clearly answer questions about it, only occasionally having difficulty in switching from one question to the next (Part II, Section 4G).

Often, therefore, such patients will supplement the story by details that are not a part of it (e.g., when narrating the story "The Hen and the Golden Egg," they may say: "A man had a large farm and sold eggs," and so on), or they mix up the meanings of fragments read to them (e.g., when narrating the story "The Jackdaw and the Pigeon" they start to incorporate into it elements of the story "The Hen and the Golden Egg" they heard previously). Just as in the case of telling the story of thematic pictures, the patients do not show the necessary critical attitude toward their mistakes and only rarely do they correct them (Part II, Section 5G).

Characteristically, patients with various forms of a frontal syndrome, who can relatively easily begin to narrate a story, are quite unable to form a plan of a story given to them. They find it impossible to pick out the important meaningful elements of the story or to inhibit irrelevant associations which spring up involuntarily and, as a special investigation (Tsvetkova, 1966) has shown, they soon begin to repeat the text directly (sometimes echolalically) instead of forming a plan for it.

From the foregoing it can be seen that, despite the fact that the analysis of a thematic picture and the understanding of the theme of a written passage are among the more complex forms of activity and the fact that they may be disturbed in patients with any brain lesion, the examination of the performance of these tasks can be used as part of the investigation for diagnostic localization of such lesions.

C. INVESTIGATION OF CONCEPT FORMATION

The investigation of the process whereby abstract ideas are formed has always occupied a central place both in the psychological study of intellectual activity and in the psychiatric study of patients, and certain authors (for example, Goldstein, 1934, 1942, 1948) have regarded it as the most important part of the experimental psychological investigation of patients with brain lesions. Those investigators who have placed such a high value on this aspect of the study of mental activity took as their starting point the fact that it is in operations with logical relationships and abstract ideas that the subject advances from the level of concrete operations to a new, specifically human level of abstract, or categorical behavior. It was felt that, because of the complexity of such operations, they are inevitably impeded by any brain lesions, the assumption being that a brain lesion nullifies the most complex forms of cortical activity. A disturbance in abstract intellectual activity has therefore come to be regarded as one of the basic signs of a functional change due to a pathological condition of the brain.

It is difficult to object to this concept as a whole, for from the descriptive point of view it correctly reflects the final result produced by brain lesions. However, the inference that a lowering of categorical intelligence arises from all brain lesions is by no means true and detracts from the correct analysis of the mechanisms lying at the root of such a defect where it occurs.

We know that although a general failure in cerebral development (oligophrenia), like a diffuse lesion of the cerebral cortex (organic dementia), does, in fact, lead to imperfect evolution or impairment of abstract intellectual activity, the overwhelming majority of cases of local brain lesions either does not lead to these disturbances or gives rise to them only secondarily. Thus, a disturbance of what Goldstein calls "categorical behavior" cannot take place with subcortical lesions or with extensive local lesions of the sensorimotor, auditory, and visual cortex and in certain other forms it must be regarded as only a consequence of other defects directly resulting from these lesions.

The range of experimental psychological methods available for studying a patient's use of logic and ability to form abstractions is very wide. These tests have been described in several textbooks (Vygotskii, 1934, 1956; Kleist, 1934; Pittrich, 1949; Pflugfelder, 1950; Bruner *et al.*, 1956; Zeigarnik, 1961; etc.), so that they will not be discussed in detail here. Only a few tests that are particularly popular in clinical practice and that can be used for the psychological investigation of patients with local brain lesions will be described.

First, tests involving *definition* are given. The patient is asked to define a series of words denoting different ideas (for example, "table," "tractor," "tree," "auto," and "island"). The investigator takes note of the patient's ability to use abstract categories in defining a particular idea: Does the patient incorporate the idea into a system of equivalent or more general concepts and then make the definition more precise (e.g., "a table is a piece of furniture on which we place dishes or books and where one sits")? Special attention is paid to those definitions that are limited to the description of the particular object and to the inclusion of a concrete situation (e.g., "a table may be for writing or eating"; "there is a table on our ward, covered with a cloth"). Naturally, a proper evaluation of the results of the tests can be made only if the patient's premorbid level of performance is known.

Other methods of investigating mental activity consist of experiments involving the *comparison and differentiation* of ideas. In these experiments the patient is given a pair of ideas to compare with a view to finding the common ground between them; they then have to be designated by a single word (e.g., "a table and a sofa—they are both furniture"). Or, the difference between them has to be discerned (e.g., "a fox is a wild animal, while a dog is a tame animal"). Particular attention must be paid to the extent to which the patient goes beyond the direct description of the two objects, i.e., the extent of generalization in his classification. If the patient cannot do this task unaided, he is given an example of the correct way to solve the problem; the investigator then looks for the transfer of this principle to other parts of the test.

The next group of tests in the investigation of intellectual activity includes experiments involving the finding of *logical relationships*. In one, the patient must relate each word in a given series to a more general category (e.g., "a table is furniture," "a chisel is a tool"), or, conversely, a general term must be related to a more particular idea, (e.g., "a flower – a rose," "a fish – a carp"). Similar operations may be carried out with different problems, for example, finding the parts of a whole (e.g., "table – leg," "knife – blade") or the whole from its parts (e.g., "wall – house," "shelf – cupboard"). A special place in this series is occupied by tests involving the finding of opposite values. The patient is given a word and he must find another, opposite to it in meaning (e.g., "healthy – sick," "high – low").

The investigator watches to see whether the patient performs the operation easily, whether he has difficulty in keeping to the required relationship—or slips off into random associations—and whether he easily switches from one given relationship to another. In this experiment, too, the investigator may give the patient a series of examples if he has difficulty in finding the necessary reply unaided. The experimenter then observes whether the patient has grasped the principle of the solution; if the patient repeats the same answer when solving the subsequent problems, he was able to grasp only the concrete elements. In a special variant the patient may be asked not to find the words unaided, but to choose the required word from three suggested words, two of which stand in different relationships to the given word. An example of this type of test is one involving the discovery of species-genus or genus-species relationships (e.g., dog [cat, sheep-dog, animal]; gun [bullet, firearm, rifle]). Another example is the test involving the discernment of the opposite relationship (e.g., high [low, thin, long]; happiness [laughter, grief, tears]). This variant of the experiment does away with the need for seeking words unaided, but it gives the patient the more complex task of selecting from a number of alternatives and inhibiting closely similar, but inappropriate associations.

Tests involving the finding of analogies are similar to the preceding group. In addition to a pair of words bearing a definite relationship to each other, the patient is given a third word for which he has to find another bearing the same relationship (e.g., high – low; good – ? [bad]; table – leg; bicycle – ? [wheel]). More difficult to carry out are: regiment – soldiers; library – ? (books); river – banks; street – ? (sidewalks). Relationships of varying degrees of complexity may be incorporated in these tests; some may be concrete and others abstract. In all these tests the investigator, having explained the task in detail by means of one or two examples, observes the extent to which the patient grasps the necessary principle, transfers it to the solution of the new problems, and, particularly important, changes from one task to another without inertly reproducing a relationship previously established.

In a special variant of the experiment the patient may be asked to choose the required word from three possible alternatives (e.g., high – low; good – ? [poor, bad, man]; regiment – soldiers; library – ? [reader, building, books]). As in the experiment already described, this variant does away with the difficulty of actively searching for the required word, but it complicates the operation by making necessary inhibition of irrelevant associations and choosing an adequate alternative.

Subsequent experiments are devoted to the analysis of the systems of association at the patient's command, the study of which leads directly to the investigation of categorical intelligence. These are concerned with the classification of objects and may be divided into two main variants.

In the first of these—the well-known classification experiments containing a "superfluous fourth"—the patient is given a drawing depicting four objects; three of these belong to the same category (e.g., articles of clothing, furniture, china), while the fourth, although bearing some outward resemblance to the rest or associated with them in a single concrete situation, does not belong to the same category (e.g., spade, saw, ax, [log]). The patient is asked to find the object that does not belong to the same group as the rest and to cover it, leaving the other objects open to view; he must explain the reasons for his choice by giving the common word descriptive of the three remaining articles. The investigator observes the extent to which the patient grasps the instruction and is able to make a true classification of objects on the basis of their relation to a definite category. He pays particular attention to grouping the objects only by their external appearance (shape, color, size) or substitution of a nother, concrete relationship (i.e., recreating a situation in which these objects could be associated together) for a definite category. Again, two or three concrete examples are given if the patient is unable to perform the necessary operations, with the investigator alert to ascertaining the patient's ability to transfer the demonstrated principle to other groups of objects. The way the patient explains what he has done is particularly instructive. The investigator must note whether the explanation is completely relevant to the task performed or whether irrelevancies are incorporated into it. This series of experiments, like the next, can of course be used only when the patient's premorbid intellectual level is relatively high.

Other experiments in the same series, developed in the course of special psychological investigations (Weigl, 1927; Vygotskii, 1934; Goldstein and Scheerer, 1941; etc.) involve the free classification of objects. In them, the patient is given a series of objects (or pictures of objects) to classify, by arranging them in several groups. The patient is usually not advised of the principle of classification; he is not given the concrete descriptive terms of the groups or told the number of groups into which the objects or pictures must be arranged. However, the very nature of the objects (among which are animals, plants, china, furniture, tools, etc.) points to their categorical classification. If, instead of grouping the objects or their pictorial representations according to the respective categories, the patient places together objects found in a single concrete situation (e.g., a table, chair, plate, knife, fork, bread, etc., are grouped together to recreate the situation of "having a meal"), the nature of the solution is explained to him and what is required is demonstrated. In this test, too, the investigator watches to see whether the principle is retained and applied to the classification of other objects. If the patient arranges the objects into a very large number of very small groups based on concrete factors (e.g., the flowers in one pile, the cereals in another, mushrooms in another, trees in a fourth), he is instructed to combine them in larger groups for the sake of generalization. After each performance, the patient is asked why he has grouped together the various articles and what is the basis of his classification.

The investigator is particularly heedful of the selectivity shown in regard to the classifying principle, making note of inappropriate, extraneous inclusions. The ease of transfer from one principle of classification to another is also relevant. In this experiment, any lowering of abstract intelligence, any deviation from selective, controlled reasoning, and any breakdown in the mobility of those nervous processes essential for the formation of the required associations readily become apparent.

In the same category are tests for the evaluation of the *formation of artificial ideas*. They were originally suggested by Vygotskii (1934), Bruner (1957), and others. Because of their complexity, however, they have only limited application to the clinical investigation of patients with local brain lesions.

A cleverly designed variant of the test used to investigate abstraction is that suggested and used by Halstead (1947), in the diagnosis of patients with brain lesions. In this test the patient is shown four figures, each placed above a corresponding key. Three of these figures are identical in a certain respect, while the fourth differs from the rest on the basis of this sign. The subject has to press the key corresponding to the discordant figure. The experiment is gradually made more difficult: The subject is given geometrical shapes divided into four parts or divisible into four parts; from some of them one part is missing. The subject has to press the key that corresponds to the serial number of the missing part. Finally, the patient is given shapes composed of different numbers of parts (from one to four), with the numbers of the keys corresponding to the number of elements drawn on the figure.

Since the principle of construction of the figures and the appropriate reaction are not revealed at once but gradually, as the result of progressive reinforcement of correct reactions, the subject must formulate the required principle by his own devices. The investigator is thus able to study both the stages in the formation of this principle and its limits and stability. The course of such an experiment is shown in Fig. 136. According to Halstead, this method is more successful than any other in distinguishing the factor disturbing abstraction and it gives valuable results in patients with *lesions of the frontal lobes*.

Various forms of organic deterioration of mental processes may be revealed by the tests used to investigate the formation of concepts; these deficiencies may be manifested as a disturbance in abstract formulations or as a lowering of the intellectual level to the simplest and most concrete type of functioning. Although such patients, extensively studied by modern psychiatrists, can still carry out tasks involving the most habitual types of logical relationships (e.g., oppositeness), these relationships may disintegrate, being replaced by those deduced from more elementary operations (e.g., concrete differences). The definition of concept frequently does not go beyond the description of the concrete properties of an object, and generalization stops at the discovery of the concrete situation in which the particular object is found. However, examination of these problems lies outside the scope of the present book.

Disturbances in abstract intellectual operations are much less frequent in patients with local brain lesions than supposed by such authorities as Goldstein (1934, 1942, 1948). They may usually be regarded as secondary results of primary defects, and the latter may be very varied in nature. Observations have shown that even though patients with *semantic aphasia* cannot grasp the meaning of complex logical-grammatical relationships, they are still able (provided that no marked general cerebral defects are present) to discover such

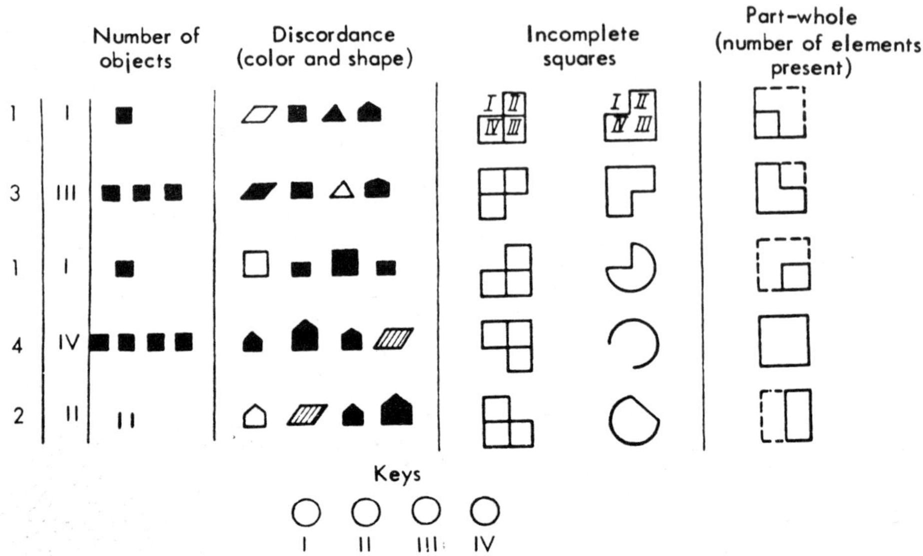

FIGURE 136 Halstead's test (1947) for investigating abstraction. The patient is shown the figures drawn in the table and he has to decide which of the four keys to press. The various principles of categorization may be ascertained from the illustration.

logical relationship as oppositeness, genus and species, and part and whole, and can still perform elementary operations of classification (e.g., identify the "superfluous fourth"). Sometimes such patients can even perform practical tasks involving object classification. The disturbance of simultaneous spatial synthesis does not prevent these patients from perceiving those logical relationships that have become ingrained from previous experience. Difficulties may arise only when these relationships begin to be expressed in complex verbal forms or when spatial synthesis is required. On the whole, however, these difficulties should not be regarded as by-products of a disturbance in categorical intellectual activity.

Those impairements in abstract intellectual activity that are based on speech, occurring in various forms of *sensory (acoustic) and motor aphasia*, are also secondary; they cannot be interpreted as a primary disintegration of abstract orientation. Observations (Part II, Sections 2F and 4H) have shown that patients with these forms of aphasia are unable to operate with complex systems of speech associations, so that those intellectual operations that are purely verbal in nature cannot be investigated. When, however, these restrictions are removed, it is found that the patients have not lost their abstract orientation or their categorical behavior. Within the narrow limits of their ability, they grasp logical relationships that, although developed on the basis of speech, have acquired some degree of independence. Difficulties arise when logical operations must be carried out by means of speech and when the evolved systems of associations become unstable because of the instability of word meanings and defects in internal speech. The defects that come to light during the comparison of ideas or during the making of analogies and classification indicate that the alterations have a speech basis and cannot be regarded as products of general dementia.

It should be noted, however, that among the many hundreds of articles published on the subject of the aphasias, hardly any deal with the investigation of the intellectual activity of aphasic subjects. Even the reports of van Woerkom (1925), Gelb and Goldstein (1920) and Goldstein (1926*b*, 1948) do not make clear to what extent the observed intellectual defects are attributable to the speech disorders present in this group of patients. For this reason, the definitive description of the intellectual disturbances arising in these cases remains to be done.

Highly characteristic disturbances in operations involving abstract relationships are revealed by patients with *frontal lobe lesions.* As mentioned (Part II, Section 5G), the basic feature of the intellectual disorder in such patients is the vulnerability of their associative processes to loss of selectivity and to the influence of irrelevant associations or inert stereotypes. Patients with a marked frontal syndrome may for a short time exhibit integrity of the processes involved in the establishment of fundamental abstract relationships (e.g., oppositeness, genus and species, part and whole, cause and effect), but the processes very quickly disintegrate, with consequent replacement of these relationships by others that are more firmly established, or are the result of random associations, or are inertly consolidated from previous operations. For this reason, these patients cannot select stable abstract associations. Although the patient sometimes gives correct answers both in the experiments on comparing and distinguishing and in the experiments on discerning abstract relationships (especially, analogies), he does not keep to them, but, having lost the discriminatory capacity, wanders off into irrelevant associations. A patient with a frontal lobe lesion, as a special investigation (Luria and Lebedinskii, 1966) showed, can thus relatively easily solve a problem of finding an analogy under ordinary conditions but is unable to do so if given several possible solutions from which he must choose the appropriate one (the "selective" variant of problem solving). Connections of all possible kinds appear with equal probability, and the patient has very great difficulty in finding the appropriate one. Hence, these patients also show deficiencies in classification. The associations arising in each patient differ very widely, and the choice of the associations defined by the task in hand consequently presents great difficulties. The specific feature of the intellectual processes of patients with lesions of the frontal lobes is thus related principally to the primary disturbances in the process of selection (a faculty under the control of the associations of the second signal system) and to a defect in the process of evaluating the relevance of the result obtained to the problem.

D. INVESTIGATION OF DISCURSIVE INTELLECTUAL ACTIVITY

In describing methods for investigating the understanding of pictorial themes and texts and the establishment of logical relationships, we mentioned only certain special forms and components of intellectual activity. However, intellectual activity assumes its most distinct and highly developed form in other operations—in discursive intellectual activity and in the solution of problems. It is in these activities that the basic structure of the intellectual processes is seen especially clearly. The person solving a problem must analyze its requirements, select the essential relationships, and discover the intermediate aims and the operations by which these aims may be secured. Only by carrying through intermediate operations of this nature can he reach a final solution to the problem.

This typical process of discussion or reasoning requires subordination of all the operations to the final goal, for otherwise they lose their purpose. It requires inhibition of all digressions from the final goal and, consequently, restriction of the whole process to a closed system, whose boundaries are determined by the conditions of the problem. For all these reasons, several authors (Bruner, 1957; Miller, Pribram, and Galanter, 1960; etc.) assert that in the solution of a discursive problem it is possible to distinguish a general "strategy" (fixation of the goal, identification of a general plan of solution) and special "tactics" devoted to the finding and execution of the corresponding intermediate operations. Whether the activity as a whole is undertaken step by step or is accomplished more directly and succinctly, the fundamental structure of the process remains the same in principle. One of the most typical examples of a discursive operation is the solution of arithmetical problems. The operations involved in this type of discursive activity are amenable to observation, and its examination has therefore been successfully used in the field of clinical psychology.

The problems used are presented in the order of increasing complexity. Usually they are of a kind that can be solved easily by a normal subject of average education and are therefore feasible for clinical psychological studies.

The experiments usually begin with *arithmetical problems of an elementary level*, which can be solved either by simple addition and subtraction or by means of a comparatively simple intermediate operation. The first type includes such problems as: "Peter had 2 apples and John had 6 apples. How many did they both have together?" "Jane had 7 apples and gave 3 away. How many did she have left?" The second type of problem requires an intermediate operation (not formulated in the proposition), for example: "Mary had 4 apples and Betty had 2 apples more than Mary. How many apples did they both have together?" The investigator observes how the patient solves these problems. If a direct answer is substituted for a composite solution, the mistake is pointed out and the results of this explanation are tested by means of another problem.

The most important part of this series of experiments is the solution of *complex* arithmetical problems at first of an easy variety, in which the subject has only to adhere to the items of the proposition and to carry out a series of consecutive operations. Then problems are given in which the intermediate operation is performed by means of special mathematical procedures acting purely as aids. The investigation ends with the solution of the most complex problems, in which the burden of the activity resides in the formulation of a series of intermediate problems.

The *first type* includes problems such as: "Some farmers had 10 acres of land; from each acre they harvested 6 tons of grain; they sold one-third to the government. How much did they have left?" It is easy to see that this problem consists of a series of consecutive solutions and that the only real difficulty is to calculate one-third of 60 tons and to subtract the result from the total amount. The *second type* includes such problems as: "There were 18 books on two shelves; there were twice (or half) as many on one shelf as on the other. How many books were there on each shelf?" The principal difficulty resides in the fact that operations with fractions must precede whole-number distribution. As a check, the patient may be given a problem similar in wording but different in solution: "There were 18 books on two shelves; there were two more (or less) on one shelf than on the other. How many books were there on each shelf?" Although similar in form, this problem is solved in a completely different manner: The two "surplus" books are first discarded and then added to the number obtained by dividing the remaining number of books by 2.

The solution of problems of this type often causes considerable difficulty, for some patients are unable to find the required method of dividing into parts and attempt to solve the problem by trial and error or, simplifying the conditions, by dividing the sum into two parts; this, though, is followed by difficulty in deciding how to set about solving the next part. When difficulty arises, the subject is told the method to be adopted for solving the problem; his retention of the principle of solving the problem is tested by similar problems in which the objects, the numbers, and the wording of the conditions are altered. In a control test a problem of the second type is given, similar in content but not requiring operations with fractions.

The *third type* consists of more complex problems whose conditions are not immediately fully apparent. The subject, therefore, must himself formulate a series of intermediate problems. An example of this type of problem is as follows: "A son is 5 years old. In 15 years his father will be 3 times as old as he. How old is the father now?" In this problem it is necessary to find how old the son will be at the end of the specified time, then to calculate the father's age at that time, and finally, to revert to the father's present age. The impossibility of solving this type of problem by a series of separate, direct operations is what puts it in the "most difficult" class.

The last type of problem successfully used in clinical psychological investigation is what is called the "conflict problem." The wording of such a problem causes a tendency toward a wrong method of solution. This type includes problems such as: "A pedestrian walks to the station in 15 minutes, and a cyclist rides there 5 times faster. How long does the cyclist take to get to the station?" The word "faster" causes a tendency to multiply, and this must be overcome in order to arrive at a correct solution. A second example is: "A workman received 30 rubles and gave his wife not 10 rubles, as he usually did, but 5 rubles extra. How much did he have left?" The wording "5 rubles extra" suggests an increase rather than a reduction in the remainder, and this misinterpretation must be overcome for the final calculation. Another problem of the same type is: "A pencil is 6 inches long; the shadow of this pencil is 18 inches longer than the pencil. How many times longer than the pencil is the shadow?" The element of conflict in this problem resides in the fact that the patient tends to leave out the intermediate stage (18 + 6) and to immediately divide 18 by 6.

During these experiments on problem solving the investigator must take note of the method of solution rather than of the final answer. The patient is asked to repeat the items in the problem and the accuracy with which he repeats them is noted. The investigator must carefully observe the degree of the patient's activity, his trials and errors, and his attitude toward him. If necessary, the patient is given leading or control questions. If the patient is unable to solve a particular problem unaided, the investigator fully explains and demonstrates the method of solving one problem; the investigator then examines the extent to which the patient has mastered the principle of solution by giving him similar problems. As previously stated, experiments involving problem solving can be used only for patients of a high enough educational level; otherwise, the results cannot be correctly evaluated.

In the course of this step-by-step method of solving problems, the investigator may observe many different—and sometimes opposite—forms of disturbance, the differences attributable to lesions situated in different parts of the brain. The main forms of these disturbances are analyzed in detail elsewhere (Luria and Tsvetkova, 1966); here I shall only dwell briefly on the most fundamental differences between the process of problem solving in patients with lesions of different parts of the brain. Lesions of the *left inferoparietal and parieto-occipital divisions* of the cortex, accompanied by manifestations of *simultaneous agnosia, constructive apraxia, and semantic aphasia,* may affect the performance of arithmetical operations and interfere with the patient's ability to survey all the conditions of the problem at the same time. Such a patient cannot, therefore, grasp the conditions at once. He therefore tends to dwell on single elements of the condition and makes remarks such as: "No, I don't understand . . . what '5 kilograms more' means. Five . . . and kilograms . . . yes, but what is the 'more' about?" and so on. Besides having difficulty in understanding the logical-grammatical structure of the problem, such a patient takes a long time to analyze the conditions, reading them out piecemeal, and laying vocal stress on their essential components. Once, however, this is completed, in the great majority of cases the general logical plan of the problem becomes sufficiently clear and the patient can frequently say what he must do in order to arrive at a correct solution. While the general plan of solution of the problem remains within his grasp in principal, the individual operations, if they require the simultaneous integration of several systems of associations, are defective. For this reason such a patient can solve the problem better if he breaks it up into consecutive parts and writes them down, but he cannot solve it mentally.

Different defects may be observed during the solution of problems by patients with *lesions of the temporal systems* and with manifestations of *acoustic aphasia*. The instability of word meanings, the ease with which their meaning is alienated, and the rapid extinction of word traces are the main obstacles in the retention of the elements of the problem and in the following of the necessary path of reasoning. For this reason, the mastery of these elements and the performance of the required chain of operations remain beyond the patient's grasp. If a patient with the amnestic variant of temporal aphasia is given a short enough problem or if its component parts are reinforced by means of concrete aids, his powers of solution are increased far more than suspected at first glance.

A completely different picture may be observed in patients with *frontal syndromes*. As a rule, these patients (except with the severest forms of this syndrome) can repeat the elements of the problem comparatively easily. But these elements cannot be analyzed properly, and the systems of associations that they incorporate do not determine the subsequent course of the operations.

Characteristically, patients with lesions of the posterior zones of the brain have difficulty in analyzing the logical-grammatical structure of the conditions of a problem, but as a rule the basic feature of the problem is always preserved. However, in patients with a frontal syndrome the picture is different. Even though they repeat the conditions of the problem correctly, these patients will very often lose the crux of the problem or replace it by echolalic repetition of another element of the condition (e.g., when repeating the problem: "There were 18 books on two shelves; there were twice as many books on one shelf as on the other; how many books were there on each shelf?" they replace the question by a different one: "How many books were there on the two shelves?" without realizing the pointedness of this question). Naturally the whole process of problem solving is defective in such patients. Although they usually manifest no appreciable defect in simple arithmetical operations, such patients, as a rule, grasp one particular fragment of the problem and, without forming a general plan of solution, start to carry out disconnected arithmetical operations with this fragment. They do not relate these operations to the ultimate goal and are quite unconcerned with the relative position occupied by them in the general structure of the problem. It follows, therefore, that the solution of the simplest problems is well within the grasp of such patients, but they have great difficulty with problems incorporating an intermediate operation not formulated in the instruction. Being unable to analyze the conditions of the problem or to plan a series of mutually interdependent operations, they do not go about solving the problem in the proper manner; instead, they simply add or subtract the numbers contained in the problem posed. More severe defects appear when such patients attempt to solve more complex problems. As explained (Part II, Section 5G), the whole process of solution is transformed into a series of impulsive, fragmentary arithmetical operations, frequently unconnected with the ultimate goal.

Patients with frontal syndromes also have considerable difficulty in solving problems with an element of conflict. They accept the external wording of these problems without proper analysis and proceed impulsively to perform whatever action is prompted by the direct impression made on them by the problems. Analysis of the mistakes made by these patients shows that, in contrast to patients with lesions of the inferoparietal (parieto-occipital) or temporal systems, as a rule they do not devote much effort to the preliminary analysis of the conditions of the problem, make no serious attempt to understand the meaning of these conditions, and proceed to act only when the principal ways of solving the problem have been made clear. Every action is impulsive and arises as a direct reaction to one element of the problem. This omission of preliminary investigation and this transformation of a complex activity into a cycle of isolated, impulsive reactions provide the key to the understanding of the discursive defects manifested by these patients. Characteristically, it is this fundamental defect that makes these patients particularly difficult to teach. Even if the solution of the problem is explained to them time and time again, they continue to apply the same method of solution as an inert stereotype, disregarding the changed conditions that have been introduced.

As Tsvetkova has shown (Luria and Tsvetkova, 1966), the retraining of such patients requires the creation of special programs in which all the successive actions which the patients must perform are included (reading the conditions, distinguishing the questions, finding out whether there is an answer to it, finding out what must be done to obtain the answer, and so on). Some of the patients (especially those with a postfrontal syndrome) can be taught successfully to solve problems with the aid of such a program; others, with a severe frontal syndrome, cannot be taught to do so even under these conditions.

Since we have already presented a detailed analysis of the intellectual disturbances in patients with frontal syndromes (Part II, Section 5G), these brief remarks will suffice for the present discussion. Naturally, the type of disturbance we have outlined will be manifested in a clearly defined form only in patients with severe lesions of the frontal lobes; however, signs of latent disturbance in these operations may also be encountered with milder forms of frontal syndrome when such patients are presented with more complicated variants of these problems. It should be noted that these remarks also apply to patients with mild or compensated frontal lobe lesions, where the aforementioned disturbances do not appear in a clearly defined form. A particularly careful analysis must always be undertaken in such cases.

Diffuse brain lesions, associated with *acutely increased intracranial pressure* or *vascular insufficiency*, may give rise to appreciable discursive difficulties. However, these disturbances—associated with instability of traces, a contraction of the range of possible operations, and a tendency to lapse into previously established, stereotyped, or fragmentary responses—are unstable in character and the actual course of the problem solving may vary significantly with the patient's general condition.

It seems apt to conclude this part of the book by repeating what was said previously, namely, that intellectual processes are so complex in composition that their disturbance in patients with brain lesions cannot always be used directly for localization. Not until the various aspects of the difficulties have been carefully analyzed is it possible either to identify the factors responsible for their production or to use the investigation of intellectual activity for the purpose of making a topical diagnosis of local brain lesions.

Conclusion

We have concluded our survey of the factual evidence pertaining to disturbances of the higher cortical functions in the presence of local brain lesions, collected in the course of our investigations over a number of years. We have attempted to describe them as systematically as possible, on the assumption that this would enable us to examine some of the important theoretical problems connected with the principles of human brain activity as well as some of the practical problems in the diagnosis of circumscribed lesions of the cerebral cortex. We adopted as our starting point the idea of a dynamic, systematic localization of functions, originally proposed by Pavlov and subsequently developed and applied to the higher mental functions of man by Vygotskii. From the standpoint of the systematic localization of functions we regard the higher cortical processes as complex, dynamically localized, functional systems that are affected differently with lesions of different parts of the cerebral hemispheres. We are satisfied that this approach is a most productive one, both for diagnostic localization of circumscribed lesions and for the analysis of the principal ways by which the disturbed functions may be restored in patients with local brain lesions (Luria, 1948).

In the course of the description of our material, we naturally came into conflict both with the naive mechanistic ideas of localization, in which mental functions are consigned to rigidly demarcated areas of the brain, and with the idealistic concept that the higher mental processes stand quite apart from the biological functions of the brain or result from the indivisible activity of the "brain as a whole." We hope that in the preceding pages we have been able to adduce sufficient arguments to prove the inadequacy of both these conceptions and the productivity of the dynamic, systematic approach to the study of human cerebral cortical function.

In concluding the book, we feel more than ever that the task of constructing a scientific theory on the activity of the human brain is still only at the beginning and that, in Pavlov's words, "... it is abundantly obvious here that, for longer than we can tell, the truth is immeasurably greater than all the tiny fragments we have so far been able to discover ...." (Luria 1947, Lecture 22).

It is with this reminder of the limited and incomplete nature of our investigations that we end our book. We have described the disturbances of the higher mental functions arising in local brain lesions, distinguishing the syndromes of the disturbances associated with lesions in different areas of the left hemisphere. We have attempted to show the role of the cortical terminations of the various analyzers in the construction of the higher mental processes and to describe the systematic disturbances arising from these lesions. However, in this book we could only outline the most general approaches to the solution of the problems with which we are concerned, for neither the clinical nor the physiological analysis of the facts we have described can be regarded as complete. We can now see particularly clearly the prospects opened up by this initial analysis of the pathology of the higher cortical functions. We could not attempt to give a full account of the whole range of higher mental malfunctioning in patients with lesions of different parts of the brain or examine fully the relationship of the disturbance to the extent or depth of the pathological process, the cerebrovascular and cerebrospinal fluid changes produced by increased intracranial pressure, and so on. Moreover, we have not touched upon the details of the clinical picture in patients with disturbances of the higher cortical functions as a result of lesions of different pathology: tumors, inflammatory processes, vascular disturbances, and trauma. We have not described the differences in the symptomatology and in the course of the manifestations appearing in patients with these lesions. We have done no more than mention the wealth and variety of the pictures observed in the numerous cases in which the pathological process is not confined to a single narrowly circumscribed area of the cortex, but is regional in character, affecting not one, but several regions of the cerebral hemispheres. We have paid very little attention to the symptomatology of lesions of the right (subdominant) hemisphere and mediobasal divisions of the cortex, although they constitute a considerable proportion of the possible cases of brain lesion, and their diagnosis may present very great difficulty. These clinical problems of local brain lesions must be made the subject of future investigation.

In describing the symptoms of disturbed higher mental processes in patients with local brain lesions, we have tried to demonstrate the great importance of their physiological analysis. However, the precise, detailed neurophysiological analysis of the mechanisms underlying these disturbances was not within the scope of this book. It would take the combined efforts of a whole generation of investigators, equipped with the latest physiological techniques, to provide sufficiently accurate answers to a whole series of questions: What changes in the dynamics of neural processes are responsible for disturbances of the higher cortical functions, what laws of nervous activity do they obey, in what varied forms can the pathological changes in the activity of the cortical divisions of the various analyzers manifest themselves, and what is the effect of a localized lesion within the cortical division of one analyzer on the activity of the other parts of the brain? We have not mentioned the group of processes related to the pathophysiological analysis of the relationship between the specific and nonspecific components of higher nervous activity in patients with local brain lesions. Investigations along these lines, which have been began only very recently, make it likely that considerable progress will be made in this direction but, at the same time, they demonstrate the enormous amount of work that will have to be done before these advances are of any practical value.

Finally, our task remains incomplete in relation to the psychological disturbances arising from local brain lesions. Our interest has been confined to the systematic disturbances of the higher cortical functions caused by local brain lesions, and we could not give adequate consideration to problems associated with a general lowering of the level of mental activity caused by practically every lesion of the cerebral hemispheres. For this reason, the integrative examination of the problem proposed by Hughlings Jackson almost a century ago, and still engaging the attention of many psychologists, has largely been omitted from this book. We have also been unable to take up the study of those disturbances of the higher level of mental processes that are based on the second signal system, also arising in patients with brain lesions. Because of the limits which we placed on this book, we have not examined the relationship between word and meaning, speech and thought, and voluntary and automatized activity in pathological brain conditions. The problem of the change in the regulatory role of speech in pathological brain conditions, which has occupied the author for many years (1932 [Eng.], 1956 [with Yudovich], 1961 [Eng.]), likewise has not received its due place in this book.

All these problems need long and careful investigation, combining clinical analysis with a detailed study of the changes in the structure of mental activity, with the aim of giving them, as far as possible, a physiological explanation. However, we hope that these references to still unsolved problems and to the prospects of future research will be no less valuable than the detailed description of what, at the time of writing, appears relatively well established and clear.

Bibliography

RUSSIAN

Abashev-Konstantinovskii, A. L. (1957): Some aspects of the clinical pathology of frontal lobe tumors. Problems in Neurosurgery. Vol. 3. (Medgiz; Kiev).

Abashev-Konstantinovskii, A. L. (1959): Mental Disturbances in Organic Brain Diseases [in Ukrainian]. (Medgiz; Kiev).

Abov'yan, V. A., Blinkov, S. M., and Sirotkin, M. M. (1948): Origin of mistakes in the speech of aphasics. *Izv. Akad. Ped. Nauk RSFSR* no. 15.

Akhutina, T. V. (1975): The Neuropsychological Analysis of Dynamic Aphasia. (Moscow Univ. Press; Moscow).

Anan'ev, B. G. (1947): Recovery of writing and reading skill in agraphia and alexia. *Uch. Zap. Mosk. Univ.* no. 111.

Anan'ev, B. G., Ed. (1959): Tactile Sensation. (Izd. Akad. Ped. Nauk RSFSR; Moscow).

Anan'ev, B. G. (1960): The Psychology of Sensory Perception. (Izd. Akad. Ped. Nauk RSFSR; Moscow).

Andreeva, E. K. (1950): Disturbance of the System of Logical Associations in Frontal Lobe Lesions [Candidate Dissertation]. (Inst. Psychol.; Moscow).

Anokhin, P. K. (1935): Problems of Center and Periphery in the Physiology of Nervous Activity. (Gosizdat; Gorki).

Anokhin, P. K. (1940): Problems of localization from the point of view of systematic ideas on nervous functions. *Nevrolog. i Psikhiat.* **9**.

Anokhin, P. K. (1949): Problems in Higher Nervous Activity. (Izd. Akad. Med. Nauk SSSR; Moscow).

Anokhin, P. K. (1955): New data on the afferent apparatus of the conditioned reflex. *Vop. Psikhol.* no. 6.

Anokhin, P. K. (1956): General principles of compensation for disturbed functions and their physiological basis. *In*: Proceedings of a Conference on Problems in Defectology. (Izd. Akad. Ped. Nauk RSFSR; Moscow).

Anokhin, P. K. (1958): Internal Inhibition as a Problem in Physiology. (Medgiz; Moscow).

Anokhin, P. K. (1968): The Biology and Neurophysiology of the Conditioned Reflex. (Meditsina; Moscow).

Anokhin, P. K. (1971): Fundamental Problems in the General Theory of Functional Systems (USSR Acad. Sci.; Moscow).

Anzimirov, K. L., Karaseva, T. A., Kornyanskii, G. P., and Simernitskaya, E. G. (1967): Hemispheric dominance and its determination. *Vop. Psikhol.* no. 4.

Apresyan, Yu. D. (1974): Lexical Semantics. (Nauka; Moscow).

Arana, L. (1961): Perception as a stochastic process. *Vop. Psikhol.* no. 5.

Artem'eva, E. Yu., and Khomskaya, E. D. (1966): Changes in asymmetry of slow waves in different functional states in normal subjects and patients with frontal lobe lesions. *In*: A. R. Luria and E. D. Khomskaya, Eds.: The Frontal Lobes and Regulation of Psychological Processes. (Moscow Univ. Press).

Asratyan, É. A. (1953): Physiology of the Central Nervous System. (Izd. Akad. Med. Nauk SSSR; Moscow).

Astvatsaturov, V. M.: Clinical and Experimental Psychological Investigations of the Speech Function [Candidate Dissertation]. (St. Petersburg).

Babenkova, S. V. (1954): Special features of the interaction between signal systems in the process of restoration of speech in various forms of aphasia. *In*: Proceedings of the Seventh Session of the Institute of Neurology. (USSR Acad. Med. Sci.; Moscow).

Babenkova, S. V. (1971): Clinical Syndromes of Lesions of the Right Cerebral Hemisphere in Acute Stroke. (Meditsina; Moscow).

Babkin, B. P. (1910): Characteristics of the acoustic analyzer in dogs. *Trans. Obsh. Russk. Vrach. v SPb:* **77**.

Balonov, L. Y. (1950): Changes in Visual Sequential Images as a Sign of Disturbance of Cortical Dynamics in Certain Psychopathological Syndromes [Candidate Dissertation]. (Leningrad).

Balonov, L. Ya., and Deglin, V. L. (1976): Hearing and Speech of the Dominant and Nondominant Hemisphere. (Nauka; Leningrad).

Baranovskaya, O. P., and Khomskaya, E. D. (1966): Changes in the EEG frequency spectrum during the action of indifferent and informative stimuli in patients with frontal lobe lesions. *In*: A. R. Luria and E. D. Khomskaya, Eds.: The Frontal Lobes and Regulation of Psychological Processes. (Moscow Univ. Press).

Baru, A. V., Gershuni, G. V., and Tonkonogii, I. M. (1964): The importance of detecting acoustic stimuli of different duration in the diagnosis of lesions of the temporal zones of the brain. *Zh. Nevropat. i Psikhiat.* im. Korsakov **64**, no. 4.

Bassin, F. V. (1956): Some debatable problems in the modern theory of localization of functions. *Zh. Nevropat. i Psikhiat. Korsakov* **56**.

Bassin, F. V. (1956): Electrophysiological analysis of the state of the problem of the set for performance of movement. *Byull. Inst. Nevrol. Akad. Med. Nauk SSSR* **1**, 21–23.

Bassin, F. V., and Bein, É. S. (1957): Use of an electromyographic technique of speech investigation. *In*: Proceedings of a Conference on Psychology, July 1–6, 1956. (Izd. Akad. Ped. Nauk RSFSR; Moscow).

Bein, É. S. (1947): The Psychological Analysis of Temporal Aphasia [Candidate Dissertation]. (Moscow).

Bein, É. S. (1947): Restoration of speech processes in sensory aphasia. *Uch. Zap. Mosk. Univ.* no. 111.

Bein, É. S. (1957): Fundamental laws of the structure of words and of the grammatical construction of speech in aphasics. *Vop. Psikhol.* no. 4.

Bein, É. S. (1964): Aphasia and Ways of Overcoming It. (Meditsina; Leningrad).

Bein, É. S., and Ioselevich, F. M. (1957): Effects of vestibular stimulation on visual-spatial perception in local lesions of the cerebral cortex. *Zh. Nevropat. i Psikhiat. Korsakov.* **57**.

Bekhterev, V. M. (1905–1907): Fundamentals of Brain Function. 7 vols. (St. Petersburg).

Bekhterev, V. M. (1906): Demonstration of a brain with a lesion of the anterior and medial parts of both temporal lobes. 19, 990.

Bekhtereva, N. P. (1974): Neuropsychological Aspects of Psychological Activity. (Nauka: Leningrad).

Bekhtereva, N. P., Ed. (1974): Neuropsychological Mechanisms of Human Psychological Activity. (Nauka; Leningrad).

Bekhtereva, N. P. (1975): The neurophysiological course of the simplest human mental process. *Vestnik Akad. Nauk SSSR,* no. 11.

Bekhtereva, N. P., Bundzen, P. V., Gogolitsyn, Yu. L., Kaplunovskii, V. S., and Malyshev, V. N. (1975): Principles of organization of the nervous code of individual activity. *Fiziologiya Cheloveka,* **1**, no. 1.

Bel'tyukov, V. I. (1956): Defects in Pronunciation of Words and Their Correction in Deaf and Deaf-Mute Pupils. (Izd. Akad. Ped. Nauk RSFSR; Moscow).

Bel'tyukov, V. I. (1960): Role of Acoustic Perception in Teaching Pronunciation to Deaf and Deaf-Mute Pupils. (Izd. Akad. Ped. Nauk RSFSR; Moscow).

Beritov, I. S. (1959): Mechanisms of Spatial Orientation in Higher Vertebrates (Izd. AN Gruz. SSR; Tbilsi).

Beritov, I. S. (1961): Nervous Mechanisms of Behavior of Higher Vertebrates. (Izd. AN SSSR; Moscow).

Bernshtein, N. A. (1926): General Biomechanics. (Izd. VTsSPS; Moscow).

Bernshtein, N. A. (1935): The problem of the relationship between coordination and localization. *Arkh. Biol. Nauk* **38**.

Bernshtein, N. A. (1947): The Construction of Movements. (Medgiz; Moscow).

Bernshtein, N. A. (1957): Some undeveloped problems in the regulation of motor acts. *Vop. Psikhol.* no. 6.

Bernshtein, N. A. (1966): Outlines of the Physiology of Movements and the Physiology of Activity. (Meditsina; Moscow).

Betz, V. A. (1870): Two centers in the cerebral cortex. Anatomical and Histological Investigations. (Medgiz; Moscow, 1950).

Betz, V. A. (1874): Two centers in the cortical layer of the human brain. *Mosk. Vrachebn. Vestn.* no. 24.

Birenbaum, G. V. (1948): Relationship between the conceptual and structural components of perception. *In*: Investigations on the Psychology of Perception. (Izd. AN SSSR; Moscow).

Blinkov, S. M. (1948): Writing disorders in parietal lobe lesions. *Izv. Akad. Ped. Nauk RSFSR* no. 15.

Blinkov, S. M. (1955): Structural Peculiarities of the Human Cerebrum. (Medgiz; Moscow).

Blinkov, S. M., Zankov, L. V., and Tomilova, M. A. (1945): Therapeutic and educational problems in connection with restoration of speech and writing in motor aphasias. *Izv. Akad. Ped. Nauk RSFSR* no. 2.

Blinkov, S. M., Zav'yalova, E. N., Mokhova, T. M., and Shif, Zh. I. (1945): Restoration of speech in a patient with aphasia and mirror-image reading and writing. *Izv. Akad. Ped. Nauk RSFSR* no. 2.

Blinkov, S. M., and Luria, A. R.: Personal communication.

Bogush, N. R. (1939): Special features of optic images in hallucinatory-paranoid and confabulatory syndromes in schizophrenics. *Nevropat. i Psikhiat.* **8**.

Boskis, R. M. (1953): Peculiarities of speech development in children with disturbances of the acoustic analyzer. *Izv. Akad. Ped. Nauk RSFSR* no. 78.

Boskis, R. M., and Levina, R. E. (1936): One form of acoustic agnosia. *Nevropat. i Psikhiat.* no. 5.

Bragina, N. N. (1966): Clinical Syndromes of Lesions of the Hippocampus and Adjacent Areas. [Doctoral Dissertation]. USSR Acad. Med. Sci.; Moscow).

Bubnova, V. K. (1946): Disturbance of the Understanding of Grammatical Constructions in Brain Lesions and its Restoration during Rehabilitation [Candidate Dissertation]. (Inst. Psychol; Moscow).

Buslaev, F. I. (1858): History of the Grammar of the Russian Language. (St. Petersburg).

Bzhalava, I. T. (1958): Toward a psychology of set in schizophrenics. *In:* Experimental Investigations on the Psychology of Set. (Tiflis).

Bzhalava, I. T. (1958): The psychopathology of epilepsy from the point of view of the psychology of set. *In*: Experimental Investigations of the Psychology of Set. (Tiflis).

Chlenov, L. G. (1934): Advances in the Study of Apraxia, Agnosia, and Aphasia. (Moscow).

Chlenov, L. G. (1938*a*): Inactivity as a manifestation of physiological inertia. *Uch. Zap. Mosk. Univ.* no. 111.

Chlenov, L. G. (1938*b*): The pathology of spatial vision. *In*: Clinical Problems and Treatment of Mental Diseases. (Moscow).

Chlenov, L. G. (1945): The problem of localization in the light of the restoration of functions. *Nevropat. i Psikhiat.* **14**.

Chlenov, L. G. (1948): Aphasia in polyglots. *Izv. Akad. Ped. Nauk* RSFSR no. 15.

Chlenov, L. G., and Bein, É. S. (1958): Agnosia for faces. *Nevropat. i Psikhiat.* **58**.

Davidenkov, S. I. (1915): The Study of Aphasias. (Kharkov).

Davydov, V. V. (1957): Initial formation of concept of number in children. *Vop. Psikhol.* no. 2.

Demidov, V. A. (1909): Conditioned (Salivary) Reflexes in Dogs Without the Anterior Halves of Both Hemispheres [Candidate Dissertation]. (St. Petersburg).

Dul'nev, G. M., and Luria, A. R., Eds. (1960): Principles of Grading Children in Special Schools. 2nd. ed. (Akad. Ped. Nauk; Moscow).

Egorov, T. G. (1953): The Psychology of Learning to Read. (Izd. Akad. Ped. Nauk RSFSR; Moscow).

Éidinova, M. B., and Pravdina-Vinarskaya, E. N. (1959): Cerebral Paralysis in Children and Methods of Overcoming It. (Izd. Akad. Ped. Nauk RSFSR; Moscow).

Él'konin, D. B. (1955): Interaction between the first and second signal systems in children of preschool age. *Izd. Akad. Ped. Nauk RSFSR* no. 64.

Él'konin, D. B. (1956): Some aspects of the psychology of learning grammar. *Vop. Psikhol.* no. 5.

Él'konin, D. B. (1960): Child Psychology. (Uchpedgiz; Moscow).

Él'yasson, M. I. (1908): Investigation of the Hearing Capacity of Dogs under Normal Conditions and after Partial Bilateral Extirpation of the Cortical Hearing Center [Candidate Dissertation]. (Military Med. Acad; St. Petersburg).

Endovitskaya, G. V. (1955): The role of speech in the performance of simple actions by children of preschool age. *Izv. Akad. Ped. Nauk RSFSR* no. 64.

Endovitskaya, G. V. (1957): The effect of organization of orienting activity on the capacity of attention in children. *Dokl. APN RSFSR* no. 3.

Endovitskaya, G. V. (1961): The development of sensation and perception in children of preschool age. *In*: A. V. Zaporozhets *et al.*, Ed: The Psychology of Children of Preschool Age.

Faller, T. O. (1948): The Neurological Symptom Complex in Craniocerebral Wounds with Splinters Situated in the Region of the Longitudinal Fissure [Candidate Dissertation]. (USSR Acad. Med. Sci.; Moscow).

Figurin, N. L., and Denisova, M. P. (1949): Stages in the Behavioral Development of Children from Birth Until the Age of One Year. (Moscow).

Filimonov, I. N. (1940): Localization of functions in the cerebral cortex. *Nevropat. i Psikhiat.* **9**.

Filimonov, I. N. (1944): Functional polyvalency of the architectonic formations of the cerebral cortex. *Nevropat. i Psikhiat.* **12**.

Filimonov, I. N. (1949): Comparative Anatomy of the Mammalian Cerebral Cortex. (USSR Acad. Med. Sci. Press; Moscow).

Filimonov, I. N. (1951): Localization of functions in the cerebral cortex and Pavlov's theory of higher nervous activity. *Klin. Med.* **29**.

Filimonov, I. N. (1957): Architectonics and localization of functions in the cerebral cortex. Textbook of Neurology. vol. 1 (Medgiz; Moscow).

Filimonov, I. N., and Vifleemskaya, Z. Y. (1945): The so-called constructive apraxia. *Izv. Akad. Ped. Nauk RSFSR* no. 2.

Filippycheva, N. A. (1952): Inertia of the Higher Cortical Processes in Local Lesions of the Cerebral Hemispheres [Candidate Dissertation]. (USSR Acad. Med. Sci.; Moscow).

Filippycheva, N. A. (1959): The study of the functional characteristics of the motor analyzer in patients with a pathological focus in the parietal lobe. *In*: Problems in Modern Neurosurgery. vol. 3. (Moscow).

Filippycheva, N. A. (1966): Neurophysiological mechanisms of disturbance of motor responses in patients with frontal lobe lesions. *In*. A. R. Luria and E. D. Khomskaya, Eds.: The Frontal Lobes and Regulation of Psychological Processes. (Moscow Univ. Press).

Fradkina, F. I. (1955): The appearance of speech in the child. *Uch. Zap. Inst. Gertsena* **112**.

Gadzhiev, S. G. (1951): Analysis of the Processes of Intellectual Activity in Patients with Frontal Lobe Lesions [Candidate Dissertation]. (Inst. Psychol.; Moscow).

Gadzhiev, S. G. (1966): Disturbance of optical intellectual activity in frontal lobe lesions. *In*: A. R. Luria and E. D. Khomskaya, Eds.: The Frontal Lobes and Regulation of Psychological Processes. (Moscow Univ. Press).

Gal'perin, P. Y. (1957): Mental activity as the basis of formation of thought and image. *Vop. Psikhol.* no. 6.

Gal'perin, P. Y. (1959): The development of investigations on the formation of mental activities. *In*: Psychological Science in the USSR. (Moscow).

Gal'perin, P. Y., and Golubova, R. A. (1933): Mechanisms of complex paraphasias. *Sovet. Psikhonevrol.* no. 6.

Genkin, A. A. (1962): The use of the method of statistical description of the duration of the ascending and descending phases of brain electrical activity to discover information in processes accompanying intellectual activity. *Dokl. Akad. Ped. Nauk RSFSR* no. 6.

Gershuni, G. V. (1949): Reflex reactions to external stimuli. *Fiziol. Zh. SSSR* no. 5.

Gershuni, G. V. (1959): Study of the activity of the human acoustic analyzer using various reactions. Problems in Physiological Acoustics. vol. 3. (Izd. AMN SSSR; Moscow).

Gershuni, G. V. (1962): Evaluation of the functional significance of electrical responses of the auditory system. *Fiziol. Zh. SSSR* **48**, no. 3.

Gershuni, G. V. (1965): The afferent flow and processes of discrimination of an external stimulus. *In*: E. A. Asratyan, Ed.: Reflexes of the Brain. (Izd. Akad. Nauk SSSR; Moscow).

Gershuni, G. V. (1968): On the mechanism of hearing. *In*: Mechanisms of Hearing. (Nauka; Leningrad).

Gilyarovskii, V. A. (1912): On the disorders of memory in certain local brain lesions. *Sovrem. Psikhiatriya*, (Moscow) February, p. 93.

Glezer, I. I. (1955): New data on the development of the cortical nucleus of the motor analyzer in man. *In*: Proceedings of the Second Conference on Age Morphology and Physiology. (Izd. Akad. Ped. Nauk RSFSR; Moscow).

Glezer, I. I. (1959): F. J. Gall and his role in the history of neurology. *Zh. Nevropat. i Psikhiat Korsarkov* **59**.

Grashchenkov, N. I. (1946): The problem of functional asynapsia. *In*: Neuropathology and Psychiatry. [Collection in honor of V. P. Osipov.] (Leningrad).

Grashchenkov, N. I. (1948*a*): Interneuronal Communication Apparatuses—Synapses and Their Role in Physiology and Pathology. (Izd. AN Belor. SSR; Minsk).

Grashchenkov, N. I., Ed. (1948*b*): Neurology in Wartime. (Izd. Akad. Med. Nauk SSSR; Moscow).

Grashchenkov, N. I., and Luria, A. R. (1945): The systematic principle of localization of functions in the cerebral cortex. *Nevropat. i Psikhiat.* no. 1.

Grindel', O. M., and Filippycheva, N. A. (1959): Lowering of the mobility of excitation in the motor analyzer in a patient with a localized pathological process in the frontal lobe. *Zh. Vyss. Nerv. Deiat.* **9**.

Grinshtein, A. M. (1946): Tracts and Centers of the Nervous System. (Medgiz; Moscow).

Grinshtein, A. M. (1956): The problem of dynamic localization of functions in experimental and clinical practice. *Zh. Nevropat. i Psikhiat. Korsakov.* **56**.

Gurevich, M. O., and Ozeretskii, N. (1930): Psychomotor Functions. 2 vols. (Medgiz; Moscow).

Gur'yanov, E. V. (1940): The Development of the Writing Skill in the Schoolchild. (Uchpedgiz; Moscow).

Ingel'der, B. (1960): From perceptive configuration to the construction of the logical operation. *Vop. Psikhol.* no. 5.

Ioshpa, A. Ya., and Khomskaya, E. D. (1966): On regulation of the temporal parameters of voluntary motor responses in normal subjects and patients with frontal lobe lesions. *In*: A. R. Luria and E. D. Khomskaya, Eds.: The Frontal Lobes and Regulation of Psychological Processes. (Moscow Univ. Press).

Istomina, Z. M. (1948): The development of voluntary memory in the preschool age child. *Izv. Akad. Ped. Nauk RSFSR* no. 14.

Ivanov-Smolenskii, A. G. (1933): Fundamental Problems in the Pathophysiology of Activity. (Medgiz; Moscow).

Ivanov-Smolenskii, A. G. (1949): Essays on the Pathophysiology of Higher Nervous Activity. (Medgiz; Moscow).

Ivanov-Smolenskii, A. G. (1951): The study of the combined working of the first and second signal systems of the brain. *Zh. Vyss. Nerv. Deiat. Pavlov* no. 2.

Ivanov-Smolenskii, A. G. (1952): Pathological changes in the combined activity of the first and second signal systems of the human brain. *Voennmed. Zh.* no. 2.

Ivanov-Smolenskii, A. G., Ed. (1956): Objective investigation of higher nervous activity, especially of the interaction between the two signal systems in certain mental diseases. *Trans. Inst. Vyss. Nerv. Deiat. Patofiziol.* **1**.

Ivanova, M. P. (1953): Disturbance of the Interaction between the Two Signal Systems in the Formation of Complex Motor Reactions in Brain Lesions [Candidate Dissertation]. (Moscow State Univ.; Moscow).

Ivanova, M. P. (1966): Disturbance of the reaction of choice in massive lesions of the frontal lobes. *In*: A. R. Luria and E. D. Khomskaya, Eds.: The Frontal Lobes and Regulation of Psychological Processes. (Moscow Univ. Press).

Kabelyanskaya, L. G. (1957): The state of the acoustic analyzer in sensory aphasia. *Zh. Nevropat. i Psikhiat. i Korsakov* **57**.

Kaidanova, S. I. (1954): Features of the auditory analyzer in children with impaired development of sensory speech. *In*: Abstracts of Proceedings of a Scientific Session of the Lesgaft State Scientific Institute. (Leningrad).

Kaplan, A. E. (1949): Visual Sequential Images during Disturbances of the Normal Activity of the Central Nervous System [Candidate Dissertation]. (Leningrad).

Karaseva, T. A. (1967): Diagnosis of Lesions of the Temporal Lobe by Quantitative Methods of Investigation of Hearing [Candidate Dissertation]. (Academy of Medical Sciences; Moscow).

Kartsovnik, I. I. (1949): The Frontal Syndrome and Its Clinical Variants in Penetrating Wounds of the Brain. (Novosibirsk).

Kaufman, O. P. (1947): Optic agraphia. Neurology in Wartime. Transactions of the Institute of Neurology. (USSR Acad. Med. Sci.; Moscow).

Kaverina, E. K. (1950): The Development of Speech in Children during the First Two Years of Life. (Medgiz; Moscow).

Khachaturyan, A. A. (1949): The precentral region. *In*: S. A. Sarkisov and I. N. Filimonov, Eds.: Cytoarchitectonics of the Human Cerebral Cortex. (Moscow).

Khodzhava, Z. I. (1957): Role of orientation in processes of reading. Proceedings of a Conference on Psychology. (Izd. Akad. Ped. Nauk RSFSR; Moscow).

Khomskaya, E. D. (1956): The role of speech in the compensation for motor reactions. *In*: A. R. Luria, Ed.; Problems in the Higher Nervous Activity of the Normal and Abnormal Child. vol. 1. (Izd. Akad. Ped. Nauk RSFSR; Moscow).

Khomskaya, E. D. (1958): Investigation of the effect of speech reactions on motor functions in children with cerebral asthenia. *In*: A. R. Luria, Ed.: Problems in the Higher Nervous Activity of the Normal and Abnormal Child. vol. 2. (Izd. Akad. Ped. Nauk RSFSR; Moscow).

Khomskaya, E. D. (1959): The mechanism of compensation of defects in local brain lesions. *In*: Abstracts of Proceedings of the First Congress of the Society of Psychologists, June 29–July 4, 1959. (Moscow).

Khomskaya, E. D. (1960): The effect of verbal instruction on vascular and psychogalvanic components of the orienting reflex in various local brain lesions. *Dokl. Akad. Ped. Nauk RSFSR* no. 6.

Khomskaya, E. D. (1961): The effect of verbal instruction on the autonomic component of the orienting reflex in various local brain lesions. *Dokl. Akad. Ped. Nauk RSFSR* nos. 1 & 2.

Khomskaya, E. D. (1965): Regulation of the autonomic components of the orienting reflex by verbal instructions in patients with various brain lesions. *Vop. Psikhol.* no. 1.

Khomskaya, E. D. (1966*a*): Autonomic components of the orienting reflex under the influence of indifferent and informative stimuli in patients with frontal lobe lesions. *In*: A. R. Luria and E. D. Khomskaya, Eds.: The Frontal Lobes and Regulation of Psychological Processes. (Moscow Univ. Press).

Khomskaya, E. D. (1966*b*): Regulation of the intensity of voluntary motor responses in frontal lobe lesions. *In*: A. R. Luria and E. D. Khomskaya, Eds.: The Frontal Lobes and Regulation of Psychological Processes. (Moscow Univ. Press).

Khomskaya, E. D. (1972): The Brain and Activation. (Moscow Univ. Press; Moscow).

Khomskaya, E. D. (1976): General and local changes in brain electrical activity during psychological activity. *Fiziologiya Cheloveka*, **2**, no. 3.

Khomskaya, E. D., and Luria, A. R., Eds. (1977): Problems in Neuropsychology. Psychophysiological Investigations. (Nauka; Moscow).

Khomskaya, E. D., Konovalov, Y. V., and Luria, A. R. (1961): Participation of the speech system in regulation of the autonomic components of the orienting reflex in local brain lesions. *Vop. Neirokhir.* no. 4.

Khoroshko, V. K. (1912): Relationship of the Frontal Lobes of the Brain to Psychology and Psychopathology. (Moscow).

Khoroshko, V. K. (1921): Clinical observations in wartime on wounds of the frontal lobes of the brain. *Med. Zh.* nos. 5–6 & 6–7.

Khoroshko, V. K. (1935): Results of personal investigations of the frontal lobes of the brain. *Klin. Med.* 13.

Kiyashchenko, N. K. (1973): Disturbance of Memory in Local Brain Lesions. (Moscow Univ. Press; Moscow).

Kiyashchenko, N. K., Moskovichute, L. I., Simernitskaya, E. G., Faller, G. O., and Filippycheva, K. A. (1975): Brain and Memory. (Moscow Univ. Press; Moscow).

Klimkovskii, M. (1961): The effect of verbal instruction on the automatic component of the orienting reflex in patients with lesions of the posterior divisions of the cerebral hemispheres. *Dokl. APN RSFSR* no. 2.

Klimkovskii, M. (1966): Disturbance of Audioverbal Memory in Lesions of the Left Temporal Lobe. [Candidate Dissertation]. (Moscow Univ. Press).

Kogan, V. M. (1947): Restoration of the conceptual aspect of speech in aphasia. *Uch. Zap. Mosk. Univ.* no. 111.

Kogan, V. M. (1961): Dynamics of aphasia and restoration of speech. *In*: Transactions of the Central Institute of Evaluation of Working Capacity. (Moscow).

Kogan, V. M. (1961): Acoustic agnosia. *In*: Transactions of the Central Institute of Evaluation of Working Capacity. (Moscow).

Kok, E. P. (1957): Investigation of Abstractions and Generalizations in Patients with Aphasia [Candidate Dissertation]. (I. P. Pavlov Inst. Physiol., USSR Acad. Sci.; Leningrad).

Kok, E. P. (1958): Disturbance of abstraction and color naming in certain local brain lesions. *Dokl. Akad. Ped. Nauk RSFSR* no. 4.

Kok, E. P. (1960): Disturbance of abstraction and spatial direction in the syndrome of the inferior parietal lesion of the dominant hemisphere. *Dokl. Akad. Ped. Nauk RSFSR* no. 2.

Kok, E. P. (1967): Visual Agnosias. (Meditsina; Moscow).

Kolodnaya, A. Y. (1949): The syndromes of spatial disturbances in brain wounds. *Uch. Zap. Mosk. Univ.* no. 111.

Kolodnaya, A. Y. (1954): Disturbance of differentiation of right and left and the role of the cutaneous analyzer in its restoration. *Izv. Akad. Ped. Nauk RSFSR* no. 53.

Kol'tsova, M. M. (1958): Formation of the Higher Nervous Activity of the Child. (Medgiz; Leningrad).

Kononova, E. P. (1940): Development of the frontal region in the postnatal period. *In: Tr. Inst. Moz.* 5.

Kononova, E. P. (1948): Development of the human frontal lobes during the intrauterine period. *Tr. Inst. Moz.* 6.

Konorskii, Y. M., and Miller, S. M. (1936): Conditioned reflexes of the motor analyzer. Tr. Fiziol. Labor. Akad. *Pavlov* 6.

Konorskii, Y. M. (1956): Effect of extirpation of the frontal lobes on the higher nervous activity of the dog. *In*: Problems in the Modern View of Physiology of the Nervous and Muscular Systems. (Tiflis).

Konorskii, Y. M. (1957): Hyperactivity of animals after removal of the frontal lobes. *In*: Problems in the Physiology of the Central Nervous System. (Leningrad).

Konovalov, Y. V. (1954): Analysis of mistakes in the diagnosis of tumors of the occipital lobe within the cerebral hemispheres. *Vop. Neirokhir.* no. 6.

Konovalov, Y. V. (1957): Difficulties in the differential diagnosis between tumors of the anterior divisions of the cerebral hemispheres and of the posterior cranial fossa. *In*: Problems in Modern Neurosurgery. vol. 1. (Medgiz; Moscow).

Konovalov, Y. V. (1960): Value of focal symptoms in the diagnosis of brain tumors. *Vop. Neirokhir.* no. 3.

Konovalov, Y. V., and Filippycheva, N. A.: Unpublished data.

Korchazhinskaya, V. I., and Popova, Ya. T. (1977): Unilateral Spatial Aphasia. (Moscow Univ. Press; Moscow).

Korolenok, K. K. (1946): Illusions of spatial orientation. *In*: Problems in General Psychopathology. (Irkutsk).

Korst, L. O. (1951): Tumors of the Parietal Region [Candidate Dissertation]. (USSR Acad. Med. Sci.; Moscow).

Korst, L. O., and Fantalova, V. L. (1959): Characteristics of disorders of certain cortical functions in patients with tumors of the temporal and occipital lobes of the brain. *In*: Problems in Modern Neurosurgery. vol. 3. (Moscow).

Kornyanskii, G. P., Karaseva, T. A., Anzimirov, K. L., and Simernitskaya, E. G. (1965): The diagnostic importance of Wada's test in clinical neurosurgery. *Vop. Neirokhir.* no. 4.

Kotik, B. S. (1975): Investigation of Interhemispheric Interaction in Auditory Processes [Candidate Dissertation]. (Moscow University; Moscow).

Kotlyarova, L. I. (1948): Significance of the Motor Factor in Tactile Sensation [Candidate Dissertation]. (Inst. Psychol.; Moscow).

Kramer, V. V. (1931): The Theory of Localization. (Medgiz; Moscow).

Krasnogorskii, N. I. (1911): Retention and Localization in the Cutaneous and Motor Analyzers in the Cerebral Cortex of the Dog [Candidate Dissertation]. (Military Med. Acad.; St. Petersburg).

Krasnogorskii, N. I. (1954): Studies on the Higher Activity of Man and Animals. vol. 1. (Medgiz; Moscow).

Krol', M. B. (1933): Neurological Syndromes. (Ukrain. Medizdat; Kharkov-Kiev).

Krol', M. B. (1934): Old and new in the study of apraxia. *In*: M. B. Krol, Ed.: Progress in the Study of Apraxia, Agnosia, and Aphasia. (Medgiz; Moscow).

Kryzhanovskii, I. I. (1909): Conditioned Reflexes after Extirpation of the Temporal Regions of the Cerebral Hemisphere in Dogs [Candidate Dissertation]. (Military Med. Acad.; St. Petersburg).

Kudrin, A. N. (1910): Conditioned Reflexes in Dogs after Extirpation of the Posterior Halves of the Cerebral Hemispheres [Candidate Dissertation]. (Military Med. Acad.; St. Petersburg).

Kukuev, L. A. (1940): Relationship Between the Motor Area of the Cortex and the Striopallidum in Mammalian Phylogenesis [Candidate Dissertation]. (Brain Inst.; Moscow).

Kukuev, L. A. (1955): Localization of motor functions in the cerebral cortex. *Zh. Nevropat. i Psikhiat. i Korsakov* **55**.

Kukuev, L. A. (1958): Relationship between the Cortical End of the Motor Analyzer and the Dominant Subcortex during Human Development [Doctorate Dissertation]. (Brain Inst.; Moscow).

Kunstman, K. I., and Orbeli, L. A. (1924): Consequences of deafferentation of the hindlimb in dogs. *Izv. Inst. Lesgafta* **9**.

Kuraev, S. P. (1912): Investigation of Dogs after Disturbances of the Anterior Lobes of the Brain [Candidate Dissertation]. (St. Petersburg).

Kvasov, D. G. (1956): The muscular apparatus of the analyzers. *Fiziol. Zh. SSSR* **38**.

Lebedinskii, M. S. (1941): Aphasia, Agnosia, and Apraxia. (Kharkov).

Lebedinskii, M. S. (1948): Disturbance of mental function in lesions of the right hemisphere. *In*: Problems in Modern Psychiatry. (Moscow).

Lebedinskii, V. V. (1966): The performance of symmetrical and asymmetrical programs by patients with frontal lobe lesions. *In*: A. R. Luria and E. D. Khomskaya, Eds.: The Frontal Lobes and Regulation of Psychological Processes (Moscow Univ. Press).

Leont'ev, A. N. (1931): The Development of Memory. (Krupskaya Acad. of Communist Education Press; Moscow).

Leont'ev, A. N. (1959): Problems in Mental Development. (*Izd. Akad. Ped. Nauk RSFSR*; Moscow).

Leont'ev, A. N. (1961): The social nature of human mental activity. *Vop. Filos.* no. 1.

Leont'ev, A. N., Ed. (1974): The Bases of A Theory of Speech Activity. (Nauka; Moscow).

Leont'ev, A. N. (1975): Activity. Consciousness. Personality. (Mysl'; Moscow).

Leont'ev, A. N., and Zaporozhets, A. V. (1945): Restoration of Hand Movements after War Injuries. (Moscow).

Levina, R. E. (1940): Defects of Reading and Writing in Children. (Uchpedgiz; Moscow).

Levina, R. E. (1951): The Study of Dumb Children (Alalics). (Izd. Akad. Ped. Nauk RSFSR; Moscow).

Livanov, M. N., Gavrilova, N. A., and Aslanov, A. S. (1966): Correlation between bio-potentials in the frontal zones of the human cerebral cortex. *In*: A. R. Luria and E. D. Khomskaya, Eds.: The Frontal Lobes and Regulation of Psychological Processes. (Moscow Univ. Press).

Lubovskii, V. I. (1956): Some aspects of the higher nervous activity of oligophrenic children. *In*: A. R. Luria, Ed.: Problems in the Higher Nervous Activity of the Normal and Abnormal Child. vol. 1. (Izd. Akad. Ped. Nauk RSFSR; Moscow).

Luria, A. R. (1939): Disturbances of perception in frontal lobe lesions (the problem of the frontal agnosias). Unpublished investigation.

Luria, A. R. (1940*a*): Temporal (Acoustic) Aphasia. [Doctorate Dissertation]. vol. 1 of: The Study of Aphasia in the Light of Cerebral Pathology. (Kiev Med. Inst.; Kiev).

Luria, A. R. (1940*b*): Parietal (Semantic) Aphasia. vol. 2. of: The Study of Aphasia in the Light of Cerebral Pathology. (Unpublished investigation).

Luria, A. R. (1943): Psychological analysis of the premotor syndrome. (Unpublished investigation).

Luria, A. R. (1945): The Pathology of Arithmetical Operations. no. 3. (Izd. Acad. Ped. Nauk RSFSR; Moscow).

Luria, A. R. (1947): Traumatic Aphasia. (Izd. Akad. Ped. Nauk RSFSR; Moscow).

Luria, A. R. (1948): Restoration of Brain Functions after War Injuries. (Izd. Akad. Med. Nauk SSSR; Moscow).

Luria, A. R. (1950): Essays on the Psychophysiology of Handwriting. (Izd. Akad. Ped. Nauk RSFSR; Moscow).

Luria, A. R. (1955): The Role of Speech in the Formation of Temporary Connections in Normal and Abnormal Development. (Izd. Akad. Ped. Nauk RSFSR; Moscow).

Luria, A. R., Ed. (1956–1958): Problems in the Higher Nervous Activity of the Normal and Abnormal Child. 2 vols. (Izd. Akad. Ped. Nauk RSFSR; Moscow).

Luria, A. R. (1957*a*): The motor analyzer and cortical organization of voluntary movements. *Vop. Psikhol.* no. 2.

Luria, A. R. (1957*b*): The development of voluntary movement. *Vop. Psikhol.* no. 6.

Luria, A. R. (1957*c*): The two types of analytic-synthetic activity of the cerebral cortex. *Trans. Odessa State Univ.* **147**. [Issued in commemoration of the 50th anniversary of I. M. Sechenov's death].

Luria, A. R. (1959): The development of speech and formation of mental processes. *In*: Psychological Science in the USSR. vol. 1. (Izd. Akad. Ped. Nauk RSFSR; Moscow).

Luria, A. R., Ed. (1960): The Mentally Retarded Child. (Izd. Akad. Ped. Nauk RSFSR; Moscow).

Luria, A. R. (1963): The Human Brain and Psychological Processes. (Izd. Akad. Ped. Nauk RSFSR; Moscow. English translation, Harper and Row; New York; 1966).

Luria, A. R. (1964*a*): Neuropsychology and the local diagnosis of brain lesions. *Vop. Psikhol.* no. 2.

Luria, A. R. (1964*b*): Brain and Mind. *Kommunist* no. 6.

Luria, A. R. (1966): Neuropsychology and its importance to psychological science. *Zh. Nevropat. i Psikhiat. i Korsakov* **16**, no. 8.

Luria, A. R., and Bzhalava, I. T. (1947): Disturbance of orientation in brain lesions. Neurology in Wartime. *In*: Transactions of the Institute of Neurology. (USSR Acad. Med. Sci.; Moscow).

Luria, A. R., Karpov, B. A., and Yarbus, A. L. (1965): Disturbance of the perception of complex objects in frontal lobe lesions. *Vop. Psikhol.* no. 3.

Luria, A. R., and Khomskaya, E. D., Eds. (1966): The Frontal Lobes and Regulation of Psychological Processes. (Moscow Univ. Press; Moscow).

Luria, A. R., Konovalov, A. N., and Podgornaya, A. E. (1970): Memory Disturbances in the Clinical Picture of Aneurysms of the Anterior Communicating Artery. (Moscow Univ. Press; Moscow).

Luria, A. R., and Polyakova, A. G. (1959): Observations on the development of voluntary action in early childhood. *Dokl. Akad. Ped. Nauk RSFSR* nos. 3 & 4.

Luria, A. R., Pravdina-Vinarskaya, E. N., and Yarbus, A. L. (1961): The mechanism of the following movements of the gaze and their pathology. *Vop. Psikhol.* no. 5.

Luria, A. R., and Simernitskaya, É. G. (1975): Functional interaction between the cerebral hemispheres in the organization of verbal-mnemic functions. *Fiziologiya Cheloveka,* 1, no. 3.

Luria, A. R., and Skorodumova, A. V. (1950): The phenomenon of fixed hemianopsia. *In*: Collection in Memory of S. V. Kravkov. (Moscow).

Luria, A. R., Sokolov, E. N., and Klimkovskii, M. (1967): On some neurodynamic mechanisms of memory. *Zh. Vyssh. Nerv. Deyat.* 17.

Luria, A. R., and Tsvetkova, L. S. (1965): The programming of constructive activity in local brain lesions. *Vop. Psikhol.* no. 2.

Luria, A. R., and Tsvetkova, L. S. (1965): Reeducation and its importance to psychology and pedagogics. *Sovetskaya Ped.* no. 12.

Luria, A. R., and Tsvetkova, L. S. (1966): The Neuropsychological Analysis of Problem Solving. (Prosveshchenie; Moscow).

Luria, A. R., and Yudovich, F. L. (1956): Speech and the Development of Mental Processes. (Izd. Akad. Ped. Nauk RSFSR; Moscow).

Lyubinskaya, A. A. Essays on the Mental Development of the Child. (Izd. Akad. Ped. Nauk RSFSR; Moscow).

Maizel', I. I. (1959): Disturbance of Intellectual Activity Following Disintegration of Active, Goal-directed Activity. (Unpublished investigation for diploma, Moscow State Univ.).

Manuilenko, Z. V. (1948): Development of voluntary movement in children of preschool age. *Izv. Akad. Ped. Nauk RSFSR* no. 14.

Markova, E. A. (1957): Disturbances of neurodynamics in amnestic aphasia. *Zh. Vyss. Nerv. Deiat. Pavlov* 8.

Marr, N. Y. (1933–1935): Selected Works, 5 vols. (State Academy of History of Material Culture Press; Leningrad).

Martsinovskaya, E. N. (1958): Disturbance of the regulating role of speech in severely mentally retarded children. *In*: A. R. Luria, Ed.: Problems in the Higher Nervous Activity of the Normal and Abnormal Child. vol. 2. (Izd. Akad. Ped. Nauk RSFSR; Moscow).

Marushevskii, M. (1959): Changes in the organization of movements in local brain lesions. *In*: Abstracts of the Proceedings of the First Congress of the Society of Psychologists, June 29–July 24, 1959. (Moscow).

Maruszewski, M. (1966): On disturbances of the simplest forms of voluntary action in local lesions of the frontal lobes. *In*: A. R. Luria and E. D. Khomskaya, Eds.: The Frontal Lobes and Regulation of Psychological Processes. (Moscow Univ. Press).

Mel'chuk, I. A. (1974): Trial of a Theory of Linguistic Models: Meaning—Text. (Nauka; Moscow).

Menchinskaya, N. A. (1955): The Psychology of Teaching Arithmetic. (Uchpedgiz; Moscow).

Meshchaninov, I. I. (1936): Advances in Language Teaching. (Sotsékgiz; Moscow).

Meshcheryakov, A. I. (1953): Disturbance of Interaction between the Two Signal Systems in the Formation of Simple Motor Reactions in Local Brain Lesions [Candidate Dissertation]. (Inst. Psychol., Acad. of Pedagogic Sci., Moscow).

Meshcheryakov, A. I. (1956): Participation of the second signal system in analysis and synthesis of sequential stimuli in normal and mentally retarded children. *In*: A. R. Luria, Ed.: Problems in the Higher Nervous Activity of the Normal and Abnormal Child. vol. 1. (Izd. Akad. Ped. Nauk RSFSR: Moscow).

Meshcheryakov, A. I. (1958): Mechanisms of disturbance of the processes of abstraction and generalization in mentally retarded children. *In*: A. R. Luria, Ed.: Problems in the Higher Nervous Activity of the Normal and Abnormal Child. vol. 2. (Izd. Akad. Ped. Nauk RSFSR; Moscow).

Meshcheryakov, A. I. (1966): Disturbance of simple motor responses in massive lesions of the frontal lobes. *In*: A. R. Luria and E. D. Khomskaya, Eds.: The Frontal Lobes and Regulation of Psychological Processes. (Moscow Univ. Press).

Meynert, T. (1884): Psychiatry. [Russian translation.] (Kharkov).

Mokhova, T. M. (1948): Restoration of speech in motor aphasia. *Izv. Akad. Ped. Nauk RSFSR* no. 15.

Morozova, N. G. (1947): Textual comprehension. *Izv. Akad. Ped. Nauk RSFSR* no. 7.

Morozova, N. G. (1953): Teaching Conscious Reading to Deaf-Mute Schoolchildren. (Uchpedgiz; Moscow).

Nazarova, L. K. (1952): The role of speech kinesthesias in writing. *Sovet. Pedag.* no. 6.

Nebylitsyn, V. D. (1960): Present state of factor analysis. *Vop. Psikhol.* no. 4.

Neiman, L. V. (1960): The Hearing Function in Deaf and Deaf-Mute Children. (Izd. Akad. Ped. Nauk RSFSR; Moscow).

Nepomnyashchaya, N. I. (1956): The psychological mechanisms in the formation of mental activity. *Vestn. Mosk. Univ.* no. 2.

New Developments in the Study of Apraxia, Agnosia, and Aphasia (1934) (Medgiz; Moscow).

Novikova, L. A. (1955): Electrophysiological investigations of speech kinesthesias. *Vop. Psikhol.* no. 5.

Orbeli, L. A. (1935): Lectures on the Physiology of the Nervous System. (Biomedgiz; Leningrad).

Ozeretskii, N. I. (1930): Technique of investigating motor function. *In*: M. Gurevich and N. Ozeretskii: Psychomotor Functions. (Medgiz; Moscow).

Pantina, N. S. (1954): Formation of the motor skill of writing in relation to the type of orientation to the task. *Vop. Psikhol.* no. 4.

Paramonova, N. P. (1956): Formation of interaction between two signal systems in the normal child. *In*: A. R. Luria, Ed.: Problems in the Higher Nervous Activity of the Normal and Abnormal Child. vol. 1. (Izd. Akad. Ped. Nauk RSFSR, Moscow).

Pavlov, I. P. (1949): Complete Collected Works. 6 vols. (Izd. AN SSSR; Moscow).

Pavlov, I. P. (1949): Pavlov's Wednesdays. 3 vols. (Izd. AN SSSR; Moscow).

Perel'man, L. B. (1946): Pharmacological treatment of motor and sensory disturbances after injury to the central nervous system. *Sovet. Med.* no. 8–9.

Pevzner, M. S. (1960): Oligophrenia. Mental Deficiency in Children. (Izd. Akad. Ped. Nauk RSFSR; Moscow). [English translation: Consultants Bureau, New York, 1961.]

Piaget, J. (1956): Problems in developmental psychology. *Vop. Psikhol.* no. 3.

Polyakov, G. I. (1938–1948): Ontogenesis of the isocortex in man. Communications 1–6. *Tr. Inst. Moz.* nos. 1–6.

Polyakov, G. I. (1956): Relationship between principal types of neurons in the human cerebral cortex. *Zh. Vyss. Nerv. Deiat. Pavlov* **6**.

Polyakov, G. I. (1959): Structural organization of the cortical representation of various analyzers in man. *Izv. Akad. Med. Nauk SSSR* no. 9.

Polyakov, G. I. (1965): Principles of the Neuronal Organization of the Brain. (Moscow Univ. Press).

Polyakov, G. I. (1966): Structural organization of the cortex of the frontal lobes in connection with its functional role. *In*: A. R. Luria and E. D. Khomskaya, Eds.: The Frontal Lobes and Regulation of Psychological Processes. (Moscow Univ. Press).

Popov, E. A. (1941): Clinical Aspects and Pathophysiology of Hallucinations. (Kharkov).

Popova, L. T. (1964): Disturbance of Mnemic Processes in the Clinical Picture of Some Local Brain Lesions [Candidate Dissertation]. (First Moscow Medical Institute).

Popova, L. T. (1973): Disturbances of Memory in Local Brain Lesions. (Meditsina; Moscow).

Pork, M. E. (1977): Investigation of Interhemispheric Asymmetry in the Process of Stereoscopic Perception [Candidate Dissertation]. (Moscow University; Moscow).

Potebnya, A. A. (1826): Thought and Language. 5th ed. (Kharkov, 1926).

Potebnya, A. A. (1888): Writings on Russian Grammar. 2 vols. (Kharkov).

Pravdina-Vinarskaya, E. N. (1957): Neurological Features of the Syndrome of Oligophrenia. (Izd. Akad. Ped. Nauk RSFSR; Moscow).

Preobrazhenskaya, N. S. (1948): Postnatal ontogenesis of the occipital region. *Tr. Inst. Moz.* **6**.

Preobrazhenskaya, N. S. (1953): Disturbance and Recovery of Visual Functions in Gunshot Wounds of the Occipital Lobes of the Brain [Candidate Dissertation]. (USSR Acad. Med. Sci.; Moscow).

Preobrazhenskaya, N. S. (1958): Disturbance and restoration of some aspects of the visual functions after injury to the occipital lobes of the brain. *Probl. Fiziol. Opt.* **12**.

Pribram, K. H. (1969). The frontal lobes of primates. *In*: Organization of Physiological Functional Systems. (Meditsina; Moscow).

Rapoport, M. Y. (1936–1941): Dislocation syndromes in brain tumors. I: *Nevropat., Psikhiat i Psikhogig.* **5**; II–V: *Vop. Neirokhir.* **2, 3, 4, 5**.

Rapoport, M. Y. (1947): Essays on the Neuropathology of Head Wounds. (Izd. Akad. Med. Nauk SSSR; Moscow).

Rapoport, M. Y. (1948): Neuropathological Diagnosis of Temporal Lobe Tumors. (Izd. Akad. Med. Nauk RSFSR; Moscow).

Rau, F. F. (1954): Role of pronunciation in teaching words to deaf-mute children. *Izv. Akad. Ped. Nauk RSFSR* no. 62.

Rozengardt-Pupko, G. L. (1948): Speech and the Development of Perception in Early Childhood. (Izd. Akad. Med. Nauk SSSR; Moscow).

Rubinshtein, S. L. (1958): Intellectual Activity and Methods of its Investigation. (Izd. AN SSSR; Moscow).

Rubinshtein, S. Y. (1944): Restoration of Working Capacity after War Injuries of the Brain [Candidate Dissertation].

Rudenko, Z. Y. (1953): Disturbance of Arithmetical Skill in Brain Lesions [Candidate Dissertation]. (USSR Acad. Med. Sci.; Moscow).

Ruzskaya, A. G. (1958): Role of orienting and investigatory activity in the formation of elementary generalizations in children. *In*: The Orienting Reflex and Inquisitive Activity. (Izd. Akad. Ped. Nauk RSFSR; Moscow).

Sapir, I. D. (1934): Aphasia, speech, and intellectual activity. *Nevropat. i Psikhiat.* **3**.

Sarkisov, S. A. (1940): Problems of localization in the light of modern information on the architectonics and bioelectrical phenomena of the cerebral cortex. *Nevropat. i Psikhiat.* **9**.

Sarkisov, S. A. (1950): Pavlov's theory of higher nervous activity and problems of brain structure. *Vop. Filos.* no. 3.

Sarkisov, S. A. (1957): Distinctive structural features of the higher divisions of the central nervous system and their physiological importance. *Zh. Nevropat. i Psikhiat. Korsakov* **57**.

Saturnov, N. M. (1911): Further Investigations of Conditioned Salivary Reflexes in a Dog Following Removal of the Anterior Halves of Both Hemispheres [Candidate Dissertation]. (St. Petersburg).

Sechenov, I. M. (1891): Physiology of the Nervous Centers 2nd ed. (Izd. Akad. Med. Nauk SSSR; Moscow, 1952).

Sechenov, I. M. (1947): Selected Works. vol. 1. (Izd. AN SSSR; Moscow).

Semernitskaya, F. M. (1945): Rhythm and its Disturbance in Various Motor Lesions [Candidate Dissertation]. (Inst. Psychol.; Moscow).

Sepp, E. K. (1945): Fundamental principles of localization of functions in the cerebral cortex. *Nevropat. i Psikhiat.* **14**.

Sepp, E. K. (1955): Localization of functions in the human cortex. *Zh. Nevropat. i Psikhiat. Korsakov* **55**.

Shakhnovich, A. R. (1961): The scanning pupillograph. *Vop. Neirokhir.*, no. 2.

Shakhnovich, A. R., and Shakhnovich, V. R. (1964): Pupillography. (Medgiz; Moscow).

Shchelovanov, N. M., and Bekhterev, V. M. (1925): The basis of genetic reflexology. *In*: Advances in Reflexology and the Physiology of the Nervous System. (Leningrad).

Shemyakin, F. N. (1940): The psychology of spatial ideas. *In*: Scientific Reports of the State Institute of Psychology. (Moscow).

Shemyakin, F. N. (1954): Investigation of topographical ideas. *Izv. Akad. Ped. Nauk RSFSR* no. 53.

Shemyakin, F. N. (1959): Spatial orientation. *In*: Psychological Science in the USSR. vol. 1. (Moscow).

Shevarev, P. A. (1959): Generalized Associations in the Learning Activity of the School Child. (Izd. Akad. Ped. Nauk RSFSR; Moscow).

Shif, Zh. I. (1948): Writing disturbances in disorders of letter recognition. *Izv. Akad. Ped. Nauk RSFSR* no. 15.

Shkol'nik-Yarros, E. G. (1945): Disturbance of Movement in Lesions of the Premotor Area [Candidate Dissertation]. (USSR Acad. Med. Sci.: Moscow).

Shkol'nik-Yarros, E. G. (1958): Efferent tracts in the visual cortex. *Zh. Vyss. Nerv. Deiat. Pavlov* **8**.

Shkol'nik-Yarros, E. G. (1966): The premotor cortex and the syndrome produced by its lesions. *In*: A. R. Luria and E. D. Khomskaya, Eds.: The Frontal Lobes and Regulation of Psychological Processes. (Moscow Univ. Press).

Shmar'yan, A. S. (1949): Cerebral Pathology and Psychiatry. (Medgiz: Moscow).

Shmidt, E. V. (1942): Syndromes of a lesion of the premotor and motor areas in gunshot wounds of the skull. *Vop. Neirokhir.* **6**.

Shmidt, E. V., and Sukhovskaya, N. A. (1954): The pathophysiology of sensory aphasia. *Zh. Nevropat. i Psikhiat. Korsakov* **54**.

Shumilina, N. I. (1949): Functional importance of the frontal divisions of the brain in the conditioned-reflex activity of dogs. *In*: Problems in Higher Nervous Activity. (Izd. Akad. Med. Nauk SSSR; Moscow).

Shustin, N. A. (1955): Disturbance of Nervous Activity after Removal of the Frontal Lobes of the Brain in Dogs [Doctorate Dissertation]. Author's abstract. (Moscow State Univ.; Leningrad).

Shustin, N. A. (1958): Pathological inertia of the process of excitation in the motor analyzer after removal of the frontal lobes of the brain. *Zh. Vyss. Nerv. Deiat. Pavlov* **8**.

Shustin, N. A. (1959): The Physiology of the Frontal Lobes of the Brain. (Moscow).

Simernitskaya, É. G. (1970): The Study of Regulation of Activity by the Evoked Potentials Method. (Moscow Univ. Press; Moscow).

Simernitskaya, É. G. (1978): Dominance of the Hemispheres. (Moscow Univ. Press; Moscow).

Simernitskaya, É. G., and Bunatyan, E. A. (1966): Disturbance of rhythmic movements in patients with tumors of the premotor area. *In*: A. R. Luria and E. D. Khomskaya, Eds.: The Frontal Lobes and Regulation of Psychological Processes. (Moscow Univ. Press).

Simernitskaya, É. G., and Khomskaya, E. D. (1966): Changes in parameters of evoked responses depending on informative value of stimuli in normal subjects and patients with frontal lobe lesions. *In*: A. R. Luria and E. D. Khomskaya, Eds.: The Frontal Lobes and Regulation of Psychological Processes. (Moscow Univ. Press).

Skipin, G. V. (1941): Analysis of higher nervous activity by the combined secretory-motor technique. *Tr. Fiziol. Lab. Pavlov.* **10**.

Skipin, G. V. (1947): The mechanism of formation of conditioned food reflexes. Soviet Science. (Moscow).

Skipin, G. V. (1956): Localization of the process of conditioned (internal) inhibition. *Zh. Vyss. Nerv. Deiat. Pavlov* **6**.

Skipin, G. V. (1958): Interaction between different forms of motor defensive conditioned reflexes in animals. *Zh. Vyss. Nerv. Deiat. Pavlov* **9**.

Smirnov, A. A. (1948): The Psychology of Memory. (Izd. Akad. Ped. Nauk RSFSR; Moscow).

Smirnov, A. A. (1966): Problems in the Psychology of Memory. (Prosveshchenie; Moscow).

Smirnov, L. I. (1946): The Pathological Anatomy of Brain Trauma. (Medgiz; Moscow).

Smirnov, L. I. (1947): The Pathological Anatomy and Pathogenesis of Traumatic Diseases of the Nervous System. (Medgiz; Moscow).

Smirnov, L. I. (1948): The Topography, Anatomy, and Histology of Brain Tumors. (Medgiz: Moscow).

Smirnov, L. I. (1951): The Histogenesis, Pathology, and Topography of Brain Tumors. (Medgiz; Moscow).

Sokolov, A. N. (1957): Speech mechanisms of mental activity. Proceedings of a Conference on Psychology, July 1–6, 1955. (Izd. Akad. Ped. Nauk RSFSR; Moscow).

Sokolov, A. N. (1959): Investigations into the speech mechanisms of intellectual activity. *In*: Psychological Science in the USSR. vol. 1. (Izd. Akad. Ped. Nauk RSFSR; Moscow).

Sokolov, A. N. (1968): Internal Speech and Intellectual Activity. (Prosveshchenie; Moscow).

Sokolov, E. N. (1957): Reflex mechanisms of reception. *In*: Proceedings of a Conference on Psychology, July 1–6, 1955. (Moscow).

Sokolov, E. N. (1958): Perception and the Conditioned Reflex. (Moscow Univ. Press; Moscow).

Sokolov, E. N., Ed. (1959): The Orienting Reflex and Problems in Higher Nervous Activity. (Izd. Akad. Ped. Nauk RSFSR; Moscow).

Sokolov, E. N. (1960): A probability model of perception. *Vop. Psikhol.* no. 2.

Sokolov, E. N., Danilova, N. N., and Khomskaya, E. D., Eds. (1975): Functional States of the Brain. (Moscow Univ. Press; Moscow).

Solov'ev, I. M. (1953): Mental activity of mentally retarded schoolchildren during arithmetical tests. *In*: Problems in the Cognitive Activity of Pupils at Special Schools. (Izd. Akad. Ped. Nauk RSFSR; Moscow).

Sorkina, E. G., and Khomskaya, E. D. (1960): Dynamics of the disturbance of visual perception in lesions of the parieto-occipital divisions of the brain. *Dokl. Akad. Ped. Nauk RSFSR* no. 6.

Spirin, B. G. (1951): Disturbances of the Mobility of Nervous Processes after Operations on the Brain [Candidate Dissertation]. (USSR Acad. Med. Sci.; Moscow).

Spirin, B. G. (1954): Speech perseverations with lesions of both the motor and the acoustic analyzer. *Zh. Nevropat. i Psikhiat. Korsakov* **54**.

Spirin, B. G. (1966): Manifestation of pathological inertia after operations on the anterior zones of the human brain. *In*: A. R. Luria and E. D. Khomskaya, Eds.: The Frontal Lobes and Regulation of Psychological Processes. (Moscow Univ. Press).

Sukhovskaya, N. A. (1958): The Study of Human Reflex Reactions in Normal and Pathological Conditions Using the Index of Functional Lability [Candidate Dissertation]. (USSR Acad. Med. Sci.; Moscow).

Talyzina, N. F. (1957): Grasping initial geometrical concepts. Proceedings of a Conference on Psychology, July 1–6, 1955. (Izd. Akad. Ped. Nauk RSFSR; Moscow).

Teplov, B. M. (1937): Inductive changes in absolute and discriminatory sensation of the eye. *Vestn. Oftal.* **11**.

Teplov, B. M. (1947): The Psychology of Musical Ability. (Izd. Akad. Ped. Nauk RSFSR; Moscow).

Teplov, B. M., Ed. (1953, 1959): Topological Features of Human Higher Nervous Activity. (Izd. Akad. Ped. Nauk RSFSR; Moscow).

Tikhomirov, N. I. (1906): A Strictly Objective Experimental Investigation of the Functions of the Cerebral Hemispheres in the Dog [Candidate Dissertation]. (St. Petersburg).

Tikhomirov, O. K. (1958): The formation of voluntary movements in children of preschool age. *In*: A. R. Luria, Ed.: Problems in the Higher Nervous Activity of the Normal and Abnormal Child. vol. 2. (Izd. Akad. Ped. Nauk RSFSR; Moscow).

Tikhomirov, O. K. (1961): Investigation of optimal methods of testing hypotheses in normal and pathological conditions. *Dokl. Akad. Ped. Nauk RSFSR* nos. 4–6.

Tikhomirov, O. K. (1964): Experience of the application of information theory to the analysis of problem solving. *Vop. Psikhol.* no. 4.

Tikhomirov, O. K. (1966): Disturbance of the programming of active search in frontal lobe lesions. *In*: A. R. Luria and E. D. Khomskaya, Eds.: The Frontal Lobes and Regulation of Psychological Processes. (Moscow Univ. Press).

Tonkonogii, I. M. (1966): Aphasias in Vascular Diseases of the Brain. [Doctoral Dissertation]. (First Leningrad Medical Institute).

Traugott, N. N. (1947): Sensory alalia and aphasia in childhood. *In*: Research Abstracts on Medicobiological Sciences. no. 1. (Izd. Akad. Med. Nauk SSSR; Moscow).

Traugott, N. N. (1973): The Mechanisms of Disturbance of Memory. (Nauka; Leningrad).

Traugott, N. N., Balonov, L. Y., and Lichko, L. E. (1957): Essays on the Physiology of Human Higher Nervous Activity. (Medgiz: Leningrad).

Tsvetkova, L. S. (1966*a*): Disturbance of constructive activity in lesions of the frontal and parieto-occipital regions of the brain. *In*: A. R. Luria and E. D. Khomskaya, Eds.: The Frontal Lobes and Regulation of Psychological Processes. (Moscow Univ. Press).

Tsvetkova, L. S. (1966*b*): Disturbance of the analysis of texts in patients with frontal lobe lesions. *In*: A. R. Luria and E. D. Khomskaya, Eds.: The Frontal Lobes and Regulation of Psychological Processes. (Moscow Univ. Press).

Tsvetkova, L. S. (1966*c*): Disturbance of solving arithmetical problems in patients with lesions of the parieto-occipital and frontal regions of the brain. *In*: A. R. Luria and E. D. Khomskaya, Eds.: The Frontal Lobes and Regulation of Psychological Processes. (Moscow Univ. Press).

Tsvetkova, L. S. (1972*a*): Rehabilitation After Local Brain Lesions. (Pedagogika; Moscow).

Tsvetkova, L. S. (1972*b*): Disturbances of Calculation in Local Brain Lesions. (Moscow Univ. Press; Moscow).

Tsvetkova, L. S., Ed. (1976): Problems in Aphasia and Reeducation. (Moscow Univ. Press; Moscow).

Ukhtomskii, A. A. (1945): Essays on the Physiology of the Nervous System. Collected Works. vol. 4. (Leningrad).

Uznadze, D. N. (1958): Experimental basis of the psychology of set. *In*: Experimental Investigations on the Psychology of Set. (Tiflis).

Vagner, V. A. (1928): Appearance and development of mental abilities. Evolution of Mental Abilities Along Pure and Mixed Lines. no. 7. (Leningrad).

Vasilevskaya, V. Y. (1960): Understanding of Educational Material by Mentally Retarded Children. (Izd. Akad. Ped. Nauk RSFSR; Moscow).

Vinogradova, O. S. (1959): Role of the orienting reflex in the formation of a conditioned link in man. *In*: E. N. Sokolov, Ed.: The Orienting Reflex and Problems in Higher Nervous Activity. (Izd. Akad. Ped. Nauk RSFSR; Moscow).

Vinogradova, O. S. (1959): Investigation of the Orienting Reflex in Children by the Method of Plethysmography. (Izd. Akad. Ped. Nauk RSFSR; Moscow).

Vinogradova, O. S. (1965): Dynamic classification of hippocampal unit responses. *Zh. Vyssh. Nerv. Deyat.* **15**, 500.

Vinogradova, O. S. (1974): Memory and the Hippocampus. (Nauka; Moscow).

Vladimirov, A. D., and Khomskaya, E. D. (1961): A photoelectric method of recording eye movements. *Vop. Psikhol.* no. 3.

Vladimirov, A. D., and Khomskaya, E. D. (1962): A photoelectric method of recording eye movements during examination of objects. *Vop. Psikhol.* no. 5.

Voronin, L. G. *et al.*, Eds. (1958): The Orienting Reflex and Investigatory Activity. (Izd. Akad. Ped. Nauk RSFSR; Moscow).

Vygotskii, L. S. (1934): Intellectual Activity and Speech. (Sotsékgiz; Moscow).

Vygotskii, L. S. (1956): Selected Psychological Investigations. (Izd. Akad. Ped. Nauk RSFSR; Moscow).

Vygotskii, L. S. (1960): Development of the Higher Mental Functions. (Izd. Akad. Ped. Nauk RSFSR; Moscow).

Yakovleva, S. V. (1958): Conditions of formation of the simpler types of voluntary action in children of preschool age. *In*: A. R. Luria, Ed.: Problems in the Higher Nervous Activity of the Normal and Abnormal Child. vol. 2. (Izd. Akad. Ped. Nauk RSFSR; Moscow).

Yarbus, A. L. (1948): Some illusions in the evaluation of visible distances between edges of objects. *In*: S. L. Rubinshtein, Ed.: Investigations in the Psychology of Perception. (Moscow).

Yarbus, A. L. (1950): Adequacy of Perception as Shown by Investigation of Optical Illusions [Candidate Dissertation]. (USSR Acad. Sci.; Moscow).

Yarbus, A. L. (1956): The perception of an immobile graticule. *Biofizika* **1**.

Yarbus, A. L. (1961): Eye movements during examination of complex objects. *Biofizika* **6**.

Yarbus, A. L. (1965): The Role of Eye Movements in the Perception of Pictures. (Nauka; Moscow).

Zankov, L. V. (1944): The Schoolchild's Memory. (Uchpedgiz; Moscow).

Zankov, L. V., Ed. (1954): Psychological-pedagogical problems in speech restoration after head injuries. *Izv. Akad. Ped. Nauk RSFSR* no. 2.

Zankov, L. V., Ed.: The disturbance of speech in head injuries and its restoration. *Izv. Akad. Ped. Nauk RSFSR* no. 15.

Zaporozhets, A. V. (1960): Development of Voluntary Movement in the Child. (Izd. Akad. Ped. Nauk RSFSR; Moscow).

Zeigarnik, B. V. (1959): Disturbances of Intellectual Activity in Mental Patients [Doctorate Dissertation]. (Moscow State Univ.; Moscow).

Zeigarnik, B. V. (1961): The Pathology of Thinking. (Moscow Univ. Press; Moscow). [English translation: Consultants Bureau, New York, 1965.]

Zhinkin, N. I. (1958): Speech Mechanisms. (Izd. Akad. Ped. Nauk RSFSR; Moscow).

Zinchenko, V. P. (1958): The formation of an orienting image. *In*: L. G. Voronin *et al.*, Eds.: The Orienting Reflex and Investigatory Activity. (Izd. Akad. Ped. Nauk RSFSR; Moscow).

Zinchenko, P. I. (1959): The psychology of memory. *In*: Psychological Science in the USSR. (Moscow).

Zislina, N. N. (1955): Disturbance of visual sequential images in lesions of the cerebral cortex. *Probl. Fiziol. Opt.* **11**.

NON-RUSSIAN

Ackerly, S. (1935): Instinctive, emotional and mental changes following prefrontal lobe extirpation. *Am. J. Psychiat.* **92**.

Adey, R. (1959): Paper presented at the meeting of the American Academy of Neurology. Symposium on Rhinencephalon, April 17, 1959.

Adey, W. R. (1958): Organization of the rhinencephalon. *In*: H. Jasper *et al.*, Eds.: Reticular Formation and Brain. (Little Brown; Boston).

Adey, W. R., and Meyer, M. (1952): Hippocampal and hypothalamic connections of the temporal lobe in monkey. *Brain* **75**.

Adey, W. R., Sunderland, S., and Dunlop, C. W. (1957): The entorhinal area: electrophysiological studies of its interrelations with rhinencephalic structures and the brainstem. *Electroenceph. & Clin. Neurophysiol.* **9**.

Ajuriaguerra, J. (1953): Langage, geste, attitude motrice "la voix." *In*: Cours international de phonologie et phoniatrie. (Paris).

Ajuriaguerra, J. (1957): Langage et dominance cérébrale, *J. Franç. Oto-rhino-laryng.* no. 3.

Ajuriaguerra, J., and Hécaen, H. (1960): Le cortex cérébral. 2e éd. (Masson; Paris).

Alajouanine, T., Ed. (1955): Les grandes activités du lobe temporal. (Masson; Paris).

Alajouanine, T. (1956): Verbal reaction in aphasia. *Brain* **79**.

Alajouanine, T., Ed. (1960): Les grandes activités du lobe occipital. (Masson; Paris).

Alajouanine, T., Ed. (1961): Les grandes activités du rhinencéphale. 2 vols. (Masson; Paris).

Alajouanine, T., and Lhermitte, F. (1960): Les troubles des activités expressives du langage dans l'aphasie. *Rev. Neurol.* **102**.

Alajouanine, T., and Mozziconacci, P. (1947): L'aphasie et la désintégration fonctionnelle du langage. (Imprimerie Molière; Lyon).

Alajouanine, T., Ombredane, H., and Durant, M. (1939): Le syndrome de désintégration phonétique dans l'aphasie. (Masson; Paris).

Albe-Fessard, D. (1964): Converging sensory inflow to thalamic and cortical zones in the monkey. *IBRO Bull.* **3**, 79.

Andersen, V. O., Buchman, B., and Lennox-Buchtal, M. A. (1962): Single cortical units with narrow spectral sensitivity in monkeys. *Vision Res.* **2**, 295.

Anton, G. (1899): Über die Selbstwahrnehmung der Herderkrankungen des Gehirns durch den Kranken. *Arch. Psychiat.* **32**.

Anton, G. (1906): Symptome der Stirnhirnerkrankungen. *München. Med. Wschr.* **53.**

Artemieva, E., and Homskaya (Khomskaya), E. D. (1973): Changes in the asymmetry of EEG waves in different functional states in normal subjects and in patients with lesions of the frontal lobes. *In*: K. Pribram and A. R. Luria, Eds.: Psychophysiology of the Frontal Lobes. (Academic Press; New York).

Ashby, W. R. (1952): Design for a Brain. (Chapman & Hall; London).

Association for Research on Nervous and Mental Disease: (1948): Frontal Lobes. *A. Res. Nerv. & Ment. Dis. Publ.* **27.**

Baddeley, A. D. (1976): The Psychology of Memory. (Basic Books: New York).

Bailey, P., and Bonin, C. von (1951): The Isocortex of Man. (Univ. of Ill. Press; Urbana).

Baillarger, J. (1865): Recherches sur les maladies mentales. (Masson; Paris).

Baldwin, M. (1956): Modifications psychiques survenant après lobectomie temporale subtotale. *Neurochirurgie* **2.**

Baldwin, M., and Bailey, P., Eds. (1958): Temporal Lobe Epilepsy. (Charles C Thomas; Springfield, Ill.).

Balint, R. (1909): Seelenlähmung des Schauens. *Monatsschr. Psychiat. u. Neurol.* **25.**

Baranovskaya, O. P., and Homskaya (Khomskaya), E. D. (1973): Changes in EEG frequency spectrum during the presentation of neutral and meaningful stimuli to patients with lesions of the frontal lobes. *In*: K. Pribram and A. R. Luria, Eds.: Psychophysiology of the Frontal Lobes. (Academic Press; New York).

Baruk, H. (1926): Les troubles mentaux dans les tumeurs cérébrales. *In*: Thèses de la Faculté de Médecine de Paris. vol. 4. (Paris).

Bastian, H. C. (1869): The physiology of thinking. *Fortnightly Rev.* **5.**

Bastian, H. C. (1880): The Brain as an Organ of Mind. (C. K. Paul; London).

Bay, E. (1944): Zum Problem der taktilen Agnosie. *Deutsche Z. Nervenh.* **156.**

Bay, E. (1950): Agnosie und Funktionswandel. *In*: Monographien aus dem Gesamtgebiet der Neurologie und Psychiatrie, vol. 73.

Bay, E. (1952): Der gegenwärtige Stand der Aphasieforschung. *Folia Phoniat.* **4.**

Bay, E. (1957*a*): Untersuchungen zum Aphasieproblem. *Nervenarzt* **28.**

Bay, E. (1957*b*): Die corticale Disartrie und ihre Beziehung zur sog. motorischen Aphasie. *Deutsche Z. Nervenh.* **176.**

Bender, M. B. (1952): Disorders of Perception. (Charles C Thomas: Springfield, Ill.).

Bender, M. B., and Jung, R. (1948): Abweichungen der subjektiven optischen Vertikalen und Horizontalen bei Gesunden und Hirnverletzten. *Arch. Psychiat.* **181.**

Bender, M. B., and Teuber, H. L. (1946): Phenomena of fluctuation, extinction and completion in visual perception. *Arch. Neurol. & Psychiat.* **55.**

Bender, M. B., and Teuber, H. L. (1947, 1948): Spatial organization of visual perception following injury to the brain. *Arch. Neurol. & Psychiat.* **58, 59.**

Benson, D. F. (1967): Fluency in aphasia. *Cortex* **3.**

Berendt, H., and Leonhard, K. (1964): Die zwei Formen des frontalen Antriebsstöreungen, *Z. Psychol.* **170,** no. 1–2.

Berger, H. (1926): Über Rechenstörungen bei Herderkrankungen des Grosshirns. *Arch. Psychiat. u. Nervh.* **78.**

Bergson, H. (1896): Matière et mémoire. (Paris).

Bernstein (Bernshtein), N. A. (1967): The Coordination and Regulation of Movements. (Pergamon Press; Oxford).

Bethe, A. (1931): Plastizität und Zentrenlehre. *In*: A. Bethe *et al.*, Eds.: Handbuch der Normalen und pathologischen Physiologie. vol. 16. (Springer; Berlin).

Bianchi, L. (1895): The functions of frontal lobes. *Brain* **18.**

Bianchi, L. (1920): La meccanica del cervello e la funzione dei lobi frontali. (Bocca; Torino).

Binswanger, L. (1926): Zum Problem von Sprache und Denken. *Schweiz. Arch. Neurol. u. Psychiat.* **136.**

Bonhöffer, K. (1923): Zur Klinik und Lokalisation des Agrammatismus und der Rechts-Linksorientierung. *Monatsschr. Psychiat. u. Neurol.* **54.**

Bonin, C. von (1943): Architectonics of the precentral motor cortex. *In*: P. C. Bucy, Ed.: The Precentral Motor Cortex. (Univ. of Ill. Press; Urbana).

Bonin, C. von (1948): The frontal lobe of primates. *A. Res. Nerv. & Ment. Dis. Publ.* **27.**

Bonin, C. von (1960): Some Papers on the Cerebral Cortex. (Charles C Thomas; Springfield).

Bonin, C. von, Garol, H. W., and McCulloch (1942): The functional organization of the occipital lobe. *Biol. Symp.* **7**.

Bonvicini, G. (1929): Die Störungen der Lautsprache bei Temporallappenläsionen. *In*: G. Alexander and O. Marburg, Eds.: Handbuch der Neurologie des Ohres. vol. 11.

Bouillaud, J. (1825*a*): Recherches cliniques propres à démontrer que la perte de la parole correspond à la lésion des lobules anterieurs du cerveau. *Arch. Gén. Méd.* **8**.

Bouillaud, J. (1825*b*): Traité clinique et physiologique de l'encéphalite. (Ballière; Paris).

Bouman, L., and Grünbaum, A. A. (1925): Experimentell-psychologische Untersuchungen zur Aphasie. *Z. Ges. Neurol. u. Psychiat.* **96**.

Brain, W. R. (1941): Visual disorientation with special reference to lesions of the right cerebral hemisphere. *Brain* **64**.

Brain, W. R. (1961*a*): The neurology of language. *Brain* **84**.

Brain, W. R. (1961*b*): Speech Disorders. (Butterworth; London).

Bremer, F. (1952): Les aires auditives de l'écorce cérébrale. *In*: Cours international d'audiologie clinique. (Librairie Maloine; Paris).

Bremer, F., and Dow, R. S. (1939): The cerebral acoustic area of the cat. *J. Neurophysiol.* **2**.

Brickner, R. M. (1936): The Intellectual Functions of the Frontal Lobes. (Macmillan; New York City).

Broadbent, W. H. (1872): On the cerebral mechanism of speech and thought, *Trans. Med. & Chir. Faculty Md.* **55**.

Broadbent, W. H. (1879): A case of peculiar affection of speech, with commentary. *Brain* **1**.

Broca, P. (1861*a*): Perte de la parole etc. *Bull. Soc. Anthrop.* **2**.

Broca, P. (1861*b*): Remarques sur le siège de la faculté du langage articulé. *Bull. Soc. Anthrop.* **6**.

Brodmann, K. (1909): Vergleichende Lokalisationslehre der Grosshirnrinde in ihren Prinzipien dargestellt auf Grund des Zellenbaues. (Barth; Leipzig).

Brown, G. (1915–1916): Studies in the physiology of the nervous system. *Quart. Journ. Exper. Phys.* **9**, pp. 81–99, 136–145; **10**, pp. 97–102.

Brown, G., and Sherrington, C. S. (1912): On the instability of a cortical point. *Proc. Roy. Soc. London (B)* **85**.

Brown, J. W. (1974): Aphasia, Apraxia and Agnosia. (Charles C Thomas; Springfield).

Brown, J. W. (1977): Mind, Brain, and Consciousness. (Academic Press; New York).

Brown, R., and McNeill, D. (1966): The tip of the tongue phenomenon. *Verb. Learn. Verb. Behav.* **85**.

Brouwer, B. (1936): Chiasma, tractus opticus, Seestrahlung und Sehrinde. *In*: O. Bumke and O. Foerster, Eds.: Handbuch der Neurologie. vol. 6. (Springer; Berlin).

Brower, C., and Abt, L. E. (1956): Progress in clinical psychology. **22**.

Brun, R. (1921): Klinische und anatomische Studien über Apraxie. *Schweiz. Arch. Neurol. u. Psychiat.* **9**.

Bruner, J. (1957): On perceptual readiness. *Psychol. Rev.* **64**.

Bruner, J., and Goodnow, A. (1956): A Study of Thinking. (Wiley; New York City).

Brutkowski, S. (1957): The effect of prefrontal lobectomies on salivary conditioned reflexes in dogs. *Acta Biol. Exp.* (Lodz) **17**.

Brutkowski, S. (1964): Prefrontal cortex and drive inhibition. *In*: J. M. Warren and K. Akert, Eds.: Frontal Granular Cortex and Behavior. (McGraw-Hill; New York).

Brutkowski, S., Konorski, J., Lawicka, W., Stepien, I., and Stepien, L. (1956): The effect of the removal of the frontal poles of the cerebral cortex on motor conditioned reflexes. *Acta Biol. Exp.* (Lodz) **17**.

Bucy, P. C., Ed. (1943): The Precentral Motor Cortex. (Univ. Ill. Press; Urbana).

Bühler, K. (1943): Sprachtheorie. (Fischer; Jena).

Burns, B. D., and Pritchard, R. (1964): Contrast discrimination by neurons in the cat's visual cerebral cortex. *J. Physiol.* (London) **175**.

Buser, P., and Imbert, M. (1961): Sensory projections to the motor cortex in cats: a microelectrode study. Sensory Communication. (MIT Press; Cambridge, Mass.).

Butler, R. A., Diamond, I. T., and Neff, W. D. (1957): Role of auditory cortex in discrimination of changes in frequency. *J. Neurophysiol.* **20**.

Campbell, A. W. (1905): Histological Studies on the Localisation of Cerebral Function. (Cambridge Univ. Press; London).

Cannon, W. B. (1929): Bodily Changes in Pain, Horror, Fear and Rage. 2nd ed. (Appleton; New York City).

Carreras, M., and Andersson, S. A. (1963): Functional properties of neurons of the anterior ectosylvian gyrus of the cat. *J Neurophysiol.* **26**.

Cassirer, E. (1923): Philosophie der symbolischen Formen. I. (Berlin).

Charcot, P. (1886–1887): Oeuvres complètes. 9 vols. (Bureau du Progrès Médical; Paris).

Chester, E. C. (1936): Some observations concerning the relations of handedness to the language mechanism. *Bull. Neurol. Inst. New York* **4**.

Chomsky, N. (1957*a*): Syntactic Structures (Mouton; s'Gravenhage).

Chomsky, N. (1957*b*): Syntactical Structures. (Mouton; The Hague).

Chomsky, N. (1965): Aspects of the Theory of Syntax. (M.I.T. Press; Cambridge, Mass.).

Chomsky, N. (1968): Language and Mind. (Harcourt Brace; New York).

Chow, K. L. (1951): Effects of partial extirpations of the posterior association cortex on visually mediated behavior in monkeys. Comparative Psychology Monographs. vol. 20. (Univ. of Calif. Press; Berkeley and Los Angeles).

Chow, K. L. (1952): Further studies on selective ablation of associative cortex in relation to visually mediated behavior. *J. Comp. & Physiol. Psychol.* **45**.

Christensen, A. L. (1974): Luria's Neuropsychological Investigations. (Munksgaard; Copenhagen).

Coghill, G. E. (1929): Anatomy and the Problem of Behaviour. (Cambridge Univ. Press; London).

Cohen, L. (1959): Perception of reversible figures after brain injury. *AMA. Arch. Neurol.* **81**.

Conrad, K. (1932): Versuch einer psychologischen Analyse des Parietalsyndromes. *Monatsschr. Psychiat. u. Neurol.* **84**.

Conrad, K. (1954): New problems of aphasia. *Brain* **77**.

Critchley, M. (1953): The Parietal Lobes. (E. J. Arnold; London).

Critchley, M. (1960): Alterations de l'organisation visuospatiale dans les lésions occipito-pariétales. *In*: Alajouanine, T., Ed.: Les grandes activités du lobe occipital. (Masson; Paris).

Critchley, M. (1964): The drift and dissolution of languages. *Proc. Roy. Soc. Med.* 57, no. 12.

Crown, S. (1951): Psychological changes following prefrontal lobectomy. *J. Ment. Sc.* **97**.

Dax, M. (1836): Lésion de la moitié gauche de l'encéphale coincidant avec l'oubli des signes de la pensée. *Gaz. Hebd. Méd.* **2**.

Déjerine, J. (1914): Sémiologie des affections du système nerveux. (Masson; Paris).

Delay, J. P. (1935): Les astéréognosies. *In*: Thèses de la Faculté de Médecine de Paris. vol. 24. (Paris).

Delgado, J. M. R. (1955): Evaluation of permanent implantation of electrodes in the brain. *Electroenceph. & Clin. Neurol.* **7**.

Delgado, J. M. R., Roberts, W. W., and Miller, N. (1954): Learning motivated by electrical stimulation of the brain. *Am. J. Physiol.* **179**.

Denny-Brown, D. (1932): Theoretical deduction from the physiology of the cerebral cortex. *J. Neurol. Psychiat.* **13**.

Denny-Brown, D. (1951): The frontal lobes and their functions. *In*: H. Feeling, Ed.: Modern Trends in Neurology. (Butterworth; London).

Denny-Brown, D. (1958): The nature of apraxia. *J. Nerv. J. Ment. Dis.* **126**.

Denny-Brown, D. (1963): The physiological basis of perception and speech. *In*: L. Halpern, Ed.: Problems in Dynamic Neurology. (Jerusalem).

Denny-Brown, D., Meyer, J., and Horenstein, S. (1952): The significance of perceptual rivalry resulting from parietal lesions. *Brain* **75**.

Descartes, R. (1686): Tractatus de Homine (Amsterdam).
Diamond, I. T., and Neff, W. D. (1957): Ablation of temporal cortex and discrimination of auditory patterns. *J. Neurophysiol.* **20**.
Dimond, S. J., and Beaumont, J. G., Eds. (1974): Hemisphere Function in the Human Brain. (Elek; London).
Dubner, R. (1966): Single cell analysis of sensory interaction in anterior lateral suprasylvian gyri of the cat cerebral cortex. *Exper. Neurol.* **15**.
Dusser de Barennes, J. G., and McCulloch, W. S. (1941): Suppression of motor responses obtained from area 4 by stimulation of area 4s. *J. Neurophysiol.* **4**.
Dunsmore, R. H., and Lennox, M. A. (1950): Stimulation and strychninization of suprocallosal anterior cingulate gyrus. *J. Neurophysiol.* **13**.
Eccles, J. C. C. (1951): Hypotheses relating to the brain-mind problem. *Nature* (London) **168**.
Eccles, J. C. C. (1953): The Neurophysiological Basis of Mind. (Clarendon Press; London).
Eccles, J. C. C., Ed. (1966): Brain and Conscious Experience. (Springer; Berlin and New York).
Ettlinger, G., Jackson, G. V., and Zangwill, O. L. (1955): Dysphasia following right temporal lobotomy in a right-handed man. *J. Neurol. Neurosung. & Psychiat.* **18**.
Ettlinger, G., Jackson, G. V., and Zangwill, O. L. (1956): Cerebral dominance in sinistrals. *Brain* **79**.
Ettlinger, G., Warrington, E., and Zangwill, O. L. (1957): A further study in visual-spatial agnosia. *Brain* **80**.
Evans, E. F., Ross, H. F., and Whitefield, I. C. (1965): The spatial distribution of the unit characteristic frequency in the primary auditory cortex of the cat. *J. Physiol.* (London) **179**.
Evans, J. P. (1953): A study of sensory defects resulting from excision of cerebral substance in humans. *A. Res. Nerv. & Ment. Dis. Publ.* **15**.
Evarts, E. V. (1965): Relation of discharge frequency to conduction velocity in pyramidal tract neurons. *J. Neurophysiol.* **28**.
Exner, S. (1881): Untersuchungen über die Lokalisation der Funktionen in der Grosshirnrinde des Menschen. (Braumüller; Wien).
Fajans, S. (1931): Die Wirkung von Erfolg und Misserfolg auf Ausdauer der Aktivität beim Säugling und Kleinkind. *Psychol. Forsch.* **15**.
Faust, C. (1955): Zur Symptomatik frischer und alter Stirnhirnverletzungen. *Z. Neurol.* **193**.
Ferrier, D. (1874): Experimental research in cerebral physiology and pathology. *West Riding Lunatic Asylum M. Rep.*
Ferrier, D. (1876): The Functions of the Brain. (Smith, Elder; London).
Fessard, A. E. (1954): Mechanisms of nervous integration and conscious experience. *In*: The Council for International Organizations of Medical Sciences: Brain Mechanisms and Consciousness. (Blackwell; Oxford).
Feuchtwanger, E. (1923): Die Funktionen des Stirnhirns. *In*: O. Foerster and K. Wilmanns, Eds.: Monographien aus dem Gesamtgebiete der Neurologie und Psychiatrie. vol. 38. (Springer; Berlin).
Feuchtwanger, E. (1930): Amusie. (Berlin).
Finan, J. L. (1939): Effects of frontal lobe lesion on temporal organized behavior in monkeys. *J. Neurophysiol.* **2**.
Finkelburg (1870): Asymbolie. *Berl. Klin. Wschr.* **7**.
Flechsig, P. (1883): Plan des menschlichen Gehirns. (Veit; Leipzig).
Flechsig, P. (1896*a*): Über Lokalisation der geistigen Vorgänge, insbesondere der Sinnesempfindungen des Menschen. (Veit; Leipzig).
Flechsig, P. (1896*b*): Gehirn und Seele. (Veit; Leipzig).
Flechsig, P. (1900): Über Projections- und Associations-Zentren des menschlichen Gehirns. *Neurol. Centralbl.* **19**.
Flechsig, P. (1920): Anatomie des menschlichen Gehirns und Rückenmarks auf myelogenetischer Grundlage. (Thieme; Leipzig).

Flechsig, P. (1927): Meine myelogenetische Hirnlehre. (Springer; Berlin).

Flourens, M. J. P. (1824): Recherches expérimentales sur les propriétés et les fonctions du système nerveux dans les animaux vertébrés. (Crevot; Paris).

Flourens, M. J. P. (1842): Examen de phrénologie. (Hachette; Paris).

Foerster, O. (1936): Symptomatologie der Erkrankungen des Gehirns. Motorische Felder und Bahnen.—Sensible corticale Felder. *In*: O. Bumke and O. Foerster, Eds.: Handbuch der Neurologie. vol. 6. (Springer; Berlin).

Foix, C. (1928): Aphasies. *In*: Nouveau traité de médecine et thérapeutique. vol. 18. (Baillière; Paris).

Frankfurter, W., and Thiele, R. (1912): Experimentelle Untersuchungen zur Bezoldschen Sprachsext. *Z. Psychol. u. Physiol. Sinnesorg. (Z. Sinnesphysiol.)* **47**.

Franz, S. I. (1907): On the function of the cerebrum; the frontal lobes. *Arch. Psychol.* **1**.

Franz, S. I. (1924): Nervous and Mental Reëducation. (Macmillan; New York City).

Freeman, W., and Watts, J. W. (1942): Psychosurgery: Intelligence, Emotion, and Social Behavior Following Prefrontal Lobectomy for Mental Disorders. (Charles C Thomas; Springfield, Ill.).

Freeman, W., and Watts, J. W. (1951): Psychosurgery: Intelligence, Emotion and Social Behavior Following Prefrontal Lobotomy for Mental Disorders. 2nd ed. (Charles C Thomas; Springfield, Ill.).

French, G. M. (1964): The frontal lobes and association. *In*: J. M. Warren and K. Akert, Eds.: The Frontal Granular Cortex and Behavior. pp. 56–74.

French, J. D., Sugar, O., and Ghusid, J. E. H. (1948): Corticocortical connections of superior bank of the Sylvania fissure in monkey. *J. Neurophysiol.* **11**.

Freud, S. (1891): Zur Auffassung der Aphasien. (Deuticke; Leipzig und Wien).

Fritsch, G., and Hitzig, E. (1870): Über die elektrische Erregbarkeit des Grosshirns. *Arch. Anat. Physiol. u. Wisse. Med.* **37**.

Froment, J. (1953): Langage articulé et fonction verbale. *In*: G. H. Roger, Ed.: Traité de physiologie normale et pathologique 2nd ed. vol. 10. (Masson; Paris).

Fuller, J. L.; Rosvold, K. E., and Pribram, K. H. (1957): The effect on affective and cognitive behavior in the dog of lesions of the pyriform-amygdala-hippocampal complex. *J. Comp. & Physiol. Psychol.* **50**.

Fulton, J. F. (1935): A note on the definition of the "motor" and "premotor" areas. *Brain* **58**.

Fulton, J. F. (1937): Forces grasping and groping in relation to the syndrome of premotor area. *Arch. Neurol. & Psychiat.* **31**.

Fulton, J. F. (1943): Physiology of the Nervous System. 2nd ed. (Oxford Univ. Press; New York City).

Fulton, J. F. (1949): Functional Localization in the Frontal Lobes and Cerebellum. (Clarendon Press; London).

Fulton, J. F., Kennard, M., and Viets, M. R. (1934): The syndrome of the premotor cortex in man. *Brain* **57**.

Fuster, J. M. (1961): Excitation and inhibition of neuronal firing in visual cortex by reticular stimulation. *Science* **133**.

Gall, F. J. (1825): Sur les fonctions du cerveau et sur celles de chacune de ses parties. 6 vols. (Baillière; Paris).

Gall, F. J., and Spurzheim, H. (1810–1818): Anatomie et physiologie du système nerveaux en général et du cerveau en particulier. 5 vols. (Schoell; Paris).

Gastault, H. *et al.* (1957): Topographical study of the conditioned electroencephalographic reactions in man. *Electroenceph. & Clin. Neurophysiol.* **9**.

Gazzaniga, M. S. (1967): The split brain in man. *Scientific American* **217**.

Gazzaniga, M. S. (1970): The Bisected Brain. (Appleton-Century Crofts; New York).

Gazzaniga, M. S., Bogen, J. E., and Sperry, R. W. (1962): Some functional effects of sectioning of the cerebral commissures in man. *Proc. Nat. Acad. Sci. USA.* **48**.

Gazzaniga, M. S., Bogen, J. E., and Sperry, R. W. (1963): Laterality effects in somesthesis following cerebral commissurotomy in man. *Neuropsychologica* **1**.

Gazzaniga, M. S., and Sperry, R. W. (1965): Observations on visual perception after disconnection of the cerebral hemispheres in man. *Brain* **88**.

Gazzaniga, M. S., and Sperry, R. W. (1967): Language after section of the cerebral commissures. *Brain* **90**.

Gelb, A., and Goldstein, K. (1920): Psychologische Analysen hirnpathologischer Fälle. (Springer; Berlin).

Gerstmann, J. (1924): Fingeragnosie. *Wien. Klin. Wschr.* **37**.

Gersuni, G. V. (1965): Organization of afferent flow of the process of external signal discrimination. *Neurologia* 3, no. 2.

Geschwind, N. (1965*a*): Disconnexion syndromes in animals and man. *Brain* **88**, nos. i–iii.

Geschwind, N. (1965*b*, 1966): Disconnexion syndromes in animals and man. *Brain,* **88, 89**.

Geschwind, N. (1974): Selected Papers on Language and the Brain. (Reidl; Dordrecht).

Goldberg, I. M., Diamond, I. T., and Neff, W. D. (1957): Auditory discrimination after ablation of temporal and insular cortex in cat. *Fed. Proc.* **16**.

Goldstein, K. (1926*a*): Das Symptom, seine Entstehung und Bedeutung für unsere Auffassung vom Bau und von der Funktion des Nervensystems. *Arch. Psychiat. u. Nervenh.* **76**.

Goldstein, K. (1926*b*): Über Aphasie. *Schweiz. Arch. Neurol. u. Psychiat.* **19**.

Goldstein, K. (1927): Die Lokalisation in der Grosshirnrinde. *In*: A. Bethe *et al.*, Eds.: Handbuch der normalen und pathologischen Physiologie. vol. 10. (Springer; Berlin).

Goldstein, K. (1934): Der Aufbau des Organismus. (Nijhoff; Haag).

Goldstein, K. (1936): The significance of the frontal lobes for mental performances. *J. Neurol. & Psychopathol.* **17**.

Goldstein, K. (1942): Aftereffects of Brain Injuries in War. (Grune & Stratton; New York City).

Goldstein, K. (1944): The mental changes due to frontal lobe damage, *J. Psychol.* **17**.

Goldstein, K. (1948): Language and Language Disorders. (Grune & Stratton; New York City).

Goldstein, K., and Gelb, A. (1924): Über Farbennamenamnesie. *Psychol. Forsch.* **6**.

Goldstein, K., and Scheerer, M. (1941): Abstract and Concrete Behavior. *Psychol. Monog.* **53**.

Goltz, F. (1876–1884): Über die Verrichtungen des Grosshirns. *Pflüger's Arch. Ges. Physiol.* **13, 14, 20, 26**.

Goodglass, H., and Quadfasel (1954). Language laterality in left-handed aphasics. *Brain* **77**.

Granit, R. (1955): Receptors and Sensory Perception. (Yale Univ. Press; New Haven).

Grasset (1907): La fonction du langage et la localisation des centres psychiques dans le cerveau. *Rev. Philos.*

Grastyan, G. (1959): The hippocampus and higher nervous activity. *In*: 2nd Macy Conference: The Central Nervous System and Behavior. (National Institutes of Health; Bethesda, Md.).

Gratiolet, P. (1861): Observations sur la forme et le poids du cerveau. (Paris).

Grünbaum, A. A. (1930): Aphasie und Motorik. *Z. Ges. Neurol. u. Psychiat.* **130**.

Grünbaum, A., and Sherrington, C. S. (1901, 1903): Observation of the physiology of the cerebral cortex of some of the higher apes. *Proc. Roy. Soc. London* **69, 72**.

Grünthal, E. (1939): Über das Corpus Mamillare und den Korsakowschen Symptomenkomplex. *Confinia Neurol.* **2**, 84.

Grünthal, E. (1947): Über das klinische Bild bei umschriebenem beiderseitigem Ausfall der Ammonhirnrinde. *Monatsschr. Psychiat. u. Neurol.* **113**.

Haeffner, H. (1955): Störungen des Plan- und Entwurfvermögens bei Stirnhirnläsionen. *Arch. Psychiat. u. Z. Neurol.* **193**.

Haeffner, H. (1957): Psychopathologie des Stirnhirns 1939 bis 1955. *Forsch. Neurol. Psychiat.* **25**.

Haller, A. (1769): Elementa physiologiae corporis humani (Lausanne).

Halstead, W. C. (1947): Brain and Intelligence. (Chicago Univ. Press; Chicago).

Harlow, J. (1868): Recovery from the passage of an iron bar through the head. *Publ. Mass. Med. Soc.* **2**.

Harlow, H. F. *et al.* (1952): Analysis of frontal and posterior association syndromes in brain-damaged monkeys. *J. Comp. Psychol.*

Harnad, S., *et al.*, Eds. (1977): Lateralization in the Nervous System. (Academic Press: New York).

Harrower, M. R. (1939): Changes in figure-ground perception in patients with cortical lesions. *Brit. J. Psychol.* **30**.

Head, H. (1920): Studies in Neurology, 2 vols. (Oxford Med. Pub.; London).

Head, H. (1926): Aphasia and Kindred Disorders of Speech. 2 vols. (Cambridge Univ. Press; London).

Hebb, D. O. (1942): The effect of early and late brain injury upon test scores. *Proc. Am. Philos. Soc.* **85**.

Hebb, D. O. (1945): Man's frontal lobes. *Arch. Neurol. & Psychiat.* **54**.

Hebb, D. O. (1949): The Organization of Behavior. (Wiley; New York City).

Hebb, D. O. (1950): Animal and physiological psychology. *Ann. Rev. Psychol.* **1**.

Hebb, D. O. (1959): Intelligence, brain functions and the theory of mind. *Brain* **82**.

Hebb, D. O., and Penfield, W. (1940): Human behavior after extensive bilateral removal from the frontal lobes. *Arch. Neurol. & Psychiat.* **44**.

Hécaen, H., and Angelergues, R. (1963): La Cecite Psychique. (Masson; Paris).

Hécaen, H., and Angelergues, R. (1964): Localization of symptoms in aphasic disorders of language. *In*: Disorders of Language. (Ciba Foundation Symposium).

Hécaen, H., and Angelergues, R. (1965): Pathologie du Langage. (Larousse; Paris).

Hécaen, H., and Ajuriaguerra, J. (1952): Méconnaissances et hallucinations corporelles. (Masson; Paris).

Hécaen, H., and Ajuriaguerra, J. (1956*a*): Agnosie visuelle pour les objects inanimés par la lésion unilaterale gauche. *Rev. Neurol.* **94**.

Hécaen, H., and Ajuriaguerra, J. (1956*b*): Troubles Mentaux au Cours des Tumeurs Intracraniennes. (Masson; Paris).

Hécaen, H., and Ajuriaguerra, J. (1959): Balint's syndrome and its minor forms. *Brain* **77**.

Hécaen, H., Ajuriaguerra, J., and Massonet, J. (1951): Les troubles visuoconstructifs par lésion pariéto-occipitale droite. *Encéphale* **40**.

Hécaen, H., Ajuriaguerra, J., Magis, C., and Angelergues, R. (1952): Le probléme de l'agnosie des physionomies. *Encéphale* **41**.

Hécaen, H., David, M., and Reeth, von C. J. (1953): Über pariétale Tumoren. *Wien. Z. Nervenh.* **8**.

Hécaen, H., Dell, M. B., and Roger, A. (1955): L'aphasie de conduction. *Encéphale* **44**.

Hécaen, H., and Garcia Badaraco, J. (1956): Sémeiologie des hallucinations visuelles en clinique neurologique. *Acta Neurol. Latino-Am.* **2**.

Hécaen, H., and Marcie, P. (1974): Disorders of written language following right hemisphere lesions. *In*: S. J. Dimond and J. G. Beaumont, Eds.: Hemisphere Function of the Human Brain. (Elek; London).

Hécaen, H., Penfield, W., Bertrand, C., and Malmo, R. (1956): The syndrome of apractagnosia due to lesion of the minor hemisphere. *AMA Arch. Neurol. & Psychiat.* **75**.

Hécaen, H., and Piercy, M. (1956): Paroxysmal dysphasia and the problem of cerebral dominance. *J. Neurol. Neurosurg. & Psychiat.* **19**.

Heilbronner, K. (1910): Die aphasischen, apraktischen und agnostischen Störungen. *In*: M. Lewandowsky, Ed.: Handbuch der Neurologie. vol. 1. (Springer; Berlin).

Henschen, S. E. (1920–1922): Klinische und anatomische Beiträge zur Pathologie des Gehirns. (Stockholm).

Hernandez-Peon, R. (1955): Central mechanisms controlling conduction along central sensory pathways. *Acta Neurol. Latinoamer.* **1**, 256–264.

Hess, W. R. (1954): Diencephalon: Automatic and Extrapyramidal Functions. Monographs in Biology and Medicine. no. 3. (Grune & Stratton; New York City).

Heygster, H. (1948): Die psychische Symptomatologie bei Stirnhirnlesionen. (Hirzel: Leipzig).

Heygster, H. (1949): Die doppelseitige Stirnhirnverletzungen. *Psychiat. Neurol. u. Med. Psychol.* **1**.

Hitzig, F. (1874): Untersuchungen über des Gehirn. (Unger; Berlin).

Hoff, H. (1929): Beiträge zur Relation der Sehsphäre und des Vestibularapparates. *Z. Ges. Neurol. u. Psychiat.* **121**.

Hoff, H. (1930): Über zentrale Abstimmung der Sehsphäre. (Karger; Berlin).

Hoff, H., and Kamin, M. (1930): Reizversuche im linken Sulcus Interparietalis beim Menschen. *Z. Ges. Neurol. u. Psychiat.* **128**.

Hoff, H., and Pötzl, O. (1930): Über die Grosshirnprojektion der Mitte und der Aussengrenzen des Gesichtsfeldes. *Jahrb. Psychiat.* **52**.

Holmes, G. (1919): Disturbances of vision by cerebral lesions. *Brit. J. Ophth.* **1**.

Holmes, G. (1938): Cerebral integration of ocular movement. *Brit. M. J.* **2**.

Holmes, G., and Horrax, G. (1919): Disturbances in spacial orientation. *Arch. Neurol. & Psychiat.* **1**.

Homskaya (Khomskaya), E. D. (1970): The frontal lobes and the regulation of arousal processes. *In*: D. I. Mostofsky, Ed.: Attention, Contemporary Theory and Analysis. (Prentice-Hall; New York).

Homskaya, E. D. (1973): The human frontal lobes and their role in the organization of activity. *Acta Neurol. Exper.* **33**.

Homskaya, E. D. (1975): Local changes of the functional states of the brain associated with mental activities. *In*: D. Ingvar and N. A. Lassen, Eds.: Brain Work. (Copenhagen), pp. 424–428.

Hoppe (1930): Erfolg und Misserfolg. *Psychol. Forsch.* **14**.

Hubel, D. H. (1960): Single unit activity in lateral geniculate body and optic tract of unrestrained animal. *J. Physiol.* (London) **150**.

Hubel, D. H., Henson, C., Rupert, A., and Galambos, R. (1959): Attention units in the auditory cortex. *Science* **129**.

Hubel, D. H., and Wiesel, T. N. (1962): Receptive fields, binocular interaction and functional architecture in the cat's visual cortex. *J. Physiol.* (London) **106**.

Hubel, D. H., and Wiesel, T. N. (1963): Receptive fields of cells in striate cortex of very young, visually inexperienced kittens. *J. Neurophysiol.* **26**.

Hubel, D. H., and Wiesel, T. N. (1965): Receptive fields and functional architecture in two nonstriate visual areas (18 and 19) of the cat. *J. Neurophysiol.* **28**, 229–289.

Humphrey, M. E., and Zangwill, O. L. (1952): Dysphasia in left-handed patients with unilateral brain lesion. *J. Neurol. Neurosurg. & Psychiat.* **15**.

Isserlin, M. (1922): Über Agrammatismus. *Z. Ges. Neurol. u. Psychiat.* **75**.

Isserlin, M. (1929–1932): Die pathologische Physiologie der Sprache. *Ergebn. Physiol.* **29, 33, 34**.

Isserlin, M. (1936): Die Aphasie. *In*: O. Bumke and O. Foerster, Eds.: Handbuch der Neurologie. vol. 6. (Springer; Berlin).

Jackson, J. H. (1869): On localization. Selected Writings. vol. 2. (Basic Books; New York City, 1958).

Jackson, J. H. (1876): Case of large cerebral tumor without optic neuritis and with left hemiplegia and imperception. Selected Writings. vol. 2. (Basic Books; New York City, 1958).

Jackson, J. H. (1884): Evolution and Dissolution of the Nervous System. Selected Papers. vol. 2. (Basic Books; New York City, 1958).

Jackson, J. H. (1931–1932): Selected Writings of John Hughlings Jackson. 2 vols. (Hodder & Stoughton; London).

Jacobsen, C. F. (1931): A study of cerebral functions in learning; the frontal lobes. *J. Comp. Neurol.* **52**.

Jacobsen, C. F. (1935): Function of frontal association area in primates. *Arch. Neurol. & Psychiat.* **33**.

Jacobsen, C. F., Wolf, J. B., and Jackson, T. A. (1935): An experimental analysis of the frontal association area in primates. *J. Nerv. & Ment. Dis.* **82**.

Jakobson, R. (1942): Kindersprache, Aphasie und allgemeine Lautgesetze. (Uppsala Univ. Arsskrift.)

Jakobson, R. (1971): Studies in Child Language and Aphasia. (Mouton; The Hague).

Jakobson, R., and Halle, M. (1956): Fundamentals of Language. (Mouton; The Hague).

James, W. (1890): Principles of Psychology. 2 vols. (Holt; New York City).

Janet, P. (1928): La psychologie du mémoire et de la notion du temps. (Paris).

Jasper, H. H. (1954): Functional properties of the thalamic reticular system. *In*: The Council for International Organizations of Medical Sciences: Brain Mechanisms and Consciousness. (Blackwell; Oxford).

Jastrowitz, M. (1888): Beiträge zur Lokalization im Grosshirn und über deren praktische Verwertung. *Deutsche Med. Wschr.* **14**.

Jung, R. (1958*a*): Excitation, inhibition and coordination of cortical neurons. *Exp. Cell Res. Suppl.* **5**.

Jung, R. (1958*b*): Coordination of specific and nonspecific afferent impulses at single neurons of the visual cortex. *In*: Reticular Formation of the Brain. (Little Brown; Boston).

Jung, R. (1961): Neuronal integration in the visual cortex and its significance for visual information. *In*: Sensory Communication. (MIT Press; Cambridge, Mass.).

Kalinowsky, L. B., and Hoch, P. K. (1952): Shock Treatment, Psychosurgery and Other Somatic Treatments in Psychiatry. (Grune & Stratton; New York City).

Katz, D. (1925): Der Aufbau der Tastwelt. *Z. Psychol. Ergebn.* **11**.

Katz, F. G. (1930): Die Bezoldsche Sprachsexte und das Sprachverständnis. *Passow-Schaefer Beitr.* **28**.

Kennard, M., Spenser, S., and Fountain, G. (1941): Hyperactivity in monkeys following lesions in the frontal lobes. *J. Neurophysiol.* **4**.

Kennard, M., Viets, H. R., and Fulton, J. F. (1934): The syndrome of the premotor cortex in man. *Brain* **57**.

Kerschensteiner, M. K., Poeck, S., and Brunner, E. (1972): The fluency–non-fluency dimensions in the classification of aphasia. *Cortex* **8**.

Kimble, D. P., Ed. (1965): The Anatomy of Memory. (Science and Behavior Books; Palo Alto, Calif.).

Kimura, D. (1961): Cerebral dominance in the perception of verbal stimuli. *Canad. J. Psychol.* **16**.

Kimura, D. (1964): Left-right dominance in perception of melodies. *Quart. J. Exp. Psychol.* **16**.

Kimura, D. (1966): Dual functional asymmetry of the brain in visual perception. *Neuropsychologia* **4**.

Kimura, D. (1967): Functional asymmetry in dichotic listening. *Cortex* **3**.

Kimura, D. (1969): Spatial organization in the left and right visual fields. *Canad. J. Psychol.* **24**.

Kimura, D. (1973): The asymmetry of the human brain. *Scientific American* **228**.

Kimura, D., and Durnford, M. (1974): Normal studies on the function of the right hemisphere in vision. *In*: S. J. Dimond and J. G. Beaumont, Eds.: Hemisphere Function in the Human Brain. (Elek; London).

Klages, W. (1954): Frontale und dienecephale Antriebsschwäche. *Arch. Psychiat. u. Z. Neurol.* **191**.

Klebanoff, S. G. *et al.* (1954): Psychological consequences of brain lesion. *Psychol. Bull.* **51**.

Klein, R. (1931): Zur Symptomatologie des Parientallappens. *Z. Ges. Neurol. u. Psychiat.* **129**.

Klein, R., and Mayer-Gross, W. (1957): The Clinical Examination of Patients with Organic Cerebral Lesions. (Cassel; London).

Kleist, K. (1907): Corticale (innervatorische) Apraxie. *J. Psychiat.* **28**.

Kleist, K. (1911): Der Gang und der gegenwärtige Stand der Apraxieforschung. *Ergebn. Neurol.* **1**.

Kleist, K. (1916): Über Leitungsaphasie und grammatische Störungen *Monatsschr. Psychiat. u. Neurol.* **40**.

Kleist, K. (1930): Die alogischen Denkstörungen. *Arch. Psychiat.* **90**.

Kleist, K. (1934): Gehirnpathologie. (Barth; Leipzig).

Klüver, H. (1927): Visual disturbances after cerebral lesion. *Psychol. Bull.* **24**.

Klüver, H. (1937): An analysis of the effects of the removal of the occipital lobes in monkeys. *J. Psychol.* **2**.

Klüver, H. (1941): Visual functions after removal of the occipital lobes. *J. Psychol.* **11**.

Klüver, H. (1952): Brain mechanisms and behavior with special reference to the rhinencephalon. *Lancet* **72**.

Klüver, H., and Bucy, P. C. (1937): "Psychic blindness" and other symptoms following bilateral temporal lobectomy in rhesus monkeys. *Am. J. Psychol.* **119**.

Klüver, H., and Bucy, P. C. (1938): An analysis of certain effects of bilateral temporal lobectomy in the rhesus monkey. *J. Psychol.* **5**.

Klüver, H., and Bucy, P. C. (1939*a*): Preliminary analysis of the temporal lobe functions in monkeys. *Arch. Neurol. Psychiat.* **47**.

Klüver, H., and Bucy, P. C. (1939*b*): Preliminary analysis of functions of the temporal lobes in monkeys. *Arch. Neurol. Psychiat.* **42**, 979

Konorski, J. (1948): Conditioned Reflex and Neuron Organization. (Cambridge Univ. Press; London).

Konorski, J. (1961*a*): Distribution of the inhibitory conditioned reflexes after prefrontal lesions in dogs. *In*: Brain Mechanisms and Learning. (Blackwell; Oxford).

Konorski, J. (1961*b*): The physiological approach to the problem of recent memory. *In*: Brain Mechanisms and Learning. (Blackwell; Oxford).

Konorski, J., and Lawicka, W. (1964): Analysis of errors by prefrontal animals in the delayed response test. *In*: J. M. Warren and K. Akert, Eds.: The Frontal Granular Cortex and Behavior. (McGraw-Hill; New York).

Krapf, E. (1937): Über Akalkulie. *Arch. Suisse Neurol. et Psychol.* **39**.

Kretschmer, E. (1949): Orbital- und Zwischenhirnsyndrome nach Schädelbasisfrakturen. *Arch. Psychiat. u. Z. Neurol.* **182**.

Kretschmer, E. (1954): Verletzungen der Schädelhirnbasis und ihre psychiatrisch-neurologischen Folgen. *Deutsche Med. Wschr.*

Krieg, W. (1942): Functional Neuroanatomy. (Blakiston; Philadelphia).

Kroll, M. B. (1910): Beiträge zum Studium der Apraxie. *Z. Ges. Neurol. u. Psychiat.* **2**.

Kronfeld, A., and Sternberg, E. (1927): Der gedankliche Aufbau der klassischen Aphasieforschung im Lichte der Sprachlehre. *Psychol. u. Med. Stuttgart* 2.

Kuenberg, M. (1923): Über das Erfassen einfacher Beziehungen an anschaulichem Material bei Hirngeschädigten. *Z. Neurol. u. Psychiat.* **88**.

Kussmaul, A. (1885): Störungen der Sprache.

Kutsemilova, A. P., Luria, A. R., and Homskaya (Khomskaya), E. D. (1964): Analisi neuropsichologica di una sindrome pseudo-frontale da tumore cerebellare. *Cortex* **1**.

Lancisi, I. M. (1739): Dissertatio de sede cogitandis anima (Venezia).

Lange, J. (1936): Agnosien und Aphasien. *In*: O. Bumke and O. Foerster, Eds.: Handbuch der Neurologie. vol. 6. (Springer; Berlin).

Lashley, K. S. (1929): Brain Mechanisms and Intelligence. (Univ. Chicago Press; Chicago).

Lashley, K. S. (1937): Functional determination of cerebral localization. *Arch. Neurol. & Psychiat.* **38**.

Lashley, K. S. (1930–1942): The mechanisms of vision. I–XVII.

Lashley, K. S. (1951): The problem of serial order in behavior. *In*: Cerebral Mechanisms in Behavior. Hixon Symposium. (New York, London).

Lassek, A. M. (1954): The Pyramidal Tract. (Charles C Thomas; Springfield, Ill.).

Le Beau, J. (1954): Psycho-chirurgie et fonctions mentales. (Paris).

Le Beau, J., and Petrie, A. (1953): A comparison of the personality changes after prefrontal selective surgery etc. *J. Ment. Sc.* **99**.

Leonhard, K. (1954): Innervatorische und ideokinetische Form motiroschen Aphasie. *Nervenarzt* **25**, 117.

Leonhard, K. (1957): Apraktische Formen vom Aphasie. *Neurol. med. Psychol.* (Leipzig) **9**, 151.

Leonhard, K. (1965): Die klinische Localisation der Hirntumoren. (Barth; Leipzig).

Levy, J. (1974): Psychological implications of bilateral asymmetry. *In*: S. J. Dimond and J. G. Beaumont, Eds.: Hemisphere Function in the Human Brain. (Elek; London).

Lewin, K. (1926): Vorsatz, Wille und Bedürfnis. *Psychol. Forsch.* **7**.

Lewin, K. (1935): Dynamic Theory of Personality. (New York City).

Leyton, C. S., and Sherrington, C. S. (1917): Observations on the excitable cortex of the chimpanzee, orang-utan and gorilla. *Quart. J. Exper. Physiol.* **11**.

Lhermitte, J. (1929): Le lobe frontal. *Encéphale* **1**.

Lhermitte, J. (1938): Langage et mouvement. *Encéphale* **33**.

Lhermitte, J., and Ajuriaguerra, J. (1942): Psychopathologie de la vision. (Masson; Paris).

Lhermitte, J., and Cambien, J. (1960): Les Perturbations Somatognostiques en Pathologie Nerveuse. (Masson; Paris).

Lhermitte, J., Lévy, G., and Kyriako, N. (1925): Les perturbations de la représentation spatiale chez les apraxiques. *Rev. Neurol.* **2**.

Lhermitte, J., Massary, J., and Kyriako, N. (1928): Le rôle de la pensée spatiale dans l'apraxie. *Rev. Neurol.* **2**.

Lhermitte, J., and Mouzon, J. (1942): Sur l'apractognosie géometrique et l'apraxie constructive etc. *Rev. Neurol.* **73**.

Libertini, E. (1895): Sulla localizzazione dei poteri inibitori nella corteccia cerebrale. *Arch. Ital. Biol.* **19**.

Lichtheim, L. (1885): Über Aphasie. *Deutsches. Arch. Klin. Med.* **36**.

Liepmann, H. (1900): Das Krankheitsbild der Apraxie. *Monatsschr. Psychiat. u. Neurol.* **8**.

Liepmann, H. (1905): Über Störungen des Handelns bei Gehirnkranken. (Karger; Berlin).

Liepmann, H. (1913): Motorische Aphasie und Apraxie. *Monatsschr. Psychiat. u. Neurol.* **34**.

Liepmann, H. (1920): Apraxie. *Brugsch's Ergebn. Ges. Med.*

Lindsley, D. B. (1960): Attention, consciousness, sleep and wakefulness. *In*: J. Field *et al.*, Eds.: Handbook of Physiology. Neurophysiology, vol. 1. (Washington, D.C.).

Lindsley, D. B., Schreiner, L. H., Knowles, W. B., and Magoun, H. W. (1952): Behavioral and EEG changes following chronic brain stem lesions in the cat. *Electroencephal. & Clin. Neurophysiol.* **2**.

Lissak, K., Grastyan, E., Csanaky, A., Kekesi, F., and Vereby, G. (1957): A study of hippocampal function in the waking and sleeping animal with chronical implanted electrodes. *Acta Physiol. et. Pharmacol. Neerl.* **6**.

Lissak, K., and Grastyan, E. (1959): The possible role of the hippocampus in the conditioning process. XIX. Internat. Congress Physiol. Sciences.

Lissauer, H. (1889): Ein Fall von Seelenblindheit etc. *Arch. Psychiat. u. Neurol.* **21**.

Loeb, J. (1886): Beiträge zur Physiologie des Grosshirns. *Arch. Ges. Physiol.* **39**.

Loeb, J. (1902): Comparative Physiology of the Brain and Comparative Psychology. (Putnam; New York City).

Lorente de Nó, R. (1938): Analysis of the activity of the chains of internuncial neurons. *J. Neurophysiol.* **1**.

Lorente de Nó, R. (1943): Cerebral cortex. *In*: J. B. Fulton: Physiology of the Nervous System. (Oxford Univ. Press, London).

Lorenz, K. (1950): The comparative method in studying innate behavior patterns. *In*: Physiological Mechanisms in Animal Behavior. Symposium of the Society of Experimental Biology, No. 4. (Cambridge).

Lotmar, F. (1919): Zur Kenntniss der erschwerten Wortfindung und ihre Bedeutung für das Denken der Aphasischen. *Schweiz. Arch. Neurol. u. Psychiat.* **15**.

Lotmar, F. (1935): Zur Pathophysiologie der erschwerten Wortfindung bei Aphatischen. *Schweiz. Arch. Neurol. u. Psychiat.* **30**.

Lotze, H. (1852): Medizinische Psychologie oder Physiologie der Seele. (Leipzig).

Luciani, L. (1913): Trattato di Fisiologie, III. (Human Physiology, London, 1915).

Luria, A. R. (1932): The Nature of Human Conflicts. (Liveright; New York City).

Luria, A. R. (1958): Brain disorders and language analysis. *Language & Speech.* **1**.

Luria, A. R. (1959*a*): Disorders of "simultaneous perception" in a case of bilateral occipitoparietal brain injury. *Brain* **82**.

Luria, A. R. (1959*b*): The directive role of speech in development and dissolution. *Word* **15**.

Luria, A. R. (1960): Verbal regulation of behavior. *In*: 3rd Macy Conference: The Cen-

tral Nervous System and Behavior. (National Institutes of Health; Bethesda, Md.).
Luria, A. R. (1961): The Role of Speech in Regulation of Normal and Abnormal Behaviour. (Pergamon; London).
Luria, A. R. (1963): Restoration of Function After Brain Injury. (Pergamon Press; Oxford).
Luria, A. R. (1964*a*): Neuropsychology in the local diagnosis of brain damage. *Cortex* **1**, no. 1.
Luria, A. R. (1964*b*): Factors and forms of aphasia. Disorders of Language. (Ciba Foundation Symposium; London).
Luria, A. R. (1965*a*): Neuropsychological analysis of focal brain lesions. *In*: B. B. Wolman, Handbook of Clinical Psychology (McGraw-Hill; New York).
Luria, A. R. (1965*b*): Aspects of aphasia. *J. Neurol. Sci.* **2**.
Luria, A. R. (1965*c*): Two kinds of motor perseverations in massive injury of the frontal lobes. *Brain* **88**, 1.
Luria, A. R. (1965*d*): Le cerveau et le psychisme. *Recherches Internationales à la Lumière de Marxisme* no. **46**.
Luria, A. R. (1966*a*): Higher Cortical Functions in Man (First English Edition). (Basic Books; New York).
Luria, A. R. (1966*b*): Human Brain and Psychological Processes. (Harper and Row; New York).
Luria, A. R. (1966*c*): L. S. Vygotskii and the Problem of Localization of Function. *Neuropsychologia* **3**.
Luria, A. R. (1967): Problems and facts of neurolinguistics. *In*: To Honor Roman Jakobson: A Collection of Essays. 3 vols. (Mouton; The Hague).
Luria, A. R. (1968*a*): Traumatic Aphasia. (Mouton; The Hague).
Luria, A. R. (1968*b*): The Frontal syndrome. *In*: P. Vinken and G. W. Bruyn: Handbook of Clinical Neurology. (North-Holland Publishing Co.; Amsterdam).
Luria, A. R. (1969): Frontal lobe syndromes. *In*: P. J. Vinken and G. W. Bruyn, Eds.: Handbook of Clinical Neurology, vol. 2. (North-Holland Publ. Co.; Amsterdam).
Luria, A. R. (1972*a*): The Man with a Shattered World. (Basic Books; New York).
Luria, A. R. (1972*b*): Aphasia reconsidered. *Cortex* **10**.
Luria, A. R. (1973): Two basic kinds of aphasic disorders. *Language* **114**.
Luria, A. R. (1974*a*): The Working Brain. (Penguin; London).
Luria, A. R. (1974*b*): Basic problems of neurolinguistics. *In*: T. Seboek, Ed.: Current Trends in Linguistics, vol. 16. (Mouton; The Hague).
Luria, A. R. (1974*c*): Language and brain. *In*: *Brain and Language* **5**.
Luria, A. R. (1975*a*): Basic problems of language in the light of psychology and neurolinguistics. *In*: E. Lenneberg, Ed.: Foundation of Language Development. (Academic Press; New York).
Luria, A. R. (1975*b*): Two kinds of disorders in the comprehension of grammatical construction. *Linguistics* **154/155**.
Luria, A. R. (1975*c*): A note on the organization of fluent speech in a semantic kind of amnestic aphasia. *Linguistics* **154/155**.
Luria, A. R. (1976*a*): Basic Problems of Neurolinguistics. (Mouton; The Hague).
Luria, A. R. (1976*b*): Neuropsychology of Memory. (Winston; Washington, D.C.).
Luria, A. R. (1977): Neuropsychological Studies in Aphasia. (Swetz and Zeitlinger; Amsterdam).
Luria, A. R. (in press): Man's Conscious Action. (Plenum Press; New York).
Luria, A. R., Blinkov, S. M., Homskaya, E. D., and Critchley, M. (1967): Impairment of selectivity of mental processes in association with a lesion of the frontal lobe. *Neuropsychologia* **5**.
Luria, A. R., and Homskaya, E. D. (1962): An objective study of ocular movements and their control. *Psychol. Beitr.* **6**.
Luria, A. R., and Homskaya, E. D. (1963): Le trouble du role régulateur de langage au cours des lesions du lobe frontal. *Neuropsychologia* **1**, no. 1.
Luria, A. R., Karpov, B. A., and Yarbus, A. L. (1966): Disturbances of active visual perception with lesions of the frontal lobes. *Cortex* **11**.
Luria, A. R., Naydin, V. M., Tsvetkova, L. S., and Vinarskaya, E. (1969): Restoration of higher cortical functions following local brain lesions. *In*: P. J. Vinken and

G. W. Bruyn: Handbook of Clinical Neurology, vol. 3. (North-Holland Publishing Co.; Amsterdam).

Luria, A. R., Pravdina-Vinarskaya, E. N., and Yarbus, A. L. (1963): Disorders of ocular movements in a case of simultanagnosia. *Brain* **86**.

Luria, A. R., Pribram, K. H., and Homskaya, E. D. (1964): An experimental analysis of the behavioral disturbances produced by a left frontal arachnoidal endothelioma (meningioma). *Neuropsychologia* **2**.

Luria, A. R., and Simernitskaya, E. G. (1977): Interhemispheric relations and the function of the minor hemisphere. *Neuropsychologia* **15**.

Luria, A. R., Sokolov, E. N., and Klimkowski, M. (1967): Towards a neurodynamic analysis of memory disturbances with lesions of the left temporal lobe. *Neuropsychologia* **5**.

Luria, A. R., Tsvetkova, L. S., and Futer, D. S. (1965): Aphasia in a composer. *J. Neurol. Sci.* **2**.

Luria, A. R., and Tsvetkova, L. S. (1967): Solution des Problemes chez les Sujets Atteints de Lesions Frontales. (Gauthier-Villard; Paris).

Luria, A. R., and Tsvetkova, L. S. (1968): The mechanisms of dynamic aphasia. *Foundations of Language* **4**.

Luria, A. R., Vinarskaya, E. N., Naydin, V. L., and Tsvetkova, L. S. (1967): Restoration of higher cortical functions. *In*: P. Vinken and G. W. Bruyn: Handbook of Clinical Neurology. (North-Holland Publishing Co.; Amsterdam).

McAdam, D. W. (1962): Electroencephalographic changes and classic adversive conditioning in cats. *Exper. Neurol.* **6**.

McCulloch, W. S. (1943): Inter-areal interactions of the cerebral cortex. *In*: Bucy, P. C., Ed.: The Precentral Motor Cortex. (Univ. of Ill. Press; Urbana).

McCulloch, W. S. (1944): The functional organization of the cerebral cortex. *Physiol. Rev.* **24**.

McCulloch, W. S. (1948): Some connections of the frontal lobe established by physiological neuronography. *A. Res. Nerv. & Ment. Dis. Publ.* **27**.

McFie, J., Piercy, M. F., and Zangwill, O. L. (1950): Visuospacial agnosia associated with the lesions of the right cerebral hemisphere. *Brain* **73**.

McKey, (1956): The Epistemological Problem for Automata. Automat. Studies. (Princeton).

McLean, O. (1959): The limbic system with respect to two life principles. *In*: 2nd Macy Conference: The Central Nervous System and Behavior. (National Institutes of Health; Bethesda, Md.).

McLean, P. D. (1955): The limbic system, etc. *Psychosom. Med.* **17**.

Magoun, H. W. (1952): The ascending reticular activating system. *A. Res. Nerv. & Ment. Dis. Publ.* **30**.

Magoun, H. W. (1958): The Waking Brain. (Charles C Thomas; Springfield, Ill.).

Malinowsky, B. (1930): The problem of meaning in primitive languages. *In*: Ogden, Ed.: Meaning of Meaning. (London).

Malmo, R. B. (1942): Interference factors in delayed response in monkeys. *J. Neurophysiol.* **5**.

Marie, P. (1906): Revision de la question de l'aphase. *Sem. méd.*

Marie, P., and Foix, C. (1917): Les aphasies de la guerre. *Rev. Neurol.* **31**.

Masserman, G. H. (1943): Behaviour and Neurosis. (Chicago Univ. Press; Chicago).

Mayer-Gross, W. C. (1935): Some observations on apraxia. *Proc. Roy. Soc. Med.* **28**.

Mettler, F., Ed. (1949): Selective Partial Ablation of the Frontal Cortex. (New York City).

Mettler, F. (1952): Psychosurgical Problems. (London).

Meyer, A. (1950): Anatomical lesions from prefrontal leucotomy. Congress Intern. Psychiatry, Paris.

Meyer, A., and Beck, E. (1954): Prefrontal Leucotomy and Related Operations. (Edinburgh-London).

Meyer, L. C. A. (1779): Anatomisch-physiologische Abhandlungen vom Gehirn. (Berlin-Leipzig).

Meynert, T. (1867): Der Bau der Grosshirnrinde. (Leipzig).

Meynert, T. (1874): Vom Gehirn der Säugethiere. (Leipzig).

Meynert, T. (1884): Psychiatrie. (Wien).
Meynert, T. (1899): Klinische Vorlesungen. (Wien).
Miller, G., Pribram, K., and Galanter, E. (1960): Plans and the Organization of Behaviour. (Holt; New York City).
Miller, G. A. (1962): Some psychological studies of grammar. *Amer. Psychologist* **17**.
Miller, G. A. (1965): The psycholinguists. On the new scientists of language. *In*: G. E. Osgood and T. A. Sebock, Eds.: Psycholinguistics, Bloomington.
Miller, G. A. (1965): Some preliminaries to psycholinguistics. *Amer. Psychologist* **20**.
Miller, G. A. (1967): The Psychology of Communication. Seven Essays. (Basic Books; New York).
Miller, G. A. (1969): The organization of lexical memory. *In*: G. A. Talland and N. Waugh, Eds.: The Pathology of Memory. (Academic Press; New York).
Miller, G. A. (1970): Four philosophical problems of psycholinguistics. *Philosophy of Science* **37**.
Miller, G. A. (1972): Lexical memory. *Proc. Amer. Phil. Soc.* **116**.
Miller, G. A., and Chomsky, N. (1963): Finitary models of language users. *In*: R. D. Luce *et al.*, Eds.: Handbook of Mathematical Psychology. (Wiley; New York).
Miller, G. A., and Isard, S. (1963): Some perceptual consequences of linguistic rules. *J. Verb. Learn. Verb. Behav.* **2**.
Milner, B. (1954): The intellectual function of the temporal lobes. *Psychol. Bull.* **51**.
Milner, B. (1956): Psychological defects produced by temporal lobe excisions. *In*: The Brain and Human Behaviour. *A. Res. Nerv. & Ment. Dis. Publ.*
Milner, B. (1964): Some effects in frontal lobectomy in man. *In*: J. M. Warren and K. Akert, Ed.: The Frontal Granular Cortex and Behavior. (McGraw-Hill: New York).
Milner, B. (1966): Amnesia following operations on the temporal lobes. *In*: C. W. M. Witty and O. L. Zangwill, Ed. Amnesia. (Butterworth: London).
Milner, B. (1968): Visual recognition after right temporal lobe excision in man. *Neuropsychologia* **6**.
Milner, B., Branch, C., and Rasmussen, T. (1964): Observations on cerebral dominance disorders in language. *In*: Disorders of Language. (Ciba Foundation Conference; London).
Milner, B., Taylor, R., and Sperry, R. W. (1968): Lateralized suppression of dichotically presented digits after commissure section in man. *Science* **16**.
Milner, B., and Taylor, L. (1972): Right-hemisphere superiority in tactile pattern recognition after commissurotomy: evidence for non-verbal memory. *Neuropsychologia* **10**.
Mishkin, M. (1954): Visual discrimination performance following partial ablation of the temporal lobe. *J. Comp. & Physiol. Psychol.* **47**.
Mishkin, M. (1957): Effects of small frontal lesion on delayed alternation in monkeys. *J. Neurophysiol.* **20**.
Mishkin, M., and Pribram, K. (1954): Visual discrimination performance following partial ablation of the temporal lobe. *J. Comp. & Physiol. Psychol.* **48**.
Mishkin, M., and Pribram, K. (1955): Analysis of the effects of frontal lesions in monkey. I. Variations of delayed alternation. *J. Comp. Physiol. Psychol.* **48**.
Mishkin, M., and Pribram, K. (1956): Analysis of the effects of frontal lesions in monkey. II. Variations of delayed response. *J. Comp. Physiol. Psychol.* **49**.
Mishkin, M., and Weisenkranz, L. (1958): Effects of delaying reward on visual discrimination performance in monkeys with frontal lesions. *J. Comp. & Physiol. Psychol.* **51**.
Mohr, J. P., Watters, W. C., and Duncan, G. M. (1975): Thalamic hemorrhage and aphasia. *Brain and Language* **2**.
Monakow, C. (1910): Über Lokalisation der Hirnfunktionen. (Wiesbaden).
Monakow, C. (1914): Die Lokalisation im Grosshirn und der Abbau der Funktionen durch corticale Herde. (Bergmann; Wiesbaden).
Monakow, C., and Mourgue, R. (1928): Introduction biologue à l'étude du neurologie et de la psychopathologie. (Alcan; Paris).
Moruzzi, I. (1954): The physiological properties of the brain reticular formation. *In*:

The Council for International Organizations of Medical Sciences: Brain Mechanisms and Consciousness. (Blackwell: Oxford).
Moruzzi, I., and Magoun, H. W. (1949): Brain stem reticular formation. *Electroenceph. Clin. Neurophysiol.* **1**.
Mountcastle, V. B. (1957): Modality and topographic properties of single neurons of cat's somatic sensory cortex. *J. Neurophysiol.* **20**.
Mountcastle, V. B. (1966): Neuronal replication of somatic sensory events. *In:* J. C. Eccles, Ed.: Brain and Conscious Experience. (Springer: Berlin and New York).
Munk, H. (1881): Über die Funktionen der Grosshirnrinde. (Hirschwald: Berlin).
Murata, K., and Kameda, K. (1963): The activity of single cortical neurons of unrestrained cats during sleep and wakefulness. *Arch. Ital. Biol.* **101**.
Natadze, R. G. (1960): Emergence of set on the bases of imaginal situation. *Brit. J. Psychol.* **51**.
Nauta, W. J. (1955): An experimental study of the efferent connections of the hippocampus. *Brain* **78**.
Nauta, W. J. (1958): Hippocampal projections and related nervous pathways to the midbrain in the cat. *Brain* **81**.
Nauta, W. J. H. (1971): The problem of the frontal lobes. A reinterpretation. *J. Psychiat. Res.* **8**.
Newell, A., Shaw, J. C., and Simon, H. A. (1958): Elements of a theory of human problem solving. *Psychol. Rev.* **65**.
Nielsen, J. M. (1944): Functions of the minor cerebral hemisphere in language. *Bull. Los Angeles Neurol. Soc.* **3**.
Nielsen, J. M. (1946): Agnosia, Apraxia, Aphasia. (Los Angeles).
Nissl von Meyendorff (1930): Vom Lokalisationsproblem der artikulierten Sprache. (Barth; Leipzig).
Nissl von Meyendorff (1941): Die aphasischen Symptome und ihre kortikale Lokalisation. (Engelman; Leipzig).
Ojeman, G. (1975*a*): Language and the thalamus, object naming and recall during and after thalamic stimulation. *Brain* **95**.
Ojeman, G. (1975*b*): Subcortical language mechanisms. *In:* H. Avakian-Whitaker and A. Whitaker, Eds.: Studies in Neurolinguistics. (Academic Press; New York).
Ojeman, G., Blick, R., and Ward, A. (1971): Improvement and disturbances of short term verbal memory with human ventrolateral thalamic stimulation. *Brain* **94**.
Ojeman, G., Fedio, P., and van Buren, J. (1968): Anomia from pulvinar and subcortical parietal stimulation. *Brain* **91**.
Ojeman, G., and Ward, A. (1971): Speech representation in the ventrolateral thalamus. *Brain* **94**.
Olds, J. (1955): Physiological mechanisms of reward. *In:* Nebraska Symposium on Motivation. (Univ. of Nebraska Press; Lincoln).
Olds, J. (1958): Selective effects of drives and drugs on reward system of the brain. *In:* Neurological Basis of Behavior. (Ciba Foundation Symposium; London).
Olds, J. (1959): Higher functions of the nervous system. *Ann. Rev. Physiol.* **21**.
Olds, J., and Olds, M. E. (1958): Positive reinforcement produced by stimulating hippothalamus. *Science* **127**.
Ombredane, A. (1945): Études de psychologie médicale. I. Perception et Langage. (Rio de Janeiro).
Ombredane, A. (1951): L'aphasie et l'élaboration de la pensée explicite. (Presse Universitaire: Paris).
Oonishi, S., and Katsuki, Y. (1965): Functional organization and integrative mechanism of the auditory cortex on the cat. *Jap. J. Physiol.* **15**.
Oppenheim, H. (1890): Zur Pathologie der Grosshirngeschwülste. *Arch. Psychiat.* **21**.
Orbach, J. (1956): Immediate and chronic disturbance of the delayed response following transsection of frontal granular cortex in monkeys. *J. Comp. Physiol. Psychol.* **51**.
Orbach, J. (1959): Functions of striate cortex and the problem of mass action. *Psychol. Bull.* **56**.

Orbach, J., and Franz, R. L. (1958): Differential effects on temporal neocortical resections on overtrained and not overtrained visual habits in monkeys. *J. Comp. & Physiol. Psychol.* **51**.

Orbach, J., and Fisher, G. (1959): Bilateral resection of frontal granular cortex. *Arch. Neurol.* **1**.

Orbach, J., Milner, B., and Rassmussen, T. (1960): Learning and retention in monkeys after amygdala-hippocampus resection. *Arch. Neurol.* **3**.

Panizza, R. (1855): Osservazioni sul nervo ottico. C. J. R. Inst. Lomb. **58**.

Papez, J. W. (1937): A proposed mechanism of emotion. *Arch. Neurol. & Psychiat.* **38**.

Papez, J. W. (1958): Visceral brain, its components and connections. *In*: Reticular Formation of the Brain. (Boston).

Paterson, A., and Zangwill, O. L. (1944): Disorders of visual space perception associated with lesions of the right hemisphere. *Brain* **67**.

Paterson, A., and Zangwill, O. L. (1945): A case of topographical disorientation associated with an unilateral cerebral lesion. *Brain* **68**.

Peele, T. L. (1954): The Neuroanatomical Basis for Clinical Neurology. (McGraw-Hill; New York City).

Penfield, W., and Evans, J. (1935): The frontal lobe in man; a clinical study of maximum removal. *Brain* **58**.

Penfield, W., and Ericson, T. C. (1945): Epilepsy and Cerebral Localization. (Charles C Thomas; Springfield, Ill.).

Penfield, W., and Jasper, H. (1954): Epilepsy and Functional Anatomy of Human Brain. (Little, Brown; Boston).

Penfield, W., and Milner, B. (1958): Memory deficits produced by bilateral lesions of the hippocampal zone. *Arch. Neurol. Psychiat.* (Chicago) **79**.

Penfield, W., and Rasmussen, T. (1950): The Cerebral Cortex of Man. (Macmillan; New York City).

Penfield, W., and Roberts, L. (1959): Speech and Brain Mechanisms. (Princeton Univ. Press; Princeton).

Peritz, G. (1918): Zur Pathophysiologie des Rechnens. *Deutsche Z. Nervenh.* **61**.

Petersen, L. P., and Petersen, D. (1962): Short-term retention of individual terms. *J. Exp. Psychol.* **58**.

Petrie, A. (1957): A comparison of the psychological effects of different types of operation on the frontal cortex. *J. Ment. Sc.* **125**.

Pfeiffer, B. (1910): Psychische Störungen bei Hirntumoren. *Arch. Psychiat.* **47**.

Pfeiffer, R. A. (1936): Pathologie der Hörstrahlung und der corticalen Hörsphäre. *In*: O. Bumke and O. Foerster, Eds.: Handbuch der Neurologie. vol. 6. (Springer; Berlin).

Pflugfelder, G. (1950): Methoden der Demenzforschung. (Basel).

Piaget, J. (1935): La Naissance de L'intelligence de L'enfant. (Neuchâtel).

Piaget, J. (1947): La Psychologie de L'intelligence. (Paris).

Piaget, J. (1955): La Logique de L'enfant et la Logique de L'adolescent. (Paris).

Piaget, J., and Inhelder, B. (1941): Le Développement des Quantités Chez L'enfant. (Paris and Neuchâtel).

Piaget, J., Inhelder, B., and Szeminska, A. (1947): La Representation de L'espace Chez L'enfant. (Paris).

Pick, A. (1905): Studien Über Motorische Aphasie. (Wien).

Pick, A. (1913): Die Agrammatischen Sprachstörungen. (Springer; Berlin).

Pick, A. (1931): Aphasie. *In*: A. Bethe *et al.* Ed.: Handbuch der Normalen und Pathologischen Physiologie. vol. 15. (Springer; Berlin).

Pittrich (1949): Denkforschung bei Hirnverletzten. Sammlung Psychiat. u. neurol. Einzeldarstellungen. (Leipzig).

Polimanti (1906): Contributi alla fisiologia e all'anatomia dei lobi frontali. (Roma).

Polyak, S. (1932): The main afferent fiber systems of the cerebral cortex in primates. *A. Res. Nerv. & Ment. Dis. Publ.* **13**.

Polyak, S. (1957): The Vertebrate Visual System. (Univ. Chicago Press; Chicago).

Poppelreuter, W. (1917–1918): Die Psychischen Schädigungen Durch Kopfschuss. 2 vols. (Voss; Leipzig).

Pötzl, O. (1928): Die Aphasielehre vom Standpunkt der klinischen Psychiatrie. Die Optisch-agnostischen Störungen. (Deutike; Leipzig).

Pötzl, O. (1930): Lokalisationsproblem der Artikulierten Sprache. (Barth; Leipzig).

Pötzl, O. (1937): Zum Apraxieproblem. *J. Psychiol. u. Neurol.* **54**.

Powell, T. P. S., and Mountcastle, V. B. (1959): Some properties of the functional organization of the cortex of the postcentral gyrus of the monkey: A correlation of findings obtained in a single unit analysis with cytoarchitecture. *Johns Hopkins Hosp. Bull.* **103**.

Pribram, K. H. (1958*a*): Neocortical Functions in Behaviour. Symposium on Interdisciplinary Research in the Behavioral Sciences. (Univ. of Wisconsin Press; Madison).

Pribram, K. H. (1958*b*): Comparative Neurology and Evolution of Behaviour. Behaviour and Evolution. (Yale Univ. Press; New Haven).

Pribram, K. H. (1959*a*): On the Neurology of Thinking. Behavioral Science **4**.

Pribram, K. H. (1959*b*): The Intrinsic Systems of the Forebrain. Handbook of Physiology. (McGraw-Hill; New York City).

Pribram, K. H. (1960): A review of theory in physiological psychology. *Ann. Rev. Psychol.* **11**.

Pribram, K. H. (1961): A further analysis of the behaviour deficit that follows injury to the primate frontal cortex. *J. Exp. Neurol.* **3**.

Pribram, K. H., Ahumada, A., Hartog, I., and Ross, L. (1964): A progress report on neurological processes disturbed by frontal lesions in primates. *In*: J. M. Warren and R. Akert, Eds.: The Frontal Granular Cortex and Behavior. (McGraw-Hill; New York).

Pribram, K., and Fulton, J. F. (1954): An experimental critique of the effects of anterior cingulate ablations in monkey. *Brain* **77**.

Pribram, K., and Krüger, L. (1954): Functions of the olfactory brain. *Ann. New York Acad. Sc.* **58**.

Pribram, K., Kruger, L., Robinson, F., and Berman, A. J. (1955–1956): The effects of precentral lesions on the behaviour of monkeys. *Yale J. Biol. & Med.* **28**.

Pribram, K. H., and Luria, A. R., Eds. (1973): Psychophysiology of the Frontal Lobes. (Academic Press; New York).

Pribram, K., and Mishkin, M. (1955): Simultaneous and successive visual discrimination by monkeys with inferotemporal lesions. *J. Comp. & Physiol. Psychol.* **48**.

Pribram, K., Mishkin, M., Rosvold, H. E., and Kaplan, S. J. (1952): Effects on delayed-response performance of lesions of dorsolateral and ventromedial frontal cortex of baboons. *J. Comp. & Physiol. Psychol.* **45**.

Pribram, K., and Mishkin, M. (1956): Analysis of the effects of frontal lesions in monkeys. III. *J. Comp. & Physiol. Psychol.* **49**.

Quensel, F. (1931): Erkrankungen der höheren optischen Zentren. *In*: Kurze, Ed.: Handbuch der Ophthalmologie. XI.

Ranschburg, P., and Schill, E. (1932): Über Alexie und Agnosie. *Z. Ges. Neurol. u. Psychiat.* **139**.

Rasmussen, T., and Wada, J. (1959): The intracarotid injection of sodium amythal for the lateralisation of cerebral speech dominance. *J. Neurosurg.*

Raven, J. C. (1939): Series of perceptual tests. *Brit. J. M. Psychol.* **18**.

Reisch, G. (1513): Margarita Philosophica.

Reitman, W. (1966): Cognition and Thought. (Wiley; New York).

Revault d'Allones, G. (1923): La schématisation. L'attention. Dumas. Traité de psychologie. Paris.

Richter, C. P., and Hines, M. (1938): Increased general activity produced by prefrontal and striate lesion in monkey. *Brain* **61**.

Richter, H. (1964): Zur Frage den idiokinetischer Form der motorischen Aphasie. *Zbl. Nervenheilk.* **183**.

Ricklan, M., and Cooper, J. (1975): Psychometric studies of verbal functions following thalamic lesions in humans. *Brain and Language* **2**.

Rose, J. E. (1950): Cortical connections of the reticular complex of the thalamus. *A. Res. Nerv. & Ment. Dis. Publ.* **30**.

Rosvold, H. E. (1959): Physiological psychology. *Ann. Rev. Psychol.* **10.**

Rosvold, H. E., and Delgado, I. M. R. (1956): The effect on delayed alternation test performance of stimulating and destroying electrical structures within the frontal lobes. *J. Comp. & Physiol. Psychol.* **51.**

Rosvold, H. E., Mirsky, A. F., and Pribram, K. (1954): Influence of amygdalectomy on social behaviour in monkey. *J. Comp. & Physiol. Psychol.* **47.**

Rosvold, H. E., and Mishkin, M. (1950): Evaluation of the effects of prefrontal lobotomy on intelligence. *Canad. J. Psychol.* **3.**

Ruch, T. C. (1946): Neural basis of somatic sensation. *In*: J. F. Fulton, Ed.: Howell's Textbook of Physiology. 16th ed. Philadelphia.

Ruch, T. C., and Fulton, J. F. (1953): Cortical localization of somatic sensibility. *A. Res. Nerv. & Ment. Dis. Publ.*

Ruch, T. C., Fulton, J. F., and German, W. I. (1935): Sensory discrimination in monkey, chimpanzee and man after lesions of parietal lobe. *Arch. Neurol. & Psychiat.* **39.**

Ruch, T. C., Patton, H. D., and Amassian, V. E. (1952): Topographical and functional determinants of cortical localization patterns. *A. Res. Nerv. & Ment. Dis. Publ.* **30.**

Rylander, G. (1939): Personality Changes After Operations on the Frontal Lobes. (London).

Salomon, E. (1914): Motorische Aphasie mit Agrammatismus und sensorischen Sprachstörungen. *Monatsschr. Psychiat. u. Neurol.* **35.**

Sapir, E. (1934): Language. (New York City).

Sapir, I. D. (1929): Die Neurodynamik des Sprachapparates bei Aphasikern. *J. Psychol. u. Neurol.* **38.**

Scheerer, M. (1949): An experiment in abstraction. *Confinia Neurol.* **9.**

Schilder, P. (1935): The Image and Appearance of the Human Body. (Kegan Paul; London).

Schuell, H., and Jenkins, J. (1959): The nature of language deficit in aphasia. *Psychol. Rev.*, **66**, no. 1.

Schuell, H., and Jenkins, J. (1964): The Nature of Language Deficit in Aphasia. (McGraw-Hill; New York).

Schuell, H., Jenkins, J., and Jimenes-Pabon, E. (1965): Aphasia in Adults. (Hoeber; New York).

Schuster, P. (1902): Psychische Störungen bei Hirntumoren. (Enke; Stuttgart).

Schuster, P., and Taterka, H. (1926): Beiträge zur Anatomie und Klinik der reinen Worttaubheit. *Z. Ges. Neurol. u. Psychiat.* **105.**

Scoville, W. B. (1954): The limbic system in man. *J. Neurosurg.* **11.**

Scoville, W. *et al.* (1953): Observation on medical temporal lobotomy and uncotomy for the treatment of psychotic states. *A. Res. Nerv. & Ment. Dis. Publ.* **31.**

Scoville, W. B., and Milner, B. (1957): Loss of recent memory after bilateral hippocampal lesion. *J. Neurosurg. Psychol.* **20.**

Semmes, J. (1965): A non-tactual factor in astereognosis. *Neuropsychologia* **3**, no. 4.

Semmes, J. (1968): Hemispheric specialization: a possible clue mechanism. *Neuropsychologia* **6.**

Semmes, J., Weinstein, S., Ghent, L., and Teuber, H. L. (1960): Somatosensory changes after penetrating brain wounds in man. (Harvard Univ. Press; Cambridge).

Shankweiler, D. R., and Studdert-Kennedy, M. (1967): Identification of consonants and vowels presented to the left and right ear. *J. Exp. Psychol.* **19.**

Sherrington, C. S. (1906): The Integrative Action of the Nervous System. (London).

Sherrington, C. S. (1934): The Brain and Its Mechanisms. (Cambridge Univ. Press; London).

Sherrington, C. S. (1946): The Endeavor of Jean Fernel. (Macmillan; London and New York).

Sherrington, C. S. (1948): Man on His Nature. (London).

Simernitskaya, E. G. (1974): On two forms of writing defect following local brain lesions. *In*: S. J. Dimond and J. G. Beaumont, Eds.: Hemisphere Function in the Human Brain. (Elek; London).

Singer, H. D., and Low, A. A. (1933): Acalculia. *Arch. Neurol. & Psychiat.* **29.**

Sittig, O. (1931): Apraxie. (Karger; Berlin).

Soemmering, S. T. (1796): Über das Organ der Seele. (Königsberg).

Spearman, C. (1932): The Abilities of Man. (London).
Sperry, R. W. (1964): The great cerebral commissure. *Scientific American* **210**.
Sperry, R. W. (1966): Hemispheric interaction and the mind-brain problem. *In*: J. C. Eccles, Ed.: Brain and Conscious Experience. (Springer; Berlin).
Sperry, R. W. (1967): Mental unity following surgical disconnection of the hemispheres. The Harvey Lecture. (Academic Press; New York).
Sperry, R. W. (1968): Hemisphere deconnection and unity in conscious awareness. *Amer. Psychologist* **23**.
Sperry, R. W., Gazzaniga, M. S., and Bogen, I. E. (1969): Interhemispheric relationships; the neocortical commissures; syndromes of hemispheric disconnection. *In*: P. J. Vinken and G. W. Bruyn, Eds.: Handbook of Clinical Neurology, vol. 4. (North-Holland Publishing Co.; Amsterdam).
Stamm, I. S. (1955): The function of the medial cerebral cortex in maternal behavior. *J. Comp. & Physiol. Psychol.* **87**.
Starr, M. A. (1884): Cortical lesions of the brain. *Am. J. M. Sc.* **87**.
Stauffenberg, V. (1914): Über Seelenblindheit. *Arb. Hirnanat. Inst.* Zürich **8**.
Stauffenberg, V. (1918): Klinische und anatomische Beiträge zur Kenntnis des aphasischen, agnostischen und apraktischen Symptome. *Z. Ges. Neurol. & Psychiat.* **93**.
Stein, H., and Weizsäcker, V. (1927): Der Abbau der sensiblen Funktionen. *Deutsche Z. Nervenh.* **99**.
Stern, W. (1927): Kindersprache. (Barth; Leipzig).
Strauss, A., and Lehtinen, L. (1946): Psychopathology and education of the brain-injured child. (New York City).
Subirana, A. (1958): The prognosis in aphasia in relation to the fact of cerebral dominance and handedness. *Brain* **81**.
Subirana, A. (1969): Handedness and cerebral dominance. *In*: P. J. Vinken and G. W. Bruyn, Eds.: Handbook of Clinical Neurology, vol. 4. (North-Holland Publishing Co.; Amsterdam).
Sugar, O., French, J. D., and Ghusid, J. G. (1948): Cortico-cortical connections of the superior surface of temporal operculum in monkey. *J. Neurophysiol.* **11**.
Sugar, O., Petr, R., Amador, L. V., and Criponissiotu, B. (1950): Cortico-cortical connections of the cortex buried in intraparietal and principal sulci of monkey. *J. Neuropath. & Exp. Neurol.* **9**.
Svedelius, C. (1897): L'Analyse du langage. (Uppsala).
Talland, G. A. (1966): Deranged Memory. (Academic Press; New York).
Teuber, H. L. (1955): Physiological psychology. *Ann. Rev. Psychol.* **9**.
Teuber, H. L. (1959): Some alterations in behaviour after cerebral lesion in man. *In*: Evolution of Nervous Control. Am. Assoc. Adv. of Sciences. (Washington).
Teuber, H. L. (1960*a*): Visual field defects after penetrating missile wounds of the brain. (Harvard Univ. Press; Cambridge).
Teuber, H. L. (1960*b*): Perception. *In*: J. Field, H. W. Magoun, and V. E. Hall, Eds.: Handbook of Physiology. Section 1. Neurophysiology. vol. 3. Amer. Physiol. Soc. (Washington, D.C.).
Teuber, H. L. (1962): The search for physiological bases of memory. *In*: F. O. Schmitt, Ed.: Molecular Specificity and Biological Memory. (MIT Press; Cambridge, Mass.).
Teuber, H. L. (1964): The riddle of frontal lobe function in man. *In*: J. M. Warren and K. Akert, Eds.: The Frontal Granular Cortex and Behavior. pp. 410–444. (McGraw-Hill; New York).
Teuber, H. L. (1965): Disorders of higher tactile and visual functions. *Neuropsychologia* **3**, no. 4.
Teuber, H. L., and Mishkin, M. (1954): Judgement of visual and postural vertical after brain injury. *J. Psychol.* **38**.
Teuber, H. L., and Weinstein, S. (1956): Ability to discover hidden figures after cerebral lesions. *AMA Arch. Neurol. & Psychiat.* **76**.
Thorpe, W. H. (1956): Learning and Instincts in Animal. (London).
Thurstone, L. (1947): Multiple Factor Analysis. (Chicago Univ. Press; Chicago).
Tinbergen, N. (1951): The Study of Instincts. (Oxford Univ. Press; London).
Tizard, B. (1958): The psychological effects of frontal lesion. *Acta Psychiat. et Neurol. Scandinav.* **33**.

Trevarthen, C. (1974): Analysis of cerebral activities that generate and regulate consciousness in commissurotomy patients. *In*: S. J. Dimond and J. G. Beaumont, Eds.: Hemisphere Function in the Human Brain. (Elek; London).

Troubezkoi, N. (1939): Grundriss der Phonologie. (Prague).

Tsvetkova, L. S. (1975): The naming process and its impairment. *In*: E. Lenneberg, Ed.: Foundation of Language Development, vol. 2. (Academic Press; New York).

Ustvedt, H. J. (1937): Über die Untersuchung der musikalischen Funktionen bei Patienten mit Gehirnleiden, besonders bei Patienten mit Aphasie. (Helsingfors).

Van Buren, J. M. (1975): The question of thalamic participation in speech mechanisms. *Brain and Language* **2**.

Van Buren, J. M., and Borke, R. C. (1969): Alteration in speech and the pulvinar. *Brain* **92**.

Vieussens, R. C. (1685): Neurographia. (London).

Virchov, R. (1858): Die Zellularpathologie. (Berlin).

Vogt, C., and Vogt, O. (1919–1920): Allgemeine Ergebnisse unserer Hirnforschung. *J. Psychol. u. Neurol.* **25**.

Vogt, O. (1927): Architektonik der menschlichen Hirnrinde. *Allg. Z. Psychiat.* **86**.

Vogt, O. (1951): Die anatomische Vertiefung der menschlichen Hirnlocalisation. *Klin. Wschr.* **78**.

Wada, J. (1949): A new method for determination of the side of cerebral speech dominance. *Med. Biol.* **14**.

Wada, J., and Rasmussen, T. (1960): Intracarotid injection of sodium amytal or the lateralization of cerebral speech dominance. *J. Neurosurg.* **17**.

Walker, A. E. (1938): The Primate Thalamus. (Univ. of Chicago Press; Chicago).

Walker, A. E. (1957): Recent memory impairment in unilateral temporal lesions. *Arch. Neurol. Psychiat.* (Chicago) **75**.

Wallon, H. (1925): L'enfant turbulent. (Alcan; Paris).

Wallon, H. (1942): De L'acte à la Pensée. (Flammarion; Paris).

Walshe, F. M. R. (1935): On the "syndrome of the premotor cortex" and the definition of terms "premotor" and "motor": with a consideration of Jackson's views on the cortical representations of movements. *Brain* **58**.

Walshe, F. M. R. (1943): On the mode of representation of movements in the motor cortex. *Brain* **66**.

Walter, W. G. (1953): The Living Brain. (Norton; New York City).

Ward, A. A., Pedan, J. K., and Sugar, O. (1946): Cortico-cortical connections in the monkey with special reference of area 6. *J. Neurophysiol.* **9**.

Warren, J. M., and Akert, K., Eds. (1964): The Frontal Granular Cortex and Behavior. (McGraw-Hill; New York).

Warrington, E., James, M., and Kinsbourne, M. (1966): Drawing disability in relation to laterality of cerebral lesion. *Brain* **89**.

Wechsler, D. (1944): The Measurement of Adult Intelligence (Baltimore).

Weckroth, I. (1961): On the Relationship Between Severity of Brain Injury and the Level and Structure of Intelligent Performances. (Iyvaskula).

Weigl, E. (1927): Zur Psychologie der sogenannten Abstraktionsprocesse. *Z. Psychol.* **103**.

Weigl, E. (1963): Deblockierung Bildagnostischen Störungen bei einem Aphasiker. *Neurologia* **1**.

Weigl, E. (1964*a*): Some critical remarks concerning the problem of so-called simultanagnosia. *Neuropsychologia* **2**, no. 3.

Weigl, E. (1964*b*): Die Bedeutung der afferenten, verbo-kinästhetischen Erregungen des Sprachapparates für die expressiven und receptiven Sprachvorgängen bei Normalen und Sprachgestörten. *Cortex* **1**.

Weisenburg, T. H., and McBride, K. E. (1935): Aphasia. A Clinical and Psychological Study. (Commonwealth Fund; New York City).

Weiskrantz, L. (1956): Behaviour changes associated with ablation of the amygdaloid complex in monkeys. *J. Comp. & Physiol. Psychol.* **51**.

Weiskrantz, L. (1964): Neurological studies and animal behaviour. *Brit. Med. Bull.* **20, no. 1**.

Weiskrantz, L., Mihailovic, L., and Gross, C. (1960): Stimulation of frontal cortex and delayed alternation performance in the monkey. *Science* **131**.

Weiskrantz, L., and Mishkin, M. (1958): Effects of temporal and frontal cortical lesions on auditory functions in monkey. *Brain* **81**.

Welt, L. (1888): Über Charakterveränderungen des Menschen in Folge der Läsionen des Stirnhirns. *Deutsches Arch. Klin. Med.* **42**.

Werner, H., and Kaplan, E. (1952): The Acquisition of Meanings. Monograph Soc. Res. Child Development. No. 5.

Werner, H. (1954): Change of meaning. *J. Gen. Psychol.* **50**.

Wernicke, C. (1874): Der aphasische Symptomenkomplex. (Cohn & Weigart: Breslau).

Wernicke, C. (1894): Grundriss der Psychiatrie. Psychophysiologische Einleitung.

Willbrandt, H. (1887): Die Seelenblindheit als Herderscheinung. (Wiesbaden).

Willis, T. (1664): Cerebri Anatome. (Flesher; London).

Wilson, S. P. K. (1908): A contribution to the study of apraxia. *Brain* **31**.

Witty, G. W. M., and Zangwill, O. L., Eds. (1966): Amnesia. (Butterworth; London).

Woerkom, W. van (1925): Über Störungen im Denken bei aphasischen Patienten. *Monatsschr. Psychol. u. Neurol.* **59**.

Wolpert, I. (1924): Die Simultanagnosie. *Z. Ges. Neurol. u. Psychiat.* **93**.

Woolsey, C. N., Marshall, W. H., and Bard, P. (1942): Representation of cutaneous sensibility in the cerebral cortex of the monkey as indicated by evoked potentials. *Bull. Johns Hopkins Hosp.* **70**.

Wundt, W. (1873–1874): Grundzüge der physiologischen Psychologie. (Engelmann: Leipzig).

Wyss, O. A. M., and Obrador, S. (1937): Adequate rate of stimuli in electrical stimulation of the cerebral motor cortex. *Am. J. Physiol.* **120**.

Zaimov, K. (1965): Über die Pathophysiologie des Agnosien, Aphasien, Apraxien, etc. (Fischer: Jena).

Zangwill, O. L. (1951): Discussion on parietal lobe syndrome. *Proc. Roy. Soc. Med.* **44**.

Zangwill, O. L. (1960): Cerebral dominance and its relation to psychological function. (Oliver & Boyd: Edinburgh).

Zangwill, O. L. (1962): Handedness and dominance. *In*: J. Money, Ed.: Reading Disabilities. (Johns Hopkins Press; Baltimore).

Zangwill, O. L. (1964): Neurological studies and human behaviour. *Brit. Med. Bull.* **20**, no. 1.

Zangwill, O. L. (1967): Speech and the minor hemisphere. *Acta Neurol. Belg.* **67**.

Zeigarnik, B. (1927): Über das Erhalten erledigter und unerledigter Handlungen. *Psychol. Forsch.*

Zucker, K. (1934): An analysis of disturbed function in aphasia. *Brain* **57**.

Subject Index

Author Index